HEALTH PROMOTION
AND AGING

David Haber, PhD, is an assistant professor in the Gerontology Department at Western Oregon University, Monmouth, Oregon. Prior to his current affiliation he worked at several institutes of higher education.

For a decade he was the John and Janice Fisher distinguished professor of wellness and gerontology at Ball State University in Muncie, Indiana. For the decade prior to that, Dr. Haber was a professor at the University of Texas Medical Branch in Galveston. Before that he served as the director of the Center for Healthy Aging, at Creighton University's multidisciplinary shopping mall–based geriatric center in Omaha, Nebraska.

His early academic and research career included positions at the University of the District of Columbia; the University of South Florida, Tampa; and the University of Southern California, where he received his PhD in sociology from the Andrus Gerontology Center.

Dr. Haber is a fellow in the Gerontological Society of America, and he is recognized for two Best Practice Awards from the National Council on Aging, the Distinguished Teacher Award from the Association for Gerontology in Higher Education, and the Molly Mettler Award for Leadership in Health Promotion from the National Council on Aging.

The third edition of this book, *Health Promotion and Aging*, was selected for the 2004 Book of the Year Award by the *American Journal of Nursing* in two categories: Gerontologic Nursing, and Community and Public Health. Dr. Haber also authored *Health Care for an Aging Society*.

Dr. Haber has authored 85 academic journal publications and has been project director or principal investigator of 20 research or demonstration grants related to health and aging. Typically, these applied projects involved gerontology and health professional students leading community health promotion ventures with older adults. Dr. Haber's current scholarly interest is life review.

HEALTH PROMOTION AND AGING

PRACTICAL APPLICATIONS FOR HEALTH PROFESSIONALS

SIXTH EDITION

David Haber, PhD

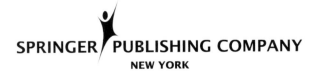

SPRINGER PUBLISHING COMPANY
NEW YORK

Springer Publishing Company, LLC
11 West 42nd Street
New York, NY 10036
www.springerpub.com

Acquisitions Editor: Sheri W. Sussman
Composition: diacriTech

ISBN: 978-0-8261-9917-1
e-book ISBN: 978-0-8261-9918-8
Instructor's Manual: 978-0-8261-9908-9

Qualified instructors may request the Instructor's Manual by emailing textbook@springerpub.com

13 14 15 16/ 5 4 3 2 1

The author and the publisher of this Work have made every effort to use sources believed to be reliable to provide information that is accurate and compatible with the standards generally accepted at the time of publication. The author and publisher shall not be liable for any special, consequential, or exemplary damages resulting, in whole or in part, from the readers' use of, or reliance on, the information contained in this book. The publisher has no responsibility for the persistence or accuracy of URLs for external or third-party Internet websites referred to in this publication and does not guarantee that any content on such websites is, or will remain, accurate or appropriate.

Library of Congress Cataloging-in-Publication Data

Haber, David, 1944-
  Health promotion and aging : practical applications for health professionals / David Haber, PhD. — 6 edition.
     pages cm
  Includes bibliographical references and index.
  ISBN 978-0-8261-9917-1 — ISBN 978-0-8261-9918-8 (e-book) — ISBN 978-0-8261-9908-9 (instructors manual) 1. Preventive health services for older people—United States. 2. Health promotion—United States. 3. Older people—Health and hygiene. I. Title.

  RA564.8.H33 2013

  362.19897′00973—dc23
                                    2012042833

Printed in the United States of America by Bang Printing.

CONTENTS

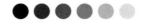

FIGURES

TABLES

FOREWORD

As a gerontological nurse who has promoted wellness for older adults for over four decades, I have been a fan of David Haber's *Health Promotion and Aging* for many years. As an author, researcher, and practitioner, I am impressed with the broad scope of his recent editions, which speak to many disciplines. The sixth edition of this book continues to provide a wealth of information to guide health care professionals whose goal is to promote health for older adults. In addition, the author's approach is refreshing and positive, as well as reality based. I particularly admire—and totally agree with—Dr. Haber's call for a "proaging movement" to challenge the common misperception that aging is primarily and necessarily associated with decline and disability. I also appreciate his emphasis on numerous, yet often overlooked, practical ways in which we as health care providers can address the many challenges inherent in aging.

Health Promotion and Aging contains many excellent evidence-based guides to essential topics such as nutrition, exercise and physical activity, nutrition and weight management, mental health concerns, complementary and alternative medicine, and numerous clinical preventive services. Dr. Haber also provides practical and well-founded guidance to health behavior change with regard to overall health promotion as well as specific topics. His approach to this topic is in stark contrast to an all too common perception that behavior change is not worthwhile or effective for people who are chronologically old. Another outstanding feature is that many aspects of diversity are addressed in the context of health promotion and current social trends. For example, Dr. Haber discusses gay aging and the influence of baby boomers on bringing issues such as same-sex marriage out of the closet, whether the closets are in community or institutional settings. In addition, the author does not shy away from addressing important but controversial topics, such as allowing physicians to prescribe life-ending medications to terminally ill patients. In this sixth edition, Dr. Haber has expanded on the following topics that are often underemphasized but increasingly important: long-term care, chronic care management, and social/emotional support. All topics are remarkably up to date and the content is relevant across many health care settings.

Dr. Haber's professional qualifications in gerontology, as delineated in the author's biographical sketch in the front matter of this book, are outstanding. All who read *Health Promotion and Aging* can benefit from the effective way in which he communicates his breadth of knowledge and helps readers apply evidence-based information to real-life situations with older adults. All content is supported by a strong and wide-ranging knowledge base, and the writing style reflects the high value that Dr. Haber places on humor and caring. Reading this book is not only enlightening and enriching but also enjoyable and sometimes even humorous. I can highly recommend *Health Promotion and*

Aging as an essential resource for those of us who have important roles in promoting health for older adults. This book provides essential tools and guidance so the terms "health" and "aging" are complementary—rather than contradictory—concepts.

Carol A. Miller, MSN, RN-BC
Clinical Nurse Specialist, Care & Counseling
Author: *Nursing for Wellness in Older Adults*
Fast Facts for Dementia Care: What Nurses Need to Know in a Nutshell
Fast Facts for Health Promotion in Nursing: Promoting Wellness in a Nutshell

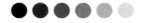

PREFACE

I was trained at the University of Southern California as a sociologist specializing in gerontology, but I spent my career implementing and evaluating health promotion projects in the community. This contradiction between training and practice has informed me on why promoting health is possible but difficult.

From a sociological perspective it is clear to me that American society is not particularly health promoting. For example, computers are increasingly promoting sedentary behavior, both at work and at play. A fast-paced society encourages us to seek convenient food and drink choices, and ubiquitous advertising—to the tune of tens of billions of dollars per year—promotes questionable foods and drinks over good nutrition. And the considerable stress engendered by a dynamic society leads to smoking, excessive drinking of alcohol, or engaging in other risky behaviors.

At the same time, however, we are becoming increasingly well educated on health matters and eager to learn more from research findings that quickly reach the Internet, magazines, newspapers, books, radio talk shows, and television news. Primarily through public education we were able to cut smoking rates in half between 1965 and 1990, and perhaps we can do the same with obesity and inactivity if we direct a similar amount of attention to these problems.

Although sociological truths are not to be denied, there is still considerable potential to empower individuals, groups, and organizations to live a healthy lifestyle. And although a vacuum of leadership has been created by mostly hands-off federal and state governments, an increasing number of local organizations are taking the initiative in health promotion: religious institutions, businesses, community centers, hospitals, medical clinics, educational institutions, shopping malls, and city governments.

As we continue our journey in the new millennium, research is providing convincing evidence that health promotion works—regardless of one's age and even after decades of practicing unhealthy habits. The findings are also providing specific ideas on what we need to do and how we ought to go about doing it. In some areas the strategies for improving health have proved a lot less onerous than we thought they had to be. For example, progressing from a sedentary lifestyle to engage in brisk walking for up to a half hour most days of the week can do your health a world of good.

Even the dreadful piece of legislation enacted in 1994, the Dietary Supplement Health and Education Act, may have some value in spite of the plethora of worthless and even harmful over-the-counter products that it allows to be promoted with ridiculous claims, such as "reverses aging." Perhaps it will be valuable in helping the American public become a bit more judicious in evaluating claims about what swallowing a pill can accomplish.

I would also like to note that the terms in the title of this book, "Health Promotion" and "Aging," are not as straightforward as they might seem. Matters relating to health, for instance, are often dominated by medical issues. And it is not clear which terms are most salient to aging people: health promotion, disease prevention, chronic disease management, health education, or some other designation.

And when does aging start? At the (supposedly) government-protected age of 40 for workers, at the AARP-eligible age of 50, at the traditional retirement age of 65, at the eligibility age of 75 for some geriatric clinics, or at the demographically significant age of 80 or 85? And how should we feel about the antiaging movement, which urges us to defy the aging process? The antiaging perspective appeals to many who have a vision of living vigorously and looking youthful for as long as possible. But what about us pro-agers, who embrace the aging process, accept its drawbacks, and creatively uncover its strengths?

This sixth edition of *Health Promotion and Aging* has been substantially revised and updated. There are multiple new subsections, topics, and terms in each chapter of this edition. To name a few, out of countless examples, there are the following new subjects: the Affordable Care Act; the future of Medicare and Social Security; the potential generational clash between boomers and millennials over upcoming health care policy; new recommendations for hepatitis C screening for boomers and new guidelines for depression and obesity screening; the utilization of complementary and alternative medicine by different age groups; new technology and its implications for older adults in the home and community; innovations in housing; rethinking retirement; and new or mostly new chapters on social/emotional support, long-term care and end-of-life care, and public health policy. In addition, all chapters have been significantly revised with topics carried over from the prior edition having been updated along with a majority of the tables and figures.

This book is focused on current research findings and practical applications, and includes detailed descriptions of two of my programs that have been recognized by the National Council on Aging and included in its Best Practices in Health Promotion and Aging. These consist of a comprehensive exercise program in the community that includes aerobics, strength building, flexibility and balance, and health education (Chapter 4); and a health contract/calendar used to help older adults change their health behaviors (Chapter 3). I have also done recent work on life reviews in the community and in educational settings, and some of that work is detailed in this edition.

This edition includes Key Terms and Learning Objectives at the start of each chapter; Questions to Ponder in each chapter; and boxes containing information to reflect upon.

I have attempted to make the book practical by including health-promoting tools, resource lists, assessment tools, illustrations, checklists, and tables; thoughtful by raising controversial issues and taking strong positions that you can agree or disagree with; and humorous, because humor is essential to health promotion. Through Springer Publishing Company there is also available an online Instructor's Manual to stimulate student thinking and suggest evaluation alternatives. **Qualified instructors may request the Instructor's Manual by emailing textbook@springerpub.com.**

ACKNOWLEDGMENTS

I would like to thank my wife, Jeanne St. Pierre, who has enriched my life in countless ways; my children, Benjamin and Rik (neé Audrey), who, like most children, taught their parents many vital lessons; my 98-year-old mother-in-law, Beatrice, who retired in her early 90s and can still beat her daughters and son-in-law in Scrabble; my cat, Maurice, for allowing me to type even when it disturbed his nap on my lap; my university, Western Oregon University, for seeing the value in hiring an older professor; and for my publisher, Springer Publishing Company, and Sheri W. Sussman and the other fine folks there who encourage me and support each new edition of this book.

1

INTRODUCTION

● ● ● Key Terms

Healthy People 2020 Initiative

libertarian paternalism

baby boomers, older adults, and older old

health promotion and disease prevention

age rectangle

chronic conditions and disability

activities of daily living

instrumental activities of daily living

centenarians

biogerontology

labor force participation rates

life expectancy and health expectancy

primary, secondary, and tertiary prevention

seven dimensions of wellness

antiaging versus proaging

compression of morbidity

health expectancy versus life expectancy

intergenerational conflict

Medicare, Medicaid, and Social Security

medical care, health care, and quality care

● ● ● Learning Objectives

- Critically evaluate the role of the federal government in promoting health
- Define libertarian paternalism
- Examine whether health promotion, disease prevention, and chronic disease management save money
- Describe the impact of sociodemographic trends on healthy aging

- Contrast the baby boomers, older adults, and the older old
- Differentiate chronic disease and disability
- Differentiate activities of daily living and instrumental activities of daily living
- Explore the future of centenarians
- Review trends in life expectancy
- Identify leading causes of death
- Examine medication utilization trends
- Identify labor force participation rates among older adults
- Contrast Internet use of boomers versus older adults
- Examine the consequences of rising educational levels on older adults.
- Describe older adult poverty
- Identify trends in older adult racial/ethnic composition
- Contrast definitions of healthy aging, and express your own definition
- Identify extraordinary accomplishments of older adults
- Distinguish among primary, secondary, and tertiary prevention
- Evaluate the antiaging movement
- Define compression of morbidity and analyze its likely future course
- Contrast health expectancy with life expectancy
- Review physical versus emotional aspects of aging
- Explore the potential for intergenerational conflict over health care
- Describe the Medicare, Medicaid, and Social Security programs
- Explain why medical care and health care are not synonymous

Youth, large, lusty, loving—youth full of grace, force, fascination. Do you know that Old Age may come after you with equal grace, force, fascination?

—Walt Whitman

Did you know that the federal government establishes goals for healthy aging? As far back as 1990, for example, the U.S. Public Health Service established the goal of increasing the number of years of healthy life remaining at age 65 from 11.8 years, as it was in 1990, to 14 years by 2000. It turned out, however, that this goal for the decade was not close to being met. Undeterred, many more goals were set during this and subsequent decades. Which raises some interesting questions: Why is the federal government doing this? Should it be doing this? Is it helping to promote healthy aging?

HEALTHY PEOPLE INITIATIVES

In 1979, one of the most influential documents in the field of health promotion, *Healthy People: The Surgeon General's Report on Health Promotion and Disease Prevention*, was published (U.S. Department of Health and Human Services [USDHHS], 1979). Over the years this report was widely cited by the popular media as well as in professional journals and at health conferences. Many attribute to it a seminal role in fostering health-promoting initiatives throughout the nation.

It was closely followed by another report, and a call to action, by the U.S. Public Health Service in 1980, *Promoting Health/Preventing Disease: Objectives for the Nation*, which outlined health objectives for the nation to achieve over the following 10 years. A decade later, in 1990, another national effort, Healthy People 2000, was initiated by the U.S. Public Health Service in an effort to reduce preventable death and *disability* for Americans by the year 2000. This was followed by Healthy People 2010 and the one for the current decade, Healthy People 2020. As you can see in Table 1.1, I have selected several measurable objectives for this decade that specifically address the health of older adults. What the table does not inform you about, is that most objectives, gerontological or otherwise, are not supported by federal funds.

On the positive side, setting health care priorities is no longer a matter of tabulating the number of deaths from a few diseases and then organizing a campaign against the most prevalent ones,

Question: What do *you* think is the most important health objective to set for older adults for the Healthy People 2020 initiative? Why? What should the federal and state governments, health professionals, and laypersons do to help achieve this objective?

TABLE 1.1 Healthy People 2020—Five Selected Older Adult Age 65+ Objectives With 10% Improvement Targets for the Decade 2010 to 2020

1. **Objective**: *Increase the proportion of older adults who are up to date on a core set of clinical preventive services*
   Baseline: 47.3% of older adults were up to date in 2008
   Target: 52.1% in 2020

2. **Objective**: *Reduce the proportion of older adults who have moderate to severe functional limitations*
   Baseline: 28.3% of older adults had moderate to severe functional limitations (age-adjusted) in 2007
   Target: 25.5% in 2020

3. **Objective**: *Increase the proportion of older adults with reduced physical or cognitive function who engage in light, moderate, or vigorous leisure-time physical activities*
   Baseline: 33.7% of these older adults engaged in these activities in 2008
   Target: 37.1% in 2020

4. **Objective**: *Increase the proportion of the health care workforce with geriatric certification*
   4a. *Physicians*
      Baseline: 2.7% of physicians had geriatric certification in 2009
      Target: 3% in 2020
   4b. *Geriatric Psychiatrists*
      Baseline: 4.3% of geriatric psychiatrists had geriatric certification in 2009
      Target: 4.7% in 2020
   4c. *Registered Nurses*
      Baseline: 1.4% of registered nurses had geriatric certification in 2004
      Target: 1.5% in 2020

5. **Objective**: *Reduce the rate of emergency department visits due to falls among older adults*
   Baseline: 5,235 emergency department visits per 100,000 older adults in 2007
   Target: 4,711 in 2020

like heart disease and cancer. The Healthy People initiatives are health oriented, not disease oriented, and as such they recognize the complexity of the socioeconomic, lifestyle, and other nonmedical influences that impact our ability to attain and maintain health.

A second major benefit of the initiatives is that they are focused on documenting baselines, setting objectives, and monitoring progress. This at least informs us on what the health problems are and whether they are getting better or worse.

The initiatives are not, however, focused on providing support to achieve these objectives. Not surprisingly, only a minority of the objectives have been achieved. According to the National Report Card on Healthy Aging (Merck Company Foundation, *The State of Aging and Health in America*, 2007), only 36% of the objectives for the year 2010 would be met, and we were falling far short of achieving the remaining target goals.

For example, in an area in which there was no financial support for encouraging change—being overweight or obese—the trend in the United States for adults between the ages of 20 and 74 has been in the opposite direction. There has been a steady increase in weight gain for Americans over the decade. There has been a similar result with respect to sedentary behavior among Americans. In the absence of financial support for encouraging change in this area, the average amount of light to moderate physical activity performed on a near-daily basis by those between the ages of 18 and 74 had not improved over the decade.

Focusing on those age 65 and over, the Merck Institute on Aging & Health cited results from the Healthy People 2010 initiative and reported many failing grades. Older Americans were falling far short of the 2010 target goals for not only physical activity and obesity, but also eating fruits and vegetables, tooth loss, and reducing hip fractures and fall-related deaths. Again, financial support for achieving target goals was largely or completely absent.

In contrast to the mere monitoring of most Healthy People 2010 target goals, financial assistance was provided to older adults through Medicare for medical screenings and immunizations. Thus, cholesterol, colorectal, and mammogram screening goals were met. (Pneumococcal and influenza vaccination goals would have been met—after all, the percentage of compliance in these two areas doubled among older adults during the decade between 1990 and 2000, meeting Healthy People 2000 target goals—but the target goals were unrealistically raised to 90% of the population for Healthy People 2010.)

Another goal, to achieve less than 12% of the older adult population smoking, also received financial support and was met. This goal received financial support from some states through the tobacco industry settlement to cover Medicaid expenses caused by smoking-related illnesses and also through coverage by Medicare (see Chapter 7, "Selected Health Education Topics").

This raises the question in the minds of those on the right of the political spectrum: conservatives and libertarians. Why should the federal government be involved at all? In the minds of liberals like myself, though, another question emerges: Should the federal government be doing *more* than setting lofty goals and monitoring data changes when it comes to promoting healthy aging?

A parallel question can be asked of state governments. The Healthy People initiatives often have a counterpart initiative at each of the state health departments. In my experience with several states, however, either this initiative establishes health baselines and, at times, monitors progress; has been ignored by the state health department altogether; or the state department accomplished a modest project more than a decade ago but did not follow up with additional activity. Many states, when given additional resources, which happened when they received tobacco settlement monies (see Chapter 7, "Selected Health Education Topics"), wound up diverting them to nonhealth purposes.

BOX 1.1	Example of Libertarian Paternalism

The author was not thrilled with the effectiveness of Healthy People 2010, but libertarian paternalists may have been. What is a libertarian paternalist, you ask?

Libertarian paternalism tries to appeal to both the libertarian (the less government intervention, the better off society will be) and the traditional liberal (there is an important role for government to play in health care).

Two former colleagues at the University of Chicago, Richard Thaler of the Graduate School of Business, and Cass Sunstein of the Law School, proposed the idea of libertarian paternalism. The libertarian component of this term suggests the allotment of no federal monies to help with implementing Healthy People initiatives. The paternalism component suggests the dissemination of vital information associated with Healthy People initiatives. What are the important health problems in America? Why are they important to recognize? What do we need to do to solve these problems?

For example, as individuals in society get heavier each year, the problem is both financial and functional for the individual (more medical bills, less mobility, and reduced quality of life) and for society (costlier health care insurance and less productive citizens). What do we need to do? Libertarian paternalists might suggest disseminating information about which health interventions work; which businesses, religious institutions, community centers, hospitals, medical clinics, academic medical centers, health plans, educational institutions, shopping malls, and city governments are doing these interventions; and what have been the benefits?

This combination pleases the libertarian (individuals are free to do what they please, and little government money is being spent) and the liberal (disseminating better data and methods about programs that work will encourage their replication). The basic premise of libertarian paternalism is that people and organizations are busy, lives are complicated, and even intelligent individuals and smart organizations can make foolish health choices. Healthy People initiatives can nudge—Thaler and Sunstein's term—people and organizations in the right direction without too much governmental intrusion and cost.

I will come back to this issue in Chapter 12, "Public Health Policy": Should the federal and state governments be involved in health promotion and, if so, should they be doing more than setting goals and monitoring data changes? In the meantime, if you are interested in the Healthy People 2020 initiative, you can access information by going to www.health.gov/healthypeople/state/toolkit.

At this time, though, I will briefly get back to the question asked at the beginning of this chapter "Does establishing federal goals help to promote healthy aging?" and give you a succinct answer: Not if you are only setting goals and monitoring.

SOCIODEMOGRAPHIC TRENDS

It has been almost obligatory over the past 30 years to begin a gerontological book or article with comments about the rapid aging of society. About 15 years ago we began to see two slight variations of this ritual: many published works began with comments about the *aging of the aged,* and an additional spate of writings were on the coming onslaught of aging *baby boomers,* born between 1946 and 1964.

Today, with the vanguard of baby boomers and very old individuals receiving considerable media attention for different reasons, both ends of the older age spectrum command our full attention. The robust baby boomers–cum–gerontology boomers make it obvious to all but the most ageist that the vitality of aging persons can remain strong. The stereotype of aging as a process synonymous with physical and mental deterioration has been convincingly challenged. Also, an increasing number of boomers are now receiving Social Security checks, and this deserves our attention as well.

At the other end of the age spectrum, among persons age 85 and older, the growth in the percentage of the very old begins to startle—about a 40% growth per decade. In 1980 there were 2.2 million Americans aged 85 and over, in 1990 about 3 million, in 2000 around 4.3 million, and in 2010 about 6 million. They are also disproportional recipients of Medicare reimbursements.

Along with the increasing breadth of the age span of Americans comes increasing complexity. Fifty-year-olds are eligible for membership in AARP (formerly the American Association of Retired Persons), but they are quite different from 70-year-olds, who in turn are significantly different from 90-year-olds. Moreover, 90-year-olds are different from one another. A few of them are pumping iron and throwing away their canes, whereas others are waiting to die. This diversity is addressed in Chapter 11.

What aging Americans have in common, be they 50 or 90, robust or frail, is a future with an intensified demand for *medical* care (euphemistically referred to in America as *health* care) and the ongoing escalation of medical care costs. Driving these demands and costs are the increasing numbers of aging persons with both chronic and acute medical conditions and an expensive, high-tech, acute care–oriented medical system.

As we entered the third millennium, this demand for costly and sophisticated medical care collided with an unpredictable federal budget. In fewer than 6 months' time during the year 2001, the United States went from a record-breaking, astoundingly huge budget surplus to budget deficits of enormous size and uncertain duration—thanks to the one-two punch of federal legislation that launched a 10-year tax cut and the surging costs of both domestic programs (and, a few years later, new programs such as Medicare Part D) and the launching of a war on terrorism.

Then, in September 2008 the United States and the rest of the world experienced the beginning of an economic meltdown unrivaled since the Wall Street crash of 1929. As retirement savings and home values plunged, a virtually unregulated financial system fueled by risky mortgage-lending practices gone bust led to many financial institutions failing, selling out, or being taken over by the government.

Paralleling the uncertainty of our overall economic future was the deterioration of Medicare finances. Medicare expenditures in 2011 totaled 500 billion—about 13% of the federal budget—and Medicare was expected to be unable to fulfill its obligations by 2017 if nothing was done. The American public's voracious appetite for medical care combined with unmanageable medical cost inflation was unsustainable.

Some argue that the solution is to encourage *health promotion, disease prevention,* and *chronic disease management*. Health promotion advocates, however, often fail to consider that prevention/promotion/management entails substantial costs in the attempt to screen and educate everyone, and many will not benefit from an intervention. And even if these interventions were to prove effective for most people, healthier individuals will live longer on tax-payer-supported Social Security and Medicare, only to die of other costly medical conditions. (Perhaps supporting the philosopher/humorist Woody Allen's contention that death is the best way to cut down on expenses.) Health promotion advocates respond to these concerns with data showing that people who are overweight and underactive are living nearly as long as those with healthier lifestyles but are much sicker for a longer period of time and require more costly interventions.

Whichever side is right, the media has taken a stand, allocating considerable time and space to the merits of promoting good health practices to improve quality of life and realize medical care cost savings. Joining the media are some federal and state government programs that have sponsored disease prevention and, to an increasing extent, health promotion and disease management; the health professions, which have proclaimed its importance in the education and training of students; the business community, which has firmly supported this approach for employees; and individuals who often discuss their attempts at these practices, both successful and otherwise.

If disease prevention, health promotion, and chronic disease management strategies have been vying for center stage in society as a way of controlling medical costs, it has been the stage of a not very prosperous community theater. The federal government plays a limited role in disease prevention and chronic disease management, and rarely subsidizes health promotion. State governments have been more concerned about dealing with the additional expenditures that the federal government has passed along to them (Medicaid, for example) than on new disease prevention, health promotion, and disease management initiatives that require funding.

Health professionals, too, have provided mostly lip service to promoting health because they have not been reimbursed for it. Health science students have received only a modicum of health promotion instruction and training, and experience in applying it is the exception rather than the rule. The business community has devoted resources to health promotion (calling it worksite wellness) but has stopped short of focusing on those who need it most—older and more sedentary employees.

And last but not least, individuals have spent more time and money on health promotion. But they also have spent more time and money at fast-food restaurants, eating larger portions of food with higher fat content; and on computers, in front of which they sit for an increasing number of hours. (Not to mention it is dangerous to walk while looking at your smartphone.)

Perhaps the disparity between the promise of health promotion, disease prevention, and chronic disease management and the associated attention shown to these activities, on the one hand, versus the lack of government resource allocation adequate to supporting them, originates in the American value of individual responsibility. Unlike medicine, where we know we are not responsible for prescribing our own drugs or conducting surgery on ourselves or our family members, we feel capable of walking briskly and eating healthfully—if we choose—without the need of experts, health programs, or taxpayer financial support. Thus, though most people are not doing as good a job as they would like at promoting their health, we tend to believe it is up to the individual to take responsibility for it.

Individual responsibility is an important American value, but individuals are imperfect and need help. If support can be provided by some combination of government, business, the media, the community, health professionals, religious institutions, family, and friends, we will be able to do much better at promoting our own health and the health of the people we love.

The following chapters of this book offer ample ideas and information on health promotion and aging to provide some basis for optimism and to inspire additional initiatives—from the individual to all major institutions of society, including family, work, government, religion, health care, and education. Sociodemographic data suggest that aging adults not only may be the leading cause of escalating medical costs, but also have the potential to lead the way in the implementation of creative and cost-effective health promotion strategies. The data reveal that the educational level of aging Americans has risen, that these individuals are increasingly health conscious, and that they are active in community health-promoting endeavors.

Much of the information in the next section is taken from summaries of data provided by sources like the U.S. Bureau of the Census, the Administration on Aging's *A Profile of Older Americans: 2011*, the National Center for Health Statistics, the Federal Interagency Forum on Aging-Related Statistics' *Older Americans 2012: Key Indicators of Well-Being, The State of Aging and Health in America* from the Merck Company Foundation, and the Centers for Disease Control and Prevention.

Population Growth Over Age 65

All but the most uninformed know that the average age of the American population has been increasing dramatically. Between 1950 and 2050 the number of Americans age 65+ increases more than six fold, with more than two thirds of that growth taking place after 2000 (Figure 1.1). The percentage age 65 and over is projected to reach 20%.

The percentages in Table 1.2 show why the population "age pyramid"—a few *older adults* at the top and many children at the bottom—is rapidly becoming an *"age rectangle."*

The Baby Boomers

The baby boomers are the 76 million persons who were born in the United States between 1946 and 1964. Most were conceived when the millions of soldiers, sailors, and marines returned home from World War II and created a surge in the number of births that started quickly—there were fewer than 2.8 million births in 1945 but more than 3.4 million in 1946—and lasted 19 years. The boomers challenged U.S. hospital capacity when they were born, the adequacy of the public school system a few years later, society

FIGURE 1.1   **Population age 65 and over and age 85 and over, selected years 1900–2010 and projected 2020–2050.**

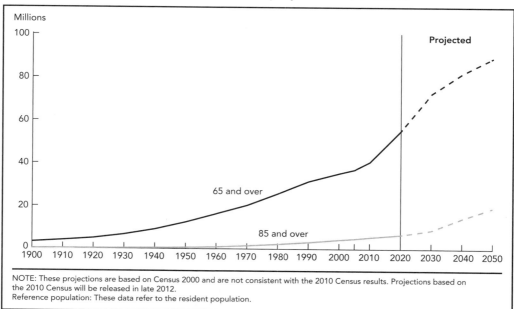

NOTE: These projections are based on Census 2000 and are not consistent with the 2010 Census results. Projections based on the 2010 Census will be released in late 2012.
Reference population: These data refer to the resident population.

Source: Data from U.S. Census Bureau. Compiled by the Federal Interagency Forum on Aging Related Statistics—Older Americans 2012: Key Indicators of Well-Being. Retrieved from www.agingstats.gov

TABLE 1.2 Becoming an Age Rectangle

YEAR	UNDER AGE 18	OVER AGE 65
1900	40%	4%
1980	28%	11%
2030	20%	20%

in general when they reached draft age and spurned the politicians intent on expanding the Vietnam War, and still later the sufficiency of available housing for raising their families.

The baby boomers' impact on society as they approach old age is still unclear. Will they be known as the spoiled descendents of the Greatest Generation or as pioneers in social reform and civil rights? Their impact on society as older persons raises an even more troublesome question, one posed by the Beatles in a song lyric that asks society if it would still need us when we're 64. If the Beatles had been more knowledgeable about aging, they would have substituted 84 for 64, as it more accurately represents a threshold to frailty and incompetence. (As far as they were concerned 64 was the same as 84: too old to differentiate.) Hopefully we will be able to answer this question in the affirmative by the time the first boomers reach age 84 in 2030.

In 2010 the number of Americans between the ages of 45 and 64 was about twice that of those age 65 and over: roughly 79 million versus 39 million. And boomers will bring into retirement not only their large numbers and a history of advocacy, but also a powerful interest in, and impact on, the solvency of the Social Security and Medicare programs. Their influence on society is likely to be dramatic and widespread as they become retirees in increasing numbers.

As eloquently stated by Frank Whittington, director of Georgia State's Gerontology Center (and paraphrased here),

> On January 2, 2008, shortly after 9 a.m., a simple bureaucratic event was the harbinger of a fundamental change in American society. Kathleen Casey-Kirschling—the first baby boomer, who had been born one second after midnight on January 1, 1946—walked into the local office of the Social Security Administration and applied for retirement benefits. She celebrated her 62nd birthday on New Year's Day and applied for early Social Security benefits at her first opportunity. Over the next couple of decades over 70 million of her peers will follow suit. We must not doubt that when Kathleen Casey-Kirschling strode up to the counter to ask for her benefits, all of our lives had begun to change.

As boomers retire they will make enormous demands on both the Social Security and Medicare programs, which, at the same time, will be supported by a shrinking taxpaying workforce. By the time the last boomer turns 65 in the year 2029, the retirees drawing Social Security and Medicare benefits will account for one in five Americans.

Will boomers be healthier than today's cohort of older adults? We do not know yet. The boomers rate their overall health status better than today's cohort of older adults, with a higher percentage reporting that their health is good to excellent. And death rates for heart disease and stroke continue to decline. But diabetes, chronic lower respiratory disease, high cholesterol, and hypertension are higher (www.bc.edu/agingandwork).

The Older Old, Chronic Conditions, and Disability

The older population itself is getting older. The percentage of persons age 85 and over is growing faster than any other age group. There was a 36% increase among Americans 85 and over from 1980 to 1990 (from 2.2 million to 3 million), a 43% increase from 1990 to 2000 (from 3 million to 4.3 million), and a 40% increase from 2000 to 2010 (from 4.3 million to about 6 million). Every decade there is another 40% increase in the number of persons aged 85 and over.

This demographic trend is significant for two reasons. On the positive side, the rapid growth of this segment of the population has made what was previously an age level rarely attained into an increasingly common stage of the life cycle. Moreover, the percentage of older adults age 75 and over who report good health or better is 66%.

Experts believe that today's 70-year-old is more like the 60-year-old of previous generations (Trafford, 2000). Older adults have the same perception about themselves. The National Council on Aging (2002) together with the Harris National Survey reported that 51% of persons between the ages of 65 and 74 and 33% of persons age 75 and over perceive themselves as middle-aged or younger! This certainly is evidence that many older adults are redefining old age as beginning later in the life cycle.

On the challenging side, for both individuals and society, is the fact that the ability of this age group to function fully is significantly less than for the younger old. *Activities of daily living* (ADL) is the standard for assessing functionality and refers to difficulties with bathing/showering, dressing, eating, transferring, walking, and toileting. As you can tell from Figure 1.2, the *older old*, those over the age of 85, have three to four times the difficulties of the younger old, those age 65 to 74.

Whereas only 6% of individuals age 65 to 69 reported difficulties with at least one ADL task, 28% of those age 85+ had such difficulties. Similarly, only 1% of persons age 65 were residents of nursing homes, but 22% of persons age 85+ were residents. The older-old person places more demands on family caregivers and societal resources.

FIGURE 1.2   **Percentage of persons with limitations in ADL by age group: 2009.**

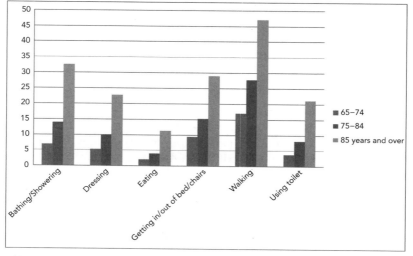

Source: A Profile of Older Americans: 2011, Administration on Aging. Retrieved from www.aoa.gov/aoaroot/aging_statistics/Profile/index.aspx.

The leading *chronic conditions* among older adults are listed in Figure 1.3. The prevalence of each condition increases in old age, and persons over age 85 often have multiple chronic conditions. The leading chronic conditions are hypertension, arthritis, heart disease, cancer, and diabetes. Women report higher levels of asthma, arthritis, and hypertension; men report higher levels of heart disease, cancer, and diabetes.

Although chronic conditions and functional limitations increase with age, disability rates for older Americans have been declining. In 1982 the disabled older population in the United States totaled 6.4 million. If the 1982 rate had continued, the number of disabled would have climbed to about 9.3 million in 1999. Instead, it rose to only 7 million—less than a quarter of the increase that might have been expected. Another way to view this change is that in 1982, 26.2% of those age 65 and over had a disability that represented a substantial limitation in a major life activity; by 1999 this percentage had fallen to 19.7%. As of 2004–2005, the rate had declined to 19%. Analysts attribute this ongoing reduction to a general rise in socioeconomic status, enhancements in medical care and rehabilitation, and improvements in lifestyle.

Another hopeful research outcome in disability trends is the conclusion that among the long-lived, even longer lives do not mean significantly more disability. As more people today are living into their 90s and beyond (the fastest-growing age segment of society in developed countries), researchers have found that the percentage who are independent changed less than expected between the ages of 92 and 100. Overall, 39% of 92-year-old Danish adults were able to care for themselves, and the same was true of 33% of those who lived to the age of 100 (Christensen, McGue, Petersen, Jeune, &

FIGURE 1.3   **Percentage of people age 65 and over who reported having selected chronic health conditions, by gender, 2009–2010.**

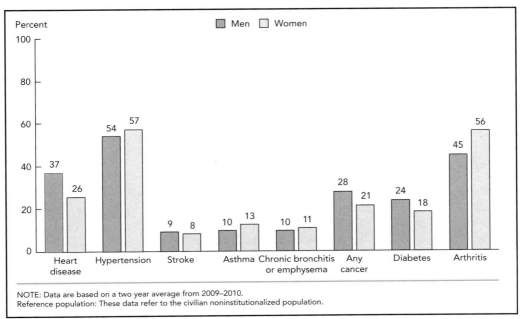

NOTE: Data are based on a two year average from 2009–2010.
Reference population: These data refer to the civilian noninstitutionalized population.

Source: Data from U.S. Census Bureau. Compiled by the Federal Interagency Forum on Aging Related Statistics—Older Americans 2012: Key Indicators of Well-Being. Retrieved from www.agingstats.gov.

Vaupel, 2008). In general, loss of independence among the very old appears to occur close to the end of life and is not significantly more severe or costly for the 100-year-old than for the 90-year-old.

Centenarians

In 2010 the Census showed that there were 53,364 people who were 100 years or older, an increase of 5.8% since the 2000 count. Some census projections forecast 15 times that many by the year 2050, when the baby boomers begin reaching age 100.

According to the *Guinness Book of World Records* (www.guinnessworldrecords.com), a French woman, Jeanne-Louise Calment, has lived the longest, reaching 122 years before she died in 1997. In 2005 the oldest living person was a Dutch woman, Hendrikje van Andel-Schipper, who had reached 115 years and who attributed her longevity to eating a piece of herring every day.

On June 9, 2005, the world's oldest living married couple had an aggregate age of 205 years. Magda Brown, age 100, attributed her 74-year union to Herbert Brown, age 105, to her taking the lead ("I am the strong one") and his following ("He is the easy-going one"). Apparently, Herbert is more than just easy-going. He survived the Nazi concentration camp at Dachau.

A USA Today/ABC News poll reported that only 25% of Americans want to live to be 100 or older. The majority of Americans are concerned that they will become disabled and a burden to their families. And yet many Americans are fascinated by the idea of an increasing number of people becoming *centenarians*. (There are also 70 verified super-centenarians—110 years or older—on the planet.)

The same holds true for scientists. One scientist, though, is not content with being a mere centenarian (or supercentenarian). Aubrey de Grey is a controversial practitioner of *biogerontology*, which focuses on the biology, physiology, and genetics of aging. He believes that the first person who will live to be 1,000 might be age 60 today. (A more credible assertion by Christensen and colleagues [2009] is that 50% of women born today in the most developed countries will celebrate their 100th birthday.) Although this Englishman's ideas are far from the scientific mainstream, he has inspired considerable interest in his theories, having been invited to deliver dozens of presentations in the United States. This interest may have been stimulated in part by his offer of a $20,000 cash prize for anyone who can disprove the scientific basis of his theories, as determined by a review panel of independent molecular biologists. His provocative ideas on increased longevity range from stem cells that can regrow diseased tissue, to implanting bacteria to clean up waste that builds up inside cells.

Life Expectancy

The *life expectancy* of Americans born in 2012 is 78.9 years, the highest it has ever been, according to a United Nations study. Before we break out the champagne, though, it should be noted that the United States was behind 49 other countries in life expectancy, with 30 of these countries having a life expectancy over age 80.

Americans' life expectancy has been rising almost without interruption since 1900, thanks to advances in sanitation, medicine, and health behavior (particularly smoking cessation). It is by no means certain whether these increases in life expectancy will continue unabated. Increases in obesity, and the related conditions of hypertension and diabetes, may reverse this trend; whereas the advent of cholesterol-lowering drugs and other advances in medicine may foster it. The future may also be determined by changes in the health behavior patterns of eating more nutritiously, exercising, and not smoking.

The longevity gender gap has been closing in the United States. Contemporary men will live to age 76.2 versus 81.3 for women. This 5-year gap is the smallest recorded since 1946. The population of men ages 85 to 94 grew by nearly half, whereas the number of women in the same age group increased by about a fifth. Medical experts speculate that women are working harder, smoking more, and undergoing more stress. The disparity between Blacks and Whites is also declining, with the gap between Black and White men being 6 years and the gap for women 4 years.

Heart disease continues to be the leading cause of death in 2009 (see Table 1.3), but during the prior 3 years the gap between heart disease and cancer continued to narrow steadily. Also during this time, respiratory diseases and strokes switched places in the rankings, and Alzheimer's disease continued to rise in the table.

Hospital Stays and Physician Visits

The average length of a hospital stay for an older patient continues to decline, from more than 12 days in 1964, to 8.5 days in 1986, to 6.5 days in 1996, to 5 days in 1999, to 4.6 days in 2007. As a percentage of overall Medicare costs, hospital expenditures declined from 32% to 24% between 1982 and 2008, and instead of being the major cost driver, it is only two thirds of the amount Medicare spends on physician/outpatient costs.

Although quickening hospital discharges over the past few decades affect all age groups, the growing numbers of older adults in the United States results in a higher percentage of older patients in the hospital. Older adults accounted for 20% of hospital stays and used one third of the total days of hospital care in 1970; by 2000 they accounted for 40% of hospital stays and almost one half of the days of hospital care (Hall & Owings, 2002).

Older persons had more than seven office visits with their doctors in 2009, compared to persons aged 45 to 65, who averaged fewer than four office visits. It is estimated that older patients occupy 50% of the time of health care practitioners, and it is predicted with near certainty that the percentage of time that health care practitioners spend with older patients will continue to increase.

Medication Use

Although hospital stays declined, medication costs among Medicare enrollees went up, from 8% of overall costs in 1992 to 16% of overall costs in 2008. Older adults constitute about 13% of the population but consume 32% of all prescription drugs and 40% of over-the-counter drugs. Accompanying the volume of drug consumption among older

TABLE 1.3 Ten Leading Causes of Death Among Older Adults Age 65+ in 2009

1. Heart Disease	599,000
2. Cancer	568,000
3. Chronic Lower Respiratory Diseases	137,000
4. Stroke	129,000
5. Unintentional Injury	118,000
6. Alzheimer's Disease	79,000
7. Diabetes	69,000
8. Influenza and Pneumonia	54,000
9. Kidney Disease	49,000
10. Suicide	37,000

Source: Centers for Disease Control and Prevention.

adults has been the burden of rising prescription drug costs over the past several years. The growth in prescription drug expenditures was double-digit every year from 1994 to 2001. The annual rate of growth in such expenditures reached an astonishing 19.7% in 1999, although it declined in 2000 (16.4%) and 2001 (15.7%) as employers increased copayments.

Medicare Part D was launched in 2006 and stimulated medication price growth that was three times the rate of inflation (see Chapter 12). The good news was that beginning a few years later, new prescriptions were increasingly being filled with lower-priced generics. Many popular medications were coming off of patent protection, and there were few expensive, patent-protected breakthroughs to drive up costs.

A nationally representative sample of community-residing individuals aged 57 to 85 years revealed at least one prescription medication was used by 81% of the sample, at least one over-the-counter medication by 42%, and at least one dietary supplement by 49%. Also, at least five prescription medications were being used concurrently by 29% of the sample (Qato et al., 2008).

By 2010 the steady increase of prescription and over-the-counter drugs rose to 17% of all health expenditures, fueled by advertising of prescription drugs on television, and an increase in the number of prescriptions written by physicians. In 2011 spending on drugs suddenly leveled off, for two reasons: (1) the use of lower-cost generic drugs increased to 80% of all dispensed prescriptions, and (2) the cumulative effects of the recession of 2008, the increase in the uninsured, and the drop in physician office visits and hospital admissions, both places where drugs are most often prescribed.

Health Habits

On the brighter side, the health habits of older adults may, on balance, be slightly superior to those of younger adults. People age 65 and over, for instance, are less likely to smoke, drink alcohol, or report high stress. They eat more sensibly than do younger adults, are as likely to walk for exercise, and are more likely to check their blood pressure regularly. Older adults continue to increase their rate of participation in medical screenings and immunizations, and adults in general increased their seatbelt use.

On the darker side, older adults are more likely to be sedentary and malnourished. And their advantage in being less stressed may be merely the result of less awareness of or less willingness to report stress. The lower percentage of smokers may be due in part to the fact that smokers are more likely to die before age 65. Also, when older adults engage in risk behaviors such as excessive alcohol consumption, sedentary behavior, poor nutrition, and failure to use seatbelts, their vulnerability to morbidity and mortality is greater.

To put things in perspective, though, few adults in the United States, young or old, live a comprehensively healthy lifestyle. National data reveal that only 3% of the population engage in all four of the following lifestyle choices: nonsmoking, healthy weight, five fruit and vegetable servings per day, and regular physical activity (Reeves & Rafferty, 2005). Among older adults, one third do not get any leisure-time physical activity, two thirds do not eat five servings of fruit or vegetables a day, and one fifth are 30 pounds or more overweight.

Perceptions of Health

Most people who are older tend to view their health positively, according to the report, *Older Americans 2012: Key Indicators of Well-Being*. Seventy-six percent of older adults, age 65 and over, rate their health as being good, very good, or excellent. Among those age 85 and over, this percentage declines to 67% who report good, very good, or excellent health. This percentage further declines to 63% among Black or Hispanic older adults age 65 and older, and to 56% among those without a high school diploma.

Volunteering

Many older adults are active and productive, and some choose to engage in volunteer opportunities. In any given year, almost one fifth of older Americans engage in unpaid volunteer work for organizations such as churches, schools, or civic organizations. In addition, an unknown percentage of older adults do other types of volunteer work, such as helping the sick or disabled, or assisting with the care of grandchildren.

Surprisingly, those who continue to work after age 65 are not less likely to volunteer than those older adults who retire (Caro & Morris, 2001). Researchers believe that the potential for increasing volunteerism among retired older adults is significant, and that "in the period immediately after retirement there is a heightened receptivity to volunteerism" (Caro & Morris, 2001, p. 349).

Marital Status

Older men are much more likely to be married, 72% versus 42%, and much less likely to be widowed, 13% versus 40%, than older women (see Figure 1.4). In absolute numbers, there were over four times as many widows (8.7 million) as widowers (2.1 million). Divorced or separated older adults represented only 12.4%, and single adults only 4.5% of the population. Both of these categories are likely to increase with the coming of the baby boomers and their greater acceptance of divorce, separation, and a single lifestyle.

Based on percentage alone, women should expect to spend all of, or part of, their later years without a husband (58%).

FIGURE 1.4   **Marital status of persons 65+, 2010.**

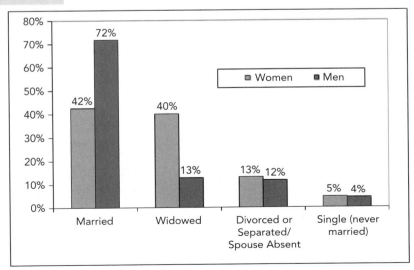

Source: *A Profile of Older Americans: 2011, Administration on Aging.* Retrieved from www.aoa.gov/aoaroot/aging_statistics/Profile/index.aspx.

Work

Labor force participation rate, that is, the percentage of a population that is in the labor force, of older men steadily declined throughout the 20th century, then began to rise in 1995 (see Figure 1.5). According to the Bureau of Labor Statistics, with the exception of the older male worker ages 55 to 61, a growing percentage of older adults are remaining in the workforce.

Among men ages 62 to 64, the participation rate increased from 45% in 1995 to 53% in 2011. Among men ages 65 to 69, the participation rate increased from 25% in the mid-1990s to 37% in 2011. Among men age 70 and over, the participation rate increased from 10% in the mid-1990s to 15% in 2011.

Labor force participation rates began to rise 10 years earlier for women than for men, around 1985 (see Figure 1.6). Also unlike for men, the greatest gains in participation for women occurred from ages 55 to 61 (men declined during this age interval), increasing from 46% in 1985 to 65% in 2011. For women ages 62 to 64, 65 to 69, and 70+, the increase in participation began in the mid-1990s, like it did for men.

The increasing labor force participation for older women reflects the aging of the huge cohort of baby boomers and the rising expectation that women will work. As the boomer women got older, the difference between the labor force participation of the sexes narrowed.

According to a 2012 Gallup survey, 81% of working people reported they thought they would work part time (63%) or full time (18%) when they reached retirement age.

| FIGURE 1.5 | Labor force participation rates of men age 55 and over, by age group, annual averages, 1963–2011. |

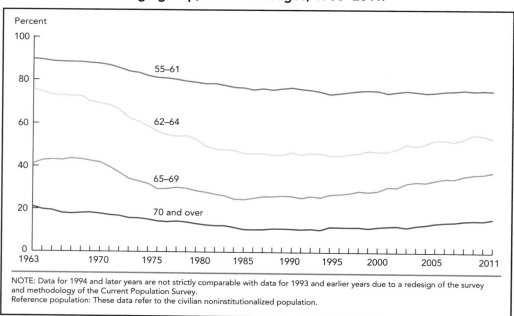

NOTE: Data for 1994 and later years are not strictly comparable with data for 1993 and earlier years due to a redesign of the survey and methodology of the Current Population Survey.
Reference population: These data refer to the civilian noninstitutionalized population.

Source: Data from U.S. Census Bureau. Compiled by the Federal Interagency Forum on Aging Related Statistics—Older Americans 2012: Key Indicators of Well-Being. Retrieved from www.agingstats.gov.

FIGURE 1.6   **Labor force participation rates of women age 55 and over, by age group, annual averages, 1963–2011.**

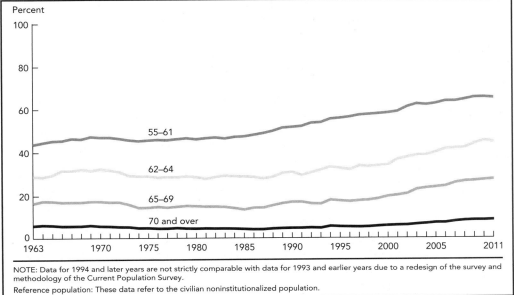

NOTE: Data for 1994 and later years are not strictly comparable with data for 1993 and earlier years due to a redesign of the survey and methodology of the Current Population Survey.
Reference population: These data refer to the civilian noninstitutionalized population.

Source: Data from U.S. Census Bureau. Compiled by the Federal Interagency Forum on Aging Related Statistics—Older Americans 2012: Key Indicators of Well-Being. Retrieved from www.agingstats.gov.

Two thirds of the part-time predictors and one third of the full-time predictors stated they would be working because they wanted to, the others because they would likely have to for financial reasons. Prior to the economic meltdown that began in September 2008, the total percentage planning to work in their so-called retirement years was 69%, considerably lower than the 81% of today. Expecting to work during one's retirement years, obviously, will not be perfectly correlated with actually working, given the challenges of finding a job, sustaining good health, and/or dealing with onerous family caregiving responsibilities.

With increasing life expectancy, workers can anticipate a longer retirement phase to save for. Complicating matters is that employees are increasingly less able to take advantage of the security and predictability of defined benefit programs (i.e., traditional pensions provided by employers) and instead must rely on defined contribution programs (i.e., do-it-yourself retirement savings plans that are subject to the whims of the stock market).

Labor force participation among older adults in the United States is considerably higher than in most other countries, including France, Germany, Italy, Sweden, United Kingdom, and Canada; although it is lower than the rate in Japan.

Educational Status

In 1965, 24% of the older population had graduated from high school and only 5% had at least a bachelor's degree or more. By 2010, 80% were high school graduates or more and 23% had a bachelor's degree or more (see Figure 1.7). When the last baby boomer reaches age 65 (replacing most of the current cohort of older adults) this percentage increases to 89% high school graduates, along with 36+% college graduates. In 2010, older men had attained two thirds of the bachelor's degrees, but if current trends hold, this percentage will be substantially reversed. Women have constituted about 57% of college matriculation for several years now.

The Sloan Center on Aging and Work at Boston College published a fact sheet in 2012 (www.bc.edu/agingandwork) that noted an important fact about the impact of education on older adults who want to continue working. The unemployment rate of workers age 65 or older who had completed 4 or more years of college was only one half that of older workers who had not completed high school.

Unfortunately, the percentage of older adults who had completed high school varied considerably by race and ethnic origin. In 2010, 84% of non-Hispanic Whites age 65 and over had completed high school, and 74% of older Asians. In contrast, 65% of older Blacks and 47% of older Hispanics had completed high school (see Figure 1.8). Regarding attainment of at least a bachelor's degree, 35% of older Asians had accomplished this along with 24% of older non-Hispanic Whites. The proportions, however, were 15% and 10%, respectively, for older Blacks and Hispanics.

The boomers in 2008 (ages 44 to 62 at that time) reached the highest educational levels: 89% were high school graduates and 34% (and counting) were college graduates. If Nola Ochs and Phyllis Turner are role models, boomers have *plenty* of time to further increase their college graduation rate.

| FIGURE 1.7 | **Educational attainment of the population age 65 and over, selected years 1965–2010.** |

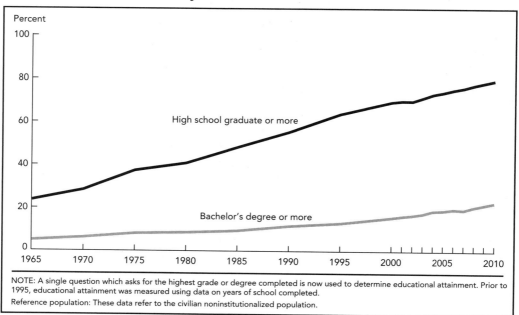

NOTE: A single question which asks for the highest grade or degree completed is now used to determine educational attainment. Prior to 1995, educational attainment was measured using data on years of school completed.
Reference population: These data refer to the civilian noninstitutionalized population.

Source: Data from U.S. Census Bureau. Compiled by the Federal Interagency Forum on Aging Related Statistics—Older Americans 2012: Key Indicators of Well-Being. Retrieved from www.agingstats.gov.

FIGURE 1.8   Educational attainment of the population age 65 and over, by race and Hispanic origin, 2010.

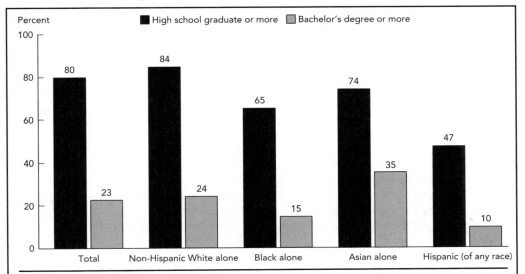

NOTE: The term "non-Hispanic White alone" is used to refer to people who reported being White and no other race and who are not Hispanic. The term "Black alone" is used to refer to people who reported being Black or African American and no other race, and the term "Asian alone" is used to refer to people who reported only Asian as their race. The use of single-race populations in this chart does not imply that this is the preferred method of presenting or analyzing data. The U.S. Census Bureau uses a variety of approaches.

Reference population: These data refer to the civilian noninstitutionalized population.

Source: Data from U.S. Census Bureau. Compiled by the Federal Interagency Forum on Aging Related Statistics—Older Americans 2012: Key Indicators of Well-Being. Retrieved from www.agingstats.gov.

Nola Ochs got her undergraduate degree from Fort Hays State University in Kansas in 2007 at the age of 95. Nola was not the only nonagenarian that year with such an impressive educational achievement. Phyllis Turner, at age 94, received her master's degree in medical science at the University of Adelaide in Australia. Not many boomers are likely to be discouraged from attending college because of their age.

By 2007 there were more than 400 *lifelong learning* programs targeted toward older adults in the United States and Canada, almost all of them linked with colleges and universities and many of them loosely associated with Road Scholar (formerly Elderhostel and Exploritas) or the Osher Lifelong Learning Institutes, funded by the Bernard Osher Foundation. There were also a variety of other lifelong learning opportunities, such as the Adventures in Learning programs at Shepherd's Centers, the educational programs at OASIS Centers, and other innovative educational options at community colleges, community centers, art museums, and hospitals (see Chapter 9, "Community Health").

As the educational level of older adults continues to rise, this may well correlate with an increase in their interest in seeking out health information and engaging in health-promoting activities in their communities.

Political Power

The Federal Election Commission reports that older adults are disproportionately likely to vote. Moreover, the percentage of voting elders has increased over the past

20 years. In 1978 older adults generated 19% of all votes cast, in 1986, 21%, and in 1998, 23%.

Older adults are more likely to demonstrate high levels of civic engagement, paying more attention to politics and public affairs than younger adults (Binstock & Quadagno, 2001). Voting differences, however, are greater among older adults than between younger and older adults, as socioeconomic class, ethnicity, gender, and religion are more important influences on voting patterns than age. One exception to this trend was when older voters in the 2008 presidential election were the only age group that gave a majority of their votes to John McCain who, coincidentally or otherwise, was the considerably older candidate (Binstock, 2009).

Internet Access

A 2012 national survey from the Pew Research Center's Internet & American Life Project, reported that more than half—a majority for the first time—of adults ages 65 and older are now online. This is due to the tech-savvy baby boomers moving into the age 65+ ranks. Internet use among those over age 75 is, in contrast, only one third. Thus, the Internet access gap between younger adults and older adults will close rapidly in the near future.

Social-networking site use among Internet users ages 65 and older grew 150% in 2 years, from 13% in 2009 to 33% in 2011. The Pew study reported that people younger than age 50 used social-networking websites to stay in touch with friends, and people older than age 50 reported that they used them to connect with family.

Gender differences in overall computer usage have disappeared, with older women as likely to use the computer as older men—though usage of social-networking sites is likely to be greater among older females than older males. Income and education levels still govern differences in computer usage.

Poverty

The poverty rate among older persons had fallen from 35% of those age 65 and over, in 1969, to 9% in 2010. Without Social Security and cost-of-living increases, the rate would have risen to 50% over this time. Thanks to a variety of sources of income—Social Security (37%), public and private pensions (19%), earnings (30%), asset income (11%), and other (3%)—the poverty rate for older adults has, seemingly, fallen below the rate for persons age 18 to 64.

The declining poverty rate for older adults may be overstated, however. The U.S. Bureau of the Census assumes that the costs of food and other necessities are lower for older adults and it does not adequately take into account the rising costs of medical care, transportation, and housing expenses. Also, there are hidden poor among the older population who reside in nursing homes or who live with relatives and are not counted in the official census statistics (Hooyman & Kiyak, 2011).

The Supplemental Poverty Measure is a U.S. Census research tool that considers previously overlooked costs, like out-of-pocket medical expenses for older adults, and estimates the poverty rate of seniors to be 16% (Schwartz, 2011). The National Academy of Science estimates the poverty rate for older Americans at 19%.

The poverty rate is almost three times higher for older Hispanics and Blacks than for older Whites, and almost twice as high for older women than for older men, according to the 2011 Profile of Older Americans, published by the Administration on Aging. Combining gender and ethnicity, the highest poverty rates were experienced among Hispanic women (40.8%) who lived alone and by older Black women (30.7%) who lived alone.

Racial and Ethnic Composition

The diversity of the older adult population in America is increasing, and will continue to increase for the foreseeable future. In 2010, non-Hispanic Whites accounted for 80% of the older adult population in the United States, but this is projected to drop dramatically to 58% in 2050 (Figure 1.9). The fastest growing minority will be Hispanic elders of any race, almost tripling in percentage between 2010 and 2050. Comparable growth, but on a smaller scale, will be the tripling in percentage of older Asians.

Although health professionals will need to become more knowledgeable about the ethnic backgrounds of their older clients, there is great diversity within ethnic groups as well. Age, gender, region, religion, English-speaking skills, income, education, lifestyle, physical disability, marital status, place of birth, and length of residence in the United States are examples of important variables to consider within each ethnic group.

There is also a continuum of acculturation that occurs among elders within each ethnic group. Acculturation is the degree to which individuals incorporate the cultural values, beliefs, language, and skills of the mainstream culture. To avoid stereotyping ethnic groups, there needs to be recognition of the many distinctive ethnic subgroups (Haber, 2005a).

| FIGURE 1.9 | **Population age 65 and over, by race and Hispanic origin, 2010 and projected 2050.** |

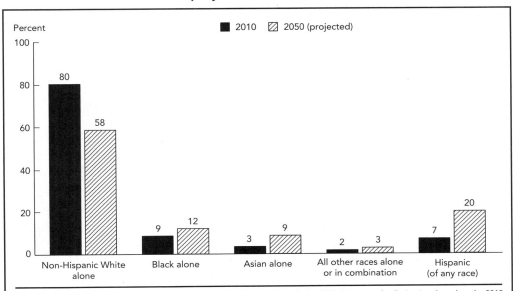

NOTE: These projections are based on Census 2000 and are not consistent with the 2010 Census results. Projections based on the 2010 Census will be released in late 2012. The term "non-Hispanic White alone" is used to refer to people who reported being White and no other race and who are not Hispanic. The term "Black alone" is used to refer to people who reported being Black or African American and no other race, and the term "Asian alone" is used to refer to people who reported only Asian as their race. The use of single-race populations in this chart does not imply that this is the preferred method of presenting or analyzing data. The U.S. Census Bureau uses a variety of approaches. The race group "All other races alone or in combination" includes American Indian and Alaska Native alone; Native Hawaiian and Other Pacific Islander alone; and all people who reported two or more races. Reference population: These data refer to the resident population.

Source: Data from U.S. Census Bureau. Compiled by the Federal Interagency Forum on Aging Related Statistics—Older Americans 2012: Key Indicators of Well-Being. Retrieved from www.agingstats.gov.

DEFINITIONS OF HEALTHY AGING

Health professionals need to be cautious about defining good health for older adults. This is the message delivered by Faith Fitzgerald in an editorial in the *New England Journal of Medicine* (Fitzgerald, 1994) cautioning against a narrow or rigid definition of health: "We must beware of developing a zealotry about health, in which we take ourselves too seriously and believe that we know enough to dictate human behavior, penalize people for disagreeing with us, and even deny people charity, empathy, and understanding because they act in a way of which we disapprove. Perhaps (we need to) debate more openly the definition of health" (pp. 197–198). Let us begin.

> **Question:** What is *your* definition of healthy aging?

The Federal Government

One such "cautious" definition of health is provided by the federal government's Public Health Service through its Health Objectives for the Nation. This broad definition of health includes the following three components:

1. Disease prevention, which comprises strategies to maintain and to improve health through medical care, such as high blood pressure control and immunization.
2. Health protection, which includes strategies for modifying environmental and social structural health risks, such as toxic agent and radiation control, and accident prevention and injury control.
3. Health promotion, which includes strategies for reducing lifestyle risk factors, such as avoiding smoking and the misuse of alcohol and drugs, and adopting good nutritional habits and a proper and adequate exercise regimen.

Extraordinary Accomplishments

The definition of good health in late life can be viewed from the unique perspective of extraordinary accomplishments by older adults.

Arts: *Falstaff*, Verdi's last opera, was composed when he was age 80. George Burns won an Oscar, his first, also at age 80. And Anna Mary Robertson, better known as Grandma Moses, had her first showing of her paintings at, you guessed it, age 80, after beginning this artistic pursuit just a couple of years earlier.

Enough with the youngsters. Herman Wouk, Pultizer Prize-winning author of *The Caine Mutiny*, published his latest novel, *The Lawgiver*, in 2012 at the age of 96. (At age 97, he is working on a new novel.) Mieczyslaw Horszowski, a classical pianist, recorded a new album at age 99. Johannes Heesters, a Dutch-born German singer–dancer–actor, was still appearing on stage at age 101. He announced at that age that he had no plans to take what he called "early retirement" because the stage was his life.

Jumping up to the age of 107, George Abbott collaborated on the revival of the musical *Damn Yankees*. George wasn't the only 107-year-old with an artistic bent. After Sadie and Bessie Delany wrote their bestseller: *The Delany Sisters' First Hundred Years*, Bessie died at age 104. Sadie then went on to author *On My Own at 107: Reflections on Life Without Bessie*. She died 2 years later at age 109.

Politics: In 2006 the average age of a United States senator was 62 years, the oldest it had ever been. Not surprisingly, the term *senate* derives from the Latin word for "old." Golda Meir became prime minister of Israel at age 71. Former Senator John Glenn completed the rigorous physical preparation necessary to become the oldest space traveler in history at age 77. Former President Jimmy Carter won the Nobel Prize as a global peacemaker at age 78.

Sports: Kozo Haraguchi ran the 100 meters in 22.04 seconds, setting a record for the 95 to 99 age group. This 95-year-old Japanese man said he had to run cautiously because the outdoor track was slick with rain. Another runner, Johnny Kelley, won the Boston Marathon twice. Even more remarkable was that he had started this annual race 61 times during his lifetime, completing the entire 26.2 miles 58 times. Mr. Kelley died in 2004 at the age of 97. Another nonagenarian, though, continued to race in 2004. Fauja Singh moved from India to England and decided to take up running at the age of 82. At the age of 92 he set a world record for his age group by running the Toronto Marathon in 5 hours and 40 minutes.

Ken Mink was a basketball player at Roane State, a junior college about 35 miles west of Knoxville, Tennessee. The 6-foot, 190-pound player was listed as a *senior* on the basketball roster. No kidding! Ken Mink was 73 years of age in 2008, more than a half-century older than his teammates. In fact, this septuagenarian was the oldest person ever to play college basketball.

Mountain climbing: Japanese mountaineer Tamae Watanabe set a world record in 2012 by becoming the oldest woman to scale Mount Everest, the tallest mountain in the world. She did this at the age of 73. She may have a couple of more decades to add to this achievement. Hulda Crooks, for instance, climbed Mount Whitney, the highest mountain in the continental United States, at the age of 91.

Work: U.S. District Court Judge Wesley E. Brown became the oldest working judge in the nation's history. Near the end of his life, he had to transfer some of his work from his Wichita, Kansas, courtroom to his bedroom at home—because of his health—where he died a few weeks later at the age of 104. Judge Brown, however, was not the oldest worker in the United States. Ray Crist still worked as a research scientist at Messiah College in Pennsylvania at the age of 104. He had earned his doctorate in chemistry from Columbia University at the age of 26 and was still putting it to good use 78 years later.

Religion: In 2009, 10 women ranging in age from 89 to 96 each memorized Hebrew in order to become a bat mitzvah, a Jewish girl who is marking the transition into religious adulthood. Unlike a bar mitzvah for a boy, a bat mitzvah was rare until the 1960s, and these women decided to make up for what they were denied as children. They met weekly for several months with a rabbi to study Hebrew to prepare for their rite of passage at the synagogue of the Menorah Park senior residence in Cleveland, Ohio. Although three used walkers and another carried a small oxygen tank to the podium, all successfully completed their deferred quest.

Birthing: A California woman named Arceli Keh lied about her age (she said she was 51 but was actually 61) in order to become eligible for a fertility program in which she was implanted with an embryo from an anonymous donor. In 1996, at age 63, she became the oldest woman on record to have a baby. Her record was surpassed in 2006 when Maria del Carmen Bousada, a 66-year-old Spanish woman, who had become pregnant after receiving in vitro fertilization treatment, gave birth to twins by Cesarean section in a hospital in Barcelona. The wisdom of this accomplishment was, however, called into question in 2009, when she died from cancer at age 69, leaving behind boys not yet 3 years old.

Bank robbing: Red Rountree, at the age of 91, became the oldest known bank robber in U.S. history in 2004. Sentenced to a 12-year term—likely a life sentence—in Texas, Red said he robbed banks for fun: "I feel good, awfully good for days after robbing a bank." After two successful heists, the third time apparently was not the charm. The teller at the third bank, responding to his demand for money, asked, "Are you kidding?"

Although I marvel at these examples of unusual achievement by aging adults, I do not use them as inspiration for older, or even younger, persons. These models are astonishing, but they do little to enhance the confidence of aging adults who do not believe they can—and perhaps do not want to—come close to achieving similar milestones.

As Betty Friedan (1993) noted in her book *The Fountain of Age*, as an older adult one may "attempt to hold on to, or judge oneself by, youthful parameters of love, work and power. For this is what blinds us to the new strengths and possibilities emerging in ourselves."

Nonetheless, I had an uproariously good time compiling these accomplishments.

Prevention

Prevention is often categorized as primary, secondary, or tertiary (Figure 1.10). *Primary prevention* focuses on an asymptomatic individual in whom potential risk factors have been identified and targeted. Primary preventive measures, such as regular exercise, good nutrition, smoking cessation, or immunizations, are recommended to decrease the probability of the onset of specific diseases or dysfunction. Primary prevention is different from *health promotion* in that it is less broad in scope and tends to be the term used by clinicians in a medical setting.

Secondary prevention is practiced with an asymptomatic individual in whom actual (rather than potential) risk factors have been identified even though the underlying disease is not yet clinically apparent. A medical screening, as an example of secondary prevention, is cost-effective only when there is hope of lessening the severity or shortening the duration of a pathological process. Blood pressure screenings, cholesterol screenings, and bone densitometry are the most widely implemented forms of secondary prevention.

Tertiary prevention, which takes place after the individual with a disease or disability becomes symptomatic, focuses on the rehabilitation or maintenance of function. Health professionals attempt to restore or maintain the maximum level of functioning possible, within the constraints of a medical problem, to prevent further disability and dependency on others.

Tertiary prevention corresponds to phase 2 (rehabilitation of outpatients) and phase 3 (long-term maintenance) of the rehabilitation of a cardiac patient (phase 1 is the care of a hospitalized cardiac patient). Randomized clinical trials with patients who had myocardial infarctions revealed that programs of tertiary prevention reduced the likelihood of cardiovascular mortality by 25%.

A focus on prevention may be more appealing to some older adults than an emphasis on health promotion. Older adults are likely to be coping with chronic conditions, and the prevention, delay, or reduction of disability and dependency is a much more salient issue for them than it is for most younger adults.

FIGURE 1.10   **Three levels of prevention.**

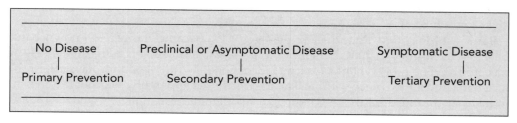

No Disease	Preclinical or Asymptomatic Disease	Symptomatic Disease
Primary Prevention	Secondary Prevention	Tertiary Prevention

Moreover, among medical professionals the relevancy of the term *prevention* is enhanced, because the costs of several prevention activities, such as mammograms, are reimbursable through Medicare. Prevention has gotten its foot in the door, so to speak, in the system of health care reimbursement, whereas the activities of health promotion have lagged considerably behind.

One advantage of the use of the term *health promotion*, however, is that it encompasses mental and spiritual health concerns. In contrast to clients and health professionals fixated on risk factors and the prevention of disease or disability, health promotion or wellness can be viewed as an affirming, even joyful, process. As health professionals who promote health, for instance, we can encourage playing with grandchildren or the joy of bird watching to an older client and not concern ourselves with its ability to prevent disease or illness.

Health promotion is also a more proactive approach than primary prevention, which tends to imply a reaction to the prospect of disease. Directing a client's anger or frustration into political advocacy work, for example, is a proactive, health-promoting enterprise that benefits both the individual and society.

Wellness

Although the term *wellness* has had many supporters in the health professions over the years (Jonas, 2000), particularly among persons who conduct health programs at large U.S. corporations (Jacob, 2002), it tends to be embraced less than the terms *health promotion* and *disease prevention*. Nonetheless, wellness conveys an important message—that good health is more than physical well-being. In fact, *seven dimensions* are usually touted among wellness advocates, as shown in Table 1.4.

Wellness sends a welcome and important reminder about the breadth of health promotion that is not conveyed by most other terms. The only limitation to the term wellness is that it tends to be identified with "alternative" activities—acupuncture, homeopathy, spiritual healing, aromatherapy—to the exclusion of more mainstream activities such as exercise and nutrition. Thus, it suggests fringe pursuits or even flakiness to some.

Antiold and Antiaging

Who is healthier, an old person or an older adult? Is this a preposterous question? Maybe not. Do the terms *old* and *older* reflect our prejudices? One of the leaders in the field of gerontological language, Erdman Palmore, thought so. Palmore suggested that

TABLE 1.4 Seven Dimensions of Wellness

Physical—Exercise, eat a well-balanced diet, get enough sleep, protect yourself.

Emotional—Express a wide range of feelings, acknowledge stress, channel positive energy.

Intellectual—Embrace lifelong learning, discover new skills and interests.

Vocational—Do something you love, balance work with leisure time.

Social—Laugh often, spend time with friends/family, join a club, respect cultural differences.

Environmental—Recycle daily, use energy-efficient products, walk or bike, grow a garden.

Spiritual—Seek meaning and purpose, take time to reflect, connect with the universe.

most of the synonyms for *old* are unhealthy in some way—words like *debilitated, infirm,* and *frail. Older adult,* on the other hand, is a more neutral term; and perhaps the term *elder* connotes an even healthier role for older persons in society (Palmore, 2000).

And yet I am reminded of an anecdote about Maggie Kuhn, the founder of the advocacy organization the Gray Panthers. She reported on an exchange that she had with President Gerald Ford at a hearing on a pension bill in Washington, DC. Once she had gotten President Ford's attention, he asked, "And what do you have to say, *young lady?*" Maggie replied, "First of all, I'm not a young lady. I'm an *old woman.*" She was making the statement that she was proud of being old, and that she had earned that label.

A related concern is the *antiaging* movement and its chief proponent, the American Academy of Anti-Aging Medicine. This professional society is "pursuing the fountain of youth with their lucrative nostrums and illusory interventions, [while] we geriatricians remain solidly in the trenches caring for our patients, the most aged, complex, frail, and vulnerable—far removed from the fantasies of eternal life, much less the fountain of youth" (Hazzard, 2005, p. 1435).

Most proponents of the antiaging movement are focused not on the most aged, but on the middle-aged and the young-old, those most concerned with combating the signs of aging. One key weapon in their arsenal is the *cosmeceutical,* a combination of the terms *cosmetic* and *pharmaceutical* that refers to a topical skin treatment formulated to eliminate the wrinkles and other signs of aging. If the cosmeceutical intervention proves insufficient, there are Botox injections, microdermabrasion, chemical peels, collagen injections, and plastic surgeries. Antiagers deliver a clear message that aging is a disease that needs to be cured—at least cosmetically and temporarily.

Another segment of the antiaging movement believe in the power of human growth hormone (HGH). A review of 31 randomized, controlled studies, however, concluded that the risks outweigh any potential antiaging benefits of HGH when taken by healthy older adults (Liu et al., 2007). Side effects may include diabetes, hypertension, hardening of the arteries, and abnormal growth of bones or internal organs. Nonetheless, government officials estimate that 25,000 to 30,000 American take injections of HGH for antiaging purposes, paying up to $1,000 a month. Although it is illegal to prescribe HGH for healthy people in the United States, speakers at the annual conference of the American Academy of Anti-Aging Medicine have told physicians in the audience how they can diagnose a mild hormone deficiency so that they can legally prescribe HGH (Wilson, 2007).

I think, however, that we need a *proaging movement,* one that emphasizes the healthy aspects of aging and the benefits that accrue with age. No longer needing to impress employers, in-laws, or peers, older adults are free to be themselves. The old have the opportunity to be not only freer, but also wiser, more conscious of the present, and more willing to be advocates for a healthy future. Maggie Kuhn certainly practiced a proaging lifestyle.

I am not the first to use the term *proaging.* Over the last few years advertisements for Dove beauty products have consistently asked the question "Are you antiage or proage?" Unfortunately, Dove's proage movement consisted entirely of selling moisturizers and other skin products. This is not what I have in mind when I talk about promoting a healthy attitude toward aging. (Not that I have anything against reasonably priced moisturizers.)

Compression of Morbidity

By definition, chronic diseases are not curable. The onset of chronic disease, however, may be postponed through the modification of risk factors. As the onset is delayed to later ages approaching the limit of the human life span, the result is a *compression of morbidity*. The goal is to live in robust health to a point as close as one can come to the end of the life span, so that one can die after only a brief period of illness. In short, spend a longer time living and a shorter time dying.

For most people, though, the prospect of living long past one's 65th birthday is a mixed blessing. With Americans living longer today than ever before, we have come to dread a prolonged period of disability and dependency in late life.

One definition of healthy aging, then, is to be able to live life fully until death. Unfortunately, very few Americans who die at age 65 or later are fully functional in the last year of life. Moreover, the longer one has lived, the longer the period of disability before death. At age 65 the average American has about 17 years left to live, with 6.5 (38%) of those years spent in a dependent state. In contrast, at age 85 we have an average of 7 years left to live, with 4.4 (63%) of those years spent in a dependent state.

Pessimists argue that the period of morbidity preceding death will lengthen in the future as a result of (a) limited biomedical research funds available to improve the physical and mental capacity of the very old; (b) the fact that some major diseases, such as Alzheimer's, do not have recognized lifestyle risk factors that we can modify; and (c) medical advances, such as dialysis and bypass surgery, that will increase the life expectancy of individuals with disease rather than prevent the occurrence of disease.

Optimists, on the other hand, claim that there will be a *compression of morbidity* (see Figure 1.11) in the future due to (a) the likelihood of advances in biomedical research that will prevent or delay the occurrence of disease and (b) the continued potential for reducing risk factors such as smoking, high blood pressure, poor nutritional habits, and sedentary lifestyles, which will result in better health.

Even as the general population further delays the onset of chronic disease due to these risk factors, the life *span* (the maximum number of years for a member of the species) is likely fixed. Thus, argue the compressionists, we will not only delay morbidity, but we will also shorten it.

Studies by Manton and colleagues (Connolly, 2001; Manton, Gu, & Lamb, 2006; Manton, Stallard, & Corder, 1998) analyzed data from the 1982 to 2004–2005 results of the National Long Term Care Survey, a federal study that regularly surveys almost 20,000 people age 65 and older. The researchers arrived at the unexpected conclusion that the percentage of chronically disabled older persons—those having impairments for 3 months or longer that impede daily activities—has been slowly falling. Whereas 26%

FIGURE 1.11   **Compression of morbidity.**

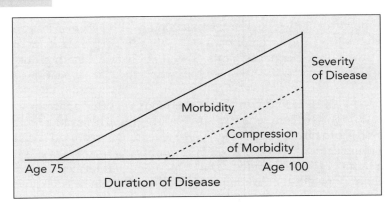

of people over age 65 reported chronic disability in 1982, only 20% reported this to be the case in 1994 and 19% did so in 2004–2005. Also, the percentage of persons over age 65 reporting no disabilities continued to rise.

Another study did not support evidence of a compression of morbidity. Over the past decade, length of life with disease and deteriorating function of mobility increased (Crimmins & Beltran-Sanchez, 2010). Although mortality rates declined, the prevalence of living with disease had increased.

Will we be able to compress morbidity? Unfortunately, we do not even know which factors most affect the compression of morbidity: Initiatives in health promotion, such as better diet, more exercise, and smoking cessation? Improved medical access and advances such as treatment for arthritis and cataracts? Increased use of devices such as canes, walkers, walk-in showers, support rails, and handicapped-accessible facilities? Societal improvements such as increased education and income levels? Improvement in any or all of these areas would be greatly welcomed by an aging population.

HEALTH PERSPECTIVES AND AGING

Health Expectancy Versus Life Expectancy

Those who live to the age of 65 are likely to live into their 80s or beyond. Of the remaining years, on average, of life after age 65, two thirds are likely to be healthy and one third will be years in which there is some functional impairment. Place yourself in the shoes of the person who has just reached age 65. Are you primarily interested in extending your life beyond the expected years you are likely to remain alive, or are you most interested in how many of these remaining years will find you healthy and independent?

Your *health expectancy*, or the number of healthy years you can expect to have left, depends to a great extent on your level of physical activity, nutritional intake, social support network, access to good medical care, health education, and utilization of health services. Health expectancy is more important to older adults than life expectancy. Unfortunately, we have not made adequate progress on this front. The goal of Healthy People 2000, for example, was to increase the number of years of healthy life remaining after age 65 to 14. It increased only to 12.2 years, an advance of only 0.4 of a year.

Physical Versus Emotional Aspects of Aging

There is a strong reciprocal relationship between the physical and emotional aspects of health. When our physical health is threatened, so typically is our emotional health. The converse is equally true.

As we age, however, it may be the case that good health becomes less dependent on our physical status than on our emotional status. Studies report shifting perspectives of health over time, with older participants expecting physical health problems because of their age and discounting them somewhat, when they do appear, because of this expectation.

A study of 85-year-olds living in the Netherlands reported that physical function was not the most important component of successful aging. These older adults were able to adapt successfully to physical limitations. The researchers reported social contacts as the most important factor in well-being, and the quality of the contacts was more important than their number (Von Faber et al., 2001). Open-ended interviews reveal more than 100 characteristics of health that are important to older adults besides physical health, including the ability to enjoy life and good personal relationships. Many older adults who are frail and sometimes disabled do *not* evaluate their health or life negatively.

Most health professionals subscribe to the notion that health is more than the absence of illness. Were this not the case, they would have to label the vast majority of older adults, 90% of whom are coping with a chronic condition, unhealthy. The chronic diseases that older persons contend with do not necessarily relate to their ability to perform daily activities. Disease, in fact, may not be evident even to the person who has it.

The presence or absence of disease, therefore, may not be a source of great concern to older adults. The ability to perform ADL, however, *is* of great concern to older adults, who desire as much independence as possible. The definition of health, especially among older adults, should not be linked with disease or its absence, as the medical model suggests, but with independence, the ability to accomplish one's goals, and the presence of satisfying relationships.

A health perspective that emphasizes the psychological status of older adults does not view health as a physical continuum ranging from disability and illness at one end, to a high level of robustness at the other. Critics of this type of health continuum argue that even a person who is functionally impaired or disabled, and thus residing at one end of the physical continuum, can focus considerable attention on a high level of wellness and psychological growth.

Finally, health professionals need to walk a fine line with older clients. On the one hand, they have been accused of ignoring the medical needs of older adults by discounting the viability of certain medical interventions due to advanced patient age. In fact, patients in their 80s can benefit as much from surgical interventions as can younger patients (Varghese & Norman, 2004). On the other hand, health professionals can unduly focus on the (reimbursable) medical needs of very old clients and neglect the personal values that inform the quality of life of the older adult and how they might shape a decision to risk surgery and its aftereffects.

Intergenerational Conflict Over Health Care?

Creating a name for a generation and then generalizing about it is fraught with complexity, and some analysts shy away from it—but many do not. I personally think it is a type of intellectual fun that analysts find hard to resist. Moreover, there is an interesting argument to be made that there will be generational conflict over health care expenditures in the future. But first, there are three generations to define.

The baby boomers refer to those born between 1946 and 1964. Many argue that people born up to two decades apart are too diverse for one label (Pruchno, 2012). In fact, some differentiate between leading-edge boomers (1946–1955) and trailing-edge boomers (1956–1964). Leading-edge boomers are 76% Caucasian, 9% never married, 38% without postsecondary education, and 29% who served in the military. Trailing-edge boomers, in contrast, are 68% Caucasian, 14% never married, 44% without postsecondary education, and 13% who served in the military (the draft ended after all the leading-edge boomers had turned age 18). Smartphone ownership of leading-edge boomers is two thirds that of trailing-edge boomers.

The boomers are differentiated from *generation X* born between 1965 and 1981 and *generation Y*, also referred to as the *millennials*, born between 1982 and 2000. Some argue that these two generations not only differ from each other but are too diverse within each generation for one label. Within each of these generations are there shared values about hard work, trust, respect for authority, teamwork, competition, privacy, independence, optimism, and so forth, as some analysts claim without much data?

In one area, though, I can see the potential for *intergenerational conflict*, and that is over health care. Let's face it, the boomers use a lot more of it (see Medicare in the next section) than generation X and the millennials. There is insufficient national wealth for all Americans to get all the medical care they desire. One can see the boomers wanting to preserve the benefits of Medicare that the current cohort of older adults gets, and to even quest for improvements in the current (and miserable) state of long-term care insurance—both of which will be costly to all taxpayers.

The younger generations, conversely, may resent the expensive cost of Medicare and other resources that older adults disproportionately use, versus education and the other needs disproportionately affecting younger adults. Young millennials, though, may have complex feelings about their boomer parents. They may resent the debt and high unemployment rate facing them, but those between ages 20 and 25 who are living with their parents increased to 43% in 2009. This could add to their resentment or mitigate it, as this is a voluntary generosity on the part of the boomer parents.

Intergenerational conflict over jobs may be *less* likely than health care. According to one study (Munnell & Wu, 2012), there is no evidence that increasing the employment of older persons reduces the job opportunities or wage rates of younger persons.

LEGISLATION

We will revisit the following pieces of legislation—Medicare, Medicaid, and Social Security, plus the Affordable Care Act, when we examine the future of these landmark legislative acts in Chapter 12, "Public Health Policy." Below, however, are overviews of these legislative acts because the reader needs to know what they are if she or he is to understand health and aging in America. Many people do not even understand the difference between Medicare and Medicaid, so we begin there.

Medicare

Medicare was enacted in 1965 to help persons age 65 or older pay for medical care. In 2010 Medicare covered almost 40 million older adults and 8 million younger persons with disabilities. Medicare is a major player in the U.S. health care system, spending $523 billion in 2010. Ironically, despite the generous reimbursements they receive through the Medicare program ($11,000 per beneficiary in 2008), older Americans spend more money out-of-pocket now (almost $5,000 per beneficiary in 2008), after controlling for inflation, than they did prior to the inauguration of Medicare. Medical care has become increasingly desired and expensive.

Medicare Part A is referred to as hospital insurance, and most people do not have to pay a monthly premium for this insurance because they are eligible through the taxes they paid while working. Part A includes hospital care ($1,156 deductible in 2012), inpatient psychiatric care (190-day lifetime maximum), skilled nursing facility care (100 days), rehabilitation or home care following a hospitalization, and hospice care for the terminally ill. There are restrictions on what kinds of conditions are covered and the length of coverage. Copayments apply as well.

Medicare Part B is referred to as medical insurance and covers physician services, outpatient hospital care, and other medical services such as physical and occupational therapy and some home health care. Part B requires a premium of $99.90 per month in 2012 and generally pays 80% of physician and outpatient services after an annual $140 deductible. Part B includes most medical screenings and clinical laboratory tests but does not cover dental services, hearing aids, eyeglasses, and most long-term care services. Chronic conditions are, for the most part, not covered by

Medicare, and prevention coverage is limited primarily to medical screenings and immunizations.

Beginning in 2007 Medicare shifted, for the first time, to *means-based testing* for Part B premiums. In 2012, only individuals earning less than $85,000 a year ($170,000 for married couples) paid the $99.90 premium; individuals who exceeded this income level had their premiums increased, based on how much additional income they earned. Use of this type of *income indexing* will continue to increase in the coming years, and some project that beneficiaries with high incomes may pay at least three times the basic premium amount.

Part C refers to private health insurance plans that provide Medicare benefits. At the time of this writing, the Affordable Care Act would soon be eliminating the additional subsidy, at taxpayers' expense, granted to private insurers during the Bush Administration, when this subsidy was unavailable for those opting for the traditional Medicare option (see Chapter 12, "Public Health Policy").

Part D refers to the Medicare Prescription Drug plan, which went into effect on January 1, 2006. This part is also administered by private health insurance companies (and will also be examined in Chapter 12).

A little over one fourth of the federal outlay for older adults is for Medicare, and these expenditures have been rising (and continue to rise) rapidly. Between 1960 (5 years before the onset of Medicare) and 1990, the proportion of the federal budget spent on programs serving older adults had doubled, from 15% to 30%. Much of this increase occurred between 1975 and 1988, when personal health care expenditures under Medicare increased an average 14.4% per year, more than twice the rate of inflation! Stated in absolute dollars, Medicare spending increased from $7.5 billion in 1970 to $114 billion in 1991, and although the rate of increase has slowed since then, annual increases have been relentless.

In 2012, the nonpartisan Congressional Budget Office (CBO) reported that even under its most conservative projections, health care spending would rise by 8% a year from 2012 to 2022, mainly as a result of an aging U.S. population and rising treatment costs. Medicare, according to the CBO, will account for about half of this projected growth. Moreover, government spending for Medicare and Medicaid will more than double over the next decade to $1.8 trillion, or 7.3% of the country's total economic output.

It is not surprising, therefore, that even though the single largest component of out-of-pocket costs for older adults is much needed long-term care, the federal government has resisted overtures to include substantial long-term care coverage under Medicare. (The CLASS act, as proposed under the Affordable Care Act, was quickly dropped as a federally coordinated long-term care program because it was not financially feasible as designed.) Even without the additional expense of long-term care, Medicare will be unable to meet its financial obligations by 2017 unless substantial cost containment is implemented (more on this in Chapter 12).

An interesting line of research has shown that Medicare spending across the country varies greatly, but health outcomes tend to be the same no matter how much money is spent in a particular region. Some argue, therefore, that Medicare costs could be reduced significantly if the entire nation could bring its costs down to match the lower-spending regions. Landrum and colleagues (2008) agree with this premise, with one caveat. Although increased area-level spending does not correlate with improved patient outcomes overall, in certain cases increased spending is beneficial. The problem is that high-spending areas also spent too much money on health care problems where little or no benefit results. The authors concluded that Medicare could save money not by capping costs, but by applying *comparative effectiveness studies*, that is, determining which treatments work best for which patients, and whether the benefits are commensurate with the costs.

The Centers for Medicare and Medicaid Services oversees all financial and regulatory aspects of the Medicare and Medicaid systems. For additional information, call 800-MEDICARE (800-6334227) or go to the Medicare website at www.medicare.gov.

Medicaid

Medicaid is different from Medicare in that it is not focused primarily on older adults; it is a state-run, not a federally managed, program; and it is funded jointly by the states and the federal government, not by the federal government alone. The most significant difference is that Medicaid is the largest source of funding for medical and health-related services for people with limited income—what used to be referred to as a welfare program—as opposed to Medicare, which is partially financed by users through payroll taxes.

Because it is state run, Medicaid policies for eligibility, services, and payment vary considerably (and thanks to the Supreme Court decision on June 28, 2012, which allows states to opt out of the Medicaid component of the Affordable Care Act, the variation will be even more extreme). One aspect of Medicaid that has not varied much across states is that costs have increased steadily throughout the years, and now constitute, on average, a quarter of each state's budget. Medicaid spending totaled $399 billion in 2011 and was projected to increase rapidly in the coming years if the economy continues to struggle.

On a gerontological note, one third of Medicaid's budget, about $130 billion, goes to fund long-term care for the frail elderly and the disabled, most of it to nursing homes. It pays for nearly 60% of nursing home care, and an increasing amount of home- and community-based, long-term care. Medicaid is based on the premise that individuals pay out of pocket until they become impoverished and eligible for coverage. Moreover, an older person cannot shelter money by giving it away to a relative within a 5-year period of qualifying for Medicaid-subsidized long-term care.

Medicaid, unlike Medicare, has no influential constituency advocating on its behalf. It is recognized by the general public as a program for low-income people and many do not feel generous with their tax dollars for supporting it. With federal deficits looming as far as the eye can see, and with Medicaid the largest cost item in most states' budgets, the pressure to reduce Medicaid expenditures is and will continue to be enormous. This is likely to have a strong and negative impact on the quality of long-term care for older adults and disabled persons.

Social Security

Few would argue that inadequate income is irrelevant to health. It is important, therefore, in a book focused on health and aging to examine Social Security. *Social Security* is a federal program designed to protect individuals and their families from loss of earnings due to retirement, disability, or death (when signed into law in 1935, it covered only retired workers). It was believed by historians that President Franklin Roosevelt was interested not only in the economic security of older adults, but in reducing the politically sensitive high unemployment rate at the time.

Social Security is a progressive benefit, replacing a higher proportion of preretirement earnings of low lifetime earners than higher lifetime earners. Additional protection was provided in 1975 when the Social Security benefit was adjusted to reflect increases in prices (the Cost of Living Adjustment or COLA).

It is an entitlement in that to receive retirement benefits, a person must contribute through payroll tax contributions for about 10 years. Workers and employers are both responsible for paying half of the payroll tax—6.2% each, with the self-employed paying the full 12.4%, up to a taxable maximum of $110,100 of earnings.

In 2012, about 56 million Americans—retired workers (64%); spouses, children, and survivors (20%); and the disabled (16%)—received Social Security benefits, including about 90% of those age 65 and older. The average monthly benefit for retired workers in 2012 was $1,231, and for disabled workers was $1,111.

In 2009, Social Security helped more than 14 million Americans aged 65 and older stay above the poverty line. Without access to Social Security, 58% of women and 48% of men above the age of 75 would be living below the poverty line. Even with Social Security being a program initially designed to be a *partial* replacement of lost income, it has become almost the entire income of many retired persons. In 2011, although it replaced 42% of past annual earnings for an average worker, more than a third of older men and half of older women relied on their Social Security check for 80% or more of their income.

Another problem is a societal one: meeting the financial obligation. In 1935 only 6% of the population was age 65 or over; present day that percentage has increased to 13%. Reflecting this increase in older adults, there were approximately 4 workers per beneficiary in the 1960s, 2.9 workers in 2012, and a projected 2.1 workers in 2036. The widening gap between those paying into Social Security and those receiving Social Security means that full benefits will be reduced in 2033 to about 75% of scheduled payments, but only if changes are not made.

QUALITY CARE, HEALTH CARE, MEDICAL CARE

In a democratic society there is stiff competition for societal resources that are taxpayer subsidized. *Health care*, however (typically referring primarily to *medical care*), has consistently maintained its status in this country as a very high priority for these limited resources. Moreover, the growth in national expenditures for health care has been nothing short of phenomenal. Spending for national health care grew from 5.2% of the gross domestic product (GDP) in 1960 to an astonishing 17.6% in 2009. This represents an increase from $27 billion in 1960 to $2.5 trillion in 2009 (see Figure 1.12).

The United States spent almost 18% of its GDP on health care in 2009, whereas other developed countries spent between 6% and 11%. Much of this discrepancy in health care costs compared to other countries began in 1980 with the rise of private health care insurers in the United States (and their profit-making motivation) and the greater use of sophisticated medical technology in this country. In the past three decades health expenditures doubled in other countries, but more than tripled here. This disparity would be even greater if we did not have almost 50 million younger Americans lacking health insurance coverage in 2012. (This will change when the Affordable Care Act takes effect in 2014, a topic we will examine in Chapter 12, "Public Health Policy.")

Although we spend more on health care than any other country, this does not necessarily mean we have the best health care. "Best" can be defined in a number of ways—for example, as access to medical care by the greatest number of citizens, or as a system that prioritizes disease prevention and health promotion, or, as in contemporary America, a system that prioritizes costly specialized medical procedures. Many of us are hoping that the Affordable Care Act makes large inroads in the first two areas, along with judicious use of the third area, without jeopardizing *quality care*.

Until then, though, the World Health Organization (WHO) and others have measured quality of health care and by most any measure we do not do well. WHO ranked

FIGURE 1.12   **Summary of national health care expenditures, population and share of the Gross Domestic Product, 1960–2009.**

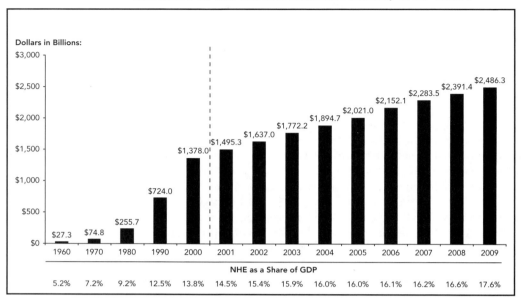

Source: Centers for Medicare and Medicaid Services, Office of the Actuary, National Health Statistics Group.

the United States 37th in the quality of health care. We are 50th in life expectancy. We just do not get enough "bang for our buck." Regarding number of *healthy* years we have to live—a more important measure of quality of life in my opinion than mere life expectancy—we spend more than double in health care expenditures per capita than Japan, but have almost 5 fewer healthy years to live than they do.

Another international study of health care quality was conducted in 2006, and the United States ranked last compared with Australia, Canada, Germany, New Zealand, and the United Kingdom. The per capita health expenditures of these five countries ranged from 33% to 53% of the United States, yet among 51 indicators—including such health promotion measures as use of mammograms, flu shots, medication reviews, and diet and exercise advice—the United States ranked last or tied for last on 27 (Monaghan, 2006).

One international study compared the United States, Australia, Canada, France, Germany, the Netherlands, New Zealand, and Britain, and suggested that the supremacy of American health care may be limited to a handful of preeminent medical centers. Although the United States does well in such important aspects of health care as providing prompt access to some of the best specialists in the world, 43% of *insured* (!) Americans skipped care at some point during the year because they could not afford the high out-of-pocket costs (Schoen, Osborn, How, Doty, & Peugh, 2009).

Health Care Versus Medical Care

It is estimated that 60% of early deaths in the United States are due to behavioral, social, and environmental circumstances, versus 10% that result from shortfalls in medical care (with genetic predisposition responsible for the remainder) (McGinnis, Williams-Russo, & Knickman, 2002). Paradoxically, however, the behavioral, social, and environmental components of health care have not constituted a high priority for the health care dollar. In fact, only about 3% of the nation's health care expenditures are targeted toward health-promoting and disease-preventing activities.

> **Question:** Why do we call medical care "health care"?

Most of that 3% goes either to the physician's office or to other clinical settings for preventive measures, such as medical screenings and vaccinations (about a third), or toward health protection in the physical environment, such as toxic agent and radiation control (also about a third). And only a portion of the remainder is spent on changing unhealthy behaviors.

Although there has been undeniable financial stinginess at the federal level in addressing unhealthy lifestyles among the American people, public attention has at least been engaged by this problem behavior ever since the publication of the landmark document *Healthy People: The Surgeon General's Report on Health Promotion and Disease Prevention* (USD-HHS, 1979). This report provided considerable credence to the idea that any major gains in health and independence in the future will likely come from personal lifestyle changes.

> **Question:** In your opinion, what are two of the most important changes we need to make to convert our medical care system into a health care system? How can we make these changes?

Dr. John Rowe, director of the MacArthur Foundation's Consortium on Successful Aging, supported this report's message by concluding that our vigor and health in old age are mostly a matter of managing how we live. A classic article in the *Journal of the American Medical Association* (McGinnis & Foege, 1993) suggested that we no longer should view death as being due to heart disease, cancer, stroke, and chronic obstructive pulmonary disease; rather, we should see it as the result of tobacco use, inactivity, poor diet, alcohol abuse, microbial and toxic agents, risky sexual behavior, motor vehicle injuries, and illicit or inappropriate use of drugs.

Even if we continue to devote most of our money to medical care, we need to focus more of our attention on health care.

2

●●●●●●●

CLINICAL PREVENTIVE SERVICES

●●● Key Terms

Guide to Clinical Preventive Services
medical screenings
accuracy, reliability, and effectiveness
prophylaxis
breast cancer
mammography
menopause
hormone replacement therapy
Women's Health Initiative
hypertension and prehypertension
osteoporosis
densitometry
cholesterol
statins
National Cholesterol Education
   Program guidelines
Pap smears
cervical cancer

human papillomavirus
colorectal cancer
colonoscopy
prostate cancer
prostate-specific antigen screening
skin cancer
hearing and vision
oral health
diabetes and prediabetes
depression
hepatitis C
influenza and pneumococcal
   vaccinations
dog screenings
shingles
aspirin prophylaxis
Polypill and Polymeal
Medicare prevention

● ● ○ **Learning Objectives**

- Summarize the *Guide to Clinical Preventive Services*
- Define accuracy, reliability, and effectiveness of screening tests
- Contrast breast self-examination, clinical examination, and mammography
- Critically evaluate the effectiveness of mammography
- Review the research on hormone replacement therapy
- Explain the Women's Health Initiative
- Define prehypertension and discuss its utility
- Define densitometry
- Differentiate osteoporosis and osteopenia
- Review the effectiveness of bisphosphonates
- Examine the cholesterol guidelines and their consequences
- Analyze the role statins play in cholesterol reduction
- Analyze the consequences of more stringent screening guidelines
- Review Pap smears, cervical cancer, and human papillomavirus
- Contrast fecal occult blood test, sigmoidoscopy, and colonoscopy
- Analyze colonoscopy compliance
- Critically evaluate routine screenings for prostate cancer
- Review screenings for skin cancer, hearing and vision problems, oral health, and depression
- Define prediabetes and its utility
- Describe the role staff plays in depression care support
- Review immunization guidelines
- Examine hepatitis C and the susceptibility of baby boomers
- Review aspirin prophylaxis
- Examine the Polypill and Polymeal
- Examine the cholesterol guidelines and their consequences
- Critically evaluate Medicare prevention coverage

MEDICAL SCREENINGS AND PROPHYLAXIS: CONSIDERABLE CONTROVERSY

For an earlier edition of this book I wrote the chapter on *medical screenings*—tests with the potential for the early diagnosis of medical problems—with a lot more certainty about the reliability of its content. I began by stating a few of the obvious successes achieved by medical screenings and subsequent interventions. For example, I noted that because of the Pap smear test, cervical cancer mortality dropped substantially during the 1970s and 1980s. I also noted that, due in part to the increased screening for—and treatment of—hypertension, the incidence of stroke and heart attack was significantly reduced.

I was not Pollyannaish about the topic, however. I reported that despite considerable support (and, in some specific screening instances, universal acclaim), medical screenings were neither systematically nor uniformly implemented by clinicians. I noted that this behavior was due in part to clinicians' and researchers' failing to agree on the effectiveness of screenings and interventions—that is, the relative benefits versus the risks (medical, psychological, and financial) to individual patients. I also reported that people with low education levels (including Medicare recipients) were less likely to discuss screening options and other health education matters with their physicians.

Obviously, none of this examination in the 1990s could predict the controversy that emerged later over both medical screenings and *prophylaxis*—defined as prevention, for example, hormone replacement therapy (HRT) and statins. After the turn of the century there was an explosion of research findings and popular articles on the effectiveness of medical screenings and prophylactic interventions. Much of the attention was on whether women should get mammograms and HRT. But there were also interesting questions raised about such screenings as bone density, blood pressure, cholesterol, and prostate cancer, plus the age at which screenings should begin and end; and whether we should be taking statins as a prophylaxis for just about everything.

Underlying many of the issues raised about medical screenings and prophylactic interventions were fundamental questions about the validity of the research that had been conducted. Before we tackle these questions, intervention by intervention, we need to lay some groundwork on what guides clinical decision making.

Guide to Clinical Preventive Services

Many physicians value an annual physical because they can address health issues before they become a problem, such as gradual weight gain. Or they can provide a yearly conversation about staying well. Also, many adults, particularly older adults, have a medical problem or a medication that warrants yearly monitoring. The problem with the annual physical arises when they are associated with annual medical screenings.

About 35 years ago, routine annual medical screenings were being replaced by periodic reviews, based on the unique health-risk factors of individual clients. In other words, based on age, gender, and other risk factors, specific medical screening recommendations could range from not at all to every 10 years, to something in between.

There is some evidence to suggest, however, that both the public (Oboler, Prochazka, Gonzales, Xu, & Anderson, 2002) and physicians (Prochazka, Lundahl, Pearson, Oboler, & Anderson, 2005) still believe in an undifferentiated approach of an annual physical examination that includes screenings. The bias toward more frequent screenings was revealed in one study of 1,266 primary care physicians. They were asked if they agreed with a hypothetical scenario of an 80-year-old patient with advanced lung cancer receiving a colorectal cancer screening. Despite the fact that the older patient would not benefit from this screening, 25% of the physicians agreed with this recommendation (Haggstrom, Klabunde, Smith, & Yuan, 2012).

The first comprehensive effort to assess not only the effectiveness but the timing of a wide array of preventive services was conducted by the Canadian Task Force on the Periodic Health Examination in 1976. It developed explicit criteria for assessing the quality of evidence in published clinical research, and establishing decision rules to guide clinicians.

A follow-up effort, beginning in 1984 by the U.S. Preventive Services Task Force (USPSTF), created the manual, *Guide to Clinical Preventive Services*. Clinician recommendations were based on a rating system that gave the most weight to research based on randomized controlled trials, followed by well-designed trials without randomization. The least weight was given to the opinions of respected authorities or expert committees, descriptive studies, and case reports.

The following categories were created: A—intervention is strongly recommended; B—intervention is recommended; C—no recommendation because of insufficient evidence for or against making a recommendation; D—intervention not recommended; and E—intervention strongly not recommended.

A and B recommendations include such interventions as mammography, Pap smear, blood pressure, dental care, colonoscopy, and influenza and pneumococcal immunizations. Occasionally, though, recommendations were withdrawn or cautions expressed. In 2002, for instance, the Task Force recommended *against* the use of combined estrogen and progestin therapy for postmenopausal women. In 2009 the American Cancer Society urged *caution* with its recommendation for mammograms, citing that a large increase in early breast cancer detection had not led to a commensurate decrease in late-stage cancer.

In the second edition of this book, I included a table from the *Guide to Clinical Preventive Services* that listed medical screenings and their recommended frequencies for persons age 65 and over. That guide is no longer in print, and that USPSTF-derived table, or a revised version of it, has not appeared in later editions of this book (though my own updated version of these guidelines appears near the end of this chapter). This is due in part to controversies that will be examined in more detail later. But it is also due to the fact that the screening tables are continually outdated, and new guidelines are now released in specific and narrow installments by the USPSTF.

Accuracy, Reliability, and Effectiveness of Screening Tests

Accuracy refers to the sensitivity and specificity of screening tests. The *sensitivity* of a screening test is defined as the percentage of persons who actually had the disease and tested positive when screened. A test with poor sensitivity will miss persons with the condition and produce a large proportion of false-negative results. Persons who receive false-negative results will experience delays in treatment.

Specificity refers to the percentage of persons without the condition who correctly test negative when screened. A test with poor specificity will result in healthy persons being told that they have the disease and will produce a large proportion of false-positive results. Persons who receive false-positive results may experience expensive follow-up tests or unnecessary treatment that might not be completely safe.

Even if the test is accurate, that is, sensitive and specific, it needs to be reliable and effective. *Reliability* refers to the ability of a test to obtain the same result when repeated. The reliability of some screenings, such as mammograms and Pap smears, has been increased due to the initiation of federal certification and annual state inspections of facilities.

Effectiveness refers to whether the test is worth the cost, time, and bother, that is, whether there is a subsequent clinical intervention for a positive finding that can prevent or delay the disease. So, even if a test has good sensitivity, specificity, and reliability, it does *not* necessarily mean the screening will be effective.

BREAST CANCER

Breast cancer is the second leading cause of death from cancer among women (after lung cancer), accounting for 40,000 deaths in 2011. An estimated 211,000 new cases of breast cancer are diagnosed annually in women (less than 1% of breast cancers are diagnosed in men). The median age at the time of breast cancer diagnosis is 61 years, with 57% of deaths from breast cancer occurring at age 65 or older.

The three screening tests for breast cancer are *breast self-examination, clinical examination,* and *X-ray mammography.* Breast self-exams have never been proven to reduce breast cancer deaths, but the American Cancer Society—along with many physicians—encourages their use on a regular basis. The encouragement is based on the belief that the procedure may be effective, and it is simple, safe, and free.

In one study, however, 266,000 women in Shanghai factories were randomly assigned to either breast self-examination or no intervention. (Mammography is not widely available in China, so self-examination is the best option available.) The breast self-examinations were supervised, and were done correctly and regularly. After 5 years there was no difference in mortality between the two groups (Thomas, Gao, et al., 2002). Although larger tumors are more likely to be discovered through self-examination, they are unlikely to be found in a timely manner, and the accuracy of self-examination overall is quite low.

An annual *clinical breast examination* for women older than 40 is recommended by the USPSTF. A thorough clinical breast examination may be as effective as mammography, but the research evidence in support of this possibility is inadequate. It is also unclear whether clinical breast examinations provide added benefit when conducted in conjunction with mammography.

Regarding *mammography*, the low-dose X-ray imaging of breasts, consensus on its utility has grown tremendously beginning in 1987. In that year only 23% of women age 65 and over had a mammogram within the preceding 2 years. By 2010, that percentage almost tripled to 64%. There was great disparity among White, Black, and Hispanic women in 1987, with the latter two groups having a little more than half the percentage of mammograms. By 2010 that ethnic difference had disappeared. The disparity still existed when socioeconomic status was considered, with 75% of middle-income women reporting having had a mammogram versus 51% for low-income women (Federal Interagency Forum on Aging-Related Statistics, 2012).

A national survey in 1985 reported that the majority of primary care physicians never recommended mammography screening to their female patients, but by 1988, 96% reported having done so. A national study of primary care physicians by the American Cancer Society in 1988 found that 80% of physicians performed more screenings than 5 years earlier.

In 1992 Medicare began offering partial coverage for routine mammograms conducted every 2 years, and Congress approved the Mammography Quality Standards Act, which regulated equipment and personnel, including technologists and physicians, and required federal certification and annual state inspections of facilities. In 1998 mammogram coverage was increased to an annual basis for Medicare-eligible women.

The specificity of mammograms, however, still left much to be desired. Fifty percent of women who have had 10 mammograms over the past decade or two will have had one false-positive result that required further testing and unnecessary stress and expense. As many as 20% of those false alarms led to a breast biopsy in which tissue was removed from the suspected tumor (Elmore et al., 1998).

The effectiveness of subsequent intervention for early detection was also a concern with some cancers. About 20% of the breast cancers being found in the 1990s, for example, were ductal carcinoma in situ (DCIS). There was evidence to suggest that indolent DCIS will not become invasive if left untreated; nonetheless, DCIS was routinely treated with surgery, radiation, and chemotherapy (Napoli, 2001).

The relatively minor controversies that the public *was* aware of—such as when breast cancer screenings should begin and how often they should be conducted—did not serve as deterrents to screening compliance. This was especially true because of the substantial federal government campaigns supporting mammograms, the expanded Medicare coverage, and the widespread endorsement of the procedure by physicians. Not surprisingly, the percentage of women age 50 and older who reported having had a mammogram in the previous 2 years went from 27% in 1987 to 69% in 1998 (Kolata & Moss, 2002). Then came the mammogram controversy, which we will tackle next.

The 2001 Mammography Controversy

Widespread use of mammography as a screening tool began in the United States in the mid-1980s, after seven large studies involving 500,000 women seemingly demonstrated the effectiveness of this screening tool. The controversies surrounding mammography over the next decade and a half were relatively minor, including whether they should start at age 40 or 50, and whether they should be annual or biannual.

On one side of the debate were the National Cancer Institute and the American Cancer Society, which recommended regular mammograms beginning at age 40. On the other side was the National Institutes of Health's (NIH) consensus panel, which recommended that decisions about starting mammograms before age 50 be left up to each woman and her physician. Taking a middle position, the American Medical Association's Council on Scientific Affairs recommended mammograms every 2 years between the ages of 40 and 49 and annually beginning at age 50.

In the 2002 issue of the *Annals of Internal Medicine*, two opposing points of view continued to be expressed. The Canadian National Breast Screening Study reported that after 11 to 16 years of follow-up, a randomized screening trial of mammography in women age 40 to 49 did *not* produce a reduction in breast cancer mortality (Miller, To, Baines, & Wall, 2002). The USPSTF, however, reviewed eight randomized controlled trials and still advised women to begin breast cancer screening at age 40 (Humphrey, Helfand, Chan, & Woolf, 2002).

The age at which mammography screenings should be terminated also generated controversy. The USPSTF recommended the discontinuation of mammogram screenings at age 69 in asymptomatic women whose results had consistently been normal on previous examinations. Other authorities and researchers recommended no discontinuation of mammographies after age 69 (McCarthy et al., 2000; McPherson, Swenson, & Lee, 2002). One study reported that mammography was not uncommon in women age 80 and older, but that 40% of the screened women were very unlikely to benefit due to limited life expectancy (Schonberg, McCarthy, Davis, Phillips, & Hamel, 2004). In 2008 the argument about when to terminate mammography emerged again between researchers who supported its benefit for women in their 80s (Badgwell et al., 2008) and those who did not (Ciatto, 2008).

These types of ongoing disagreements in the field generate little public notice, even in 2000 when two Danish researchers published a report questioning the effectiveness of mammography *at any age* (Gotzsche & Olsen, 2000). Perhaps public awareness was muted because the majority of researchers criticized the methodology and conclusions of the Danish researchers. When the report was reissued in October 2001, however, and substantiated with additional statistical analysis (Olsen & Gotzsche, 2001), considerable attention was paid to it by both researchers and the general public. The report challenged the long-prevailing orthodoxy on whether mammography was helpful at any age, and not just the uncertainty of the decade between age 40 and 50.

The conventional wisdom up to this point was that the seven previously mentioned studies were convincing and that mammography helped save women's lives by detecting tumors early enough to be treated. The Danish researchers, however, concluded differently. They reported that five of the seven studies were too flawed to be credible, and the remaining two studies showed that mammography did not save, or even prolong, lives. Their conclusions were endorsed by the *Lancet* and by an expert group sponsored by the National Cancer Institute.

Other researchers, though, took exception to their findings (Duffy, Tabár, & Smith, 2002a; Tabar et al., 2001), and an analysis in Sweden reported that mammograms may reduce deaths from breast cancer by as much as 45% (Duffy et al., 2002b).

The surrounding publicity following Olsen and Gotzsche's report in 2001 was nothing short of astonishing. Major professional organizations and experts expressed uncertainty, or they argued either for or against mammograms. In February 2002, Tommy Thompson, Secretary of Health and Human Services, declared by fiat that if you are a woman age 40 or older, you need to get screened for breast cancer with mammography every year. A not irrelevant fact was that Secretary Thompson's wife was a breast cancer survivor whose tumor was detected by mammography.

Peter Gotzsche, the original Danish researcher who started the mammography controversy, came out in 2009 with another review of the literature (Gotzsche & Nielsen, 2009). He concluded that breast cancer mortality is reduced by 15% through mammography, but that for every woman who has her life prolonged there are 200 healthy women who experience the distress of false-positive findings, and 10 healthy women who have been treated unnecessarily and sometimes with negative consequences.

Also, there are cancers that do not need to be found because they will do no harm if left alone, but that can create harm by being unnecessarily treated through biopsies and other procedures. Conversely, lethal breast cancers tend to grow quickly and even an annual mammogram (and its cumulative radiation) will do no good. Doubters of mammography suggested that perhaps the decline in breast cancer death rates was not due mostly to early detection, but to the increasing effectiveness of treatments like the drug tamoxifen.

So what is a woman to do?

2009 Mammography Update

The American Cancer Society, which has long been a staunch defender of cancer screenings, unexpectedly announced in October 2009 that American medicine has overpromised when it comes to mammograms. This announcement followed the USPSTF's latest evidence-based recommendations:

1. Women without risk factors should undergo screening beginning at age 50 instead of age 40. The risks of mammograms before age 50 exceed the benefits of early detection.
2. Women age 50 to 74 without symptoms or risk factors (e.g., family history) should undergo mammography every other year rather than annually. For every breast cancer death averted in this age group, 838 women must undergo screening for 6 years, generating thousands of screens, hundreds of biopsies, and many cancers treated as if they were life threatening when they are not.

> **Question:** What would you say to a client who is asking you for advice on whether to get a mammogram? Why would you answer that way?

3. There is insufficient evidence either for or against a screening recommendation for women age 75 and over.
4. Physicians should stop teaching patients to perform breast self-examinations because there is no evidence they are effective.

Task force members concluded that widespread screening has increased the detection and treatment of small, slow-growing tumors that may never cause harm—and in some cases may even disappear—while failing to detect aggressive tumors because they arise between screenings and grow quickly. There is also a small risk posed by repeated radiations.

Dr. Otis Brawley, chief medical officer at the American Cancer Society, reported that "the overwhelming majority of folks over age 75 should not be getting cancer screenings." Nonetheless in 2011 among women 75 to 79 years old, 62% received a mammogram in the past 2 years, as had 50% of women age 80 and older (Bellizzi, Breslau, Burness, & Waldron, 2011).

There was different news at the other end of the age spectrum. After the 2009 USPSTF recommendations were made discouraging women in their 40s from getting a routine mammogram, there was a 6% decline in that age group in the United States in 2010. That is a small decline, but it occurred despite the backlash by the American Cancer Society and many physicians vociferously supporting annual examinations beginning at age 40.

A European meta-analysis of 12 million women, 26 screening programs in 18 countries, supported the conclusions of the USPSTF. The chance of saving a woman's life and minimizing the negative effects of overscreening and false positives are best with screenings every 2 years between the ages of 50 and 69, with follow-up to age 79 (Euroscreen Working Group, 2012).

MENOPAUSE AND THE HRT CONTROVERSY

There is no definitive medical screening for *menopause*. The average age of menopause in the United States is 51, and its existence is primarily documented by the onset and eventual termination of a variety of symptoms. These symptoms typically include irregular menstrual cycles, hot flashes, changes in mood and cognition, insomnia, headache, and fatigue.

Some women do not view their menopausal symptoms as a medical problem and do not seek a consultation with a physician. At the other end of the spectrum, menopause may be viewed as an estrogen-deficiency disease. There is considerable cultural variation in attitudes toward, and the definition of, menopause.

At the turn of the new millennium, however, the debate over the use of HRT to relieve the symptoms of menopause and prevent disease may have even surpassed the controversy over the use of mammography. And, once again, there were serious questions about the validity of the research that had been conducted over the past couple of decades.

The early reports that provided optimism about HRT were based on observational studies in which large groups of women were tracked for years. In these studies, the patients themselves decided whether to take HRT. We later found out that the sample populations for these studies were more affluent, better educated, younger, thinner, and more likely to exercise, and they had greater access to health care than women in general. In other words, the sample populations were healthier and had better health habits than other women, and the outcomes they had may have been due more to this sampling bias than to the intervention of HRT.

Under the leadership of Bernadine Healy, the first woman to head the NIH, the *Women's Health Initiative* was launched in the 1990s and it included the Heart and Estrogen/Progestin Replacement Study (HERS) and its follow-up (HERS II). Using a more rigorous methodology, HERS and HERS II produced surprising results by correcting the previous sampling bias through a placebo-controlled clinical trial with random assignment. This type of randomized study is considered the gold standard in medical research, but it is much more expensive to conduct, and ethical questions are raised when some persons have to be randomly assigned to a placebo-control group.

To the surprise of many people, the randomized clinical trials did not agree with several decades of consistently positive results from observational studies. Even more surprising, the HERS studies reported that there was an *increase* in heart attacks, strokes, breast cancer, and blood clots in the legs and lungs among healthy women taking HRT, compared with those on the placebo. In 2001 the American Heart Association reversed its support of HRT, and for women with cardiovascular illness a recommendation was made to avoid the therapy. In 2002 NIH became sufficiently convinced about the problems associated with HRT to send letters to the 16,000 women participating in the HERS II study, recommending that the therapy be terminated. This announcement had broader implications. On June 21, 2002, there were 379,581 prescriptions filled for Prempro, a popular HRT; on September 20, 2002, only 211,249 prescriptions were filled (Elliott, 2002), a decline of 44% in 3 months.

Even prior to the termination of this study, most women who opted for HRT were not staying on it for long. Between 1993 and 1995, 53% of 900 HRT users in one study had discontinued the therapy, and two thirds had done so by the following year (Reynolds, Walker, Obermeyer, Rahman, & Guilbert, 2001). Those who discontinued HRT cited the fear of cancer and side effects. Physicians were also becoming more cautious with HRT, using lower doses and focusing on menopausal symptoms, and reassessing its effectiveness after a few years. For disease prevention, there appeared to be better options than HRT for heart disease (e.g., statins or aspirin) and osteoporosis (e.g., Fosamax or Actonel).

2012 HRT Update

In 2012, 20% of postmenopausal women in America reported having ever used HRT compared to 40% in 2002. As later revisions to the Women's Health Initiative appeared (this study continues after 15 years and involving more than 160,000 women), though, the HRT decline stopped because of the low-risk probability and the strong need some women have to treat menopausal symptoms such as hot flashes, night sweats, and vaginal dryness. Given the updated studies, many argue that HRT is a better option for the disruptive effects of menopause than the use of alternative treatments that have turned out to be comparable to placebos.

Alternative options for alleviating menopausal symptoms have not been promising. Although over-the-counter herbal supplements like black cohosh are becoming more popular for alleviating symptoms, there is no supporting research on its effectiveness beyond its placebo effect. Black cohosh and a variety of soy products (i.e., weak plant-based estrogens) result in the alleviation of symptoms in up to 40% of menopausal women; but this is about the same percentage of improvement that placebos elicit!

A 2012 analysis by a federal task force has updated recommendations about when HRT should be used (Nelson, Walker, Zakher, & Mitchell, 2012). Women who are past menopause

> **Question:** What would you say to a client who is asking you for advice on whether to start hormone replacement therapy? Why did you answer that way?

and healthy should not use HRT, as once thought, to ward off bone fracture, heart disease, or dementia. Also, there are some increased risks, most slight, in blood clots in the legs and lungs, gallbladder disease, urinary incontinence, stroke, and dementia. For women on estrogen alone, there appears to be a small measure of protection against breast cancer, but only women who have had hysterectomies can take estrogen alone (versus estrogen–progestin) because it has been linked to uterine cancer.

The 2012 North American Menopause Society guidelines can be summarized as follows:

- HRT is an acceptable choice for women age 50 to 59 or within 10 years of menopause, and healthy women who are bothered by moderate to severe menopausal symptoms.
- The decision to use HRT at any age should be decided on a case-by-case basis.
- Low-dose estrogen alone is recommended for women with only vaginal dryness or discomfort during intercourse.
- Progesterone and estrogen are recommended for women who still have a uterus to prevent uterine cancer. Estrogen alone is sufficient for women without a uterus.
- HRT increases the risk for blood clots in the legs and lungs; this risk is rare in women 50 to 59 years old.
- Breast cancer risk increases when HRT is taken continuously for 5 years—and possibly earlier. The risk declines when HRT is stopped.

BLOOD PRESSURE

In 2012 the Centers for Disease Control and Prevention reported that 67 million Americans had high blood pressure, but only 31 million of them were being treated with medicines or lifestyle changes that reduced their blood pressure to a safe level.

High blood pressure is defined, regardless of age, as a systolic blood pressure of 140 mmHg or higher, or a diastolic blood pressure of 90 mmHg or higher. Systolic and diastolic blood pressures tend to increase until age 60; after that, systolic pressure may continue to increase, whereas diastolic pressure stabilizes or even decreases (Beers & Berkow, 2000). A few decades ago, clinicians distinguished between *hypertension*, or readings over 160/95, and high blood pressure, or readings over 140/90. Now the terms are used interchangeably and the lower threshold applies.

Moreover, researchers are making the case that the threshold should be lowered. High-normal blood pressure (130/85) is associated with elevated risk for heart disease and stroke (three times more in women, two times in men), particularly among older persons (Vasan et al., 2001). In 2001, the National Kidney Foundation lowered the blood pressure target for people with diabetes to 130/85 or below.

In 2003 a panel of experts from the NIH issued new federal guidelines stating that readings of 120 to 139 mmHg systolic and 80 to 89 mmHg diastolic should be considered *prehypertensive*. The NIH panel believed there was solid evidence that damage to blood vessels begins at lower pressure levels. Although hypertension quadruples the risks of heart disease and stroke, prehypertension doubles the risks.

Heart disease and stroke are not the only problems with hypertension. Uncontrolled hypertension leads to reduction in cognitive function, specifically short-term memory and verbal ability, as one gets older (Brady, Spiro, & Gaziano, 2005). As systolic blood pressure rises, the risk of dementia later in life increases as well (Freitag et al., 2006). Elderly patients with mild to moderate hypertension are at increased risk of dementia (Skoog et al., 2005).

Researchers associated with the Framingham Heart Study of the National Heart, Lung, and Blood Institute reported that Americans age 55 with normal blood pressure levels face a 90% chance—let me repeat that, a 90% chance—of developing hypertension over the remainder of their lives (Vasan et al., 2002). Complicating the problem of a greater incidence and prevalence of high blood pressure than previously thought is the undertreatment of the problem by physicians, especially among older patients, perhaps up to 75% of them (Hyman & Pavlik, 2001; Oliveria et al., 2002).

In one study more than 4,000 hypertensive patients were randomly assigned to take a blood pressure medication or a placebo. Consistent adherence to the blood pressure medicine for more than 4 years added about 1 day each month of extra life, or almost 2 years of extra life for someone who started treatment at age 40 (Kostis et al., 2011).

The good news about blood pressure is that it has widespread awareness. It is estimated that three out of four adults, perhaps 90% of older adults, have had their blood pressure measured within the preceding year (see Figure 2.1). The bad news is that among those with high blood pressure, 54% are not being treated successfully. Some are unaware of their hypertension, but the majority either choose to do nothing or are being treated and still do not achieve adequate blood pressure control.

Nonpharmacologic therapies such as exercise, sodium restriction, weight reduction, decreased alcohol intake, smoking cessation, and stress management are promising in lowering mildly elevated blood pressure (Appel et al., 2003; Elmer et al., 2006), but these lifestyle changes can be complicated by biological factors (e.g., hypertensives who are not salt-sensitive) and behavioral factors (e.g., ability to maintain weight loss or sustain an exercise program).

Medicare does not provide specific coverage for blood pressure screening (though it is considered part of the overall care covered by Medicare), despite the fact that uncontrolled high blood pressure among older adults is widespread, with costly consequences. If Medicare coverage of periodic blood pressure screenings with counseling was instituted, it would provide more attention to the problem, encourage more reliable screenings than the ones currently available at many community sites, and allow for appropriate follow-up counseling in a timely manner (Haber, 2001a, 2005b).

One precaution rarely taken is to measure the blood pressure level in both arms. A difference of even 10 millimeters is enough to detect the risk of peripheral vascular disease.

| FIGURE 2.1 | Nursing student teaching older adult to take a blood pressure reading in one of the author's health education classes. |

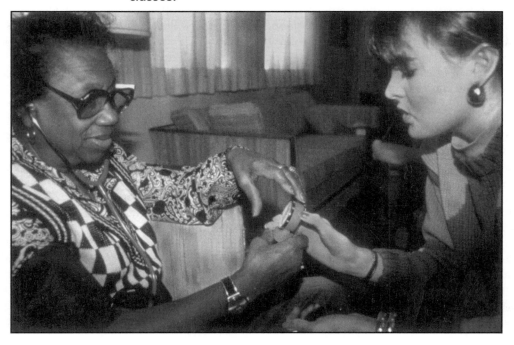

Different blood pressure readings in two arms is a sign of the narrowing or hardening of a person's arteries on one side of the body (Clark, Taylor, Shore, Ukoumunne, & Campbell, 2012).

As with other medical screenings, there is the question of an upper age limit. Although blood pressure screenings have been recommended over the entire adult life cycle for many years, there has been increasing discussion over whether screenings and counsel might be discontinued at age 80 due to uncertain impact on morbidity or mortality (Gueyffier et al., 1999; Rigaud & Forette, 2001; Staessen et al., 1998). One study reported that treatment of hypertension in patients age 80 and older is beneficial (Beckett et al., 2008). Yet other studies suggest we think twice before initiating drug therapy with persons age 85 and over with hypertension. In these studies, the systolic blood pressure associated with the *lowest mortality rate in those 85 and over was in the hypertensive range*, and attempts at decreasing hypertension can lead to increased mortality (Finestone, 2009; Rastas et al., 2006).

OSTEOPOROSIS

Osteoporosis affects more than 28 million Americans, 80% of whom are women, and causes 1.5 million fractures each year. Almost half the fractures are vertebral (700,000), followed by hip and wrist (300,000 each). Half of all women over age 50 will have an osteoporosis-related fracture in their lifetime.

Osteoporosis is a condition in which the bones are thin, brittle, and susceptible to fracture. Without intervention, about 5% to 10% of trabecular bone is lost during the first 2 years after menopause—up to 20% in the 5 to 7 years following menopause—followed by a more gradual loss after that. Osteoporosis is technically defined as a bone density that is 2.5 or more standard deviations below the young-adult peak bone density. *Osteopenia* is a weakening of the bones and can be considered a warning on the way to osteoporosis. It is technically defined as 1 to 2.5 standard deviations below the young-adult peak bone density.

A study of more than 200,000 allegedly healthy women age 50 and older found osteoporosis in 7% of the women, and osteopenia in another 40% (Siris et al., 2001). The fracture rate of women with osteoporosis in the following year was four times higher than for the women with normal bones, and two times higher in women with osteopenia. These study results were surprising not only in detecting the widespread prevalence of osteopenia, but also in the researchers' ability to detect, within a year, a significant increase in fracture rate.

It should be noted that the study used a noninvasive imaging technique (with very low levels of radiation) called single-energy X-ray *densitometry* on peripheral bone sites, rather than the more accurate double-energy X-ray densitometry that is done on the spine and hip. The authors reported, however, that the fracture prediction rates were not compromised much by the use of the quicker and less expensive single-energy X-ray readings.

Surprisingly, studies that identify osteoporosis in women report that detection does not necessarily lead to follow-up intervention. Only 24% (Andrade et al., 2003) and 46% (Feldstein et al., 2003) of those who had suffered an osteoporosis-related fracture in each of two independent samples received drug treatment for osteoporosis within a year and 6 months, respectively, following the fracture. Another problem stems from the fact that the disease goes undiagnosed in more than half of the cases (Stafford, Drieling, & Hersh, 2004). Women who are most in need of bone-density testing—women age 75 and over—are the least likely to get it. In the 3 years after Medicare reimbursement for osteoporosis screening began, 27% of women age 65 to 70 were tested, but fewer than 10% of women age 75 and over were tested (Neuner, Binkley, Sparapani, Laud, & Nattinger, 2006).

In one review of the research literature, close to 90% of women with osteoporosis were not being diagnosed with the condition, and only about one third with the diagnosis were offered treatment for the disease during the 1990s (Gehlbach, Fournier, & Bigelow, 2002). Diagnosis and treatment are increasing a decade later, though, due to the growing popularity of bone density screenings and also because of Medicare coverage for women at risk for osteoporosis. Unfortunately, the definition of risk for osteoporosis was not made immediately clear by Medicare when reimbursement was first instituted in 1998, and physicians were initially uncertain about whether their older patients would be reimbursed by Medicare for their screenings.

If almost half the women age 50 and older have osteoporosis or osteopenia, one can argue that by age 65 a significant majority of women are at risk, and therefore all women 65 and over on Medicare should be screened. The USPSTF recommended routine screening at age 65 for all women, first in their 2002 updated guidelines and again in 2011. Medicare reimbursement for densitometry is now consistent. But it is still not known how often women should undergo screenings, though some USPSTF panel members recommended every 2 or 3 years. There was no consensus at what age—or even if—they should be discontinued.

Although Medicare pays for a bone density test every 2 years, some researchers believe the frequency of testing has been oversold. Bone loss and osteoporosis develop so slowly in most women whose bones test normal at age 65, they suggest many can safely wait as long as 15 years before having a second bone density test (Gourlay et al., 2012).

Others recommend an alternative and more traditional approach, by adding the number of risk factors for osteoporosis for a specific woman before recommending screening. The risk factors in addition to age and female gender are being of Caucasian or Asian race; slender build; bilateral oophorectomy prior to natural menopause; early-onset menstruation; smoking; alcohol abuse; physical inactivity; the use of steroid hormones to treat a variety of medical conditions; and obtaining too little calcium or too much caffeine, protein, or salt from the diet.

Interventions for reducing or reversing bone loss include an increase in dietary calcium, calcium and vitamin D supplementation, weight-bearing exercise, and medication, particularly bisphosphonates such as Fosamax, Actonel, Boniva, and Reclast.

Fosamax (alendronate sodium), a medication approved by the Food and Drug Administration (FDA) in 1995, reverses osteoporotic bone loss. It increased bone density 3% to 9% in one sample of postmenopausal women, whereas a placebo group lost bone (Liberman et al., 1995). This study also reported that women with osteoporosis who took Fosamax were only half as likely to break a hip as women who did not take it.

In 2006 the first generic (i.e., no longer patented, and therefore low-cost) version of Fosamax was approved. Boniva and Reclast became generic afterward and about the time that this edition is being published, Actonel is expected to be generic as well. All substantially reduce the incidence of new vertebral fractures. For women who do not tolerate oral dosing well, intravenous injections are available.

The FDA, however, has recently cautioned against the long-term use of bisphosphonates (Black, Bauer, Schwartz, Cummings, & Rosen, 2012). The agency's analysis found little if any benefit from the drugs after 3 to 5 years of use for two thirds of women—the primary exceptions being women who have a history of spinal fracture or an existing fracture. The concern is that long-term use may actually lead to weaker bones in certain women, including femur fractures and osteonecrosis of the jaw. After a 3- to 5-year interval, one should consider taking a break from the drugs for a year or perhaps permanently.

CHOLESTEROL

At one time *cholesterol* guidelines were a rather simple affair. In an earlier edition of this book, I reported that a total blood cholesterol level of 240 mg/dL or higher was considered abnormal because it had a substantial association with coronary heart disease, and that about 27% of American adults had levels this high. I was also able to report on an increasing awareness of cholesterol levels, with the percentage of adults who had their cholesterol level checked increasing rapidly from 35% to 59% of the population between 1983 and 1988.

A more complicated issue at that time was whether cholesterol screenings were recommended after the age of 70. It had not been determined whether the association between higher cholesterol concentrations and atherosclerotic coronary artery disease, for instance, may weaken *or* strengthen with age. If the association remains the same or strengthens with age, it is an important and modifiable risk factor among older persons. If it weakens with age, cholesterol testing with older adults would not be an effective screening.

An informal survey of several hundred physicians revealed that the majority considered age 70 the approximate threshold for effective treatment of an elevated cholesterol level. Most expressed some concern about initiating treatment through drugs or diet with patients over age 70. The concerns regarding the prescribing of hypolipidemic drugs related to their cost, side effects, and potential interaction with other medications.

Dietary therapy and follow-up by physicians, dietitians, or nutritionists appeared to be effective in reducing dietary fat intake and serum cholesterol in adults of all ages. Dietary recommendations typically consisted of reducing fat intake to less than 30% of total calories, saturated fat (fat that is solid at room temperature, e.g., butter, cheese, fat in red meat) to less than 10% of total calories, and cholesterol intake to less than 300 mg/dL/.

The major concern with dietary recommendations for the lowering of cholesterol levels was that it may foster malnutrition in highly compliant older clients (see Figure 2.2). Malnutrition is not an uncommon issue when it comes to older adults, and cholesterol or fat avoidance that triggers malnutrition is a legitimate concern (see Chapter 5, "Nutrition and Weight Management").

At the turn of the century, guidelines became more aggressive for cholesterol screening and treatment. Although these changes have been motivated by medical concerns, there are health education and financial consequences as well. The *National Cholesterol Education Program* (NCEP) III guidelines that were published in 2001 were more demanding and complicated than previous guidelines (Expert Panel on Detection, Evaluation, and Treatment of High Blood Cholesterol in Adults, 2001). Determining risk involved more than the simple calculation of a total blood cholesterol level; it involved the calculation of several measurements: total cholesterol level, high-density lipoprotein (HDL) cholesterol level, systolic blood pressure, the 5-year age category that one is in, smoking status, abdominal obesity, diabetes, and a family history of heart disease.

A 2004 update to the NCEP guidelines was even more aggressive in terms of low-density lipoprotein (LDL) level. Low-risk patients (zero or one risk factor) should be below an LDL level of 160 mg/dL, as before, but moderately high-risk patients (two or more risk factors) should be below 130 mg/dL. For high-risk patients (i.e., coronary heart disease patients or its risk equivalent such as diabetes), an LDL below 100 mg/dL was now recommended, rather than the previous 130. And for a subset of very high-risk patients the recommendation was less than 70. Not surprisingly, it was recommended that a physician be consulted for expert advice on one's risk factors—hypertension, cigarette smoking, HDL below 40 mg/dL (however, a score over 60 mg/dL *removes* one

FIGURE 2.2   The late Elizabeth "Grandma" Layton took her first art class at age 68, and she drew a picture of her husband, Glenn, on a bathroom scale when he was concerned about weight loss and malnutrition.

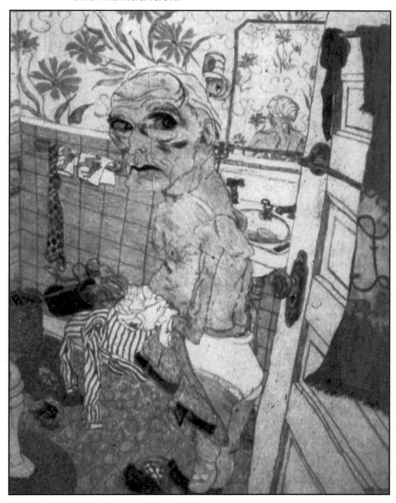

risk factor from the total count), a family history of premature coronary heart disease, and age (men over 45 and women over 55)—before determining which LDL category is acceptable.

In addition, this aggressive approach increases the number of persons who are being recommended to take the new cholesterol-lowering medications—from 13 million under the 1993 guidelines, to 36 million under the 2001 guidelines, to 43 million under the 2004 update. This may be reassuring from a medical perspective, but it raises some nonmedical issues. How many adults can afford the $1,200 a year in medication costs? If society cannot afford the estimated $48 billion annually that may be needed for cholesterol-lowering medications (Ansell, 2002), should only the well-off be privileged to get them (Gambert, 2002)? What are the long-term effects of treating younger persons more aggressively and having them on cholesterol-lowering medications for 40 years or more?

Paralleling the aggressive new NCEP guidelines, the USPSTF released new guidelines for cholesterol screening, and eliminated its upper age limit of 65 for routine cholesterol screening. The clinical evidence, however, was more supportive for treating hyperlipidemia in older adults than it was for routine screening and primary prevention (Hall & Luepker, 2000; Oberman & Kreisberg, 2002). Another study raised the question whether screening and treatment for patients over the age of 80 is effective with lowering mortality rate (Foody et al., 2006).

Another concern with the latest NCEP panel guidelines was that although the experts mention diet and lifestyle recommendations, they come close to proclaiming medication as the *only* way to achieve major cholesterol reduction (Fedder, Koro, & L'Italien, 2002). Because the majority of the NCEP panel of experts have links to the major pharmaceutical companies that produce statins, it makes one wonder whether their perspective has been influenced by this association. When dietary recommendations *are* made by the panel, they seem to be particularly harsh, for example, reducing the daily limit on dietary cholesterol to less than the amount in the yolk of a single large egg. This is tantamount to avoiding, for the most part, not only a second egg, but also meats, poultry, and cheese. Overly compliant older adults may run the risk of malnutrition.

Statins

Cholesterol levels fell markedly over the past quarter-century due in large part to the introduction in the late 1980s of *statins*, a class of drugs that lower cholesterol. By 2011, 21 million patients in the United States were prescribed statins. Not so coincidentally, annual deaths from heart disease in the United States dropped from nearly 800,000 in the late 1980s, to 599,000 in 2009. Statins, such as Lipitor, Zocor, and Pravachol, substantially reduce levels of LDL cholesterol, the kind that clogs arteries and leads to heart attacks and strokes.

Interestingly, a nationally representative sample of tens of thousands of Americans over the last 2 decades reported that cholesterol levels fell among adults *not* taking lipid-lowering medications. The authors speculated that in addition to statins, declines in trans fat, smoking, and carbohydrate consumption may be as, or more, influential than statins (Carroll et al., 2012).

The target goal of Healthy People 2010 was for no more than 17% of American adults to have a total cholesterol level of 240 mg/dL or higher, and it had been met by 2004. By 2006, for the first time in almost 50 years, the average cholesterol level in America dropped to just under 200 (to 199), which is considered to be in the ideal range (though most shun the use of total cholesterol levels for screening). The annual sales of statin drugs soared, reaching $14 billion in the United States in 2004, and $22 billion in 2006. Since then most statins have lost their patent protection, giving way to lower-cost generics, beginning with Zocor in 2006 and now including the other best-selling statins such as Lipitor, Mevacor, Pravachol, and others, thereby slowing the overall growth in profits.

When the cholesterol-lowering drugs referred to as statins were first subjected to an onslaught of research studies, they were touted to not only reduce blood cholesterol by as much as 60%, but to benefit a wide range of conditions like osteoporosis and colon cancer (Ansell, 2002; Scranton et al., 2005; "Statin Drugs," 2001), heart disease and strokes (Altman, 2001; Heart Protection Study Collaborative Group, 2002; Landers, 2001; LaRosa et al., 2005; Nissen et al., 2006; Ramasubbu & Mann, 2006), breast cancer (Ricks, 2001), cataracts (Klein, Klein, Lee, & Grady, 2006), and dementia or Alzheimer's disease (Jick, Zornberg, Jick, Seshadri, & Drachman, 2000; Masse et al., 2005; Simons, Keller, Dichgans, & Schulz, 2001; Yaffe, Barrett-Connor, Lin, & Grady, 2002).

This initial optimism has been reined in by several studies showing that statins do not appear to reduce the risk of incident dementia or Alzheimer's disease (Li et al., 2004; Rea et al., 2005; Zandi et al., 2005), incident colorectal cancer (Jacobs et al., 2006), or cancer in general (Dale, Coleman, Henyan, Kluger, & White, 2006). Moreover, in 2012 the FDA announced that there was an increase in blood sugar levels in some patients who took statins, leading to an increase in a person's chance of developing diabetes by 9%. There was also evidence of some memory loss, though cognitive ability returned to normal once the medication was stopped. These risks prompted the FDA in 2012 to issue a change in the safety information mandated on the labels of statins, warning of its side effects.

> **Question:** There has been a trend toward lowering the threshold for intervention from medical screenings such as blood pressure, blood glucose, and cholesterol. This can allow people to take action before the problem gets too serious. It can also lead to more people being on medications and the greater medicalization of health care. What do *you* think?

Most, if not all, of the first wave of studies did not involve randomized clinical trials, raising questions about their validity. Also, statins may be more efficacious (i.e., likely to succeed in studies) than effective (i.e., likely to succeed in practice) because noncompliance rates increase over time in routine care settings (Benner et al., 2002; Elliott, 2001a; Jackevicius, Mamdani, & Tu, 2002), with out-of-pocket costs being a major contributing factor (Ellis et al., 2004). There is also a clinical advisory on the safety of statins regarding the risk for myopathy, a neuromuscular disorder (Pasternak et al., 2002); liver disease (LaRosa et al., 2005); and incidence of hip osteoarthritis (Beattie, Lane, Hung, & Nevitt, 2005).

Undaunted, and on the bright side, new research touts yet new benefits for statins, such as a reduction in depression (Otte, Zhao, & Whooley, 2012). Stay tuned!

Efforts to sell cholesterol-lowering statin drugs over the counter were defeated by the FDA. There were concerns raised not only about the ability of people to self-determine whether they should take a statin, but also about the serious side effects among a minority of users.

CERVICAL CANCER

Until the 1940s, more American women died of *cervical cancer* than any other type of malignancy. However, the Pap test, named for its creator, George Papanicolaou, reduced the death rate from cervical cancer by 70%. Consequently, cervical cancer deaths are much less prevalent in the United States than in countries that perform far fewer screenings. Yet there are still about 11,000 new cases of cervical cancer each year in the United States, and 4,000 cervical cancer deaths.

A *Pap smear*—the collection of cells from the cervix—is recommended for women beginning at the age at which they first engage in sexual intercourse, and it should be repeated every 3 years after they have had at least two normal annual screenings. For women age 65 and over who have had regular normal Pap smears, the USPSTF concludes that the harms of continued routine screening, such as false-positive tests and invasive procedures, outweigh the benefits and recommends against screening.

Many older women, however, have not had adequate screening; nearly half have never received a Pap test, and 75% have not received regular screening. Older women are least likely to have had Pap smears, in part because they no longer visit gynecologists, the physicians most likely to recommend the test.

Pap screening for older women is important. Recognizing this fact, Congress mandated in 1990 that Medicare cover Pap smears triennially. In 1992 federal clinical laboratory regulations were established. In 1998 benefit coverage improved considerably when the full claim for Pap smears became reimbursable. In 2001 Medicare covered cervical cancer screening every 2 years for women not at high risk for uterine or vaginal cancers (though research suggested a 3-year interval may be more appropriate [Sawaya et al., 2003]) while continuing to cover annual tests for women at high risk.

In 2009 a new DNA test for *human papillomavirus* (HPV), the primary cause of cervical cancer, was sufficiently promising that the USPSTF in 2012 recommended HPV screening in combination with Pap testing for women ages 30 to 65 on a routine basis every 3 to 5 years. An 8-year study in India involved almost 132,000 healthy women, and a single screening with the HPV DNA test significantly outperformed the Pap smear (Sankaranarayanan et al., 2009).

In 2006 an HPV vaccine named Gardasil was approved by the FDA. In tests, the vaccine was effective in blocking viruses that cause 70% of cervical cancer cases (Lehtinen & Paavonen, 2004). The vaccine works best when given to girls before they begin having sex, and preferably between the ages of 11 and 26. The vaccine is administered in three shots over 6 months and, after a catch-up campaign, will be recommended on a routine basis for all 11- and 12-year-old girls. In 2012, the Centers for Disease Control and Prevention (CDC) recommeded Gardasil for boys as well.

A report from the CDC concluded that the safety profile of Gardasil has been similar to that of other vaccines (Haug, 2009). However, it is still not certain that the effect of Gardasil will be beneficial 20 to 40 years in the future. Thus, the decision to vaccinate is still a personal one to be worked out with one's physician. In 2010 about one in four girls got the vaccine.

The $360 cost for this vaccine is expensive and was a barrier for American women who lacked health insurance (still a problem with states that do not cooperate with the expanded Medicaid program implemented through the Affordable Care Act [ACA]—see Chapter 12, "Public Health Policy"). It is an even bigger financial barrier in the developing world, where the incidence of cervical cancer is much higher than in the United States.

Some conservative Christians negatively view the cervical cancer vaccine as a tacit license for the young to engage in sexual activity. One study reported that HPV vaccinations did not lead to increased sexual activity among adolescent and young women (Liddon, Leichliter, & Markowitz, 2012). Libertarians object to all government mandates for vaccinations.

COLORECTAL CANCER

There were 143,000 new cases of *colorectal cancer* and 51,000 deaths in 2012, making it the second leading cancer (after lung cancer) and cause of cancer-related death. Risk for colorectal cancer increases with age, with most new cancers affecting persons age 75 and older. Although the USPSTF did not recommend one screening method over another, it strongly recommended some type of screening for colorectal cancer for persons age 50 and over.

The Task Force recommended annual *fecal occult blood testing*—stool is placed on a chemically treated card to determine whether blood is present, though it should be noted that it produces a high percentage of false positives (5% to 10%). *Digital* (finger) *rectal examinations* are of limited value since few colorectal cancers (about 10%) can be detected by this procedure.

In the absence of adequate research, expert opinion recommends a *sigmoidoscopy*— insertion of a flexible tube connected to a fiberoptic camera—every 4 years for average-risk patients older than 50 (USPSTF, 2000). A sigmoidoscopy, however, examines only about 40% of the colon (about 2 feet), and research supports the need for a *colonoscopy*, which examines the entire length of the colon (about 5 feet).

Colonoscopies are the gold standard of colorectal screening. They are most effective when done by high-volume gastroenterologists (who perform multiple examinations each day) and who are skilled at recognizing flat and indented polyps or serrated lesions in the right side of the colon. In patients tracked for as long as 20 years, the death rate from colorectal cancer was reduced by 53% in those who had the test and whose doctors removed precancerous growths, known as adenomatous polyps (Zauber et al., 2012).

Medicare covers a fecal occult test annually, a flexible sigmoidoscopy every 4 years, and a colonoscopy every 10 years. There is no upper age limit to sigmoidoscopy or colonoscopy coverage, though researchers suggest this test may be discontinued at age 80 with minimal loss in life expectancy (Lin et al., 2006; Rich & Black, 2000). Beginning at age 70, life expectancy and comorbidity become factors in whether the risks of colorectal cancer screening (such as the perforation of intestinal lining or invasive follow-up procedures) outweigh the benefits (Ko & Sonnenberg, 2005).

Although Medicare coverage for colorectal cancer screening has expanded, compliance has not improved significantly. Only 25% of Medicare patients received recommended screening (Cooper & Kou, 2007). A 2-year campaign by a California health maintenance organization to encourage patients to get any of three screenings for colon cancer led to only a 26% compliance rate (Ganz et al., 2005). The tests are uncomfortable (particularly the cleansing process) and, for some, embarrassing.

There was a 20% increase in colorectal cancer screenings over a 9-month period, however, after Katie Couric, then the host of the morning TV show *Today*—whose husband died of colorectal cancer—had the procedure done live on television in March 2000 (Cram et al., 2003). This increase in screenings—referred to as the *Couric effect*—was a temporary one.

Some of the discomfort of colon cancer screening may be eliminated through a "virtual" colonoscopy, a scanner that takes hundreds of X-rays at different angles from the outside, and then uses sophisticated software to combine the data to produce a 3-D image of the colon. At the current level of technology, however, this type of scan misses growths identified by the traditional colonoscopy, and abnormal results still require a follow-up with the traditional colonoscopy.

Another approach to colorectal screening involves the swallowing of a small camera to scan from the inside (Hara, Leighton, Sharma, & Fleischer, 2004). Patients do not have to worry about returning the camera; the capsule in which the camera is placed will do what food does. Another test looks for abnormal DNA in stool samples (Ahlquist et al., 2000), and researchers at the Mayo Clinic in Minnesota believe a simple stool test may detect not only colon cancer, but stomach, pancreatic, bile duct, and esophageal cancer as well. A pilot test in 2009 at the Mayo Clinic detected 100% of colorectal and stomach cancers. Funded research is also underway to develop a blood test to determine colon cancer risk. These strategies are in the experimental stage, and a high rate of compliance for colon cancer screening is likely to be dependent on the success of one of them.

PROSTATE CANCER

More than half of all men over age 60 are bothered by benign prostatic hyperplasia, a gradual enlargement of the prostate that occurs with age. A much more serious diagnosis, *prostate cancer*, is a disease that is second only to lung cancer in accounting for cancer deaths in men. About 242,000 men in the United States were diagnosed with prostate cancer in 2012, and about 30,000 died from it.

Prostate-specific antigen screening (PSA) is a blood test discovered in the 1980s that measures elevated protein levels made by the prostate and that might be an indicator of cancer. Although the test is recommended for routine use by the American Cancer Society, the American College of Radiology, and the American Urology Association, it is not recommended by the more scientifically based (and less financially influenced)

USPSTF. In fact, in 2012, the USPSTF went from no recommendation to recommending against routine screening.

The task force found that one man in every 1,000 given the PSA test may avoid death as a result of the screening, whereas another man for every 3,000 tested will die prematurely as a result of complications from treatment *and* up to 43 men per 1,000 will be seriously harmed. Prostate biopsies can cause pain, infection, and emotional distress, whereas a cancer diagnosis typically leads to surgery or radiation treatment that can render a man impotent and/or incontinent but not necessarily extend longevity.

Although autopsy studies indicate that prostate cancer is present in about 70% of men at age 80, only 3% of men die from it. A large proportion of prostate cancers are latent, unlikely to produce clinical symptoms or affect survival. Moreover, many men may live with slow-growing prostate cancers that never cause any problems; but removing them, or radiating them, can cause urinary or bowel incontinence, impotence, painful defecation, or chronic diarrhea without providing any benefit.

A case-control study of patients at 10 Veterans Affairs medical centers reported that a PSA screening is not an effective tool for predicting prostate cancer risk (Concato et al., 2006). Another study reported that 29% of prostate cancers in White men and 44% of prostate cancers in Black men that are detected by PSA may represent overdiagnosis, which is defined as the detection of a prostate cancer that otherwise would not have been detected within the patient's lifetime (Etzioni et al., 2002). An examination of PSA testing in Cambridge, United Kingdom, reported substantial overdiagnosis of men with prostate cancer who would otherwise not have been diagnosed within their lifetimes (Pashayan, Powles, Brown, & Duffy, 2006). Another study similarly concluded, "Most men with prostate cancer detected by PSA screening will live out their natural span without the disease ever causing them any ill effects" (Parker, Muston, Melia, Moss, & Dearnaley, 2006).

Two rigorous studies—one involving 182,000 men in several European countries (Kolata, 2009) and the other 77,000 men at 10 medical centers in the United States (Andriole et al., 2009)—reported that routine prostate cancer screening saved few lives. Interestingly, routine prostate cancer screening is still highly promoted in the United States despite the negative research findings, along with the continued promotion and implementation of mass prostate cancer screenings at fairs, workplaces, and shopping malls, whereas in Europe it is not widely recommended.

Given that (1) media publicity portrays PSA testing as unequivocally beneficial, and that 80% of patients in one sample believed that "doctors are sure that PSA tests are useful" (Chan et al., 2003); and (2) 90% of men with early-stage prostate cancer still choose immediate treatment with surgery or radiation in the United States, and many of these men are left with impotency or incontinence, it is important to find ways to temper overenthusiasm for routine screening and treatment when no one has yet demonstrated that finding prostate tumors early from routine screenings saves lives or improves health.

Perhaps a summary of yet one more research finding is prudent. The Prostate Cancer Intervention Versus Observation Trial randomly assigned men with early-stage disease to either surgical removal of the prostate (there are about 110,000 radical prostatectomy surgeries each year in the United States) or to an observation group (Wilt et al., 2012). By the end of the 15-year study there was no statistical difference in overall mortality rates between the two groups, with most men dying from a cause other than prostate cancer.

There are other aspects of PSA testing that need further examination. Not only is it questionable whether high PSA scores are predictive of prostate cancer mortality, but people with low PSA scores—about 15% of patients who score below the standard 4.0 ng/mL threshold—may nonetheless have prostate cancer (Thompson et al., 2004).

The study by Wilt et al. (2012) did a secondary analysis (notoriously unreliable as the research design was not set up for posthoc analysis) and found there may be a group for which surgery may benefit men with early-stage disease—those with a PSA value higher than 10 ng/mL.

Another promising line of research in the field focuses on the rapidity with which the PSA level increases in the year before a cancer diagnosis (Loeb, Metter, Kan, Roehl, & Catalona, 2012). Twenty-eight percent of the men whose PSA level increased by more than 2.0 ng/mL during the year before diagnosis of prostate cancer died within 7 years—about 10 times the predictive value for prostate cancer death compared with the absolute PSA level (D'Amico, Chen, Roehl, & Catalona, 2004). However, one group of researchers report that the methods of calculating PSA velocity at this stage of the research process do not yet lead to accurate predictions, but would lead to unnecessary biopsies (Vickers, 2011).

Treatment options for benign and malignant prostate problems vary, and include drug therapy, surgery, heat, freezing, herbs, and vaccines. The increasing use of saw palmetto, a plant-based remedy for benign prostate problems, was deemed promising, providing mild to moderate improvement in earlier studies. A subsequent study, however, reported that there was no significant difference between saw palmetto recipients and placebo recipients (Bent et al., 2006).

A vaccine called Provenge was approved by the FDA in 2010 after it produced promising results regarding prostate cancer during a clinical trial. This vaccine does not prevent disease, but it may accelerate the body's own immune system to fight cancer after it has developed. The results were controversial (since you would expect it to extend life by being effective in those under age 65 who were more immunocompetent, but in fact it was more beneficial to those over age 65) and the vaccine is expensive—$93,000!

An even more expensive option, proton beam radiation, at a cost of up to $100,000 per patient, does not produce any better results than less expensive options (Chen et al., 2012). In fact, these proton-treated men had more stomach-related side effects. Nonetheless, its appealing high-tech dazzle has led to hundreds of millions of extra Medicare expenses (see Chapter 12, "Public Health Policy"). The ACA will attempt to deal with technologies that drive up costs without additional benefits in comparison to less expensive treatments.

SKIN CANCER

Skin cancer is the most common form of cancer in the United States, affecting about one in seven Americans at some point during their lifetime. More than half of all skin cancer–related deaths occur in people over age 65. All the years of sun exposure, exacerbated during an earlier time by an ignorance of the danger of sunburn and the absence of sunscreen protection, makes the older adult a prime candidate for skin cancer.

Basal (65% to 85% of cases) and *squamous* (15% to 30% of cases) cell cancers are the most common malignant skin tumors, increasing in incidence with age, but highly treatable. *Melanoma* (about 3% of cases) is the most lethal type of skin cancer, and it too increases in incidence with age. It can be cured if detected early, but if it persists to metastatic melanoma it is usually fatal. In 2008 the American Cancer Society estimated 62,000 new cases in the United States, with about 8,400 deaths. The mortality rate for melanoma in the United States increased by 29% from 1975 to 2000, perhaps due to the reduction in the ozone layer from pollution and the increased intensity of ultraviolet light (Elliott, 2007).

The key for all malignant skin tumors is to not ignore a suspicious mole, wart-like growth, area that bleeds easily, persistent sore that won't heal, or a rough and scaly red spot. Any of these signs warrants a trip to the dermatologist. Prevention consists of applying and reapplying sunscreen, wearing a protective hat and clothing, and avoidance of sun during midday hours.

The American Academy of Dermatology recommends a one-time melanoma screening for all persons age 50 and older, and suggests that it is cost-effective and comparable to other cancer screening recommendations. The USPSTF, however, found insufficient evidence for or against this recommendation. The type of prospective randomized controlled trial that provides the highest level of evidence, and has brought many other screening methods into widespread use, has not been conducted for skin cancer.

The USPSTF also concluded that: (1) primary care counseling had only a minor impact on increasing sun-protective behaviors and the modest results may not be clinically meaningful, and (2) sunscreen use had no clear protective affect on melanoma risk (Lin, Eder, & Weinmann, 2011).

HEARING AND VISION

It is estimated that about a third of Americans age 60 and older have *hearing* loss, rising to 80% above age 80. Yet only 14% of older adults who need hearing devices actually have them. Barriers include cost—it is not covered by Medicare, and the typical range is from $1,000 to $4,000 per ear; vanity; denial of a problem; dissatisfaction with past devices; and fear of technology, which has become quite sophisticated for hearing devices.

Future cohorts of older adults may have worse hearing problems thanks to the popularity of headphones for music and cell phone conversations at too high a volume or too long an exposure (Fligor & Cox, 2004). Yet, when researchers conducted the first study to examine generational differences in hearing loss, they tentatively concluded that baby boomers retain good hearing longer than previous generations (Zhan et al., 2010). The researchers suggest that offsetting the negative influences are fewer noisy jobs, a decline in smoking, and better medical care.

Presbycusis is age-related hearing loss that results in the inability to register higher-frequency sounds. Consonants with higher-frequency sounds blend together, and a hearing aid that merely amplifies will not be effective. Interventions for hearing loss, though, have improved markedly over the last several years. Digital hearing aids have a precision enabling them to selectively enhance frequencies that older analog models cannot, and are able to create a signal that is more finely tuned to the hearing loss of older adults.

For instance, sophisticated digital hearing aids have directional microphones that prioritize sound from where the person is looking. Sound is amplified in front and is dampened from behind and to the sides, which helps in a room with a lot of background noise, like restaurants. A 2011 survey by the former American Association of Retired Persons (now known simply as AARP) and the American Speech-Language-Hearing Association found that 82% of Americans older than age 50 were satisfied with their hearing aids, a large increase from a decade ago.

Hearing tests are inexpensive and effective, with no known drawbacks except the financial one for obtaining it. Yet in 2012 the USPSTF did not advise for or against screenings for hearing loss. The Task Force noted that there was only a single study that reported that adults who tested positive for hearing loss were more likely to use a hearing aid 1 year later (Yueh et al., 2010). The study was flawed in that most participants already knew they had a hearing problem before they were tested.

It is important to deal with hearing loss because a National Council on Aging study reported that those with hearing loss are more susceptible to depression, worry, anxiety, paranoia, lower social activity, and emotional insecurity than those who get help

("Time to Deal," 2002). In addition, memory and other cognitive functions are impaired with the extra processing required from hearing-impaired individuals attempting to comprehend words (McCoy et al., 2005). Recently, a Johns Hopkins University study suggested that hearing loss can upset a sense of balance and triple the chances of a fall (Lin & Ferrucci, 2012).

Before buying a hearing aid, clients should consider having a physician's evaluation (preferably by an otolaryngologist or otologist in a soundproof room). After this initial screening, consumers can access an audiologist or licensed hearing-instrument specialist to evaluate hearing loss and recommend an appropriate device. Unfortunately, some practitioners who dispense hearing aids may receive a commission from a hearing-aid maker, affecting their objectivity in choosing the most appropriate aid for a client ("Age, Hearing Loss," 2000).

Because Medicare and most health insurers do not pay for hearing aids, it may be helpful to contact Hear Now (800-648-HEAR), which can provide hearing aids to persons whose income level qualifies them for assistance. The Better Hearing Institute (800-EAR-WELL) may also help persons obtain financial aid in their local area.

Although less common than hearing impairment, blindness is one of the most-feared disabilities. Impaired visual acuity can lead to blindness; it is common among older adults, and there are effective treatments available. Nonetheless, the USPSTF does not recommend routine visual screening for older adults, because there is no direct evidence yet that screening in primary care settings is associated with improved outcomes (Chou, Dana, & Bougatsos, 2009).

Presbyopia, a universal age-related change in *vision*, begins in most persons in their 40s. Despite age-related changes, visual acuity in the absence of disease should be correctable to 20/20 even in very old persons.

Macular degeneration, the loss of central vision (see www.macular.org), is the leading cause of blindness among older adults and can be self-detected by looking at a grid with a dot in the middle of it. Approximately 25% of persons over age 65, and 33% of those over 80, have signs of macular degeneration. Though damage from macular degeneration cannot be reversed, early detection may help slow the progression of the disease. The National Eye Institute's Age-Related Eye Disease Study reported that antioxidant vitamins with zinc may slow the progress of macular degeneration in certain subsets of people with the disease ("Preserving Your Sight," 2002). A vitamin E supplement by itself, however, does not appear to slow the progress of macular degeneration (Taylor, Tikellis, Robman, McCarty, & McNeil, 2002).

In 2012, University of California–Irvine ophthalmologists implanted tiny telescopes into the eyes of two patients (ages 85 and 94) suffering from age-related, end-stage macular degeneration, and the devices restored limited vision by projecting an image onto the undamaged section of the retina. The patients were able to recognize faces, read, and perform daily activities.

A *cataract* is a clouding of the lens that reduces visual acuity. In patients over age 75, 52% have visually significant cataracts (Lee & Beaver, 2003). Most cataracts can be successfully dealt with through changes in corrective lenses, and more advanced cataracts can be successfully removed through surgery. Surgery should be performed when desired activities cannot be performed, rather than on the basis of which stage of maturation the cataract is in (Beers & Berkow, 2000). The surgery can be performed under local or topical anesthesia, has very low morbidity and almost no mortality, and 92% report improved visual function after surgery (Lee & Beaver, 2003).

Glaucoma is a condition that occurs when fluid in the eye does not drain and the increased pressure damages the optic nerve. Half of the 3 million Americans afflicted by this disease, however, do not know they have it because they do not have their eyes tested often enough. Tests should preferably be done every year or 2. As of January 1, 2002, Medicare covers an annual dilated eye examination for persons at high risk of glaucoma. "High risk" is defined as having diabetes, having a family history of glaucoma, or being African American. Glaucoma is five times more likely to occur in African Americans.

There are a wide variety of low-vision aids available, such as large-type books, talking clocks, high-intensity lamps, magnifiers, and computer adapters. These devices are not covered by insurance. If you are age 65 or older, you may qualify to have a volunteer ophthalmologist perform a comprehensive medical eye exam and provide up to 1 year of care at no out-of-pocket cost. Visit EyeCareAmerica.org.

ORAL HEALTH

The surgeon general has reported that Americans' mouths have shown steady improvement. For instance, there has been a steady decline in the level of edentulism (loss of all teeth) among successive cohorts of older adults. Nonetheless, about 25% of U.S. citizens over the age of 65 were still edentulist in 2012, increasing to 33% among those age 85 and over. Income level is the major divider, though, according to the report, *Older Americans 2012: Key Indicators of Well-Being.* Among those living above the poverty level, 22% are edentulist, but this percentage almost doubles, to 42%, among those living below the poverty line.

As the American population ages, visits to physicians increase, but visits to dentists decrease. Only 43% of older Americans reported a dental visit in 2004. The lack of reimbursement by a third-party payment system for dental care is no small factor in this neglect. As older adults retire they lose employer-based dental insurance and, at the same time, deal with a reduction in income.

The CDC reported in 2008 that there were widespread *oral health* problems among low-income older persons, including 41% with untreated dental caries, versus an overall rate of 22% among older adults. Older adults are seven times more likely to have oral cancer, and older adults with periodontal disease are 53% more likely to have experienced weight loss than those with healthy gums and teeth (Weyant et al., 2004).

Professional oral health care may be particularly important in nursing homes. A study of older residents in two nursing homes reported that professional oral health care given by dental hygienists was associated with a reduction in the prevalence of fever and fatal pneumonia (Adachi, Ishihara, Abe, Okuda, & Ishikawa, 2002). Other researchers suggest that aggressive oral care might reduce nursing home pneumonias by as much as 40% (Terpenning, 2005).

One public policy initiative that could benefit older adults is the promotion of water fluoridation in the 31% of communities (as of 2006) that were not yet treating their public water supplies. A study of more than 3,000 women age 65 and older reported that fluoridation not only enhanced the prevention of dental caries, but also appeared to increase bone density in the hip and spine and to slightly reduce the risk of fractures at these sites (Phipps, Orwoll, Mason, & Cauley, 2000).

Interestingly, dental X-rays can show the beginnings of low skeletal bone mineral density (Taguchi, Ohtsuka, Nakamoto, & Tanimoto, 2006). A woman may be more likely to take a trip to the dentist's office than get checked for osteoporosis by her physician.

DIABETES

Type II diabetes (previously called adult-onset diabetes until it started showing up as early as the teenage years) is the form of the disease related to obesity and inactivity.

According to the Administration on Aging's *Profile of Older Americans: 2011*, the prevalence of diabetes among Americans age 65+ is 27%. The two strongest influences on the increasing prevalence of diabetes in late life are the steady increases in obesity over the past few decades and the increase in the number of older people from minorities (Asians, Hispanics, and African Americans) with higher incidence rates. The more poorly managed the disease, the greater the physical deterioration as well as the greater decline in mental function (Yaffe et al., 2011).

The American Diabetes Association (ADA), with the endorsement of the NIH, has recommended that Americans over age 45 have their blood sugar screened every 3 years. A USPSTF update concluded, however, that there is insufficient evidence to recommend for or against routine screening for diabetes mellitus in asymptomatic adults. Less controversial was the decision by the ADA to lower the blood sugar screening threshold for diabetes from 140 to 126 milligrams of glucose per deciliter of blood.

Prediabetes refers to the range between 100 to 125 mg/dL, with an estimated 41 million Americans falling within this range. This new level can detect many more cases in which diet and exercise can prevent or delay the disease. Through diet and exercise, prediabetics can reduce by 60% their chances of eventually developing diabetes.

One study compared diet, exercise, and weight loss with use of the drug metformin (Glucophage) for preventing the onset of diabetes. Changing lifestyle habits was nearly twice as effective as using the medication, particularly in people age 60 and over, who were helped little by the drug (Knowler et al., 2002). Another study also concluded that type II diabetes can be prevented by changes in lifestyle among high-risk older subjects (Tuomilehto et al., 2001). Once diabetes is diagnosed, high-intensity resistance training improves glycemic control in older persons (Dunstan et al., 2002).

One program that has been around for more than a decade is the YMCA's Diabetes Prevention Program (DPP). This lifestyle intervention program operates in 25 states and caters to prediabetics with a physician's referral. Prevention programs like this, which have demonstrated positive results, may be expanded through monies allocated for prevention in the ACA (see Chapter 12, "Public Health Policy").

Medicare prevention policy does not routinely cover diabetes screening, consistent with the recommendation of the USPSTF. In practice, however, it does reimburse most older adults for an annual screening because it covers those who are overweight; have a family history of diabetes; or have hypertension, dyslipidemia, or prediabetes. Also, for those with prediabetes, screening can occur every 6 months; and patients with diabetes can receive outpatient self-management training that includes nutrition and exercise education.

DEPRESSION

Lifetime prevalence of depressive disorders in the United States ranges among surveys from 5% to 17% (Williams et al., 2002a), and *depression* is projected to become the second leading cause of disability worldwide by the year 2020. Despite its prevalence and economic impact, studies show that usual care for depression by primary care physicians fails to identify 30% to 50% of depressed patients.

The USPSTF issued an updated guideline advising that physicians begin screening adults for depression in the clinical setting. This revises the Task Force's previous recommendation, which encouraged clinicians to remain alert for signs of depression but did not recommend for or against regular formal screening. The Task Force's update concluded that there was good evidence that screening improves the accurate identification of depressed patients in primary care settings, and that treatment of depressed adults identified in these settings decreased clinical morbidity.

The USPSTF found little evidence to recommend one screening method over another, and recommended that clinicians choose the method they prefer based on their patient population and their practice setting. Asking two simple questions may be as useful as administering longer instruments: "Over the past two weeks have you (a) felt down, depressed, or hopeless; or (b) felt little interest or pleasure in doing things?" An affirmative response to these questions may indicate the need for more in-depth diagnostic tools. The optimum interval for screening for depression is unknown.

Screening adults for depression should take place only when adequate diagnosis, treatment, and follow-up are in place. Treatment and follow-up are based on the availability of *staff-assisted depression care supports*. This term refers to clinical staff that assist the primary clinician by providing some direct depression care, such as care support or coordination, case management, or mental health treatment.

The minimum level of staff-assisted support consists of a screening nurse who advises the physician of positive screening results and implements a protocol that facilitates referral to behavioral treatment. Treatment may include antidepressants, cognitive-behavioral therapy, other types of brief psychosocial counseling, or a combination of these interventions.

HEPATITIS C

According to the CDC, 1 in 30 baby boomers has been infected with hepatitis C, and most do not know it. *Hepatitis C* is a blood-borne virus that is spread through shared needles, blood transfusions (that took place before routine screening), and other exposures to infected blood. The virus can also be spread through sexual contact. Hepatitis C causes serious liver disease, such as liver cancer and cirrhosis, and contributed to more than 16,000 deaths in 2009. It was also the primary cause of liver transplants in the United States.

In 2012, the CDC recommended testing for every person born between 1945 and 1965 (roughly comparable to baby boomers, who were born between 1946 and 1964). The CDC states that routine blood tests can address the largely preventable consequences of the disease, especially in light of newly available and highly effective antiviral therapies that can cure around 75% of infections.

Chronic infections from this disease may cause no symptoms for 30 or 40 years, but then people may see symptoms from liver disease after that. And once symptoms of liver disease appear, such as jaundice, there is already significant damage to the liver.

If hepatitis C is a virus most often transmitted via blood and body fluids, why does the CDC recommend screening all boomers rather than just those who had a blood transfusion before 1992 or engaged in risky behavior in the '60s? Because a person in his or her 60s may not have perfect memory of what happened in his or her youth, and because baby boomers probably account for 2 million of the 3.2 million Americans who are infected with this blood-borne disese. The CDC estimates that if all boomers were screened there would be found an estimated 800,000 cases of hepatitis C, and 120,000 deaths would be prevented.

ARE SCREENINGS GOING TO THE DOGS (AND CATS)?

In 1989 two London dermatologists described the case of a woman asking for a mole to be cut out of her leg because her dog would constantly sniff it. One day the dog tried to bite it off. It turned out that she had a malignant melanoma that was caught early enough to save her life. Similar cases have been reported by a variety of other physicians in regard to dogs detecting skin cancer.

The dog's hypersensitive nose appears to detect changes in blood sugar levels as well. When blood sugar levels fall to dangerously low levels and the person is about to have a hypoglycemic attack, dogs react by whining, barking, licking, or performing some other agitated display (O'Connor, O'Connor, & Walsh, 2008). Dogs are currently being trained in Britain to warn diabetic owners that their blood sugar level has fallen to a dangerously low level. Trained animals are certified as Diabetic Hypo-Alert dogs, and are dressed in a red jacket in order to identify themselves as working assistance animals (www.msnbc.msn.com/id/31486267/ns/health-diabetes/, accessed June 22, 2009).

An experiment was set up to determine whether dogs could correctly select urine from patients with bladder cancer. The dogs were briefly trained and were able to identify the cancer 41% of the time, compared with 14% expected by chance alone (Willis et al., 2004). In another experiment using breath samples, dogs were accurate in identifying lung cancers 99% of the time and breast cancers 88% of the time (McCullough et al., 2006). Cancer tumors exude tiny amounts of alkanes and benzene derivatives not found in healthy tissue, and it is believed that a dog's sense of smell is generally more than 10,000 times better than that of a human being.

Dogs have also been trained through operant conditioning methods over a 24-month period to sniff urine for early detection of prostate cancer. When half of a sample had prostate cancer and the other half did not, the sensitivity and specificity rates were both 91% with 66 patients (Cornu, Cancel-Tassin, Ondet, Girardet, & Cusseno, 2011).

Nonetheless, if your dog starts sniffing you repeatedly in a specific area, it is probably not a good idea to begin chemotherapy right away. I would suggest taking a bath first, and if that does not work, head for an open-minded physician and see whether a biopsy is recommended.

Finally, as a cat lover, I must end with Oscar the Cat, a feline who was able to screen for impending death. When Oscar was alive he had an uncanny ability to predict death at the nursing center where he resided. He presided over the deaths of 25 residents on the third-floor dementia unit at the Steere House Nursing and Rehabilitation Center in Providence, Rhode Island. His presence at the bedside or on the bed of a particular patient was viewed by physicians and nursing home staff as an indicator of impending death. It usually meant that the patient had less than 4 hours to live.

Every day Oscar would make his own rounds, just like the doctors and nurses. When Oscar would sniff the air and decide to curl up on the bed of a resident, the first attending staff person who noticed this would grab the medical chart and quickly make phone calls to notify family members. The priest would also be called to deliver last rites. If there was no family, Oscar provided companionship for those who otherwise would have died alone. After the death of a resident, Oscar would quickly depart.

A geriatrician at this facility, David Dosa, wrote about this phenomenon in *The New England Journal of Medicine* (Dosa, 2007). On the wall of the Rehabilitation Center where Oscar did his work is a commendation from the local hospice agency, with this inscription on a plaque: "For his compassionate hospice care, this plaque is awarded to Oscar the Cat."

IMMUNIZATION

The CDC estimates that influenza deaths vary widely from year to year, from 3,000 to 49,000, depending on influenza strains and the accuracy or propensity of death certificates (i.e., attributing death to influenza versus attributing it to a primary medical condition). Pneumonia deaths are typically higher, about 50,000 in 2010, with 300,000 people hospitalized. What is consistent is that about 90% of the deaths from flu and pneumonia occur in people age 65 and older.

Researchers report that widespread use of the *influenza and pneumococcal vaccinations* can prevent up to 60% of these deaths among older persons (Nordin et al., 2001). One study reviewed data from 286,000 persons over the age of 65 and found that an older person's chance of being hospitalized for heart disease or stroke is sharply reduced during the flu season that followed a vaccination (Nichol et al., 2003). Also, in elderly patients hospitalized with community-acquired pneumonia, prior pneumococcal vaccination reduced respiratory complications, decreased time spent in the hospital, and improved survival (Fisman et al., 2006).

The *pneumococcal vaccine* should be administered to persons 65 and older at least once during their lifetime, with possible revaccination for older persons with severe comorbidity after 5 years. Vaccinations increased dramatically in the 1990s due largely to Medicare reimbursement. Only 10% of older adults in the community had received the pneumococcal vaccination in 1989; by 1997, 46% of Medicare beneficiaries had received the vaccine. The vaccination rate had increased to 60% in 2010—still well short of the Healthy People 2010 goal of 90%.

There was considerable racial disparity. In 2010, 64% of White older adults had received a pneumonia vaccination, compared with 46% of Blacks, and 39% of Hispanics (Federal Interagency Forum on Aging Related Statistics, 2012).

The *influenza vaccine* should be administered annually to all persons age 65 and older, although an advisory panel at the CDC recommended that flu shots be administered beginning at age 50. Two years after this recommendation (in 2002), only about a third of individuals in the age group 50 to 64 were vaccinated. Health care providers working with high-risk patients should also receive the influenza vaccine. In 2004, however, only 36% of health care workers received a flu shot. Unvaccinated workers can be a major threat to the health of children (6 to 23 months old), older adults, and the chronically ill. In nursing homes where staff who had contact with patients were vaccinated against influenza, resident deaths from influenza decreased significantly (Hayward et al., 2006). A recent Cochrane review, however, found the evidence unpersuasive that vaccinating health care workers who work with the elderly reduces influenza or pneumonia deaths (Rabin, 2012).

> **Question:** What do you believe accounts for the racial disparity in immunization rates, and what can be done about it?

Again, the immunization rate for influenza, similar to pneumonia, increased dramatically in the 1990s due to the advent of Medicare reimbursement. Only 20% of older adults in the community were receiving influenza vaccines in 1989, but this percentage increased to 65% by 1999.

In 2010, the influenza vaccination rate was 63%, with significant racial disparity. Sixty-six percent of Whites had a flu shot, compared with 52% of Blacks, and 54% of Hispanics (Federal Interagency Forum on Aging Related Statistics, 2012).

To increase the compliance rate, the federal government approved "standing orders" for annual flu and pneumonia vaccinations in nursing homes, hospitals, and home health agencies that serve Medicare and Medicaid beneficiaries. "Standing orders" means that the shots can be administered by a nurse without the need for a physician to write a new order. Also, influenza and pneumococcal vaccinations became mandatory for nursing home residents (unless contraindicated or refused by the resident) but, unfortunately, not for nursing home care workers.

Beginning in 2005 the NIH became interested in strengthening flu shots for the elderly, either through higher vaccine doses or adding immune-boosting compounds. These revved-up versions of the flu vaccine for older adults were inspired by preliminary evidence suggesting that the standard flu vaccine each year was less effective in the people who need it most—less healthy seniors (Jackson et al., 2006; Jefferson et al., 2005). One study reported that an experimental high-dose influenza vaccine (up to four times the normal dose) stimulated better antibody response in older adults and was safe and well tolerated (Keitel et al., 2006). This higher-octane vaccine is now available as high-dose Fluzone.

The *tetanus vaccine* is an immunization recommended for adults of all ages. The disease is sometimes called lockjaw, because the first symptom is often a contraction of muscles around the mouth. After a primary series of three doses of the tetanus–diphtheria toxoid, a booster shot should be administered at least once every 10 years. Medicare does not cover tetanus immunization, as there are only about 50 tetanus cases reported each year in the United States. About 70% of cases leading to death, however, occur in persons over age 65.

Shingles, also called herpes zoster, is a painful skin rash and blistering on the trunk, but can also affect the face and other areas of the body. Among adults who previously had chickenpox (about 95% of adult Americans), roughly 30% are afflicted with shingles. About a million cases of shingles are reported annually in the United States. The risk for shingles increases with age; for those over age 85, the risk is close to 50%.

A vaccine called Zostavax, roughly equivalent to 14 doses of the pediatric chickenpox vaccine, was approved by the FDA in 2006 to reduce the risk of shingles in people age 60 and older. The vaccine reduced the occurrence of shingles by about 50% in patients age 60 and older. In 2008 the CDC's Advisory Committee on Immunization Practices recommended that nearly everyone age 60 and older should be vaccinated, except for those who are allergic to the vaccine or those who have a compromised immune system.

The shingles vaccine is partially covered by Medicare under Part D, but many argue that, like the influenza and pneumococcus vaccines, it should be covered under Part B, which would reimburse more of the $200 price. Although about 60% receive an annual influenza shot or a one-time pneumonia vaccination, just 10% received the one-time shingles vaccine despite the fact that among those who got the vaccine, the rate of shingles was 55% lower than in those who did not (Tseng et al., 2012).

ASPIRIN PROPHYLAXIS

The USPSTF reports that there is insufficient evidence to recommend either for or against routine *aspirin prophylaxis* for the primary prevention of myocardial infarction in asymptomatic persons. Although aspirin reduces the risk of heart attack in men 40 to 84 years of age, there are significant adverse effects, and the balance of risk versus benefit is uncertain. Side effects are gastrointestinal upset and bleeding disorders, gout, and kidney stones.

Nonetheless, the use of aspirin at least every other day by healthy individuals older than age 35 increased by 20% between 1999 and 2003 (Ajani, Ford, Greenland, Giles, & Mokdad, 2006). There also appeared to be an interesting difference in the effect of regular aspirin use on men versus women. Men were more likely to reduce the risk of heart attack, whereas women were more likely to reduce the risk of stroke (Berger et al., 2006). For a subset of women who were 65 and older, though, aspirin appeared to lower the risk of heart attack as well.

Unexpectedly, researchers found in two studies that after 3 years of daily aspirin use, the risk of developing cancer was reduced by almost 25% when compared with a control group; after 5 years the risk of dying of cancer was reduced by 37%; and daily aspirin use reduced the risk of cancer progressing to metastatic disease (Algra & Rothwell, 2012; Rothwell et al., 2012).

Because of the risk of gastrointestinal bleeding and hemorrhagic strokes, no one should start taking low-dose aspirin on a regular basis without first consulting a physician. One study reported that for every 162 people who took baby aspirin on a preventive basis, the drug prevented one nonfatal heart attack, but caused about two serious bleeding episodes (Seshasai et al., 2012). Consequently, USPSTF recommends aspirin therapy should be decided on a case-by-case basis depending on risk factors and family history.

THE POLYPILL

Much controversy was created by a proposal from Wald and Law (2003) for a single daily pill to be recommended for all persons age 50 and over. This would contain a statin, three half-dose antihypertensives, aspirin, and folic acid. The authors suggested that such a pill, universally implemented for older adults, even those without a history of cardiovascular disease, could reduce the risk of both cardiovascular disease and stroke with minimal adverse side effects. Their formulation was based on the results of meta-analyses of randomized trials and cohort studies. They concluded that the *Polypill* would be acceptably safe and "with widespread use would have a greater impact on the prevention of disease in the Western world than any other single intervention."

After several years of hypothesizing, the researchers had a chance to implement a study and evaluate it. The health implications were impressive. In a placebo-controlled, cross-over trial (each person took the Polypill for 3 months, and a placebo for 3 months, in random sequence), an estimated 28% of the participants would have avoided or delayed a heart attack or stroke during their lifetime, according to the researchers (Wald & Wald, 2012). The researchers also estimated that even if only 50% of the population of the United Kingdom (where the research took place) took the Polypill, about 94,000 heart attacks and strokes would be prevented each year. Although single studies can be promising, they are far from conclusive.

An alternative argument could be made that interventions affecting lifestyle would be even more powerful and have no side effects. Interventions to increase physical activity and to improve dietary habits, along with public policies regarding food (e.g., banning junk food and vending machines in public schools) and sedentary behaviors (e.g., urban planning to encourage sidewalks and attractive places to walk to) could provide a nonmedical alternative for the prevention of disease and the promotion of health (see Chapter 12, "Public Health Policy").

A team of researchers from the Netherlands suggested that a *Polymeal* would be even better than a Polypill (Franco et al., 2004). The long title of their article provided a good summary of it: "The Polymeal: A More Natural, Safer, and Probably Tastier (than the Polypill) Strategy to Reduce Cardiovascular Disease by More than 75%." The Polymeal consists of wine, fish, dark chocolate, fruits, vegetables, garlic, and almonds.

Proponents of nonmedical approaches believe that government policies and research funding for the promotion of health have been inadequate to date. Opponents argue that nonmedical approaches have been tried and proved to be inadequate at best (Green, 2005). This same argument—medical versus lifestyle perspective—plays out in the policy arena of Medicare prevention.

MEDICARE PREVENTION

If you review the USPSTF recommendations inserted into the specific screening summaries in this chapter, you will undoubtedly conclude that the USPSTF recommendations and *Medicare prevention* are often out of sync. Much of the content of Medicare prevention

TABLE 2.1 Medicare Prevention

One-Time "Welcome to Medicare" Physical

Within 6 months of initial enrollment; no deductible or copayment

Physician takes history of modifiable risk factors (coverage makes special mention of depression, functional ability, home safety, falls risk, hearing, vision); height and weight, blood pressure, electrocardiogram (EKG)

Annual Wellness Visit

Personalized prevention plan services, similar to Welcome to Medicare, except on an annual basis

Annual basis, no deductible or copayment

Cardiovascular Screening

Every 5 years; no deductible or copayment

Ratio between total cholesterol and HDL, triglycerides

Cervical Cancer

Covered every 2 years; no deductible or copayment

Pap smear and pelvic exam

Colorectal Cancer

Covered annually for fecal occult test; no deductible or copayment

Covered every 4 years for sigmoidoscopy or barium enema; no deductible or copayment

Covered every 10 years for colonoscopy; no deductible or copayment

Densitometry

Covered every 2 years; no deductible or copayment

Diabetes Screening

Annually, those with prediabetes every 6 months; no deductible or copayment

Not covered routinely, but includes most people age 65+ (if overweight, family history, fasting glucose of 100–125 mg/dL [prediabetes], hypertension, dyslipidemia)

Mammogram

Covered annually; no deductible or copayment

Prostate Cancer

Covered annually; no deductible or copayment

Digital rectal examination and PSA test

Smoking Cessation

Two quit attempts annually, each consisting of up to four counseling sessions. No deductible or copayment

Clinicians are encouraged to become credentialed in smoking cessation

Immunization

Influenza vaccination covered annually; pneumococcal vaccination covered one time, revaccination after 6 years dependent on risk; no deductible or copayment

(continued)

TABLE 2.1 Medicare Prevention *(continued)*

Other Coverage

Diabetes outpatient self-management training (blood glucose monitors, test strips, lancets; nutrition and exercise education; self-management skills: 9 hours of group training, plus 1 hour of individual training; up to 2 hours of follow-up training annually)

Medical nutrition therapy for persons with diabetes or a renal disease: 3 hours of individual training first year, 2 hours subsequent years

Glaucoma screening annually for those with diabetes, family history, or African American descent

Persons with cardiovascular disease may be eligible for comprehensive prevention programs developed by Drs. Dean Ornish and Herbert Benson: coverage for 36 sessions within 18 weeks, possible extension to 72 sessions within 36 weeks

Abdominal aortic aneurysm, one-time screening by ultrasound for men aged 65–75 years who have ever smoked

Obesity screening and intensive behavioral therapy; face-to-face counseling weekly for a month by a medical provider in a primary care setting, then five more monthly sessions, and then six additional monthly sessions if progress is being made

Depression screening, annually, if in a primary care setting that can provide follow-up treatment and referrals

Alcohol misuse counseling, annually; if screened positive in a primary care setting by a qualified provider, up to four brief face-to-face counseling sessions annually

Frequency and Duration

The following are *estimates* of what researchers recommend, relying most heavily on the USPSTF recommendations, but not exclusively on them:

Blood pressure: Begin early adulthood, annually, ending around age 80

Cholesterol: Begin early adulthood, every 2 or 3 years, ending around age 80

Colorectal cancer: Begin age 50 (age 45 in African Americans), every 10 years for colonoscopy, ending around age 75

Mammogram: Begin age 50, every other year, no consensus after age 75

Osteoporosis: Begin early adulthood for women (no frequency recommended); no consensus after age 65

Pap test: Begin with female sexual activity, two normal consecutive annual screenings, followed by every 3 years; two normal consecutive annual screenings around age 65, then discontinue

Prostate cancer: Do not do routinely, except if there is a family history or African American heritage

Definitions

Hypercholesterolemia: LDL above 160/130/100 (depending on risk factors), HDL below 40, ratio (total/HDL) 4.2 or above

Diabetes: fasting glucose 126 mg/dL and above; prediabetes, 100–125 mg/dL

High blood pressure: over 140/90; between 120/80 and 140/90 is prehypertensive

Osteopenia: 1 to 2.5 standard deviations below young-adult peak bone density

Osteoporosis: 2.5 standard deviations or more below young-adult peak bone density

interventions (see Table 2.1) appears to have been influenced as much by medical lobbyists advocating for specific segments of the medical industry (e.g., oncology, urology, orthopedics) than by policy derived from evidence-based medicine (Haber, 2001a, 2005b).

Nonetheless, the expansion of Medicare prevention has been consistent over the years, with major improvements in 1998 and 2005 and in 2010 when the ACA was enacted. The ACA eliminated all cost sharing for prevention services, that is, deductibles and copayments, to maximize access.

Although the expansion of Medicare prevention undoubtedly benefits older Americans, the bottom-line question remains: What is the most effective and cost-effective way to promote health and prevent disease through the Medicare program? How do you get the most bang for your buck? The present system, although consistently improving, still falls far short of ideal.

Mammogram screening is an example of a benefit unduly influenced by medical lobbyists. This screening benefit was increased to *annually* for all Medicare-eligible women age *40* and older. The USPSTF noted, however, that the more frequent (i.e., annual) than recommended mammogram screenings, reimbursed without an upper age limit, would be expensive, would not result in reduced mortality, and would increase risk of unnecessary additional intervention. The Task Force raised the prospects of more false-positive results and additional biopsies as a consequence.

Bone mass screening procedures covered by Medicare every 2 years is also unnecessarily frequent and expensive. In women whose bones test normal at age 65, many can safely wait more than a decade due to potential bone loss and osteoporosis that develops so slowly in most women.

Little criticism can be leveled at the Medicare benefits for colorectal cancer screenings for all Medicare-eligible individuals 50 and over, now that the colonoscopy has been included. One could argue, though, that the sigmoidoscopy, barium enema, and fecal occult test are not worth the expense. However, the most relevant issue—how to increase the exceptionally low compliance rate for colorectal cancer screening—is not being addressed by Medicare policymakers.

Another example of the effects of lobbying is the coverage for an annual prostate cancer screening for Medicare-eligible men over age 55. This coverage is made available despite the lack of evidence that early detection among older men improves survival. Prostate screening also carries a strong risk of screening results leading to expensive and invasive interventions, whereas the original condition may have posed no harm during the individual's life expectancy. The USPSTF does not recommend routine screening; yet Medicare prevention allows for annual screening.

The expansion of Medicare prevention benefits for 3 million Medicare beneficiaries with diabetes is not controversial, and begins moving policy into the risk-reduction counseling area. Diabetics receive outpatient self-management training services, and the program has been expanded to include up to 10 hours annually to help control blood sugar, though only 1 of the 10 hours is targeted at nutrition education.

An estimated 4.5 million Medicare recipients with diabetes (and 110,000 persons with kidney disease) are eligible to receive additional individualized medical nutrition therapy to help them eat better. Medicare recipients are now able to meet with a registered dietitian to discuss food intake and exercise, review lab tests, and set goals for making dietary changes. Health promotion advocates were hoping this benefit for diabetes patients would pave the way for routine nutrition counseling for other Medicare recipients.

Another example of medical lobbying influence is the coverage of an initial EKG, following a USPSTF 2004 update conclusion that it is inconclusive in terms of how it would change the course of treatment, and that false positives leading to unnecessary invasive procedures and overtreatment outweigh any benefit of the test.

In general, there are two criticisms about the cost-effectiveness and effectiveness of Medicare prevention: (1) there are no upper age limits and overly frequent routine medical screenings are permitted, which are unnecessarily costly, and can lead to unintended consequences; and (2) there needs to be a better balance between overly generous medical screenings versus inadequate counseling for risk reduction.

Other analysts have argued that given limited prevention resources, we should reexamine policy that is so heavily focused on medical screenings (Mason, 2001; Napoli, 2001). I noted in 2001 and 2005 that perhaps it would be more effective—and cost-effective—to focus on counseling in the areas of sedentary behavior, inadequate nutrition, smoking and tobacco use, and alcohol abuse (Haber, 2001a, 2005b). Since that time several positive steps have been implemented, most of them a product of the ACA:

1. An initial physical examination that includes prevention counseling;
2. Annual wellness visits;
3. Smoking cessation—no longer limited to those who have an illness caused by or complicated by tobacco use;
4. Comprehensive health promotion programs developed by Dean Ornish and Herbert Benson, for beneficiaries with heart problems;
5. Screening and intensive behavioral therapy for obesity;
6. Depression screening in a primary care setting that can provide follow-up and referral;
7. Alcohol misuse counseling sessions, up to four per year, in a primary care setting with a qualified provider; and
8. Elimination of deductibles and copayments for prevention services to enhance access.

| BOX 2.1 | Medicare Prevention and Sex |

Medicare was developed by men and began with a sex bias. Older women are more likely to be afflicted with debilitating arthritis, osteoporosis, and other conditions that lend themselves to chronic care. Women are also likely to live longer than men with these debilitating conditions. Older men are more likely to encounter life-threatening acute conditions that require hospitalization. Thus, Medicare, with its emphasis on hospital coverage and neglect of chronic-care support services, favors older men.

In addition to reimbursement biases, a review of Table 2.1, Medicare Prevention, reveals differences in counseling content that could be differentiated by sex. For instance, only a small minority of men have breast cancer or osteoporosis, and health education messages in these areas might be tailored primarily to women. When it comes to smoking-cessation counseling, women have different concerns than men—for example, they have greater anxiety about gaining weight if they should stop smoking. Although prostate cancer is a male disease, the consequences of treatment on sexual capacity affect female partners as well.

Finally, America is made up of many cultures (see Chapter 11, "Diversity"), and in some cultures there are differences in the way female and male patients should be communicated to, as well as the way the body may be examined.

The next steps are to consider (1) judicious expansion of prevention to both exercise and nutrition counseling, and (2) to publicize all prevention programs. "Welcome to Medicare" physical exam, for instance, is a good idea, but an even better idea if we can increase the 13% of eligible older adults who took advantage of this opportunity in 2011.

A FINAL WORD

Medical screenings and immunizations are undeniably important tools for disease prevention, but the data collected by the USPSTF years ago resulted in a surprising—at the time—conclusion: The most effective interventions available to clinicians for reducing the incidence and severity of the leading causes of disease and disability in the United States are not clinical activities such as diagnostic testing, but rather those that address the personal health practices of patients. Counseling and patient education need to be a central role of the clinician.

To be fair to clinicians, a study reported that the average patient in a family practice waiting room needs 25 preventive services (Yarnall, Pollak, Østbye, Krause, & Michener, 2003). Using a base of 2,500 patients, the researchers conservatively estimate that 7.4 hours a day would be needed to provide the recommended preventive care in a typical practice. The authors recommended a team approach toward prevention, involving health educators and other practitioners in the clinic and collaboration with health-promoting practitioners in the community.

Even if these collaborative recommendations are pursued, disease prevention and health promotion interventions require prioritizing among the many available medical screenings, immunizations, and risk-reduction counseling areas. The next chapter focuses on risk-reduction communication, counseling, and intervention.

3

●●●●●○○

HEALTH EDUCATORS:
COLLABORATION, COMMUNICATION,
AND HEALTH BEHAVIOR CHANGE

●●○ **Key Terms**

collaboration

clients versus patients

client-centered versus
professionally centered
relationships

empowerment

medical encounter versus health
encounter

health literacy

Put Prevention into Practice

andragogy

interpersonal effectiveness

information processing

social and behavioral support

cruising the Internet

web deception

electronic newsletters

communication barriers

jargon and elderspeak

health risk appraisal and reflective
health assessment

health coaches

stages of change

health contract and calendar

PRECEDE

motivation

measurable and modest goals

positive thoughts

reinforcement

environmental support

stress management

social support

problem solving

behavioral and cognitive
management

healthy pleasures and
self-monitoring

food behavior diary

social cognitive theory and
  self-efficacy

chronic disease self-management
  program

health locus of control

health belief model

theories versus concepts

● ● ● Learning Objectives

- Examine ways to improve collaboration
- Explain the importance of empowerment
- Identify U.S. Preventive Services Task Force recommendations for patient education and counseling
- Explore ways to make a profession more health promoting
- Apply health-promoting ideas to the medical clinic
- Examine health education and health literacy
- Review likely sources of health promotion in the community
- Define and give examples of andragogy
- Review personality characteristics of a health educator who is a collaborator
- Examine communication skills associated with interpersonal effectiveness, informational processing, and social and behavioral support
- Assess the credibility of health information on the Internet
- Describe Internet deception
- Review health-promoting resources on the Internet
- Identify communication barriers between health professionals and older clients
- Examine the five spheres of influence on early deaths
- Evaluate health risk appraisals and reflective health assessments
- Describe stages of change, and precontemplation in particular
- Describe the health contract technique
- Apply a health contract to an older adult
- Describe the PRECEDE model
- Apply the 10 tips for changing a health behavior
- Differentiate among behavior management, cognitive management, healthy pleasure, social cognitive theory, health locus of control, and health belief model
- Analyze the impact of a food behavior diary
- Examine the importance of self-efficacy
- Distinguish between efficacious and effective chronic disease self-management programs
- Contrast theories versus concepts

This chapter is focused on health educators, regardless of disciplinary background. In the *medical clinic*, this could be a nurse, physician, health educator, social worker, gerontologist, or even a well-trained receptionist. One staff person with a substantial focus on health education makes a valuable contribution to the medical clinic. If this person is a clinician, it will be more cost-effective if she or he facilitates a *group* of patients with similar health challenges, such as arthritis patients, and mixing newly diagnosed patients with long-term patients willing to share their coping experiences. If this person is a lower-cost health educator, one-on-one counseling is more financially feasible.

In the *community*, it is important that health educators have an awareness of the older participants' medical histories, and to know that exercise, nutrition, smoking cessation, and other community health programs can affect medication usage and other medical concerns. Too often health education in the community operates in a world parallel to what is going on in the medical care of an older individual, a particularly troubling duality given the comorbidities and multiple medications typical of older adults.

COLLABORATION

The art of medicine consists of amusing the patient while nature cures the disease.
—Voltaire, French physician and author

Voltaire knew that most medical conditions are self-limiting, and that benignly amusing the patient is often all that is needed. Benign amusement, however, is not enough support to provide older clients who want to collaborate with health educators on health promotion or disease prevention goals.

I prefer to use the term *client* in this book, and restrict the use of *patient* to medical settings. The term *patient* is derived from a Latin word meaning "to suffer," and suffering is an appropriate adjective for some patients. Patients are also associated with another adjective—*passive*. Passivity is no longer appropriate for older patients. When it comes to managing chronic conditions or engaging in health promotion or prevention, aging persons are better off participating in the decision-making process and becoming collaborative clients, rather than patients who passively comply with the decisions of medical professionals.

In order to collaborate, clients must understand the choices available to them. These choices may be profound, such as deciding whether to combine chemotherapy with visualization techniques; or mundane, such as helping to decide on the timing of a treatment plan. Research has shown that client participation, even in mundane choices such as the timing of chemotherapy treatment, can result in fewer side effects. Similarly, nursing home residents receive health benefits when encouraged to make choices about their environment. In a classic study, residents who made decisions became more sociable, showed improvement in mental health, and even lived longer than residents who adopted a passive lifestyle in an institutional setting (Rodin & Langer, 1977).

Another example of the benefits of participating in decision making is demonstrated by clients who improve adherence to their drug regimen after participating in the choice of which medication to take. Clients may make this choice knowing that they are able to live more easily with the side effects of one medication than those of another; or clients who take multiple medicines may choose a less challenging medication schedule because they know that it will improve adherence in a lifestyle that is already challenged by a busy calendar and a faulty memory.

In contrast, many medical decisions are made as a consequence of physician priority (and specialty) rather than client preference. For example, the selection of the best treatment for prostate cancer—surgery, radiation, or some other option—is often difficult to make. The choice, however, can depend on whether a patient visits a urologic surgeon, a radiation oncologist, or another provider. Ranging from an invasive procedure to watchful waiting, your choice depends on whom you choose to communicate with and then, preferably, whom you collaborate with.

Willingness to Collaborate

National surveys report that doctors do not involve patients enough in treatment decisions. One survey sponsored by the American Board of Family Practice reported that earlier cohorts of older persons have been less likely to take an active role in the professional–client relationship, but present and future cohorts of older adults have significantly higher educational levels than their predecessors. Higher educational levels correlate with client willingness to collaborate with a health professional.

Even older adults with less formal education, however, are more likely than previous cohorts of older adults to be exposed to health information from television, radio, newspapers, magazines, and the Internet. This type of access to informal health education also correlates with client willingness to collaborate with a health professional.

Regardless of educational level, clients may differ significantly in the degree to which they want to actively collaborate in a health care encounter. Some clients want to give up responsibility to the practitioner; others want an active part in the decision-making process. These two perspectives, however, may not be as contradictory as they appear. A focus group study of coronary artery disease patients, for instance, reported that older patients were likely to prefer that doctors make *certain* decisions for them. This deference may not mean they preferred to be passive about making *all* decisions, but either the patient or the physician was trying to simplify a particularly complicated or uncertain decision-making process (Kennelly, 2001).

Regarding recently diagnosed metastatic colon cancer, only 44% of older patients in one study wanted complete information about their condition (Elkin, Kim, Casper, Kissane, & Schrag, 2007). They were also willing—older women in particular—to leave treatment decisions partially or completely to their physician. Interviewed separately, physicians could predict with only modest success their older patients' preferences in these matters.

Practitioners also vary in their willingness to collaborate with patients. The same practitioner may relate to different patients in different ways. One study of patients at primary care clinics, for example, reported that physicians were less willing with patients age 65 and older than they were with younger patients to ask about changing a health behavior habit or to provide them with health education or counseling (Callahan et al., 2000). Patients older than age 60 with high blood pressure are less likely than younger patients to receive advice from their physicians about lifestyle modifications that can help lower their blood pressure (Viera, Kshirsagar, & Hinderliter, 2007).

Philosophical orientations among practitioners vary as well. Some health practitioners want a *professional-centered relationship* with patients. They want to be in total control of the interaction and prefer brief responses to their questions. This approach is guided by highly structured questions to patients. Others are more *client centered*. They ask open-ended questions, value information on the psychosocial aspects of the health problem, restrict the use of jargon, elicit the client's perception of the health problem, and encourage clients to participate in the decision-making process.

The theoretical middle position is for the health professional to assess each client's willingness to be active in his or her health promotion and medical care decision making, and then match his or her strategy with the level of participation desired by the client. Although this approach can theoretically reduce client stress level and enhance communication, it is based on an untested assumption—that the health professional can accurately assess the client's willingness or potential to be active in health decisions.

Another option is to encourage clients to be more involved in their health care, regardless of their initial enthusiasm toward this prospect. This stance can be justified on the basis that in this age of managing chronic health problems and promoting health over long periods of time, it is in the best interests of clients that we encourage them to be informed and involved.

Client Empowerment Versus the Passive Patient

From the client's perspective, *empowerment* means having the opportunity to learn, discuss, decide, and act on decisions. From the perspective of the health professional, empowerment of clients means not only to provide service to them, but also to collaborate with them, to encourage their decision-making ability.

> **Question:** The term empowerment can easily be viewed as a buzzword (thrown around a lot, signifying much but meaning little). Do you feel that way? Can you give an example of how you or someone you know became a more empowered student, teacher, practitioner, patient, or client?

The role of the *passive patient* evolved from the belief that health care is too complex to be understood or controlled by the layperson, that the doctor knows best. In the past, when acute care medicine reigned supreme, the patient came to the physician only when seeking a cure, and this attitude was deemed valid.

Today, however, acute care diagnosis and treatment are but two of many important health care activities. Other high-priority health activities include health maintenance, rehabilitation, disease prevention, health promotion, and health advocacy. The one element common to these areas is persistence: one cannot maintain, rehabilitate, prevent, promote, or advocate successfully except on a long-term basis. The passive-patient role, extended over time, can be dangerous to one's health.

Health educators frequently encounter older clients who could benefit from education if they were more assertive about improving their health and the health care system in which they participate. Following are some typical examples:

- An older client with unhealthy lifestyle habits expresses the desire to eat less and get more exercise, but no health professional has helped galvanize this client to action.
- A chronically impaired older client, or a member of this client's family, is disgruntled by the lack of some service, such as home care or respite, that could enhance the client's independence or the family caregiver's mental health; however, this service is not covered by Medicare or a Medigap insurance policy, and the family cannot afford it as an out-of-pocket expense.
- An older client who is recovering from a stroke (or heart attack, cancer surgery, etc.) appears to be isolated and discouraged. This client could benefit from interacting with people who are coping with similar challenges.
- An older client who takes multiple medications on an ongoing basis is having trouble complying with the medication regimen and needs help in managing the medication schedule and monitoring possible interactive effects.

The passive client or family member has little hope of rectifying any of the aforementioned situations, and health professionals cannot solve all problems for all clients. Health educators can, however, motivate, educate, refer, and follow up. These interventions can empower the older client or family member.

How to Collaborate

The U.S. Preventive Services Task Force recommendations for patient education and counseling are applicable to fostering collaboration with a client. These recommendations are liberally paraphrased as follows:

1. Consider yourself a consultant and help clients remain in control of their own health choices.

2. Counsel all clients, and especially reach out to those who differ from you in age, educational level, gender, and ethnicity.
3. Make sure your clients understand the relationship between behavior and health. Understand that knowledge is necessary, but not sufficient to change a client's behaviors.
4. Assess clients' barriers to change, including their lack of skills, motivation, resources, and social support.
5. Encourage clients to commit themselves to change, involving them in the selection of risk factors to eliminate.
6. Use a combination of strategies, including behavioral and cognitive techniques, the identification and encouragement of social support, and appropriate referrals.
7. Monitor progress through follow-up telephone calls and appointments.
8. Be a role model.

> **Question:** Select a profession of interest to you that traditionally does not include health promotion and that has older adults among its clients (a car salesman, for instance). What could you do in that role to promote health? (Hint for car salesman: Think safety.)

Health promotion takes place primarily in one's home, neighborhood, or as part of a community health program. Should it also be a part of an individual's medical care? Arguing against this is that physicians and other clinicians have their hands full taking care of medical needs. Time is at a premium for getting medical work done; is it wise to hastily include health promotion, perhaps at the tail end of a *medical encounter*? Added to the lack of time is the fact that many clinicians are not particularly well trained in health promotion or inclined to participate in this type of activity.

I argue that health promotion can, and should, be a part of most medical visits. In response to lack of time, a meta-analysis of 34 clinical trials showed that even brief physician advice, perhaps 3 minutes, can impact on smoking cessation, dietary changes, and exercise promotion (Egede, 2003; Kottke, Battista, DeFriese, & Brekke, 2000). Also, as people age, they visit a medical clinic more frequently; this provides an ongoing opportunity to briefly encourage health promotion and to follow up with advice. In addition,

BOX 3.1   Health-Promoting Occupations

It is not much of a leap in imagination to construct a health-promoting role for a nurse or physician, even if the person's current position makes such additional activity difficult. But what about a profession that is not known for being health promoting, or is known for having a narrow perspective on health promotion?

Take the profession of a minister, for example. Clearly, the health-promoting focus is on the specific dimension of spiritual health. How could the minister take a broader approach and include other dimensions of health promotion? The minister could provide free space in his church for an Alcoholics Anonymous (AA) or drug-free support group. The religious institution might be a more trusting and supportive environment for this type of behavior change than an alternative site. The minister could encourage a church-based exercise class or nutrition program, perhaps run by a qualified congregation member. Or the minister could launch a Parish Nurse program. Or the minister could arrange for periodic sermons on Bible-related topics such as "the body as God's temple," or any topic on physical, emotional, or social health care that relates to the spiritual dimension.

health promotion and medical care should not be mutually exclusive domains. Exercise and diet, for instance, can affect medication usage.

Changing Medical Encounters Into Health Encounters

Although some persons may enthusiastically discuss health issues with a nurse, physician, or other health professional, many do not. Individuals may simply wish to resolve only their immediate medical problem with a health professional. They may not view health promotion as a personal priority, much less an issue to be discussed during an illness-related visit. Moreover, persons who *are* interested in health-promoting practices may not think of their health professional as an authority in this area.

If health professionals are interested in promoting health, what should they do to encourage a collaborative relationship? First, they can inform clients at their first visit that health promotion is part of their job. Second, it helps to have an ample supply of health-related materials readily available: health articles posted on bulletin boards, a stock of updated health education materials in the waiting area, and relevant health materials given directly to clients. Third, office personnel such as receptionists need to be trained to distribute and explain health information and health assessment forms to waiting clients. Fourth, hire a trained health educator.

It is uncommon for a nurse, physician, or other health professional to turn an office waiting room into an environment that is conducive to health education. Surveys of medical clinic waiting rooms have found ample numbers of commercial magazines for patients, but few health education materials within easy reach. If health materials are provided, *health literacy* must be considered, that is, the degree to which individuals have the capacity to obtain, process, and understand the basic health information and services needed to make appropriate health decisions.

A study of patients age 65 and older found that those who could not understand basic written medical materials were much more likely to die within 6 years than those who had no problem understanding the materials (Baker et al., 2007). One option for low-literate patients is television programming. *AccentHealth* provides healthy lifestyle television programming, produced by CNN, and delivered to physician offices nationwide, educating a growing number of patients in waiting rooms.

An Office System for Implementing a Health Promotion Practice

Several researchers have presented ideas on how to incorporate health promotion into a medical practice (Haber & Looney, 2000; PPIP, 2000; Stock, Reece, & Cesario, 2004). A summary of these ideas and practices can be grouped into four components: leadership, goal setting, intervention, and evaluation and feedback.

Leadership inspires office staff to accomplish a health goal. The goal may be simply stated as "We want to promote health by encouraging our patients and staff alike to take health-promoting action most days of the week." Leadership must also let office staff know what is expected of them and how they will be held accountable. Leadership need not be limited to clinicians. A proactive receptionist can take a leadership role, from referring to a website or making a follow-up phone call to see if an action has been pursued.

Goal setting can be done on an individual basis, with each patient completing a brief health assessment. A more practical strategy is to determine a *specific* health goal for all patients, based on, for example, an unusually low rate of influenza vaccinations or colorectal cancer screenings, or a high percentage of smoking or overweight patients. Goals should be bound by time, perhaps 6 months, to maximize staff energy and to assess results.

Intervention has several subcomponents. How will patients be contacted: in person, through the mail, or through fliers that are posted? How will contacts and results be *tracked*? There are a variety of effective tracking systems, including chart inserts, flow sheets, and office computer systems that can facilitate systematic follow-up of clients' attempts to change or maintain health habits. *Location* of the intervention can be patient determined, perhaps carried out by telephone; or clinic based, possibly a group intervention; or referral to a community health program, perhaps with the aid of a community resource directory that is developed over time.

Evaluation and feedback can be multifaceted. A periodic inquiry with staff and patients can determine whether the intervention appears to be working as intended. Health results from patients can be calculated, such as a percentage increase in mammogram screenings. Feedback should be given to staff, with successes celebrated and a follow-up discussion on what to do next. Feedback should also be given to patients, preferably in person or through telephone calls, and perhaps supplemented with written feedback. The more ambitious the behavior-change goal (e.g., smoking cessation), though, the more frequent the follow-up contact needs to be.

Put Prevention Into Practice

Put Prevention Into Practice (PPIP) was developed by the U.S. Public Health Service's Office of Disease Prevention and Health Promotion to improve the delivery of clinical preventive services on a national level. PPIP clinical sites in the community are designated to provide annual health risk assessments to patients and to target risk reduction and health promotion through screening, examination, immunization, counseling, and education (Melnikow, Kohatsu, & Chan, 2000). Primary care sites throughout some states are offered support for implementing prevention services through consultation, protocols, and grants provided by the state health department (Haber, 2002a).

If a health professional is interested in assessing readiness for incorporating prevention into a clinic, as well as developing a protocol and evaluating its impact, PPIP offers a manual: *A Step-by-Step Guide to Delivering Clinical Preventive Services: A Systems Approach*. It can be downloaded from the Agency for Healthcare Research and Quality website (www.ahrq.gov), obtained through AHRQ Publications Clearinghouse (800-358-9295), or requested through e-mail (ahrqpubs@ahrq.gov).

Community Health Promotion Programs

Assisting older clients with promoting health and preventing disease is an important component of the health professional–client relationship, but the amount of time available for this endeavor is typically severely limited. It is important, therefore, for the health professional to learn more about the health resources and programs available in the community and to make appropriate referrals.

Past decades have witnessed a proliferation of low-cost or free educational opportunities for older adults within the community. Except in isolated rural areas, a considerable number of health education opportunities for older persons are available. These opportunities may include programs sponsored by the local senior center, YMCA/YWCA, hospital, religious institution, AARP (formerly American Association of Retired Persons), health professional association, health advocacy group, support group, university or community college, Road Scholar program, mall-walker program, or corporate

Question: How familiar are you with the health-promoting resources in your community? Find one that you are unfamiliar with but that you believe may be important for older persons. Summarize it sufficiently to answer most questions that older adults might have about it.

retiree" wellness program, to name a few possibilities (see Chapter 9, "Community Health").

After identifying relevant community health organizations or resources, additional considerations come into play. Cost, transportation access, and instructor competency with older persons are obviously important factors in community health education. It is also important to be knowledgeable about which community health services and programs may be best suited for a particular client. To effectively refer a client it is important to gather feedback from older participants and health practitioners on the effectiveness of community health programs.

Community health programs are likely to be more successful with older clients if based on andragogical principles. *Andragogy* is the art and science of teaching adults, versus *pedagogy*, the education of children. Andragogy is based on a different set of assumptions about learning than are found in traditional pedagogy. These assumptions, which have received limited empirical examination, are twofold:

1. *Active involvement.* Active involvement on the part of older persons is preferable to the more traditional passive student role. Older adults learn best when actively participating in an experience, such as helping to set goals, individualizing instruction to meet their needs, and helping to assess their own progress.
2. *Peer interaction.* Andragogy is fostered when age peers provide support, information, and assistance to one another. Community health education programs that allow for peer interaction and support may be more effective than those that rely primarily on didactic educational techniques.

Personality Characteristics of a Health Educator Who Is a Collaborator

Certain personality characteristics, such as patience, tolerance, and a positive attitude, enhance the health educator's chances for collaborating successfully on a health goal. Encouraging health change requires *patience*; client progress tends to be slow, incremental, and characterized by lapses or reversals. Health educators are unrealistic if they expect to achieve health goals with their clients in the same time period required for the reversal of most acute care problems.

Tolerant health educators are nonjudgmental about the health habits of clients. These habits should no more be viewed as character weaknesses than a physical illness would be. If a client senses self-righteous judgment on the part of a health professional, even though it may not be verbally expressed, any mutual health endeavor is doomed to fail.

Health educators with a *positive attitude* begin any health endeavor by identifying the personal assets of clients that will facilitate a change in health behavior. If, for instance, a client has a receptive attitude toward health, the educator should acknowledge it. It is also important to acknowledge past successes in a health area; positive personality traits, such as persistence or a sense of humor; the support of a spouse or friend; or the educational and financial resources that will help the client access community health resources or education programs.

Which brings us to the next important component of effective health education—communication.

COMMUNICATION

Collaboration between health professionals and clients is dependent upon good communication. Open-ended inquiries and empathic listening skills are important aids to the health educator, increasing the likelihood of good communication with clients.

Taking the time to explore the values and beliefs of clients can help the professional overcome *communication barriers* erected by differences in educational attainment, cultural beliefs, socioeconomic status, religion, gender, and age.

Given the limited amount of time within which most clinicians and patients operate, however, it is not surprising that health professionals who are similar to their patients or clients are viewed as better communicators and more participatory. Physicians, for example, get rated highest on participatory decision-making style when they and their patients are of the same gender and race. One study reported that African American patients who visit physicians of the same race rate their medical visits as more satisfying and participatory (Cooper et al., 2003).

Overall, though, there is limited research on the importance or the effectiveness of patient–physician similarity. When writing a prior edition of this book, I documented websites that had been created to help patients search for physicians of a particular race, religion, or sexual sensitivity (Adams, 2006). At the time of this writing, however, none of the websites remained active.

Regardless of patient and provider similarity, there are fundamental communication issues that need to be addressed between health providers and older clients. Primary among them is time. Clinicians, for example, often want their older patients to focus, to get to the point. Older patients want their clinicians to listen to them more. Communication takes time. Busy health professionals need to be part of a team effort, and some member of the team, perhaps even a nonclinician (e.g., health educator, office staff person, peer support group member, or trained paraprofessional), needs to allow the client adequate time to communicate.

Time and caring work together. Caring may be enhanced through the use of appropriate touch and the acceptance of patient reminiscences during the clinical exchange. Health professionals who are unable to communicate warmth and unwilling to spend time with older clients put themselves at a disadvantage for motivating and encouraging behavior change (Street, Gordon, Ward, Krupat, & Kravitz, 2005).

One study reported that attire may be influential. Four hundred patients were shown photographs of physicians wearing either professional attire with white coat, surgical scrubs, business outfit, or casual dress. Seventy-six percent favored the physicians dressed in white coats, and stated they would more likely trust those persons, share sensitive information with them, and return for follow-up (Rehman, Nietert, Cope, & Kilpatrick, 2005).

To help an older patient communicate more effectively with a physician, the National Institute on Aging disseminates a 30-page soft-covered book entitled *Talking with Your Doctor: A Guide for Older People*. The book provides tips for good communication with any health professional, not just a physician. To get free copies, call the NIA Information Center (800-222-2225) or order via e-mail (niaic@jbs1.com), and ask for NIH Publication No. 94-3452.

The Gerontological Society of America (GSA) publishes *Communicating with Older Adults*, which includes tips for communicating with older adults, older patients, and older adults with dementia. Contact GSA at www.geron.org; 202-842-1275.

Communication Skills

A health professional's message can be viewed as a therapeutic agent, similar to a prescription of medicine or a surgical intervention. The positive expectations and good communication skills of a person considered to be trustworthy, expert, and powerful should not be underestimated as a therapeutic tool.

Conversely, poor communication skills by health providers are significantly more likely to be associated with patient lawsuits. In one study, 40 seconds of speaking was sufficient to distinguish surgeons with prior malpractice claims from those without (Ambady et al., 2002). Surgeons with histories of malpractice claims were significantly more likely to demonstrate dominant and hostile voice tones, whereas those without such histories were more likely to demonstrate warmth, interest, concern, and sincerity.

The following questions are designed to help assess communication skills. Some were stimulated by a presentation made by Kate Lorig, a health educator at Stanford University, some borrowed from other health educators, and the rest based on my personal experience.

Interpersonal Effectiveness

1. Do you make eye contact?
2. Do you have a caring but not condescending tone of voice?
3. Are you and your clients comfortable with touching? If so, will this enhance rapport?
4. Do you engage in reciprocity of information by self-disclosing when useful?
5. Do you let your clients talk enough, or provide someone who will listen, or refer them to a support group that will listen?
6. Are you well informed about clients' religious or cultural restrictions regarding privacy, touching, speaking to a woman alone, or engagement in other types of intimate interactions?
7. Cross-cultural issues are not just racial, religious, or ethnic in nature. We all interpret our health and diseases uniquely (i.e., we try to make sense of things within our belief system). Do you try to be sensitive to your client's unique "cultural interpretation"?
8. Are you able to resist the urge to counter clients' beliefs that are not harmful and instead just add to them? "Yes, the sin you stated you committed may be contributing to your pain, but pain is also caused by other factors." Do you give clients power by adding to their data bank, rather than contradicting it?
9. Is it possible to gain insight into a client's lifestyle by making a home visit or getting feedback from someone who has?

Informational Processing

1. Do you know if your clients understand what you said—can they paraphrase it back to you?
2. Do you know what your clients mean—can you paraphrase it back to them?
3. Do you supplement your verbal instructions with clear written instructions?
4. Do you ask your clients to write down their questions between visits and bring the questions with them on their next visit?
5. Do you encourage your clients to bring along a helpful family member or friend to help with communication? Do you talk directly to your client and not primarily to his or her support person?
6. If appropriate, have you screened for cognitive impairment?
7. Are you aware of the impact that medication side effects may have on your client? Do these side effects interfere with his or her ability to communicate?
8. Do your clients have interest in the science (e.g., the anatomy and physiology) of their medical problem, or are they just interested in practical skills and knowledge?
9. Do you provide data in a manner that is preferred and easily understood?

Social and Behavioral Support

1. Do you motivate through positive incentives, rather than rely exclusively on fear tactics such as warning your clients about morbidity or mortality risks?
2. Do you rely exclusively on talk to change client behaviors, or do you combine talk with other strategies, such as behavioral management techniques?
3. Do you involve the client's social support system, such as family and friends, in the plan to change or maintain a health behavior?
4. Do you have an adequate reminder system to provide timely follow-up support for clients attempting to make health behavior change?
5. Do you make appropriate referrals to community health programs or services when necessary and, equally important, do you seek feedback from clients for the benefit of other clients and to help decide about future referrals?
6. When making referrals, do you consider programs and resources that are offered at culturally relevant and supportive sites, such as neighborhood churches?
7. Do you ascertain client goals, see the underlying importance of these goals even if seemingly grandiose or trivial, and help your client redefine them to make them more achievable?
8. If you refer clients to support groups with lay leaders, do you know if they are receiving appropriate information in these groups? Do the groups invite professional expertise, and are you interested in contributing health education to these groups?

CRUISING THE INTERNET

Face-to-face communication with health professionals has become increasingly limited in our health care system. Consumers, therefore, rely on other sources of health information. For a few decades, Americans have relied on television as their primary source of health information, followed in priority by physicians, magazines, and journals. It is not surprising that television has been the primary source of health information. A survey of 122 local news stations in the top 50 markets reported that 40% of television broadcasts contained at least one segment on health (Pribble et al., 2006). The researchers also noted, however, that an alarming number of stories included factually incorrect information, and sometimes dangerous advice was offered as well. Time limitations may have been responsible for some of the distortions aired on television—a problem shared by newspaper coverage, with its limited space.

The source of health information that is fastest growing in popularity, however, is the Internet. A 2012 national survey from the Pew Research Center's Internet & American Life Project, reported that more than half of adults ages 65 and older are, for the first time, now online. More than 80% of these users have sought information on health topics. This modality of access will increase among older adults in the future. A survey reported in the *AARP Bulletin* (December 2008, p. 4) revealed that boomers age 50 to 64 were twice as likely as persons age 65+ to use the Internet to research information.

Merely accessing online consumer health information is insufficient; consumers also need to be savvy about the source of such information. Internet health information is often not the result of peer-reviewed, high-quality research; finding information that is accurate, timely, relevant, and unbiased is a daunting challenge to all web surfers. It is important to know the credentials of any contributor to a website and whether the contributor has a financial stake in the products or information presented. For instance, a comparison of websites offering nutrition services managed by registered dietitians revealed differences from sites managed by nondietitian nutrition consultants.

Websites controlled by registered dietitians ranked higher in accuracy, inclusion of professional resumé, and inclusion of a privacy policy regarding contact with commercial interests (Hires, Ham, & Forsythe, 2005).

A review of the privacy policies, though, of the 21 most trafficked health sites on the Internet concluded that few sites followed their own privacy policies. Most sites shared the personal health information that they collected from visitors, without the visitors' knowledge or permission ("Personal Data on Websites," 2000). Accuracy may also be a problem. Ten of 19 websites on Lyme disease had no inaccurate information, but the other nine sites did contain inaccurate information (Cooper & Feder, 2004).

Case Study in Web Deception: drkoop.com

During his 8 years as U.S. surgeon general (1981–1989), Dr. C. Everett Koop became one of the most trusted and recognizable public figures in the area of public health. He was best known for leading campaigns to deter cigarette smoking and to raise AIDS awareness. In June 1999, a decade after leaving office, Dr. Koop cashed in on his fame and reputation and launched an online health information website. The initial public offering of drkoop.com sold 9 million shares and earned close to $90 million. A bull market for e-health stocks at the time resulted in a start-up value of more than $500 million for this website. By August 1999 it was the most visited health website, with about 3.5 million users.

It was downhill from there, unfortunately, due to a series of ethical lapses. Millions of dollars were made by Dr. Koop and his investment partners when they sold shares of their stock soon after the initial public offering, in direct violation of securities law (Biesada, 2000). Nor did visitors to the site know that 14 hospitals that were described on the site as "the most innovative and advanced health care institutions in the country" had actually paid a $40,000 fee to be included on this list (Noble, 1999). Repeated examples of the site's inability to distinguish between advertising and health education continued to surface.

By the time I accessed the site in May 2002, questionable dietary supplement formulas were being peddled by "the Doctor you KNOW you can trust," and free psychic readings were being promoted. A few months later drkoop.com filed for bankruptcy ("Dr. Koop to Cease Operation," 2002), and in July 2002 its assets were sold for a paltry $186,000 to a company that sells discount vitamins. At one time drkoop.com had been valued at $1 billion. Drkoop.com was not alone. Medscape Inc., worth $3 billion in February 2000, was sold to WebMD Corp. for $10 million in December 2001. WebMD Corp., in turn, worth $20 billion in May 1999, dropped in value to $1.4 billion in August 2002.

According to one investigative reporter, WebMD, which regained its dominance in web-based medical information, earned revenues of $504 million in 2010, primarily by becoming a front for the Big Pharmacy industry (Heffernan, 2011). Heffernan found that WebMD drove consumer traffic to pharmaceutical companies. For instance, she plugged "headache" and "Mayo Clinic" into Google, and was directed to information on fostering healthy habits, finding effective nondrug treatments and, later on, using medications appropriately. She then plugged "headache" and "WebMD" into Google and was quickly referred to medications to prevent or stop headaches.

Websites

Potential problems aside, more and more health consumers are finding the Internet to be an incredibly useful tool. Free online health information is available in all forms, including continuing education, consumer education, journal articles, discussion groups, magazine and newspaper articles, book reviews, chat rooms, web reviews, databases, and so forth. Back in 2000, one person estimated there may be as many as 50,000 websites devoted to health (Gearon, 2000).

I have attempted to categorize below a few of the more interesting web addresses that I have accessed. Generally speaking, government sites (.gov), nonprofit groups (.org), and educational institutions (.edu) are more trustworthy than commercial sites (.com). Two other cautions: (1) these sites are very interesting and you might find yourself lost in cyberspace for hours; and (2) on one site I read about a condition labeled *cyberchondria*, referring to a malady among people who increase their anxiety about their health by going online.

To access the websites listed below, first type www. (except where noted):

Government

- healthfinder.gov (considered by many to be the premiere site for health information, including publications, clearinghouses, databases, websites, self-help or support groups, etc.)
- nih.gov (National Institutes of Health, with links to more than 100 government databases and a list of consumer health publications)
- medlineplus.gov (a database with references to 4,000 medical journals, a medical encyclopedia and dictionary, a drug reference guide, and hundreds of links to reputable health organizations)
- fda.org (U.S. Food and Drug Administration provides the latest information on new drugs and recently identified risks)
- odphp.osophs.dhhs.gov (Office of Disease Prevention and Health Promotion provides fact sheets and links to publications)
- ahcpr.gov (Agency for Health Care Research and Quality provides information on the best treatments for specific health problems)
- clinicaltrials.gov (details on 5,200 clinical trials, most of them government funded)

Wellness

- drweil.com (Dr. Weil is director of integrative medicine at University of Arizona; this site is broad in scope but focuses on dietary supplements)
- wholehealthmd.com, healthy.net, healthtouch.com (all three sites focus on complementary and alternative medicine)
- welcoa.org (Wellness Councils of America focuses on worksite wellness programs and products)
- nationalwellness.org (the National Wellness Institute offers conferences, programs, and wellness assessment tools)
- nccam.nih.gov (National Center for Complementary and Alternative Medicine)
- quackwatch.org (identifying dubious alternative health care claims)

Professional Organizations

- n4a.org (National Association of Area Agencies on Aging)
- cancer.org (American Cancer Society)
- americanheart.org (American Heart Association)
- diabetes.org (American Diabetes Association)
- lungusa.org (American Lung Association)
- nof.org (National Osteoporosis Foundation)

- geron.org (Gerontological Society of America, focus on research)
- aghe.org (Association for Gerontology in Higher Education [AGHE], focus on education)
- ncoa.org, asa.org (National Council on Aging and the American Society on Aging sponsor many community service and educational programs, including a joint conference)
- nhpco.org (National Hospice and Palliative Care Organization will help you find a hospice near you and draft a living will)
- research.aarp.org/general/geo (AARP Policy and Research Information for professionals in aging)
- cfah.org (Center for the Advancement of Health examines behaviors, biology, emotions, and social context to promote practical health care solutions)
- agingstats.gov (Federal Interagency Forum on Aging-Related Statistics is a collaborative effort among 12 federal agencies that produce or use statistics on aging)
- hrsonline.isr.umich.edu (do not precede with www) (Health and Retirement Study surveys more than 22,000 Americans age 50 and older every 2 years on physical and mental health and related topics; data products available at no cost)
- infoaging.org (American Federation for Aging Research focuses on disease, biology, and healthy aging)
- agingsociety.org (National Academy on an Aging Society provides data profiles and issue briefs about older Americans, with emphasis on public policy research on population aging)

Specific Health Content Areas

- nfcacares.org (National Family Caregivers Association provides education, support, and advocacy for caregivers)
- aahperd.org (American Alliance for Health, Physical Education, Recreation, and Dance)
- acefitness.org (American Council on Exercise provides certification for training and fitness continuing education)
- active.com (event locator for individual and team sports, and park and community activities)
- eatright.org (American Dietetic Association offers daily nutrition tips and reliable answers to nutrition questions, including where to find a dietitian)
- wheatfoods.org (Wheat Foods Council provides everything you want to know about grains)
- cspinet.org/nah (Center for Science in the Public Interest, and publisher of Nutrition Action Health Letter)
- healthletter.tufts.edu (Tufts University Health & Nutrition Letter)
- niaaa.nih.gov (National Institute on Alcohol Abuse and Alcoholism)
- nida.nih.gov (National Institute on Drug Abuse)
- samhsa.gov (Substance Abuse and Mental Health Services Administration)
- adec.org (Association for Death Education & Counseling)

Older Consumer

- aarp.org (AARP provides health news, information on a wide range of activities, and links to other sites)
- aarp.org/internetresources (directory of 900+ Internet sites by and for older adults: caregiving, health, aging organizations, Medicare, community services, etc.)

- seniornet.org (teaches adults age 50 and older to use computers, with links to 600 discussion groups)
- thirdage.com (tips on a wide variety of topics, from retirement savings to clothing colors that flatter gray hair)
- seniorjournal.com (daily news stories on topics of interest to older adults)
- assistedlivingstore.com (lists devices for assisted living)
- webmd.com (wide range of health and medical topics)
- roadscholar.org (lists nearly 8,000 educational tours sponsored throughout the United States and in 90 other countries)
- berkeleywellness.com (University of California–Berkeley Wellness Letter)
- healthandage.com (Novartis Foundation for Gerontology provides articles and information on a wide range of health and medical topics)
- mayohealth.org (Mayo Clinic covers a wide range of health topics)
- graypanthers.org (intergenerational advocacy group on a wide range of issues)

Electronic Newsletters

Aging Means Business
Quarterly newsletter that identifies the potential for businesses to target baby boomers and older adults as consumers, provides effective marketing strategies: geron.org/Publications/E-Newsletters/aging-means-business-e-newsletter.

Aging Opportunities News
A monthly e-newsletter for academic gerontologists and geriatricians seeking news on the latest research, education, workforce training, and demonstration outcomes in the aging field. To subscribe, e-mail agingopportunities.com.

Civic Engagement in an Older America
Bimonthly newsletter that provides information on supporting older adults as a civic resource: agingsociety.org/agingsociety/Civic%20Engagement/cenewsarchive.htm.

Human Values in Aging
Edited by Rick Moody, this monthly e-newsletter contains items of interest about humanistic gerontology, including late-life creativity, spirituality, the humanities, arts and aging, and lifelong learning. For a sample copy or free subscription: hrmoody.com/newsletters.html.

News From the Geriatric Mental Health Foundation
The Foundation is dedicated to raising awareness of psychiatric and mental health disorders affecting the elderly, and to promoting healthy aging strategies. For a free subscription, e-mail web@GMHFonline.org.

Over 65
A project of the Hastings Center, written by and for seniors who are seeking health care solutions. To subscribe, contact www.over65.thehastingscenter.org

Positive Aging

Psychologists Ken and Mary Gergen edit this *electronic newsletter* devoted to positive approaches to aging. This newsletter not only offers a uniquely positive perspective, but summarizes a variety of research that is useful to practitioners. For a free subscription: taosinstitute.net/positive-aging-newsletter.

Public Policy and Aging

Bimonthly newsletter that highlights key developments in the field of aging policy: agingsociety.org/agingsociety/publications/public_policy/PPAR_ENewsletter.html.

Soul of Bioethics

Edited by Rick Moody, this monthly e-newsletter focuses on ethics and aging, including long-term care, end-of-life decisions, and holistic dimensions of caregiving. For a sample copy or free subscription: hrmoody.com/newsletters.html.

Teaching Gerontology

Examines gerontological teaching content and provides references to instructional resources for those who teach courses in aging. AGHE sponsors and publishes this newsletter: hrmoody.com/newsletters.html.

Today's Research on Aging

Published by the Population Reference Bureau with the goal of increasing awareness of research results and their application to public and private decision making: prb.org/TodaysResearch.aspx.

Selected Communications

Ageline Database

Abstracts of social gerontology and aging-related articles, books, and reports, with free access through www.research.aarp.org/ageline/home.html.

Agency for Healthcare Research and Quality

Updated prevention recommendations from the U.S. Preventive Services Task Force (see Chapter 2) for the years 2001–2005 were compiled into two loose-leaf binders as well as a CD, available for purchase for $30. Topics include medical screenings and behavior-change counseling. E-mail ahrqpubs@ahrq.gov, or call AHRQ Publications Clearinghouse at 800-358-9295. Single copies can be accessed free at www.ahrq.gov/clinic/pocketgd.htm.

Current Awareness in Aging Research

E-clippings on aging in the United States and around the world. For free access on a daily basis, contact jsolock@ssc.wisc.edu.

Health and Aging

A 2004 selected annotated bibliography entitled Health and Aging, in *AGHE Brief Bibliography: A Selected Annotated Bibliography for Gerontology Instruction*. The CD-ROM is available from the Association for Gerontology in Higher Education, 1030 15th St. NW, #240, Washington, DC 20005.

COMMUNICATION BARRIERS BETWEEN HEALTH PROFESSIONALS AND OLDER CLIENTS

Cross-Cultural Communication

Some managed-care organizations are recognizing the importance of helping health professionals communicate more effectively with minority patients. In Southern California, for instance, Kaiser Permanente has a medical anthropologist on staff to help health professionals work more successfully with minority patients and to develop special programs for minority members.

Cross-cultural communication, however, is not simply an issue of race or nationality. Many cultural differences that emerge between health professionals and clients are based on differences in age, gender, religion, ethnicity, socioeconomic class, and education. Every health professional must deal with these types of cross-cultural issues.

Open-ended questions can help the health professional understand the client's point of view: How would you describe your health problem? Why do you think this problem occurred? Do you have sources of relief that I don't know about? Apart from me, who do you think can help you get better? Has anyone made recommendations to you? Did you try any of them? (For more cross-cultural questions, organized by content area, see Haber [2005a].)

For those interested in the topic of racial and cultural biases in the health care setting, and the improvement of communication skills between health professionals and clients, the American Academy of Family Physicians provides a CD (#724) or a video (#723) entitled Quality Care for Diverse Populations (call 800-274-2237).

Communicating to Client Companions

Studies report that in primary care practices, about one third of patients bring a companion to the doctor's office, and 16% have the companion come into the exam room (Schilling et al., 2002; Wolff & Greenberg, 2012). A majority of physicians, and an even higher percentage of patients, find this arrangement to be helpful. The two major drawbacks are with patient confidentiality and patients' possible reluctance to reveal necessary information when someone close to them is in the room. Older men are less likely than women to bring a companion when visiting a doctor, but if they do bring a companion to the clinic they are more likely to bring that companion into the examining room to help them communicate with the doctor. Older women tend to bring companions primarily for transportation or companionship, visiting with the doctor alone.

A client's companion can provide a vital service to both the health professional and the client, serving as an independent monitor of a person's condition and providing helpful feedback on client collaboration with treatment regimens. A companion can make sure that questions are asked and answers are understood. On the other hand, health professionals can be seduced into communicating with younger and more articulate companions and ignoring their older clients. Problems that may stem from coalition formation (between two of the three participants) have not been examined as yet.

Health Professional Barriers

The satisfaction of older clients is positively associated with the length of their visits with physicians, and with physicians' support of topics initiated by the clients. Using audiotapes and other tools, however, researchers have found that doctors seem reluctant to discuss psychosocial and prevention issues with older clients and are less receptive to these issues when raised by older clients than when raised by younger ones (Callahan et al., 2000; Kennelly, 2001).

Physicians give older clients considerably less cardiac risk-reduction advice
regarding diet, exercise, weight control,
smoking, stress management, and work
than they give younger clients. Thus,
older clients are systematically denied
the opportunity to lessen their risk of
future heart problems by adopting the behavioral advice of the physician.

> **Question:** Describe an example of ageism that you witnessed in a health professional–client or teacher–student encounter. What made it ageist?

How well do nurses communicate with older patients? A meta-analysis of 34 studies reported that more patients were satisfied with care from a nurse practitioner than
they were with care from a physician. Some of the studies reported that the nurse practitioner gave more time, information, and advice on self-care and management of disease (Horrocks, Anderson, & Salisbury, 2002). However, the key difference between
nurse practitioners and physicians—the amount of time spent with patients—may be
diminished in the future as nurse practitioners find themselves with less time to spend
with patients.

A survey of 552 pharmacists in Indiana reported that 88% were willing to participate
in continuing education courses to learn more about health education and promotion.
Despite this willingness to learn, though, the pharmacists reported persistent barriers to health education in the pharmacy setting, such as lack of time, reimbursement,
privacy, training, and management support (Kotecki, Elanjian, & Torabi, 2000).

Jargon and Elderspeak

Jargon is language—often technical or obscure—used by people who work in a particular profession or area of interest. The lower the educational level of the client, the
fewer the terms he or she will understand. The reasons health providers continue to
use incomprehensible language may be habit; the belief that comprehension of a medical problem might increase the client's stress level; the fact that hard-to-understand
terms may be conversation stoppers, making more time available for other clients; or
the belief that the use of jargon elevates one's apparent status and authority. Transcripts
of 86 conversations between medical residents and standardized patients reveal that a
large number of jargon words are still being used by residents and that they impede
patient understanding of cancer screening tests (Deuster, Christopher, Donovan, &
Farrell, 2008).

Clients, obviously, prefer health professionals who are willing to listen, communicate clearly, and show warmth and concern. When these expectations are met, clients
are able to offer more significant diagnostic details, have greater trust, and litigate less.

Elderspeak (the counterpart to baby talk) is a term some use to describe the sweetly
belittling or infantilizing form of addressing older adults, usually involving the use of
terms such as "Sweetie" or "Dear," or addressing an unfamiliar older adult by his or
her first name. One study reported that elderspeak inspired resistance to care in older
adults with dementia in nursing homes, whereas those who were addressed normally
were more cooperative (Williams, Herman, Gajewski, & Wilson, 2009).

Communication training has been shown to reduce the use of elderspeak among
nursing staff and other care providers. Many providers believe that it conveys a caring
attitude and is easier to understand, without realizing that elderspeak conveys the message that older adults are incompetent and baby-like. This may be particularly upsetting to early-stage dementia patients who are losing cognitive abilities and trying to
maintain their personhood. Older adults without cognitive problems may also feel they
are being addressed in an infantile manner and find it upsetting.

Four Common Reasons for Health Professionals Not to Communicate About Health Promotion to Older Clients

1. I do not think most of my clients want to communicate about health promotion.

   This statement may be true, given the dry way in which health education is often presented. But many clients become more enthusiastic about health promotion when they are encouraged to identify benefits that are meaningful to them—such as more energy, less arthritic pain, better sleep, or more strength. Clients also appreciate help in identifying the best pathway for accomplishing the health goal of their choice.

2. I am not skilled in doing it.

> **Question:** Examine the major barriers preventing health professionals from engaging in client education. What is your opinion on how significant these barriers will be 10 years from now, and why?

   Not all nursing, medicine, allied health, and health science students receive adequate knowledge, skills, and especially practice in providing health promotion and education to older clients during the course of their student training. However, given the wealth of continuing health education opportunities for health professionals available online and in the community, the major barrier to becoming more skilled at practicing health promotion and education with clients is not lack of opportunity, but insufficient motivation.

3. I do not have the time for it.

   Limited time is a major concern that permeates the managed-care environment. This barrier, though, can be circumvented in several ways. Many ideas and techniques can be presented effectively to clients in a brief period of time, trained office staff and health educators can assist with providing health education, and informed referrals can be made to appropriate and effective community health programs and support groups.

4. I am not paid to do it.

   Health professionals who do not specialize in prevention and charge for their services rarely benefit monetarily from offering health promotion and education to clients. But they do receive the gratitude of clients who stop smoking, start exercising, lose weight, or reduce stress. This, in turn, provides most health professionals with tremendous mental health benefits, not to mention more client referrals from the family and friendship networks of satisfied clients.

HEALTH BEHAVIOR CHANGE

In their article "The Case for More Active Policy Attention to Health Promotion," McGinnis and colleagues (2002) examine the impact of five spheres of influence on early deaths in the United States. Using the best available data, their estimates are as follows, in ascending order:

Environmental exposures (5%)
Shortfalls in medical care (10%)
Social circumstances (education, poverty) (15%)
Genetic dispositions (30%)
Behavioral patterns (40%)

McGinnis and colleagues observe that behavioral patterns are not only the most important contributors to early death, but also to quality of life as well. They noted that "what we choose to eat and how we design activity into (or out of) our lives have a great bearing on our health prospects" (McGinnis et al., 2002, p. 82).

Yet more than 95% of the $2.3 trillion we spent on health care in America in 2008 went toward medical care; less than 5% went to prevention, and only a minuscule amount of that was allocated to improve health behavior patterns. This budgetary allocation may seem out of balance to the health-conscious reader; but it is undeniably good for certain businesses and practitioners, such as medical institutions, medical professionals, pharmaceutical companies, tobacco growers, alcohol producers, food manufacturers, and advertising companies.

The health education profession, in contrast, is a modest industry with practitioners who toil away in relative obscurity. There are few millionaires, and few lobbyists who seek concessions from congressional leaders. As a consequence, the health care industry in America is primarily a medical care industry dominated by medical practitioners. In this section, however, I will focus on the role of health educators in the health care industry—and, most important, their potential role in changing health behaviors. The topics that will be examined are health behavior assessments, interventions, and theories.

HEALTH BEHAVIOR ASSESSMENTS AND INTERVENTIONS

Health Risk Appraisals

Unlike the *specific* medical screenings detailed in the last chapter, and which tend to be the focus of research studies and clinical interventions, *health risk appraisals* (HRAs) and other health behavior assessments are typically *comprehensive* in scope and are implemented in *nonmedical settings* in the community. Health promotion advocates in the community believe that a comprehensive health behavior assessment gives clients a broad, holistic perspective and a sense of the priority areas that they may want to work on.

This big picture, though, may also discourage persons who discover an array of lifestyle risk factors that need attention. A good health assessment may be broad in scope, but it also has to guide the client, who must be able and willing to start with one achievable health behavior change.

The most common example of a comprehensive health assessment is the HRA instrument that began in work settings and is now implemented in a variety of community settings. HRAs became accepted in the workplace in the 1970s and continue to inspire widespread utilization. During the 1970s and 1980s the HRAs were used primarily by employers to give feedback to their employees on their major health risks. Some companies demonstrated cost savings through the utilization of HRAs. By the 1990s, it was estimated that about 30% of workplaces utilized HRAs, and the number of available instruments had grown to several dozen.

Eventually, HRAs were adapted to the characteristics of older adults in the community. A program like Senior Healthtrac, based in San Francisco, reached out to 300,000 individuals nationwide who were 55 and older through Blue Cross and Blue Shield plans and Medicare supplemental coverage programs. It distributed a Senior Vitality Questionnaire and followed up with a Personal Vitality Report that included an individual's "vitality age," which may be younger or older than an individual's chronological age. The Vitality Report noted an individual's risk for cancer, heart disease, emphysema, cirrhosis, and arthritis compared to that of other persons of the same gender and chronological age, and then suggested lifestyle changes to increase one's vitality age if it was found to be lower than one's chronological age.

One study of 3,000 Canadians reported that providing coronary risk profiles to narrow the gap between an actual age and a reduced "cardiovascular age" led to some individuals achieving modest success with improving lipid control (Grover et al., 2007). When there was no gap, participants were less motivated to change.

The applicability of HRAs to older adults, though, was unresolved (RAND, 2003). Risk calculations based on younger and middle-aged adults were not as accurate for older adults. Also, HRAs tend to focus on premature mortality, which is less relevant to older adults than how their lifestyle risk factors lead to the progression of illness and disability. The process of evaluating the suitability of HRA instruments for older populations is still in development.

I reviewed summaries of 20 HRAs, including ones from such well-known organizations as the National Wellness Institute and Johnson & Johnson Health Management. They were being used in work and other community sites, and all claimed to have versions of their instrument that were appropriate for, or adaptable to, specific age groups, ranging from high school to older adults.

Among the instruments that I reviewed I noted the following:

1. They were computerized and available for commercial use. Most offered individual and aggregate reporting, immediate individual feedback, and data security.
2. At minimum, they included medical questions involving such measures as blood pressure and cholesterol level, and health habits such as smoking, exercise, and nutrition.
3. There was no consensus on length. Some instruments were deliberately short, about 15 questions; others included upwards of 150 questions.
4. They were quantifiable, comparing actual age with an earned age. The apparent assumption is that learning whether your days are running out faster or slower than expected is motivating to clients.
5. They used outdated or debatable scientific evidence. This is not surprising, because research results are changing more rapidly than patented HRA instruments.
6. They had a health education component to motivate individuals to change undesirable health behaviors in order to reduce specific risk factors. In most instances, this health education component relied on tailored written resource materials, although some provided follow-up by a health educator. In some cases the specific risk factors identified by the HRA were linked to appropriate health programs in the work or community setting.

RAND research institute reviewed 267 studies of HRAs, eventually paring them down to 27 controlled studies, 13 of which were randomized controlled trials. They concluded that about 44% of HRA interventions reported positive health outcomes. Among these studies, the more limited the feedback and support to participants, the more limited the beneficial results. Feedback and support ranged from general written materials to personalized written materials, to incentives, to counseling, and finally, to the opportunity to participate in a health program. Few interventions involved vulnerable or minority populations, and most HRA methodologies designed for older adults were not tested for effectiveness on that population (RAND, 2003).

A Reflective Health Assessment

In contrast to specific responses to a series of focused risk-reduction questions posed by HRAs, Dr. Andrew Weil at the University of Arizona's Integrative Medicine Clinic offers his patients a unique health assessment tool that encourages patient reflection and initiative ("Broadening Your View," 2000). Dr. Weil begins with the following questions: What does good health mean to *you*? How do *you* attain it? Additional questions include: Does your life have meaning to you? Are you happy?

Dr. Weil also asks clients unique questions about specific content areas: What is your relationship with food? What is your relationship with exercise? Do you have satisfying personal relationships? How do you deal with your stress?

When you complete these questions, it is time for you to reflect on your answers. You may never have examined your health in this way. You will explore your attitudes toward your health, identify your health goals, recognize the obstacles to achieving your goals, and discover the personal resources you can assemble to accomplish them.

Reflecting on your answers may give you a better understanding of what is contributing to your health problems. You may be more aware of what kind of support you would like from your family, friends, and health care providers. Also, defining terms for yourself, assessing your own priorities, and designing self-tailored strategies to achieve your health goals may help you feel more empowered.

Another type of *reflective health assessment* is delivered by *health coaches* in a business setting. Health coaches encourage employees to improve their health behaviors by helping them reflect on their risk factors and ways to change them. The goal of health coaching for the employer is to reduce absenteeism and medical care costs, and improve productivity (Dolan, 2007a). Some health coaching is offered at reduced rates in the employer setting, but rarely is it coordinated with the employee's primary care physician.

Huffman (2007) believes health coaching is based on three principles: (1) asking open-ended questions, (2) affirming the client's strengths and building his or her confidence, and (3) listening carefully and demonstrating you have listened. She also encourages health coaching to be used in the home health care setting with older clients.

Stages of Change

Another type of health assessment, one that is typically *not* comprehensive in scope, is the *"stages of change"* instrument, also referred to academically as the transtheoretical model. This popular assessment tool was developed by Prochaska and colleagues (2009) to help health professionals assess an individual's readiness to change a *specific* health habit. The specific stages of change are as follows:

1. Precontemplation—no intention to change behavior in the foreseeable future
2. Contemplation—awareness that a problem exists but no commitment to action
3. Preparation—intention to take action in the next month, typically accompanied by unsuccessful action taken in the past year
4. Action—modification of behavior, experiences, or environment for a time period ranging from 1 day to 6 months in order to overcome a problem
5. Maintenance—an indeterminate period, perhaps a lifetime, in which to actively prevent relapse

The authors report that relapsing and recycling through the stages of change is the rule rather than the exception, and this process could be viewed as a spiral rather than a linear model. If individuals become more aware of the relapsing phenomenon, they might feel less guilt, embarrassment, and discouragement after an unsuccessful attempt. If health professionals become more aware of the relapsing process, they might be more patient with their clients' attempts at change.

Persons who are in the precontemplation stage are, by definition, not ready for action-oriented programs. A study of 20,000 people found that only 20% of the population is ready to make a specific behavior change (Health Promotion Interchange, 1997). So what happens to those who are *not* ready? According to Prochaska, DiClemente, Velicer, and Rossi (1993), they can be helped through the stages by giving them stage-matched messages and support. Precontemplators, for instance, are denied immediate support (justified on the basis of limited personnel resources) and are offered literature in the hope that someday they may be more ready to make a behavior change. Contemplators, however, receive both information about the pros and cons involved with changing a behavior, and the support to increase confidence and to explore ways to overcome barriers.

Despite the enormous popularity of the stages-of-change framework in the psychology literature, not everyone is a true believer. One analyst reports that the vast majority of studies testing this model are cross-sectional rather than longitudinal. As a consequence there have been serious flaws in the assignment of an arbitrary time period to a particular stage, the overlap in the definition of the different stages, and the overpromotion of meager and inconsistent results (Sutton, 2001).

One behavioral scientist questioned the ethics of too quickly ignoring reputed precontemplators, or postponing interventions with them, when they constitute the section of the population with the greatest need. She suggested that this model may lead to discrimination against those who are poor, less educated, and frail (Whitehead, 1997).

An interesting variation on the stages-of-change framework is to focus on specific aspects of a particular behavior change. A team of researchers examined the topic of weight loss, and instead of asking people whether they were ready to make changes leading to weight loss, the researchers asked which changes they were most interested in making. Six aspects of weight loss were targeted: decreasing dietary fat, improving portion control, increasing vegetable intake, increasing fruit intake, increasing physical activity, and implementing an exercise regimen. The researchers found that respondents may have been precontemplators in some aspects of weight loss, but they were ready to make a change in at least one area (Logue, Sutton, Jarjoura, & Smucker, 2000).

A similar strategy with a much broader focus is to present older persons with different categories of potential behavior change goals to choose from. Presented with sufficiently diverse options, older adults may be more motivated to choose one behavior

---

| BOX 3.2 | Perhaps There Are No Precontemplators? |

My first reservation with the stages-of-change framework occurred when I was interviewing several older people in an African American church. They reported to me that they were not interested in exercise and also not interested in joining my soon-to-be-launched church-based exercise program (Looney & Haber, 2001). Had I allowed this initial report of disinterest to result in my labeling them "precontemplators," I would have offered them literature and moved on to seek other people who may have been ready to join my exercise program.

Instead, a few days later, along with several of my health science students, I gave a 20-minute demonstration of the exercise program to a group of older adults who met weekly at that same church. Accompanied by church music, easy banter, humor, and scripture that I read ("to take care of God's temple [the body]" and "above all else, guard your heart for it provides health to a man's whole body"), many people signed up for, and then successfully completed, the 10-week program—including the several alleged precontemplators!

change that is of high priority to them (Haber, 1996). Here is a partial list of diverse health promotion categories that I have presented to older adults, accompanied by a brief and individualized health assessment in each of the categories (Haber, 2001b):

1. Complete one of several (listed) medical screenings or immunizations.
2. Increase physical activity level; begin a brisk walking program; join an aerobics, yoga, or Tai Chi class; start a strength-building program; or begin a flexibility routine.
3. Decrease dietary fat, implement portion control, increase vegetable or fruit intake, or increase fluid consumption.
4. Initiate a stress management routine.
5. Establish a sleep hygiene routine.
6. Implement a fall prevention or home safety plan.
7. Join a smoking cessation program.
8. Enroll in a memory improvement course.
9. Join one of the peer support groups in the area.
10. Implement an alcohol-in-moderation plan.

Among 48 older adults who were presented an array of health promotion options, 44 were able to select a health goal. Using the technique of a health contract, 75% achieved substantial success with their goal (Haber & Looney, 2000).

Question: Are you willing to write a health contract for a 2-week period of time? What techniques are you going to employ to increase your likelihood of completing it successfully? At the end of the 2 weeks discuss your success, or lack thereof, with others.

An interesting new wrinkle on stages of change is to target individuals who have had a *recent and serious* medical diagnosis, such as heart disease or diabetes. When these individuals are contacted at this propitious time, they are more likely to quit smoking or, to a lesser extent, lose weight (Keenan, 2009). It may prove advantageous if businesses or health care systems could target, in a timely fashion, those individuals who may be particularly ready to make a health behavior change.

Health Contracts

A health assessment and intervention tool that I use with older adults is a health contract (Figure 3.1) and health calendar (Figure 3.2). It is based on a self-management application of *social cognitive theory* (Bandura, 1977), which will be examined in more detail shortly.

Self-management refers to clients who, with the help of a health educator, can choose an appropriate behavior-change goal and create and implement a plan to accomplish that goal. The statement of the goal and the plan of action can be written into a health contract format. A health contract is alleged to have several advantages over verbal communication alone, especially when the communication tends to be limited in direction (i.e., mostly from health professional to client). The alleged advantages of a health contract, which still need additional empirical testing, are that it:

1. is a formal commitment that enhances motivation,
2. clarifies goals and behaviors and makes them explicit,
3. requires the active participation of the client,
4. enhances the therapeutic relationship between provider and client,

5. provides a structured means for involving significant others (family, friends, etc.) in a supportive role,
6. provides a structured means of problem solving around barriers that previously interfered with the achievement of a goal, and
7. provides incentives to reinforce behaviors.

The health contract includes a set of instructions that help older adults state a health goal (see Table 3.1), identify benefits that provide motivation, establish a plan of action that helps the older adult remember to perform new behaviors and to elicit social support for them, and identify potential problems to achieving the health goal and encourage solutions to overcome these barriers. The contract is signed by the older adult and a support person. Progress is typically assessed after 1 week, and the success of the contract is reviewed at the end of a month (Haber, 2007; Haber & Looney, 2000; Haber & Rhodes, 2004). Health contracts have been applied with varying degrees of success to a wide variety of behaviors, such as drug use, smoking, alcohol abuse, nutrition, and exercise.

Health contracts can be uniquely designed. A weight loss contract developed by Joseph Chemplavil, a cardiac endocrinologist in Hampton, Virginia, consists of the following: "I, (patient's name), hereby promise to myself and to Dr. Chemplavil, that I will make every effort to lose my (agreed-upon) weight, and I will pay $1 to Dr. Chemplavil's Dollar for Pound Fund, for every pound of weight that I gain, on each visit to the office, by cash. I also understand that I will receive $1 from the same fund for each pound of weight that I lose." Dr. Chemplavil paid out $1,044 to 118 patients and received $166 from 30 patients, with two patients breaking even (Kazel, 2004).

FIGURE 3.1   **Health contract.**

Health contract.

My **health goal** is: _____

My **motivations** for my health goal are:

1._____

2._____

3._____

My Plan of Action

For social or emotional **support** I will...

To **remind** me of new behaviors I will...

Problems that may interfere with reaching my health goal and solutions:

My **signature** / date   Support person's **signature** / date

FIGURE 3.2   **Health calendar.**

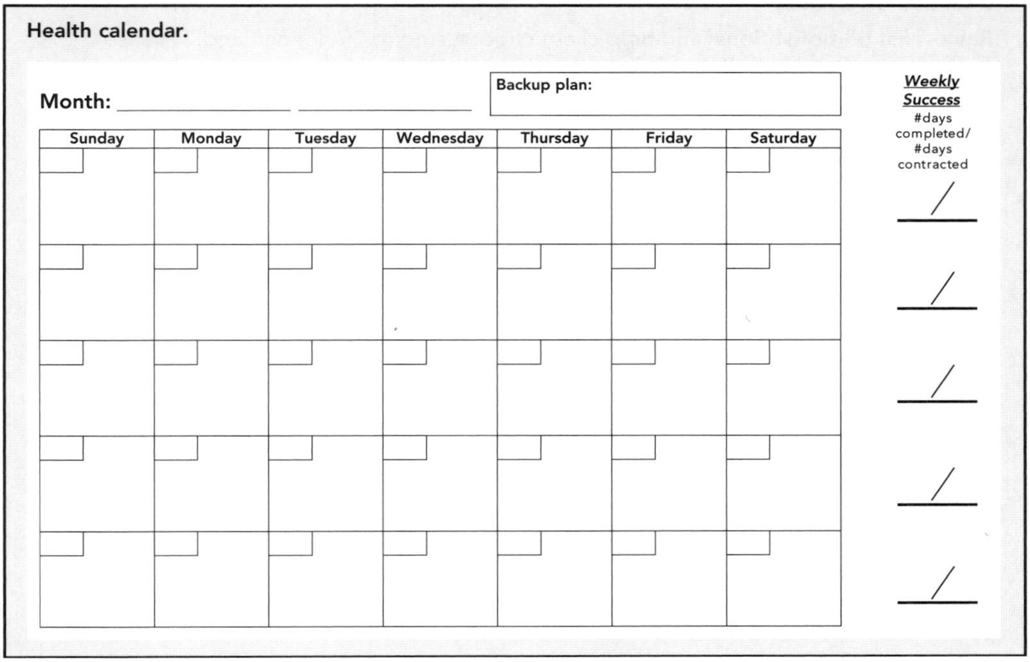

Health calendar.

Month: _____ _____				Backup plan:			Weekly Success

Sunday	Monday	Tuesday	Wednesday	Thursday	Friday	Saturday	#days completed/ #days contracted
							/
							/
							/
							/
							/

Research on health contracts has been limited (and often marred) by small sample sizes, lack of random assignment to treatment and control groups, and lack of replication. In addition, there are several uncertainties about the effectiveness of health contracts in terms of ability to identify which components work best (e.g., health education, social support, the professional–client relationship, memory enhancement, motivation building, contingency rewards, etc.), whether contracts work better with one type of client than another, and determining the content and amount of training that is required for health educators or clinicians to administer health contracts effectively.

Even without a definitive body of research, health contracts are widely used. They are simple to administer, time efficient, and cost-effective, particularly when high-priced medical personnel are not involved. The health contract can also be effectively taught to students in the classroom and applied in the community (Haber, 2007).

PRECEDE

The *PRECEDE* framework (Green & Kreuter, 1999) offers a conceptual guideline that can also be used for assessing the readiness of adults to change or maintain a health behavior. PRECEDE is an (awkward) acronym for *p*redisposing, *r*einforcing, and *e*nabling *c*onstructs in *e*ducational/ecological *d*iagnosis and *e*valuation.

Predisposing factors are the knowledge, attitudes, and beliefs a person holds about a health behavior. For instance, if an older woman believes exercise will aggravate her arthritis or cause her unnecessary fatigue, exhortation to exercise will be ineffective. Because older adults, especially minority older adults or those over age 80, frequently have lower formal educational levels than adults in general and may be prone to act on less information or on misinformation, it is necessary that health professionals ascertain the barriers to changing health behaviors.

TABLE 3.1 Health Contract Directions for Exercise

Exercise motivation

Review list of motivations, and help client choose among "function" and "disease prevention" motives. Record up to three on the health contract.

Encourage the client to write down one motivation and keep it in his or her wallet or pocketbook, or post it in a conspicuous place. The client may want to state the motivation out loud on a daily basis.

Exercise modality

Review list of exercise modalities, help client choose one before working on a health goal (e.g., community exercise program, aerobic options in the home, walking alternatives, increasing physical activity, strength-building, flexibility/balance, etc.).

Exercise baseline

If the client is sedentary, set a minimum goal; if the client is not sedentary, assess the client's baseline. Review the last week for exercise/physical activity frequency, duration, and intensity. If last week was not typical, substitute a typical week.

Frequency and duration should be assessed by number of days per week and total minutes each day. Moderate intensity level should be assessed by asking the client to be aware of increases in body warmth and breathing rate during exercise and physical activity. Establish a goal of slightly above baseline for the first week, gradually increase it over the remaining weeks, and set a modest goal for the last week of the month.

Health goal

Write a specific statement about what the client will do by the end of the first month, and include the following information: how often (days/ week), how much (duration/ day), and how intense (light/medium).

The goal should be modest and measurable—no more than 5 days a week, a half-hour a day, one unit over baseline for the first week, with week-by-week gradations until the health goal is reached during the last week of the first month. A client may choose to exceed these parameters, but not as part of the stated health goal.

Reassess the health goal at the end of the first week. Determine then whether the health educator will contact the client during the remaining part of the first month. Set a day and time to meet at the end of the first month to assess progress and possible change for the next month; record the meeting on the health calendar.

Plan of action

Social support. Review list of social support possibilities. The client should select socially supportive people, the ways support is to be given, and the frequency of support desired.

Reminders. Attach health contract to the refrigerator. Have friend or family member call to remind. Associate new behaviors with an established habit, such as engaging in brisk walking just before dinner. Keep exercise-related reading materials visible around the house. Keep work-out shoes by the door. Exercise at the same time each day. Hang a picture on the wall that shows the client or others exercising.

Problems/solutions

Consider problems that arose when similar goals were set in the past, or anticipate new problems that might arise in the coming month.

(continued)

TABLE 3.1 Health Contract Directions for Exercise (*continued*)

> *Positive thoughts.* A solution for the negative thinker is to deliberately verbalize positive thoughts about achieving the health goal on a daily basis. The positive thought can also be written on paper and read—something like "I am confident of success, though not perfection."
>
> *Reinforcement.* Seek praise. Swallow modesty; tell people about successes and solicit additional praise from them. Seek internal motivation: Pay attention to the signs of feeling better. Seek external motivation: Buy theater tickets or enjoy another (non-edible) treat if success is achieved at the end of a week or month.
>
> *Environmental support.* Alter immediate surroundings. Place walking sneakers by the front door, distribute exercise-related literature around the house, place exercise band on the coffee table, keep pictures on the wall of healthy people exercising.
>
> *Stress management.* Stress can sidetrack a person from the goal. To manage stress, consider: deep breathing, muscle relaxation, meditation, prayer, listening to music, playing with a pet, taking a walk. Schedule these things on a regular basis.
>
> *Problem solve.* Brainstorm about problems that arose from past attempts at behavior change. Brainstorm about problems that might arise in the future. Find solutions. Be especially attentive to issues of pain and fatigue. Record under Problems/solutions.
>
> **Signatures**
>
> The client signs the contract, along with someone who will be offering support and willing to sign contract. If no one comes to mind, the health educator can sign it.
>
> **Health calendar**
>
> Follow directions for recording activities on the health calendar.

Often it is better not to change a belief, but to add a new one. If older persons believe, for example, that God will take care of their health, the health professional can agree with this assertion and then simply add Sophocles's declaration, "Heaven never helps the man who will not act" (Lorig, 1992).

Predisposing factors can be determined by finding out what clients know about the health area of concern, whether they believe they have a problem, whether they have cultural habits that need to be taken into consideration, and whether they believe behavior changes will help. Older adults, for instance, may believe (or claim) that because of their age it is too late to change or to do themselves any good. It may be helpful to respond with specific data on how rapidly health improvements can take place after the age of 65. A significant number of older adults may believe they get all the exercise they need when in fact, according to indicators of exercise frequency, intensity, and duration, they do not.

Enabling factors are those resources necessary for engaging in health-related activities—specifically, access and skill level. Before making recommendations to clients, health professionals need to determine whether there are appropriate programs with experienced leaders who are trained to work with older adults, whether these programs are accessible to those with limited transportation and financial means, whether clients have the necessary skills for modifying their behavior, whether recommended materials needed by older adults are affordable and available, and whether older adults perceive their environment to be safe enough to implement a program.

Practitioners need to be resourceful; it may be necessary to help older adults find accessible programs or gain necessary skills. It is also important that health professionals facilitate ways in which older persons can help themselves, rather than solve problems for clients and thereby foster dependency.

Reinforcing factors refer to the peers, significant others, and health professionals who can support the continuation of new health behaviors. Older adults may be widowed, uninvolved in former occupational groups, and relatively isolated from other persons who are interested in maintaining health. Practitioners ought to consider whether their clients have sufficient family, peer, or professional support to reinforce health behavior changes.

TEN TIPS FOR CHANGING HEALTH BEHAVIORS

After years of working with health science students to help older adults change health behaviors, it would be wonderful if I could offer the reader a simple formula for increasing the probability of success. Unfortunately, I fall victim to the "kitchen sink" syndrome that I think also afflicts the PRECEDE model just described. There are many factors that can influence the success or failure of an individual's attempt to change a health behavior, and research has not helped us much in understanding which factors are more important for which types of people.

Over the years, therefore, I developed my own framework for helping older adults make a desired health behavior change. "Model" is too sophisticated a word to describe this framework, so I refer to it as the 10 tips. With each older client willing to attempt a behavior change, a review of the 10 tips is likely to produce strategies that will help the person succeed. From personal experience and pilot research projects, I believe this approach will be helpful. If you examine the health contract/calendar technique previously summarized, along with the directions for completing it, you will notice that the 10 tips are incorporated into this technique.

In order to make these ideas more practical, I will focus on the specific goal of increasing exercise or physical activity. This also happens to be the health goal most likely to be chosen by older adults when given a choice among many options (Elder, Williams, Drew, Wright, & Boulan, 1995; Haber & Looney, 2000).

If you work with older adults to change a health behavior and want to commit these 10 tips to memory, it may be helpful to note that the first four start with the letter *M*, the next five form the acronym PRESS, and the 10th one can be abbreviated as P.S., as for a postscript in a letter you are writing.

1. Motivation
2. Modest
3. Measurable
4. Memory
5. Positive thoughts
6. Reinforcement
7. Environmental support
8. Stress management
9. Social support
10. Problem solve

Motivation

It is obvious that a person must be motivated to change a health behavior. I have found, however, that the first motivation identified by an older adult is not necessarily the one that lights up his or her eyes with authenticity. Those contemplating a reason for overcoming their sedentary ways may first come up with a politically correct motivation that elicits the approval of others, including the health educator they are working with, rather than one that is heartfelt.

For instance, avoiding heart disease may truly be the most motivating reason for someone to take on the challenge of a new exercise routine. Or it may not be. With a little probing on the part of the health educator, it may come to light that the person is more passionate about achieving better sleeping habits, or regularity in bowel habits, or additional energy in order to play longer with the grandchildren. It is best to spend a sufficient amount of time discussing what motivates the client and to examine the client's facial expressions for clues to what is of importance.

To help in this regard, I present the client with a list of possible motivations to choose from. This list includes disease categories that the client may want to avoid or alleviate, such as arthritis, stroke, obesity, hypertension, heart disease, peripheral vascular disease, diabetes, osteoporosis, colon cancer, and depression; and areas of potential functional improvement, such as constipation, forgetfulness, low energy, sleeplessness, stress management, imbalance, muscle weakness, stiffness, and fall prevention. Once you feel confident that the primary motivation has been identified, write it down (on the health contract if that is the technique of choice), and encourage clients to remind themselves about their motivation on a regular basis.

Also, if the goal is exercise, which type: brisk walking, joining an aerobics class, increasing physical activity over the course of the day, or something else the client is likely to stick with? Motivation is enhanced by choosing an intervention a person enjoys, or at least by avoiding the more burdensome options.

Modest

No one is ever disappointed if he or she meets or exceeds the goal he or she has established. Yet, it is an uncommon event when an older adult initially declares a goal that is modest enough to elicit the health educator's confidence that it can be achieved or exceeded. It is more common for someone to state an overly ambitious goal, like exercising *every* day. It is important to make one's goal modest. If a client sets a goal to exercise four times a week and meets or exceeds that goal, motivation will be sustained. But if the goal is to exercise every day, 4 days is a failure, and motivation may be compromised.

If the person establishes 60 minutes of daily walking as the goal, reduce it by half and give "extra credit" (perhaps in the form of more praise) for exceeding that goal. Encourage the sedentary client to build up to the 30-minute goal by establishing a target of 10 minutes of walking for the first week, 20 minutes for the second week, and 30 minutes for the third and fourth weeks. Allow clients to walk a *cumulative* 30 minutes a day if they choose, rather than limit them to 30 consecutive minutes.

The opposite problem can also reduce motivation: the client's setting a goal that is too easy and then losing interest in it. This is an unusual occurrence in my experience, especially if the person has identified the appropriate motivation. Once you understand what motivates a client, help that person modify his or her goal during the first month so that it is neither grandiose nor undemanding.

Finally, a modest goal is short term. I have had success with the 1-month time period—hence the monthly contract/calendar. One month does not extend too far into the future, and with the use of the 1-month calendar, the end is in sight. It is also a long enough period of time to allow for adjustment of the goal, or the behaviors to achieve the goal, in the first week in order to increase the likelihood of success. Even if the goal turns out to be less motivating than was initially thought, the client may still have a good chance of successfully completing it in 1 month and carrying over that confidence to another, more motivating health goal the following month.

Measurable

Measurability has several components. With exercise, how much will the older adult be doing—how many minutes of exercise and on how many days of the week? How intensely will the person be doing it—will he or she establish a brisk walking pace that is twice the pace of normal walking? Will he or she monitor his or her breathing, making sure that he or she achieves sufficient intensity to produce deep breathing, but not so much intensity that talking while walking becomes difficult? Will he or she monitor intensity level, building up in the beginning and slowing down near the end?

Measurability also implies recordkeeping, which is another reason the contract/calendar technique is appealing. People are used to recording on their calendars the activities that they need to be reminded of. I encourage clients to measure and compare the number of days they actually complete the contracted behavior each week with the number of days they had contracted for. Monitoring weekly success can lead to greater confidence, or to the periodic need to revise the health goal.

Memory

Habits take up a large part of the day. We give little thought to many of the activities that constitute our daily routines, and at the same time we rarely forget them. How do we switch to a new behavior, one that is a bit challenging to adopt, and make it a new habit? The answer is by enhancing our memory in as many ways as possible.

What cues can be established to help remind us? For example, we can place our walking shoes by the front door; place the health contract on the refrigerator door; ask a family member or a friend to remind us or check on us; associate the new behavior with an established one, like walking before dinner every night (perhaps adding a well-placed cue—a note near the dinner table that reads, "Did you walk yet?").

Positive Thoughts

Substitute positive and hopeful thoughts for negative, self-defeating ones. For each negative thought like "I've never been able to maintain exercise routines before," substitute a positive argument like "It may be difficult, but this time I will persist and accomplish my goal." It may be helpful to record affirmations and place them in conspicuous locations. Other avenues of positive support are to find books or magazines that inspire clients, encourage them to associate with persons who model what they are attempting to accomplish, and have them seek friends or acquaintances who are willing to be supportive of their goal.

For those who like irony and want to use negative reinforcement to promote positive thinking, keep a rubber band unobtrusively around your wrist, and when a negative thought about the health goal occurs, snap the band and replace the negative thought with a positive one.

Reinforcement

Most psychologists rely on positive rather than negative reinforcement. If success is achieved at the end of the first week, for instance, encourage clients to treat themselves to a movie or purchase a book. If success is observed at the end of the month, perhaps the spouse will take over one of your errands. Reinforcements tend to be more effective when they fall in close proximity to achievement.

External reinforcement does not necessarily involve spending money. Praise can be an important reinforcement. Encourage clients to speak highly of themselves when they are doing well with their goal, and ask them to be a bit immodest in their solicitation of praise from others. External incentives are helpful to some people but not to others.

If the motivation to achieve a goal is strong, the successful efforts themselves may be sufficiently rewarding. External incentives may, in fact, distract from internal rewards.

Though most psychologists prefer positive reinforcement to negative reinforcement, I heard of a diabolically clever form of punishment that I will pass along. Identify an issue about which a person feels strongly (e.g., euthanasia) and then have the client make out several small checks to an organization that promotes a belief *contrary* to his or her own. When punishments are to be administered, the checks are mailed to the offending organization by someone other than the client.

Environmental Support

Another term for environmental support is *stimulus control*. The best example of this applies to weight management. If you want to contribute to weight maintenance or loss, make sure that the client does not keep junk food in the house.

Exercisers also have options in this regard. Placing sneakers by the front door is an example of environmental support. Locate the stair-stepper in front of the television set. Keep the elastic exercise band on the coffee table as a visible reminder.

Stress Management

It is the rare person who does not feel stress these days. Not only do we live in a fast-paced society, but we are also likely to contend with the automobile driver who is releasing road rage, cope with a frustrating physical disability, struggle with a personal loss, or encounter countless other hassles and annoyances. Stress is a common barrier to achieving a health goal. If possible, build into the plan of action a few stress management techniques that can be practiced on a regular basis, preferably daily.

My favorite stress management technique is deep breathing. I combine that with an everyday activity (and stressor for me), driving—which is typically done too fast and too aggressively. (It's hereditary, as I was born into a family of fast-driving New Yorkers.) Most times when I am driving a car, therefore, I prompt myself to take periodic deep breaths. This not only helps control my stress, but it also has a wonderful side effect—I am much more likely to drive sanely.

Social Support

I suggest that some thought be given to social support for every client. For many, but not all, older adults, social support is desirable, perhaps essential. It may be a good idea to build social support into the statement of the health goal itself.

Ideally, a person has multiple sources of social support. Perhaps a health educator, a spouse, a friend, a physician or nurse, a pastor, or a neighbor. Suggest to your client that he or she announce the health goal to others in general, even acquaintances, to increase the chances that additional people will offer support and approval.

Clients who unexpectedly find the social support of a spouse or friend inconvenient (they do not always want to walk when I want to walk), unreliable (they do not always show up), or overly critical will need to seek other sources of social support. Clients who have a physician who does not muster enthusiasm for their health goal may at least consider the prospect of finding another, more health-oriented health care professional. Clients needing more social support than is currently available to them may need to explore the option of joining a class in the community.

A community class that has a leader of the same age and gender as the client may provide a better role model. Fellow classmates who are also peers in age, gender, disability, or other relevant variables may provide extra social and emotional support for behavior change and maintenance.

Problem Solve

Finally, chances are good that the client has tried to achieve this exercise goal or a similar one before. It typically takes multiple efforts to achieve a goal. Explore what might have gone wrong in the past, or what might go wrong in the immediate future. Spend a little time identifying likely barriers and ways to overcome them.

An example of a problem to be solved is an older adult who lives in Oregon (me, for example) who likes to walk briskly outside. Either learn to love the rain or find a backup plan, like walking in a shopping mall; turning on music and substituting dancing alone in one's living room; or dragging out the vacuum cleaner to do some energetic sweeping.

Another problem—quite common among older adults attempting to increase their exercise level—involves working around aches, pains, and fatigue. The solution may be to modify an exercise, change the exercise modality, or alter the time that the exercise is to be performed. The challenge is to identify problems from the past, imagine possible problems in the future, brainstorm solutions, and increase the chance of success.

HEALTH BEHAVIOR THEORIES

Theories can help us understand what influences health behaviors, and thus help us plan effective interventions. Theories may focus on different levels (e.g., psychological, social, institutional, or community) and are subject to change based on new evidence. They may also be applied singly or in combination in order to address behavior-change challenges.

A few well-known behavior-change theories, along with models and concepts, will be presented after three brief definitions. A *theory* of behavior change attempts to explain the processes underlying learning. A *model* draws on a number of theories to help people understand a problem. A *concept* is the primary element of a theory or model.

Behavioral and Cognitive Management

Operant conditioning, B. F. Skinner's (1953) model of behavior control, is based on the premise that behavior is determined by its consequences, that is, the kinds of rewards and punishments that follow behavior. Behaviors followed by rewards will increase in frequency, whereas behaviors followed by punishments will decline.

Operant conditioning has spawned a number of principles. Immediate rewards and punishments are more effective than delayed ones. Intermittent reinforcement is more resistant to extinction than constant reinforcement. Careful observation of conditions that promote or discourage behavior can help shape future success.

Cognitive conditioning—unlike operant conditioning, which focuses on external behaviors—deals with internal changes in thoughts and feelings. Cognitive-conditioning advocates assert that behavior and feelings are influenced not by their consequences, but by antecedent thoughts.

The first step toward cognitive restructuring, therefore, is the identification of undesirable and unrealistic thoughts. The next step is the substitution and regular repetition of positive thoughts in order to shape future behavior. Once we have positively restructured our thoughts, we engage in fewer cognitive distortions, experience less emotional distress, and perform fewer maladaptive behaviors (Burns, 1980).

Because operant and cognitive conditioning are practiced universally, they do not appear to constitute a formal learning model. All of us use praise and punishment to influence the behavior of others as well as ourselves, and we often substitute positive thoughts for negative ones. Unlike informal methods for influencing others or ourselves, however, formal *behavioral and cognitive management* techniques are applied systematically and typically include these three steps:

1. *Clear definition of the problem.* A need to exercise is vague. The ability to climb the steps in one's home without having to stop to rest is clear.
2. *Implement a systematic and measurable response to the problem.* To exercise as often as possible is vague. To exercise three times a week, 30 minutes at a time, and periodically assess one's perceived exertion level at moderate intensity is both systematic and measurable.
3. *Implement scheduled evaluations.* To feel one is making progress is vague. To assess the effectiveness of a health plan on a monthly basis and alter the plan of action or the health goal as necessary is explicit.

Healthy Pleasures

In contrast to the behavioral and cognitive management theories, which are based on structure and self-discipline, is the theory of *healthy pleasures.* Advocates of this theory propose that healthy behaviors will be sustained when these behaviors are based on joy, intuition, and self-trust. Advocates suggest that a growing reliance on one's ability to listen to the body's internal cues for feeling good can replace behavior-change decisions based on scientific guidelines. For additional ideas on this topic, read *Healthy Pleasures* (Ornstein & Sobel, 1989).

My own bias is that healthy pleasures and management techniques are not an "either/or" proposition. Joyful and intuitive activities may be consistently practiced, even if not always in their spontaneous form, and a disciplined routine may be temporarily relieved by spontaneous and joyful forms of exercise. Whatever sustains motivation for a healthy lifestyle is the way to go.

Self-monitoring can be viewed as a strategy that borrows from both the healthy pleasures and management strategies. It consists of systematically recording one's own pattern of behavior for a specific period of time (management technique), but only for the purpose of awareness and without an effort to conform to a pattern of behavior (healthy-pleasures technique).

One example of self-monitoring is to keep a written record, or food diary, of everything you eat and drink (see Table 3.2). During a 3-day period (including a weekend day if your weekend eating pattern differs from that of weekdays), record what you eat, how much you eat, the quality of what you eat (which corresponds to the rings of the nutrition bull's eye to be described in Chapter 5, "Nutrition and Weight Management"), where you eat, with whom you eat, what you are doing while you eat, and how you feel when you are eating. Make no effort to control this pattern of behavior, and make no effort to not control it. Just be aware of what you are doing and how you are feeling, and record it.

> **Question:** Complete a food-behavior diary for 3 days. What did you learn about your eating and drinking habits? Did the monitoring process lead to changes in your eating pattern? If so, did these changes occur easily and naturally, or through discipline?

When you carefully monitor your eating behaviors, you not only increase your awareness of what triggers unhealthy eating patterns, but you also often begin to modify them as part of the self-awareness process. One study reported that people who kept daily food diaries lost twice as much weight as those who kept no records (Hollis et al., 2008).

TABLE 3.2 Food Behavior Diary

What is a food behavior diary?

The diary is for recording and monitoring the foods and drinks that you consume each day, so that you can understand what, how, and why you consume what you do.

What information do I put in my food behavior diary?

✓ **What** foods or drinks did you consume?

✓ **How much** did you eat? (not enough, ok amount, too much)

✓ **Quality** of food you ate? (refers to the three rings of the Nutrition Bull's-Eye in Chapter 5: 1—foods in bull's-eye; 2—in middle ring; 3—in outer ring)

✓ **Where** did you eat? (home, office, restaurant, school, car, etc.)

✓ **Who with?** (family member, friend, business colleague, alone, etc.)

✓ What were you **doing?** (activity)

✓ What was your **emotional state?** (happy, sad, anxious, angry, etc.)

FOOD/DRINK	AMOUNT	QUALITY	WHERE	WHO	ACTIVITY	MOOD
Oatmeal	Ok	1	Living room	Son	Watching TV	Energetic
Skim milk	Ok	1				
Grilled cheese	Too much	3	Kitchen table	Son	Reading newspaper	Anxious
Water	Not enough	1				
Chips	Too much	3	Living room	Alone	On the phone	Tired
Pepper steak	Too much	2	Restaurant	Family	Dinnertime/ Talk	Excited, happy
Brown rice	Ok	1				
Skim milk	Not enough	1				

By monitoring food intake you might realize, for instance, that you eat automatically, and in greater quantity, in front of the television set and when you socialize in certain settings, even when you are not hungry. You may choose to eliminate the former because it provides no extra pleasure, but maintain the latter—allowing yourself to indulge at parties that serve food because they happen infrequently and are more enjoyable.

Social Cognitive Theory

One broad learning perspective, referred to as social cognitive theory, has a lengthy history (Bandura, 1977, 1997; Rodin, 1986; Rotter, 1954). It addresses both the psychosocial dynamics underlying health behavior and the methods of promoting behavior change. This perspective actually encompasses a wide range of learning concepts that include role-modeling, guided mastery of tasks, verbal persuasion, physiological state, and *self-efficacy*. The last one is the most applied component, perhaps a theory unto itself.

Role-modeling is an important component of social cognitive theory. It is most effective when the role model shares many characteristics with the participant, such as age, race, physical impairment, gender, and socioeconomic status. Professional leaders of health education classes who are not role models in this sense should consider sharing teaching responsibilities and problem-solving strategies with class members who are. McAuley and Courneya (1993) suggest that role modeling with older program participants "may be particularly salient. In such cases it is common to look to other people, especially those that bear similar physical characteristics to ourselves, for motivation and information regarding our own prospects of success" (p. 73).

Guided mastery involves learning and practicing appropriate behaviors through the assignment of small, graded (i.e., increasingly challenging) tasks that are to be accomplished in a specific period of time. Achieving mastery over a difficult or previously feared task through guided personal experience may be the most potent source of self-efficacy (this will be discussed in more detail in the next section).

Persuasion is another social cognitive strategy, one that is probably more popular than effective. Persuasion is most effective when health providers and educators ensure that it is accompanied by realistic goals and includes supervision of tasks on a step-by-step basis. It is also important that messages be positive and direct ("you can do it," not "try and do it") and delivered by a respected source. Persuasion focuses on identifying the risk along with the intervention that can reduce the risk, and convincing clients that they can successfully engage in the intervention and have a positive outcome.

Physiological state can provide information that affects performance. High physiological arousal, for instance, can impair performance. People are more likely to expect failure when they are tense or agitated prior to starting something new. Someone experiencing fatigue, aches, or pains just before starting an exercise session is likely to question the effort needed to perform. Easing of physiological arousal may enhance the ability to perform.

Self-Efficacy

Self-efficacy may be the most widely utilized and tested concept in social cognitive theory. It is a belief in one's capabilities to implement a course of action. Self-efficacy is synonymous with having *confidence* about behavior change or maintenance within a specific behavioral domain (Bandura, 1997).

Self-efficacy can be manipulated experimentally with success. In one classic study, psychological tests were administered to a group of volunteers in a smoking cessation program. Half the subjects were then randomly assigned to a treatment group and told that in their tests they had demonstrated great potential to quit smoking. The other half were told the truth, which was that they had been *randomly* assigned to a control group. Fourteen months after treatment, smoking frequency had been reduced by 67% within the efficacy-enhanced group and by 35% within the control group (Blittner, Goldberg & Merbaum, 1978).

After reviewing the literature, McAuley and Courneya (1993) concluded, "If practitioners and clinicians fail to organize, present, and develop their programs in such a way as to cultivate efficacy beliefs, participants are likely to perceive the activity negatively, become disenchanted, discouraged, and discontinue. On the other hand, adequately organizing [programs] in a manner such that a strong sense of personal efficacy is promoted will result in the individual displaying more positive affect, evaluating their self-worth more positively, embracing more challenging activities, putting forth more effort, and persisting longer. In short, they will be in a position to successfully self-regulate their behavior" (p. 72).

The relationship between self-efficacy and behaviors is interactive, not unidirectional. Just as enhancing self-efficacy beliefs may increase the likelihood of sustaining a new health behavior, ongoing adherence to a new health behavior may continue to increase self-efficacy. Extreme optimism regarding one's self-efficacy, however, may relate *inversely* to successful performance (Rakowski, Wells, Lasater, & Carleton, 1991).

Other cautions apply as well. Self-efficacy is limited to an individual's belief in a *specific*, not a general, ability. People may, for example, perceive themselves to possess the self-efficacy to implement a walking program but not to follow through on a diet. Self-efficacy in one area of behavior does not necessarily carry over to another. Also, the perceived ability to change a health habit or adopt a new health behavior does not guarantee that a person has the necessary skill level, role model, peer or professional support, or access that might be required. Self-efficacy may be a necessary, though not a sufficient, condition for clients attempting to improve a health behavior.

Self-efficacy was an important part of the Arthritis Self-Help (ASH) course (Lorig, Chastain, Ung, Shoor, & Holman, 1989) developed at Stanford University in 1978 by Kate Lorig, a nurse and health educator, and physicians Halsted Holman and James Fries. More than 100,000 persons with arthritis completed the ASH course, usually in groups of 15 individuals or less and typically led by trained nonprofessionals with arthritis. During the 12-hour program, students were taught about arthritis and how to (1) design an exercise program around their limitations, (2) manage pain through relaxation techniques, (3) improve nutrition, (4) fight depression and fatigue, and (5) communicate more effectively with physicians. Participants who completed the program reported a 15% to 20% reduction in pain, were more active, and visited a physician less frequently. Among those who were depressed when starting the program, fewer depressive symptoms were reported by the end of the program.

The researchers were surprised to find that although changes in behavior, such as exercise and stress management, occurred as a consequence of the program, the factor most closely linked to outcomes (improvements in pain control, depression management, and activity level) was an increase in self-efficacy. In one group of successful patients, self-efficacy was still 17% higher 4 years after they completed the course (Lorig et al., 1989).

The ASH program and the follow-up *Chronic Disease Self-Management Program* (see Chapter 9, "Community Health") were developed and evaluated by Kate Lorig and colleagues at the Stanford University Patient Education Research Center. These programs have demonstrated effective management of chronic disease through reductions in fatigue, emotional stress, and—most important to insurers—visits to physicians and emergency rooms (see http://www.ahrq.gov/research/elderdis.htm). Similar chronic disease management programs, however, have generated controversy.

Health Locus of Control

Health locus of control refers to the idea that health can be controlled through the individual's ability to control his or her own behavior (internal locus), or through powerful others or luck (external locus). One's health-locus-of-control orientation, similar to perceived self-efficacy, is of limited utility when individuals do not place much value on their health. Also, medical practices and outcomes, unlike health practices, may not be within one's sphere of influence. Therefore, it is important that health professionals who encourage their clients to take personal responsibility for their health practices discourage them from overestimating their personal control over medical events. It may be necessary to help clients differentiate between the realistic goals—increasing energy, reducing stress, enhancing feelings of well-being, and increasing knowledge and decision-making ability—and the less realistic goal of staving off a deteriorating medical condition.

BOX 3.3   Chronic Disease Self-Management Programs

In medicine, efficacy measures how well an intervention works in clinical trials or laboratory studies when researchers exert a considerable amount of control over the experiment. Effectiveness, however, relates to how well a treatment works in the real world on a large-scale basis.

Chronic disease management programs have raised questions about whether these types of programs are effective, or just efficacious when researchers utilize small samples and exert a good deal of control over the intervention (and, some argue, the evaluation). A number of researchers report, for instance, that the results of chronic disease management programs in general have been equivocal or negative (Buszewicz et al., 2006; Chodosh et al., 2005; Newbould, Taylor, & Bury, 2006).

For instance, Medicare funded a chronic disease management pilot program that had nurses periodically check on whether patients were taking their drugs and seeing the right doctors, as well as monitor their lab results (Abelson, 2008). Not only were there no savings to Medicare, but the program was hard pressed to even be budget-neutral. A meta-analysis reported that 13 of 15 Medicare demonstration programs designed to improve chronic care, communication, and patient adherence through nurse monitoring and patient education did not yield net Medicare savings (Peikes, Chen, Schore, & Brown, 2009).

Conversely, though, a nurse-led disease management program with early-stage heart failure patients cost about $2,200 per patient, but this was offset by savings of about $2,400 per patient in lower hospitalization (Hebert et al., 2008). A randomized controlled trial examining a chronic care model, called Guided Care, where nurses focus on the sickest and most complex older patients, cost health insurers 11% less than the control group (Leff et al., 2009). Guided Care patients had 24% fewer hospital days, 37% fewer skilled nursing facility days, 15% fewer emergency visits, and 29% fewer home health care episodes. The program realized annual net savings of $75,000 per nurse.

Some of these chronic disease management programs use clinicians, whereas others use lay persons; some take place over the telephone, others in medical settings or in community settings; some report low attrition rates and others high rates; some link the efforts of medical and community staff, whereas others do not; some focus on patients with complex diseases and comorbidity and others do not; and some use well-validated and reliable measurement tools and others do not.

An excellent program producing consistent benefits may be quite efficacious; but when taken out into the real world with a large and diverse patient and provider population, and different health goals or cost objectives are applied, it may not be effective. This type of research takes plenty of time and money before convincing results can be obtained. Do we have that type of commitment in the United States?

One's health locus of control may become more external with age (Lachman, 1986). Older patients are more likely than younger ones, for instance, to prefer that health professionals make health-related decisions for them (Woodward & Wallston, 1987). This increased externality among older adults, however, may be due to *cohort factors* such as (1) the cultural orientation of specific older cohorts who believe in an authoritarian health professional role, or (2) the lower education levels of the oldest cohorts, which lead to reluctance to engage with health professionals in a dialogue they might not understand.

Increasing externality with age, though, may also be due to maturational factors. For example, the increased physical vulnerability that occurs with age may, over time, diminish an individual's sense of personal control. Conversely, an external health locus of control may correlate with a positive attitude toward the future. A belief in powerful others, such as physicians, who can influence the course of an illness may lead older patients to become more hopeful about the future.

Information seeking does not necessarily lead to better adjustment. Information about an illness can both raise and lower anxiety. When combined with the adoption of a relaxation technique, however, information seeking may lead to a more desirable outcome.

One classic study matched subjects by their health-locus-of-control profiles. Internals in self-directed programs and externals in peer support groups were more satisfied and lost more weight than nonmatched subjects (Wallston, Wallston, Kaplan, & Maides, 1976). However, another possible (and perhaps more powerful) explanation was not examined—that combining both internal *and* external sources of support may lead to better perceptions and results. The success of AA, for example, may be attributable to its reliance on both internal and external sources of control. On the one hand, AA members must take responsibility for their problem; on the other hand, they are required to acknowledge their inability to control alcoholism without the help of a higher power and the other members of AA.

Related to the study of locus of control is the topic of personal control. Two landmark studies in personal control reveal that seemingly insignificant opportunities to control events can affect both physical and mental health. In one study, the residents of two floors of a nursing home were given responsibility for such activities as taking care of a plant, deciding on when to see a movie, and rearranging furniture. The residents of the other two floors were also beneficiaries of a plant, weekly movie, and furniture, but were given no control over these activities; the staff took care of the plants, decided when the movie would be shown, and rearranged the furniture.

Despite the fact that the residents were similar in physical health, mental health, and prior socioeconomic status, the residents with personal control were physically and mentally healthier, and 18 months later only 15% of those with enhanced control had died, versus 30% of those without (Langer & Rodin, 1976; Rodin & Langer, 1977).

Schulz's (1976) experiment with residents of a retirement home revealed that student visits to residents led to more active, happier lives among the residents. However, unlike the nursing home experiments in which personal control opportunities for residents were on a continuing basis, the removal of the students from the retirement home precipitated a significant decline in health.

The rationale underlying the desirability of internal health locus of control is that decisions and actions will more likely produce advantageous outcomes. Studies show that perceived internal control is associated with reduced stress, increased motivation, improved health, and enhanced performance. Perceived internal control, however, can have negative effects under certain conditions—for example, when perceived internal control or confidence exists without sufficient information or skill to support a positive outcome; when excessive demands are made on a person's time, effort, and resources; and when individuals accept responsibility for complex medical problems or blame for medical outcomes outside of their control.

Health Belief Model

One model of health behavior change focuses on perceived threats, benefits, and barriers. The *health belief model* was developed during the early 1950s by a group of social psychologists at the U.S. Public Health Service to explain why people did not participate in screening tests for the early detection of asymptomatic disease (Rosenstock, 1990).

The researcher reported that individuals chose to take or not take preventive action depending upon their perception of threats, benefits, and barriers.

Perceived threats refer to the individual's perception of his or her *susceptibility* to a particular condition and the degree of *severity* of the condition that the individual fears. Persons who perceive no threat lack a reason to act. Perceived susceptibility to, and severity of, a condition together produce fear. For instance, when heart patients see a scan showing plaque accumulation in their own arteries, their adherence to a lipid-lowering drug regimen increases significantly. Moreover, the more severe the plaque accumulation, the more likely the patient is to stay on the medicine (Kalia et al., 2006).

Fear is an effective motivator, yet the optimal level of fear for motivating client behavior is unknown. Too little fear may not motivate, but too much can lead to denial and inaction. An important consideration in fear-inducing interventions is that fearful individuals, regardless of their motivation, may lack the necessary skills or confidence to change their health behaviors.

Perceived benefits refers to the belief that specific actions on the part of an individual will reduce the threat of negative outcomes or increase the chance of positive outcomes. Perceived benefits must outweigh perceived barriers before a person will initiate an action. *Perceived barriers* may include financial considerations, inconvenience, lack of transportation, lack of knowledge, or potential pain or discomfort.

Evaluations of the health belief model conducted exclusively with older persons have been limited. One such study, though, assessed health beliefs related to osteoporosis—specifically, the likelihood that the older adults in the study would adopt exercise behaviors and increase their calcium intake (Kim, Horan, Gendler, & Patel, 1991). The authors concluded that it is important to focus on overcoming the perceived barriers of older adults, such as their difficulty with changing old habits and the difficulty of incorporating new habits into a daily routine.

Each of these belief measures—susceptibility, severity, benefits, and barriers—has a significant but limited relationship to subsequent preventive behaviors, such as participation in flu vaccination, breast self-examination, tuberculosis skin tests, and smoking cessation activities. The predictability of the model is limited because of the uncertainty surrounding how *rationally* a person will act in a given circumstance. In addition, beliefs in and of themselves are not sufficient conditions for action. Additional factors that may need to be considered are physiological dependency, economic limitations, environmental influences, skill development, and self-efficacy.

Other Theories

The *theory of reasoned action* focuses on attitudes that precede potential behaviors (Fishbein & Ajzen, 1975). One aspect of this theory is its focus on taking into account what a person's relevant others think that person should do. An older person may finally relent and join a smoking cessation program based on the perception of his or her physician's or spouse's wishes. The *theory of planned behaviors*, an extension of the theory of reasoned action, has an additional focus on the perceived ease or difficulty of performing a behavior (Ajzen, 1988). The older smoker may intend to quit but does not believe there is access to a program that will provide the skills to quit.

There are theories that focus on *individual empowerment*, which most practitioners endorse, but the outcomes of individual-empowerment theories may not conform to practitioner values. Theresa Harvath (2008) recounts her nursing experiences and reports that empowered older adults may choose to remain in their homes, despite repeated falls and injuries, rather than transfer to a safer nursing home environment.

Also, empowered older adults with dysphagia may choose textured foods, despite the risk of aspiration, because these foods play such an important role in their lives.

There are also *community empowerment* theories that emphasize collective education and social action to promote the participation of people, organizations, and communities in gaining control over their lives (Wallerstein & Bernstein, 1988). Community empowerment initiatives to address health problems usually must surmount challenging cultural, social, and historical barriers.

Community-oriented primary care (COPC) is another community-level theory that encourages clinicians to view their patient populations, not just individual patients, and to involve other community organizations and community leaders to help with population-based behavior change (Nutting, 1987). Examples of applying COPC in the community are provided in Chapter 9, "Community Health."

A surprising article, at least to sociologists like myself, reports that, in general, well-funded large-scale programs designed to change the larger community in which people live—in order to get individuals to improve their health behaviors—have not turned out to be successful (Syme, 2003).

THEORIES VERSUS CONCEPTS

You may be asking at this point (granted, the likelihood is quite small): Why are health behavior theories placed near the end of this chapter? Should you not start with them, as they help shape the health assessments and interventions to follow? I can only answer this by offering a personal, and perhaps politically incorrect, view. I do not think that the behavior-change theories are sufficiently powerful to stimulate the shaping of a health intervention. Instead, I believe that several concepts embedded in different theories may be useful once a health intervention has entered the development phase.

> **Question:** If you were writing a grant proposal to help older adults exercise more in the community, which two health behavior concepts described in this chapter would you find most helpful for guiding your intervention? Explain your answer.

Theories, moreover, are too rich for my research blood. A theory attempts to relate a set of concepts systematically to explain and predict events and activities. Concepts, however, are the primary elements of theory; and each theory has a concept or two that is particularly well developed and helpful to me in guiding a community intervention and evaluation.

Therefore, I began my community health education projects based on the following questions, raised from my community experience rather than theory. How was a health promotion directory being utilized by older adults (Haber & Looney, 2003)? How effective was a health contract/calendar for behavior change (Haber, 2007; Haber & Looney, 2000; Haber & Rhodes, 2004)? Were African American churches good sites for exercise programs (Looney & Haber, 2001)? How effective were health science students as exercise leaders (Haber, Looney, Babola, Hinman, & Utsey, 2000)? How effective was a health promotion intervention with older adults (Haber, 1986; Haber & Lacy, 1993)? At some point after project development has begun, I examine key concepts from different theories and refine my interventions and evaluations accordingly.

4

EXERCISE

Learning Objectives

- Explain the basic principles endorsed by the surgeon general's report
- Review the benefits of brisk walking and the dangers of sitting
- Recognize the importance of access-by-walking neighborhoods
- Review research on the beneficial effects of exercise on disease and functional impairment

- Examine the importance of exercise for weight management
- Examine the basic components of a model exercise program
- Differentiate between aerobic and anaerobic exercise
- Contrast target heart rate with the Borg technique
- Recognize the importance of music for exercise
- Contrast elastic bands, free weights, machine weights, and isometrics
- Define the Valsalva maneuver, and explain the need to avoid it
- Contrast yoga with flexibility movements
- Explore Tai Chi, swimming, and other exercise options
- Identify balance exercise options
- Recognize different benefits for different exercises
- Describe the activity pyramid
- List exercise precautions and safety measures
- Respond to exercise excuses and barriers
- Contrast health club, home, and religious settings
- Evaluate personal trainers and online exercise options
- Examine Wii-hab as an exercise technique
- Recognize the importance of a health educator in the medical clinic

SURGEON GENERAL'S REPORT ON PHYSICAL ACTIVITY AND HEALTH

In her exercise video "Shopping for Fitness," Joan Rivers espouses walking the malls for aerobic conditioning, lifting shopping bags for weight training, and trying on jeans that are one size too small to motivate oneself for weight reduction. According to Rivers, "Everybody's got a tape out, Buns of Steel, Breasts of Iron and Bunions of Teflon. They just don't get it, that it should be fun." Although many of her comments on the video are satirical, much of the *Surgeon General's Report on Physical Activity and Health* supports what she espouses. More on that later.

The report represented a collaborative effort between the Centers for Disease Control and Prevention (CDC) and the President's Council on Physical Fitness and Sports. It was the most comprehensive review of the research up to that time—1996, and for that matter, up to the present time—on the effects of physical activity on people's health. According to the surgeon general's report, regular exercise and physical activity improved health in a variety of ways, including a reduction in heart disease, diabetes, high blood pressure, colon cancer, depression, anxiety, excess weight, falling, bone thinning, muscle wasting, and joint pain.

However, 60% of adults did not achieve the recommended amount of physical activity, and 25% of adults were not physically active at all. Inactivity increased with age; by age 75, 36% engaged in no physical activity (see Figure 4.1). Inactivity was more common among women and people with lower income and less education. (A 2010 update by the Federal Interagency Forum on Aging Related Statistics reported that this is still the case with inactivity increasing with age, and it is more common among women and those with low educational levels.)

Surgeon general reports mostly go unnoticed but sometimes they matter. A previous report of the surgeon general on the health hazards of tobacco, published in 1964,

FIGURE 4.1   **Prevalence of no leisure-time physical activity increases as Americans age.**

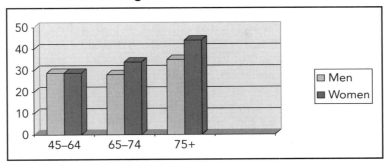

Source: CDC: Behavioral Risk Factor Surveillance System.

had a major influence on public awareness, the policies of government and business, and the percentage of Americans who smoked. The report on physical activity and health also had a major influence on public awareness and the practices of fitness teachers, but *not* on the percentage of Americans who engaged in regular exercise and physical activity. Nonetheless, as the acting surgeon general at that time, Audrey F. Manley, stated, "This report is nothing less than a national call to action. Physical inactivity is a serious nationwide public health problem, but active and healthful lifestyles are well within the grasp of everyone."

The report agreed with Ms. Rivers that most sedentary Americans are not going to rigorously pursue buns of steel, and of those who do, all will fall short of the goal. Instead, it is important to make the first step for most Americans achievable; and to do so requires a large degree of modesty in setting goals and at least a small degree of enjoyment. Hence, the emphasis on being more active, perhaps by shopping—as Joan suggested—while walking briskly, rather than narrow adherence to a rigid exercise regimen.

One of the basic premises of the surgeon general's report was that Americans should get at least 30 minutes of physical activity, most days of the week. This statement provided a major perspective shift from previous recommendations by government and exercise leaders. Instead of raising exercise intensity level to a target heart rate for a specific period of time, three times a week, the report recommended that Americans become more concerned about expending calories on a near-daily basis, through physical activity and exercise.

Also, instead of fixating on measuring target heart rate to assess intensity level, just raising one's respiratory and heart rate each day is sufficient—and these physiological changes are apparent to the participant through quicker breathing rate and body warmth increase.

The report also suggested not being rigid about the length of a physical activity or exercise session. It was no longer deemed essential to obtain 30 consecutive minutes of exercise. For Americans, the large majority of whom are not too active, accumulating shorter activity spurts throughout the day may be more accessible. Got a spare few minutes? Then briskly walk the shopping malls with Joan or climb a few stairs.

A review of the research literature concluded that accumulating several 5- or 10-minute bouts of physical activity over the course of the day provides beneficial health and fitness effects (Murphy, Nevill, Neville, Biddle, & Hardman, 2002). Moreover, if you time these bouts of activity just right, you can also use them to gain the added benefit of replacing junk-food snack breaks.

One study reported that "fractionized" exercise may be more effective than continuous exercise (Angadi et al., 2012). Three bouts of 10-minute walking led to lower average 24-hour blood pressure readings than one 30-minute session. Many older Americans will find a 10-minute session less daunting to initiate than a longer exercise period. Even more good news is that only one or two of those 10-minute sessions per day may produce significant results. A study of 416,000 Taiwanese over 12 years reported that as little as 15 minutes a day of physical activity reduced all-cause mortality compared to those who were inactive (Wen et al., 2012).

Regarding exercise itself, it is difficult for adults to go from inactivity to an exercise routine. Thinking about how to accumulate short bouts of activity is a useful way to get started on better health and fitness. For example, wax your car or wash your floor more briskly than you normally do (even if it means doing it in segments throughout the day), or put more energy into raking leaves, mowing the lawn, gardening with enthusiasm, or dancing by yourself to music on the radio.

Question: The principles of the 1996 Surgeon General's Report on Physical Activity and Health were widely accepted, though the percentage of Americans who engaged in regular physical activity and exercise has not appreciably increased since that time. Can you suggest an effective dissemination plan to policymakers, providers, and consumers that would lead to more Americans practicing what this surgeon general's report preached?

To repeat one of the surgeon general's conclusions, Americans need to be active most days of the week. Therefore, aim for the habit of everyday exercise, but do not allow the occasional lapse to discourage you. Making exercise a near-daily routine is more likely to become an enduring habit than the previously recommended three times per week.

This topic is more than just a health issue, it is a financial one as well. One study of more than 20,000 people over two decades, beginning with an average of age 51, and ending with an average age of 72, reported that participants who exercised routinely had 38% lower medical costs measured by Medicare and other insurance claims than those who failed to exercise regularly. The authors suggested that perhaps people who are able to document regular exercise should be able to share in the financial benefit gleaned by their insurers (Bachmann et al., 2012).

THE MOST POPULAR ACTIVITY: WALKING

Older adults need not become triathletes or engage in other high-intensity activities to reap the benefits of exercise. For most older adults, a brisk walking program will provide sufficient intensity for a good aerobics program. A landmark 8-year study of more than 13,000 people indicated that walking briskly for 30 to 60 minutes every day was almost as beneficial in reducing the death rate as jogging up to 40 miles a week (Blair et al., 1989). The authors of a study of 1,645 older adults reported that simply walking 4 hours per week decreased the risk of future hospitalization for cardiovascular disease (LaCroix, Leveille, Hecht, Grothaus, & Wagner, 1996).

The Nurses' Health Study is a long-term research project, spanning three decades and involving 122,000 nurses. A prospective study of 72,000 of these nurses over an 8-year period revealed that brisk walking 3 hours a week offered as much health benefit as engaging in vigorous exercise. Brisk walking is defined as about 3 miles per hour (twice the normal pace), and 3 hours a week comes to about 30 minutes per day, most days of the week. Among the brisk walkers, the incidence of coronary events (nonfatal myocardial infarction or death from coronary disease) was reduced between 30% and 40% (Manson et al., 1999). A subset of this sample containing 5,100 diabetic walkers produced a similar reduction in heart disease risk (Hu et al., 2001).

The National Center for Health Statistics reported that walking has much greater appeal for older adults than high-intensity exercise. A smaller percentage of persons age 65+ (27%), in comparison to the general adult population (41%), engaged in vigorous activities, whereas people of all age groups (41%) were equally likely to walk for exercise.

Brisk walking is the most popular aerobic activity for older adults. As the acting surgeon general emphasized in her report, most Americans can benefit from activities like brisk walking and not concern themselves about target heart rate. Many older adults *are* concerned about unfavorable weather, though, and may abandon their walking routine as a consequence. Prolonged hot or cold spells may sabotage a good walking program. Rather than discontinue this activity because of the weather, adults may choose to walk indoors at their local shopping malls. Many shopping malls—about 2,500 nationwide—open their doors early, usually between 5:30 and 10:00 a.m., for community residents, whether they shop or not.

Expanding out from the narrow perspective of shopping malls, there is a relationship between *neighborhood* and *health*. Residents who are dependent on a car to get to most places and have few sidewalks for safe walking are likely to be more obese and have chronic medical conditions that affect health-related quality of life (Booth, Pinkston, & Poston, 2005; Sturm & Cohen, 2004). For every extra 30 minutes commuters drive each day they have a 3% greater chance of being obese; and as for people who live within walking distance of shops, they are 7% less likely to be obese (Frank, Andresen, & Schmid, 2004). Older persons who believe their neighborhoods are accessible by walking are up to 100% more physically active (Li, Fisher, Brownson, & Bosworth, 2005a; King et al., 2003).

Living in an urban area where commercial spaces are near residential areas leads to more frequent and lengthier durations of walking among all age groups, including older residents (Gauvin et al., 2012). Another group of researchers surveyed 2,285 adults age 45 to 84 and found that one third of them lived in healthy neighborhoods, defined as neighborhoods with easy access to nearby walking, visibility of other residents walking in the neighborhood, availability of exercise facilities, and access to fresh produce (Auchincloss et al., 2009). Over a 5-year follow-up, 10% of participants developed type II diabetes, but those living in healthy neighborhoods were 38% less likely to develop diabetes than those who did not.

A sedentary person is estimated to walk about 3,500 steps a day, and the average American about 5,130 steps. Many advocates believe Americans should aim for 10,000 steps a day, or about 5 miles. Workplace physical activity, particularly among blue-collar occupations, helps some people reach the 10,000-step target, leaving retired older adults and sedentary workers most likely to be at risk (McCormack, Giles-Corti, & Milligan, 2006).

A *pedometer* is a small device that is usually attached at the waist and is used to count steps. Pedometers first appeared in Japan in 1965 under the name Manpo-meter (manpo in Japanese means 10,000 steps). Their introduction into America took another few decades, but they have been rapidly increasing in popularity—even McDonald's distributed them several years ago as part of an adult Happy Meal called Go Active (salad, bottled water, and a pedometer for $4.99).

In general, studies have been supportive of the benefits of using a pedometer to motivate individuals and increase physical activity. A meta-analysis of 26 studies (8 randomized controlled trials and 18 observational studies) with 2,767 participants (mean age 49) reported significant increases in physical activity and significant decreases in body mass index and blood pressure (Bravata et al., 2007). Having a step goal (such as 10,000 steps per day) was a significant influence on individual outcomes. Whether these individual improvements were durable over the long term went uninvestigated.

Groups of people—families, friends, church members, and so on—who want help adding 2,000 steps a day to their daily routine can access information and guidelines offered by the national organization, America on the Move, at www.americaonthe-move.org. Another option for older adults is to join a noncompetitive walking or hiking club, or participate in a nearby walking or hiking event. Two such possibilities are the American Volkssport Association at www.ava.org; and a local Sierra Club chapter, with the national headquarters at 415-977-5500, or at www.sierraclub.org.

Traveling to another city can also be an excuse not to exercise, or it can be an opportunity to gather information from the local newspaper or chamber of commerce about the city's walking tours. These can be an enjoyable way to get exercise and a unique way to learn about offbeat aspects of a city's history. Most, if not all, big cities have walking tours, and some sound particularly intriguing—like Oak Park, Illinois's self-guided walking tours of Frank Lloyd Wright homes (708-848-1976, www.gowright. org); Big Onion walking tours of New York City's ethnic communities and restaurants (212-439-1090, www.bigonion.com); or e-book walking tour guides and maps for the cities of Detroit, Chicago, New York, Seattle, Traverse City (northern Michigan), and Paris (www.spectacularstrolls.com).

Walking is so popular that it has spawned many magazines, newsletters, and books. It may appear that there is not much to walking—we have been doing it, after all, since we were toddlers—but proper technique improves benefits and reduces injuries. Good walking technique involves proper posture (head erect, chin in, shoulders relaxed, and back straight), a bent-arm swing, and a full natural stride. Good walking shoes should have flexible soles, good arch supports, and roomy toe boxes. Shoe inserts, called orthotics, may be helpful for cushioning impact or to prevent the feet from turning in or out.

THE MOST POPULAR INACTIVITY: SITTING

Unfortunately, sitting is more popular than walking. Americans now sit more than they sleep, spending an average of 10 hours a day in a car, or at work or home—in front of a computer screen or television set (Pope, 2012). Older adults are the most guilty, with the highest rates of sedentary behavior and the fewest hours of leisure-time physical activity. Research now shows that daily exercise is not enough protection from the harmful effects of too much sitting.

A study of 17,000 Canadians, ages 18 to 90, revealed that the greater the amount of sitting time, the greater the probability of death from all causes, and cardiovascular disease in particular (Katzmarzyk et al., 2009). What was most interesting about the results was that the findings held up regardless of the amount of leisure-time physical activity people got.

Researchers have concluded that the amount of time you sit, independent of exercise time, is a factor for heart-disease risk and all-cause mortality (Dunstan et al., 2012; Stamatakis, Davis, Stathi, & Hamer, 2012). In fact, running 35 miles a week combined with excessive sitting burns fewer calories and entails greater cardiovascular risk than people who have no actual "exercise program" but engage in much lower levels of sitting over the course of a day.

EXERCISE FOR DISEASE PREVENTION AND FUNCTIONAL IMPROVEMENT

As previously noted, the surgeon general's report documented the many benefits of regular exercise. Just prior to the publication of this report, the American Heart Association (AHA) added physical inactivity as a risk factor to its list, joining hypertension, smoking, and high blood cholesterol. It was the first new risk factor the AHA had added in almost 20 years.

The AHA recommended routine screening of all patients for inactivity. If the physician had time constraints, the AHA recommended that exercise counseling be coordinated through a nurse, allied health professional, or other type of health educator. As a number of gerontologists have noted, if exercise could be encapsulated in a pill, it would be the single most powerful medication a physician could prescribe.

In 2004 I was a member of an expert panel reviewing evidence-based outcomes of exercise in older adults. This CDC-funded project was led by Thomas Prohaska of the University of Illinois at Chicago. Dr. Prohaska and his research team reviewed 2,334 studies published in peer-reviewed journals between 1980 and 2000. This review concluded that exercise was beneficial in all the areas that were reviewed: heart disease, arthritis, chronic obstructive pulmonary disease (COPD), endurance, strength, mobility/balance, mortality, disability, and mental health.

Although this comprehensive evaluation was too detailed to adequately summarize here, I report below—unsystematically—on studies showing evidence that exercise demonstrates considerable promise for older adults in the areas of disease prevention and improved physical and cognitive function.

Cardiovascular Disease

Inactivity is the most powerful predictor of mortality from cardiovascular disease among healthy persons, surpassing smoking, hypertension, and heart disease (Myers et al., 2002). However, studies report that activity as simple as brisk walking is associated with a reduced risk of coronary heart disease for elderly men and women. Although walking by itself is sufficient to lower the risk of cardiovascular disease, brisker walking lowers the risk more (Manson et al., 2002), and more vigorous exercise lowers the risk further (Tanasescu et al., 2002).

Exercise is also a major prognostic factor in patients with existing cardiovascular disease. Patients who are physically active after a first heart attack had a 60% lower risk of a fatal heart attack or a second nonfatal heart attack than those who did not become active (Steffen-Batey et al., 2000). For a number of years, exercise was contraindicated for patients with chronic heart failure (CHF). Subsequently, exercise was recommended for CHF patients, provided the heart problem was stable (Gielen, Schuler, & Hambrecht, 2001). Exercise also appears to provide protection against in-hospital mortality in elderly patients with acute myocardial infarction (Abete et al., 2001).

Though aerobic conditioning has been considered the exercise of choice for improved cardiorespiratory function, other forms of exercise have proved beneficial as well. Tai Chi (Lan, Chen, Lai, & Wong, 1999) and resistance exercise (Tanasescu et al., 2002; Vincent et al., 2002a), for example, may provide cardiorespiratory benefits. Resistance exercise, in fact, appears to reduce blood pressure level (Kelley & Kelley, 2000) and cholesterol level (Kraus et al., 2002), which previously was believed to be only achieved through aerobic exercise interventions.

A study of peripheral vascular disease (PVD) reports what may seem incongruous to some—that an effective treatment for clogged or narrowed arteries of the legs is aerobic walking (Stewart, Hiatt, Regensteiner, & Hirsch, 2002). Walking increases muscle metabolism and may improve circulation to the legs, allowing more oxygen to get to tissues otherwise starved by blockages. The two caveats to walking interventions for PVD are to avoid extreme pain and to avoid exercise if pain continues when legs are at rest (Peripheral vascular disease, 2000).

In the Framingham Heart study, people who participated in moderate physical activity starting at age 50 lived 1.1 years longer free of heart disease, and 1.3 years longer overall; people who participated in high levels of physical activity lived 3.2 years longer free of heart disease, and 3.5 years longer overall (Franco et al., 2005). These gains were similar for both men and women.

Cancer

Epidemiological findings have established an association between the risk of cancer and physical activity and exercise. Higher levels of adult physical activity, for example, appear to afford modest protection against breast cancer or enhance survival after breast cancer (Holmes, Chen, Feskanich, Kroenke, & Colditz, 2005), perhaps by reducing body fat where carcinogens accumulate (Dirx, Voorrips, Goldbohm, & van den Brandt, 2001), or by lowering the level of estrogen in the blood (McTiernan et al., 2002). Also, women with substantial leisure-time physical activity had a 27% lower incidence of ovarian cancer (Cottreau, Ness, & Kriska, 2000). In comparison to more sedentary men, those who exercised correlated with a 24% reduction in the risk of prostate cancer and a 62% reduction in the risk of upper digestive and stomach cancer (Wannamethee, Shaper, & Walker, 2001).

High activity level is also associated with a substantial reduction, up to 50%, in colon cancer risk (Zhang et al., 2006). Although the mechanisms by which exercise protects against colon cancer are not known, it is speculated that exercise speeds food through the bowel and shortens the time carcinogens in fecal matter spend in contact with cells that line the colon. There is no research, however, that supports an association between constipation and cancer risk.

There is no agreement on a single theory that accounts for the positive association between exercise and physical activity and the risk of cancer. Several possibilities have been explored, and they tend to differ with the varying types of cancer. The theories range broadly and include the immune, nervous, and endocrine systems.

Diabetes

Exercise appears to have an impact on type II diabetes, in terms of both prevention of the disease and the risk of mortality among those who already have it. The onset of diabetes may be delayed or prevented when high-risk individuals make lifestyle changes that include increased exercise. Finnish researchers investigated 522 people over a 4-year period; the incidence of diabetes was 11% among those who received exercise instruction and other counsel, and 23% among controls—a significant difference (Tuomilehto et al., 2001).

A study of 70,000 female nurses who did not have diabetes at baseline documented almost 1,500 incidents of type II diabetes over an 8-year period. There was a substantially reduced risk of obtaining it, however, among those who exercised regularly, even among those who engaged in moderate-intensity physical activity such as brisk walking (Hu et al., 1999).

Being active also increases the chances that a person with diabetes will stay alive. Researchers studied 1,263 men with diabetes over an average of 12 years, and reported that the physically inactive had a 70% greater chance of dying than did men who reported being physically active. The overall risk of death shrank as the level of fitness rose (Wei, Gibbons, Kampert, Nichaman, & Blair, 2000). Another study of 2,803 men with type II diabetes reported that physical activity was associated with reduced risk of cardiovascular death and total mortality (Tanasescu et al., 2003).

High-intensity resistance training also improves glycemic control in older patients with type II diabetes (Dunstan et al., 2002). The study authors were surprised at the magnitude of the effects, as they equaled those typically seen with drugs for diabetes. They noted that muscles are major clearance sites for circulating glucose.

Depression

Exercise may be just as effective as antidepressant medication in treating some cases of depression (Lawlor & Hopker, 2001), although medication may initiate a more rapid therapeutic response than exercise. After 16 weeks of treatment, though, exercise was equally effective in reducing depression among patients with major depressive disorder (Blumenthal et al., 1999). Another study reported that, conversely, individuals who stop exercising lose the long-term mood-enhancing effects (Kritz-Silverstein, Barrett-Connor, & Corbeau, 2001).

A study by Singh and colleagues (2001) reported that supervised weightlifting exercises significantly benefited depressed older adults, in comparison to control persons who attended health lectures. (I suppose one could argue that if the older weightlifters had been subjected to boring health lectures as well, both groups would have remained depressed!) What was interesting about this study was that the antidepressant benefits were sustained even after exercise supervision was terminated and the participants were on their own. After 26 months, one third of the elderly exercisers were still regularly weightlifting.

At the other end of the time continuum, a single exercise session can boost the mood of mildly to moderately depressed persons (Bartholomew, Morrison, & Ciccolo, 2005). Just 30 minutes of brisk walking can immediately boost one's mood, giving a benefit similar in magnitude (to near-normal mood levels) and time (up to an hour) to what some persons seek through cigarettes, caffeine, or binge eating.

A weekly Tai Chi class, combined with an antidepressant, improved the outcomes of treating depression in older adults compared to a health education class and the use of the same antidepressant (Lavretsky et al., 2011). The participants also demonstrated better memory and cognition, and reported a higher overall level of energy.

Cognition

Studies of physical activity or exercise among older adults report that those with higher physical activity or exercise levels were less likely to experience cognitive decline (Head, Singh, & Bugg, 2012; Weuve et al., 2004). Another study of 349 healthy adults 55 and older reported that older adults with higher levels of fitness—as measured by a standard treadmill exercise test—experienced a slower rate of cognitive decline over a 6-year period (Barnes, Yaffe, Satariano, & Tager, 2003).

Leisure-time physical activity at midlife is associated with a decreased risk of dementia later in life (Rovio et al., 2005). In nondemented older adults, a modest amount of exercise—as little as 15 minutes 3 times weekly—is associated with a 32% reduced risk for developing dementia over the next 6 years (Larson et al., 2006). (Dementia is a broader term than, and not equivalent to, Alzheimer's disease—see Chapter 8, "Mental Health.")

One study examined the relationship between aerobic fitness and in vivo brain tissue density. High-resolution magnetic resonance imaging scans from 55 older adults revealed that declines in brain tissue densities, as a function of age, were substantially reduced as a function of fitness, even when other relevant variables were statistically controlled (Colcombe et al., 2003).

Exercise may not only stem a decline in cognitive functioning, it may improve it as well. Researchers found that older men and women who engaged in aerobic exercise improved the higher mental processes of memory and executive functioning—such as planning and organizational abilities—that are based in the frontal and prefrontal regions of the brain (Khatri et al., 2001). A randomized controlled research study found that 12 months of once-weekly or twice-weekly resistance training improved executive cognitive function (i.e., an improved ability to make accurate decisions quickly) in community-dwelling women age 65 to 75 (Liu-Ambrose et al., 2010). A later study conducted by some of the same researchers focused on a sample of women with mild cognitive impairment and reported that resistance training led to even more improvement in brain function than those who performed aerobics (Nagamatsu, Handy, Hsu, Voss, & Liu-Ambrose, 2012).

Bone Density

Both weight-bearing aerobic exercise and resistance training increase bone density in older women (Jakes et al., 2001; Rhodes et al., 2000). Of most relevance to older adults, in terms of achievability, is a study reporting that even low-impact aerobic exercise such as brisk walking can increase bone mass. A review of 24 studies that examined aerobic exercise and bone mineral density in women reported a 2% bone mass gain among exercisers versus nonexercisers, and that walking was the most common form of exercise used in these studies (Kelley, 2001).The Nurses' Health Study of 61,200 postmenopausal women concluded that moderate levels of activity, including walking, are associated with substantially lower risk of hip fractures (Feskanich, Willett, & Colditz, 2002).

A study of healthy older persons who engaged in 6 months of resistance training showed 2% greater bone density in the hip area, and showed signs that bone metabolism had shifted toward generating more bone than was being lost (Vincent & Braith, 2002). Another study reported that resistive back-strengthening exercises reduced the incidence of vertebral fractures among postmenopausal women (Sinaki et al., 2002).

Fall Prevention

Home-based exercise programs result in significant fall reduction and related *safety* benefits. One individually tailored exercise program in the home improved physical function, reduced falls, and decreased injuries in a sample of women aged 80 years and older. Over a 1-year period, persons in the exercise program reduced falls by 46%, compared with a control group that received an equal number of social visits instead of exercise sessions (Campbell et al., 1997). Another home-based exercise program with older adults age 70 to 84 reported significant fall reduction in comparison to groups that received home hazard management and treatment of poor vision (Day et al., 2002).

A meta-analysis of seven trials of an experiment titled Frailty and Injuries: Cooperative Studies of Intervention Techniques (FIC-SIT) revealed that a variety of exercise interventions—examined by way of randomized, controlled clinical trials—led to a reduction in falls among elderly patients (Province et al., 1995). Subjects in the seven trials were older adults, ages ranged from 60 to 75 years, and were mostly ambulatory and cognitively intact. The exercise interventions were successful even though they varied in duration, frequency, intensity, and content. The diversity in content among the interventions included endurance training, resistance training, flexibility training, and Tai Chi.

Not only can starting an exercise program lower an elderly woman's risk of falling, but the benefit can be lasting. Ninety-eight women aged 75 to 85 with low bone mass participated in one of three types of group-based exercise programs—strength training, agility exercise, or stretching exercise—and reduced their risk of falls between 37% and 43% (Liu-Ambrose et al., 2005). Apparently these interventions acted as a catalyst for ongoing physical activity, because the reduction in fall risk was maintained for at least 18 months.

Osteoarthritis

People with osteoarthritis of the knee often experience progressive deterioration in the cartilage of the knee joint until they reach the point of being disabled. Both aerobic and resistance exercise with patients who have osteoarthritis of the knee reduced the incidence of disability in activities of daily living by about 50% (Penninx et al., 2001). Another sample of older adults with knee osteoarthritis experienced significant improvement in physical function and reduced pain as a consequence of a strength-training program (Baker et al., 2001).

Another simple home-based exercise program significantly reduced knee pain from osteoarthritis (Thomas et al., 2002); and an exercise program combined with medication for knee osteoarthritis was more effective than medication alone for improving physical function and reducing activity-related pain in a sample of older persons (Petrella & Bartha, 2000).

Even a modest amount of exercise—fewer than 30 minutes per day of moderate activity—may prevent disability from arthritis, and those with arthritis show improvements in mobility with modest exercise (Feinglass et al., 2005).

Sleep

Older adults with sleep complaints improved self-rated sleep quality by completing a moderate-intensity exercise program. Exercising subjects reported significant improvement in subjective sleep quality, reduced sleep latency (average time in minutes needed to fall asleep), and increased sleep duration (average number of hours of actual sleep per night) (King, Oman, Brassington, Bliwise, & Haskell, 1997). Even a sample of healthy older adult caregivers who had not initially reported sleep complaints, but who engaged in stressful caregiving with family members, reported improvements in subjective sleep quality after they completed a moderate-intensity exercise program (King, Baumann, O'Sullivan, Wilcox, & Castro, 2002).

Another study focused on older residents in assisted living facilities. The researchers concluded that a regular yoga practice over several months improved the quality of sleep compared to residents who did not participate (Chen et al., 2010).

Other Conditions

Exercise appears to be beneficial for a wide range of other medical and functional conditions. Some examples follow: a reduction in stress among older female caregivers (King et al., 2002), a reduction in the symptoms of chronic fatigue syndrome (Powell, Bentall, Nye, & Edwards, 2001), increased function in COPD patients (Hernandez et al., 2000), a reduction in stroke risk (Hu et al., 2005) and the improvement in motor function among stroke survivors (Duncan et al., 1998), improvement in mental health status (S. P. Cheng et al., 2009), relief from lower back pain and dysfunction (Sherman, Cherkin, Erro, Miglioretti, & Deyo, 2005); relief from musculoskeletal pain (Bruce, Fries, & Lubeck, 2005), and acceleration of wound healing among older adults (Emery, Kiecolt-Glaser, Glaser, Malarkey, & Frid, 2005).

Caution

It takes an act of supreme skepticism to deny the overwhelming evidence supporting the benefits of exercise. Nonetheless, I have met such skeptics who disparage the rigor upon which most exercise research studies are based. Though I most happily do not side with these cynics, the evidence on the benefits of exercise does need to be viewed with a degree of caution. Many studies, for instance, are epidemiological in nature and reveal correlation rather than causality. In other words, exercise may be more the product of being in good health than a contributor to it. Some of these observational studies attempt to compensate for this limitation by employing analytical controls on several baseline variables.

> **Question:** What has been *your* major barrier when it comes to engaging in a well-rounded exercise program on a regular basis, and have you attempted to overcome it? If so, how?

Other methodological limitations are also common among exercise studies. Many of these studies utilize unrepresentative samples, often relying on volunteers; lack randomization between treatment and control groups; do not restrict awareness of who is in the treatment versus control group (i.e., they are unblinded studies); employ inadequate measurement tools, especially a reliance on self-reports; and report high dropout rates or do not include dropouts in the data analysis (this would be a more rigorous type of study called intention-to-treat analysis). Exercise interventions, therefore, may not be as miraculous as some of these studies seem to indicate.

Nonetheless, the breadth and depth of research on exercise interventions with older adults—including more than 200 rigorous randomized clinical trials that were included in the Prohaska-led meta-analysis that I referred to earlier—can only lead one to conclude that exercise is an astonishing health intervention, and no amount of methodological nitpicking will seriously challenge its credibility.

EXERCISE FOR WEIGHT MANAGEMENT

It has been said that man does not live by bread alone. It can also be said that man does not control his weight by nutrition alone. Restricting the number of calories consumed without exercising can result in quick, dramatic weight loss. Unfortunately, it can also result in quick, dramatic regaining of weight. About half the initial weight loss will be water, which will be regained, and muscle, which will make one weaker. Dieting without exercise also lowers our metabolic rate (the amount of energy used for physiological processes), causing a reduction in our fat-burning capacity. This not only slows weight loss, but when the dieting ends, the weight is gained back faster than ever.

Exercise, in contrast, assures that weight loss will come primarily from fat, not water and muscle. Exercise may also increase metabolic rate so that our body burns calories more efficiently and over a longer duration. Because muscle tissue is metabolically more active than fat, it burns more calories.

A study of more than 8,000 dieters who lost 10% of their starting weight and kept it off for at least a year reported that their number-1 successful weight loss maintenance strategy—cited by 81% of respondents—was exercise (Dieting, 2002). The most common form of exercise was walking, followed by increasing physical activity in their daily routine. A surprising finding from this study was that an unexpectedly high 29% of respondents reported that they added weight lifting to their exercise regime.

The vital role of exercise, however, appears to apply more to the maintenance of weight loss than to losing weight in the first place, where changing your eating patterns is the most important behavior change. A meta-analysis of U.S. studies on long-term weight loss maintenance concluded that exercise or a high level of physical activity is one of the two most important ingredients of maintaining weight loss (along with restricted caloric intake) (Anderson, Konz, Frederich, & Wood, 2001). Researchers reported that their findings were in agreement with the National Weight Control Registry study: Exercise and physical activity are essential for most people in maintaining weight loss over the long term.

Exercise as a weight maintenance strategy, however, may become less effecient as we age. Researchers monitored the fat and carbohydrate breakdown for older and younger participants who pedaled 60 minutes on stationary bikes. Measurement of oxygen consumption indicated how hard they were able to exercise. Then the study subjects pedaled at speeds that made them consume identical amounts of oxygen. Older participants oxidized less than a third as much fat as their younger counterparts. In other words, older adults appeared to burn less fat than younger adults while doing equivalent exercise. Paul Williams of the Lawrence Berkeley National Laboratory concluded that runners would have to substantially increase the amount of mileage they run each decade in order to stay at the same weight.

The best exercises for weight control are a combination of aerobics and strength building. The aerobic activity should involve the large muscle groups like the quadriceps. Also, longer duration and higher intensity accelerate progress, but are likely to increase the likelihood of dropping out of an exercise routine. Strength building will increase muscle mass and boost the metabolic rate, which may allow the individual to burn calories longer, not just when exercising.

Can we be fit and fat? Yes, according to the research of Stephen Blair and his colleagues at the Cooper Institute for Aerobics Research. Their data reveal that exercise can reduce disease risk even if body weight remains high. There is lower cardiovascular as well as all-cause mortality risk among persons who are overweight and fit, versus those who are normal weight and unfit (Heroux et al., 2009). However, a study by researchers from the Harvard School of Public Health qualified these findings. You are better off fit and fat than just fat, but fitness does not counter all the risk of excess weight (Hu et al., 2004). Also, when it comes to diabetes, exercise may not fully counter the effects of excess body fat, because fat tissue may release substances that affect the metabolism of insulin (Weinstein et al., 2004).

Unfortunately, many Americans believe you can get fit without much physical effort, as proclaimed on commercials and infomercials on television. Instead of accenting the physical effort it takes to lose weight, viewers learn that weight reduction is the consequence of buying a particular product that does not require much physical exertion to use. Over a period of several years, for instance, *electrical muscle stimulators* were a popular product purchased by consumers. By passing currents through electrodes applied to the skin you contract muscles and, allegedly, can either build them or reduce them. These devices tend to focus on the abdomen. By placing an electronic "exercise belt" around your waist and pushing a button, you can develop "washboard abs." After more than $100 million worth of the devices were sold in 2002, the Federal Trade Commission took three of these companies to court.

Adults spend about $3 billion a year on exercise equipment for home use. For a large but unknown percentage of persons who purchase exercise equipment to use while watching television, though, television viewing rather than exercising continues to be the leisure activity of choice.

THE FOUR COMPONENTS OF MY EXERCISE CLASS

The four components of a community exercise class that I coordinated for about a quarter century are *aerobics, strength building, flexibility and balance,* and *health education.* In a typical 60-minute class, I began with 25 minutes of aerobic exercise, warming up for the first few minutes and cooling down the last few minutes. I began with aerobics in order to warm up the muscles, not only for higher-intensity aerobic levels, but also for the subsequent periods of strength building (15 minutes) and flexibility and balance (10 minutes). These three components—aerobics, strength building, and flexibility and balance—typically lasted 50 minutes; the final 10 minutes of class was devoted to health education.

With the aid of students in health science classes, I implemented this exercise class for about 25 years, continually refining it during this time (see Figure 4.2). This exercise program was selected for the *Best Practices in Health Promotion and Aging* directory, compiled by the Health Promotion Institute of the National Council on Aging (NCOA). To obtain the manual with its brief summaries of selected best practices around the country, contact the NCOA at www.ncoa.org or call 202-479-1200.

The Aerobics Component

Aerobics has been defined as a series of strenuous exercises that help convert fats, sugars, and starches into aches, pains, and cramps. A more conventional definition is that aerobic means "with oxygen." An aerobic activity moves large volumes of oxygen, employs large muscle groups like the arms and legs, and is sustained at a certain level of intensity over a period of time. Aerobic exercise is rhythmic, repetitive, and continuous,

FIGURE 4.2   **The end-of-the-semester photograph of one of the author's exercise classes, taught by occupational therapy students.**

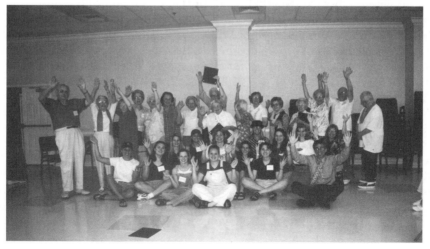

and includes such popular activities as brisk walking (about twice one's normal speed), swimming, and bicycling.

Aerobic activity can be contrasted to anaerobic ("without oxygen") activity, which depends on short bursts of energy (like a 50-meter sprint or barbell press), quickly depletes energy resources, and has limited cardiovascular benefit. This type of activity is, however, essential for strength-building purposes.

Aerobic capacity, or maximum oxygen uptake (VO_2 max), is the maximum amount of oxygen that an individual can utilize during strenuous exertion. Aerobic capacity is considered to be the best measure of cardiorespiratory fitness, and although it tends to decrease with age, aerobic capacity can be increased through a regularly practiced aerobic regimen.

Most aerobic exercise programs are designed to stimulate the heart and lungs for a sufficient period of time to produce an increased and sustained heart rate. Traditional programs encouraged participants to sustain exercise for a minimum of 20 to 25 minutes and to gradually raise the normal heartbeat, about 60 to 80 beats a minute, to the "target zone" of the individual, the upper and lower limits of which are based on age (see Table 4.1).

The target zone typically refers to between 60% and 75% of the estimated maximum heart rate, which is calculated by subtracting a person's age from 220 and multiplying the remainder first by 60% and then by 75%. The target for the beginning exerciser should be near the 60% level (or less if the person leads a sedentary lifestyle), and gradually increases to the higher level over succeeding months. Individuals can assess the intensity of their aerobic exercise program by counting their pulse beats for a 10-second period and multiplying by 6. Many aerobics instructors ask their students to conduct this assessment at periodic intervals.

The advantage to calculating target heart rates for some older adults is that they believe this is the most scientific approach and prefer this method. The disadvantages are (1) a significant percentage of older adults have difficulty obtaining a pulse count, (2) medications like beta-blockers can limit maximum heart rate intensity, and (3) there is controversy in the literature over whether the commonly used equation to estimate maximal heart rate (220 minus age) is valid for older adults (Tanaka, Monahan, & Seals, 2001). The formula for the target heart rate may be inappropriate for 30% to 40% of adults. These persons have hearts that beat faster or slower than the age-predicted maximum.

My own experience with exercise programs with older adults has led me to appreciate Fries's comment (1989): "We generally find this whole heart rate business a bit of a bother and somewhat artificial. There really are not good medical data to justify particular target heart rates. You may wish to check your pulse rate a few times to get a feel for what is happening, but it doesn't have to be something you watch extremely carefully" (p. 69). Typically, I implemented periodic checking of target heart rates during the

TABLE 4.1 Target Heart Rate by Decades

AGE	TARGET HEART RATE* (60%–75% OF MAXIMUM)	MAXIMUM HEART RATE* (220 – AGE)
50	102–128	170
60	96–120	160
70	90–113	150
80	84–105	140

*Beats per minute.

first or second class, and then encouraged those who are receptive to it to periodically check their heart rates on their own.

The technique that I use throughout the aerobic *and* strength-building components of my exercise class is my version of the Borg (1982) technique, a subjective assessment of how hard one is working. Most older adults prefer the Borg technique. It has the advantage of being easy to gauge, and it serves another purpose: It encourages older adults to become more aware of their bodies and how they feel (see Table 4.2). One study of more than 7,000 men (mean age 66 years) reported that the individual's perceived level of exertion is a better predictor of risk of coronary heart disease than of whether he or she met current activity recommendations (Lee, Sesso, Oguma, & Paffenbarger, 2003).

Ideally, the inactive older adult should seek an intensity level of very light, about 1 on the modified Borg scale, or about 50% of maximum heart rate. The active older person should be about 8 on the scale, or approximately 70% of maximum heart rate. Generally speaking, we tell participants that the exercise level should be of sufficient duration and intensity for them to break into a sweat (indicating a rising internal body temperature), but not so intense that they are unable to conduct a brief conversation (if desired) while exercising.

Regardless of whether target heart rates or perceived intensity levels are utilized, exercise is discontinued immediately if shortness of breath, chest pain, dizziness, light-headedness, confusion, or pain occurs.

My exercise classes were led by health science students after they completed a brief period of training. Regarding the aerobics component of the class, we offered the students and the older adults two options, with the second option used periodically to boost student interest.

1. A series of arm and leg movements that gradually increase, and then decrease, intensity level. I usually come up with funny names for the movements (my favorite was the Haber Hula—I'll leave that one up to your imagination) and make sure that all parts of the body are moved. If students run out of movement ideas, I encourage them to draw ideas from one of several memory-jarring techniques. For example, (1) playing one of a number of imaginary musical instruments (drums, trombone, violin, etc.) and pretending to generate the music that is playing in the background,

TABLE 4.2 Modified Borg Scale of Perceived Exertion

LEVEL	PERCEIVED EXERTION	PHYSICAL SIGNS
1	Very light	None
2		
3	Fairly light	Breathing rate increased
4		
5	Somewhat hard	Warmth, slight sweat, breathing rate increased
6		
7		
8	Hard	Sweat
9		
10	Very hard	Heavy sweat, difficult to talk

(2) mimicking an activity of daily living (drying one's back with a towel, vacuuming the rug, weeding the garden, etc.), and (3) mimicking a movement in a sport (boxing, throwing a baseball or swinging a bat, etc.).

2. An imaginary trip is acted out, perhaps a cruise to Spain, or attendance at a local baseball game. The cruise might include climbing up the boat (taking big steps in place with knees raised high), putting away clothes in one's cabin, dancing that evening with an imaginary heartthrob, getting off the boat (more big steps), visiting a bullfight, becoming the matador, and so forth. The baseball game may entail fans walking to the stadium (walking around the room, sometimes in a haphazard fashion to promote social interaction), doing the wave, being unexpectedly called upon by the manager to pinch hit (swinging an imaginary bat in both directions), or to do some relief pitching (using right and left arms).

The class was not targeted to older adults at a particular fitness level, and participants ranged from wheelchair bound (or walker dependent) to the very fit. One student typically led the frail or less fit participants, sometimes from a seated position; another student led the more fit participants; and the remaining students were free to roam and to individualize movements for older persons with special needs or to promote safety among participants.

If the older adult has a specific health problem like Parkinson's disease, stroke, an orthopedic condition, or mild confusion, the roaming students paid particular attention to helping them keep movements simple, avoid quick action, and encourage caution with twisting movements. Before the first class, students met one-on-one with older adults to find out if additional cautions needed to be observed and, if relevant, to discuss the importance of timing medications for maximal effect during classes.

Deconditioned older adults in the class were encouraged to perform at 1 or 2 on the modified Borg scale, or at 50% of the maximum heart rate for their age. Fit older adults were encouraged to perform at 8 on the Borg scale, or at 70% of the maximum heart rate. The majority of older adults were at the 5 or 6 level, which is equivalent to the moderate effort required for brisk walking. People tended to be reliable self-raters using the Borg scale.

The emphasis in the class, however, was on having fun, and only secondarily on moving up the scale to higher intensity levels. Studies have supported the surgeon general's findings that even activities of low- to moderate-intensity level not only improve the aerobic capacity of older adults, but also are less likely than more vigorous activities to result in injury, and are more likely to be maintained as a routine over time. And though low- to moderate-intensity activity does not provide the fitness benefits of higher-intensity exercise, it can be sustained over a longer exercise period because it depletes only fat, the body's richest store of energy. Higher-intensity exercise depletes carbohydrates, and cannot be sustained as long.

Older adults in classes that meet only two or three times a week need to be encouraged to comply with the surgeon general's advice and engage in aerobic exercise on most of the other days of the week as well. On days when there was no class, therefore, older adults were encouraged to engage in longer sessions of walking, swimming, cycling, dancing, gardening, yard work, or other activities that could be performed at low- or moderate-intensity level for a half hour or longer.

Finally, aerobic movement in our classes was always accompanied by *music*. One small study reported that music can promote better adherence to a regular exercise routine by adding to the enjoyment of the activity (Bauldof, Hoffman, Zullo, & Sciurba, 2002). The power of music can not only motivate, but also improve emotional and cognitive functioning as well. One study of stroke patients compared those who regularly listened to music with those in a control group who did not. The music listeners improved mood (e.g., reduced depression) and cognitive function (e.g., less confusion) in comparison to the control group (Sarkamo et al., 2008).

About two thirds of the musical selections in our exercise class, such as Big Band music, were targeted toward the preferences of older adults. The students chose the remaining music, though, with an eye toward eclecticism (rock, rap, theater music, international music, etc.). Musical variety not only promoted greater interest in attending the class, but also generated humorous discussions about the quality of the musical selections by young people.

We started and ended the class with slow-tempo music, and picked up the pace in between. When the musical cadence was faster, the slower-moving older adults were encouraged to time their physical movements to every other beat. Occasionally students chose soft background music to accompany the strength-building and flexibility and balance components of the class.

The Muscular Strength or Endurance Component

Experts did not always believe that strengthening exercises were as important for older adults as other components of exercise (Fries, 1989, p. 66), and many geriatric exercise manuals ignored strengthening exercises altogether. Now, experts and community health leaders realize the importance of strength building for maintaining an independent lifestyle with age. Preserving leg strength allows an older adult to get up from a chair in a restaurant, or help regain balance before falling. Preserving arm strength allows an older adult to carry groceries, pick up household items, twist off jar lids, and make minor repairs.

Experts, therefore, have developed resistance-training guideline recommendations for older adults (Porter, 2000). And though strength-building exercise programs are still the exception rather than the norm, the popularity of including a strength-building component into an aerobics exercise class grew quickly over the past two decades. Overall, however, the CDC estimated in 2004 that only 11% of adults 65 and older regularly performed any sort of strength training.

Muscular strength or *endurance* is the ability of the muscle to exert force (strength) or to repeat actions over time without fatigue (endurance). As people age, lean muscle tissue tends to decrease, and the percentage of body fat increases. Thus, muscle strength and endurance tend to decline with age, and bones tend to weaken. Strength training, however, will increase muscle mass, functioning ability, and bone density. When the skeletal frame is strengthened, the likelihood of bone fractures resulting from osteoporosis is reduced (Vincent & Braith, 2002).

In the spring of 1990, attitudes toward strength building for older adults began to change. A strength-exercise program captured the media headlines, which previously in the health arena had been dominated by popular aerobic activities or unusual aerobic accomplishments—such as the exploits of Johnny Kelley, who completed the Boston Marathon race 58 times and ran his last one as an octogenarian.

This highly publicized strength-exercise program, however, captured attention because it involved 10 (including one dropout) frail, *very old* nursing home residents who, after completing an 8-week training program, almost tripled their leg strength, expanded their thigh muscles by more than 10%, and were able to walk 50% faster (Fiatarone et al., 1990). The participants ranged in age from 87 to 96 years! One 93-year-old participant reported, "I feel as though I were 50 again. Now, I get up in the middle of the night and I can get around without using my walker or turning on the light. The program gave me strength I didn't have before. Every day I feel better, more optimistic. Pills won't do for you what exercise does!" Another resident who at first could not rise from a chair without using his arms was able to do so after the training, and two others no longer needed canes for walking. Less dramatic results are found in community-dwelling octogenarians, however, because they begin with higher baseline strength levels than institutionalized elders, and have less potential for improvement (Slivka, Raue, Hollon, Minchev, & Trappe, 2008).

Most community exercise classes do not have the luxury of providing weights or exercise machines to older participants. That was the case with my exercise class as well. I had found that the most affordable and perhaps safest option for strength building to be *elastic bands* (such as the Thera-Bands or Dyna-Bands sold by Fitness Wholesale; go to www.fwonline.com or call toll-free 888-396-7337), and *gravity-resisting exercises* like modified push-ups, raising arms to shoulder level and making circles, half-squats, toe raises, and others.

Elastic bands are a good alternative to *free weights*, which are associated with more injuries, and to resistance machines, which are less accessible. In addition to being safe and portable, they are inexpensive. By buying elastic bands in large rolls and cutting off four-foot strips, I provided bands to older students for less than $2 apiece.

I typically included four or five different upper-extremity exercises to strengthen different muscles such as the triceps (see Figure 4.3), biceps, deltoids, trapezius, pectoralis, and latissimus. I followed up with three or four lower-extremity exercises to strengthen the quadriceps, hamstrings, and/or gastrocnemius. The elastic band manufacturers provide the buyer with a range of illustrated exercises to follow. The booklets also include tips such as warming up, practicing smooth and slow movements in both eccentric and concentric directions, breathing while exercising, and emphasizing technically correct movements over quantity of movements.

Elastic bands come in increasing resistance levels. Typically, I started most older adults at the pink level of the Dyna-Bands, and increased repetitions and sets before I considered moving up to the green, or next intensity, level. Although the bands can be utilized at increasing levels of intensity, they are less precise than free weights or weight machines for measuring improvement.

I chose the resistance level that allowed the participants to perform about 12 repetitions of an exercise. A larger number of repetitions (using less resistance) would place greater emphasis on endurance, a smaller number of repetitions (using more

FIGURE 4.3   **Horizontal triceps press performed in one of the author's exercise classes.**

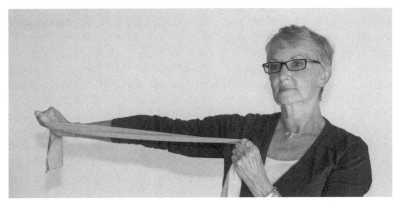

resistance) would emphasize strength. When it comes to repetitions, most older persons should err on the side of endurance over strength as it is likely to lead to fewer injuries. Moreover, researchers at McMaster University in Hamilton, Ontario, reported on preliminary evidence that older adults who performed high repetitions of 30% of maximum load (i.e., low resistance) may not only lead to fewer injuries, but may build strength that is equivalent to low repetitions at 80% of maximum load (i.e., high resistance) (Mitchell, 2012).

In my class, the number of different strength-building exercises and number of sets per exercise (usually two sets) were chosen to fit within a 15-minute exercise period. I did not try to fit all the strength-building exercises into one 15-minute component of the class, but instead offerred a few basic exercises each time, plus a few new exercises.

The elastic band fits easily into a pocket and is convenient to take to class, or anywhere else for that matter. A potential disadvantage to the band is that it can be hard to grip with arthritic fingers. This limitation can be overcome by buying handles, or tying the band into a circle and exerting power through wrists or forearms. Another disadvantage to the band is that eventually it will break (which can be startling, to say the least, when it occurs mid-exercise), and it needs to be kept out of sunlight and replaced in a regular and timely fashion.

The preferred schedule of activity for improving or sustaining strength or endurance for older adults is 2 or 3 days a week, with at least 1 day of rest between workouts. One study reported that muscle strength gains achieved during a 12-week progressive resistance-training program can be maintained by resistance training of only once per week thereafter (Trappe, Williamson, & Godard, 2002). Another study reported that even *light resistance* can help older adults get stronger while simultaneously reducing the possibility for injury (Vincent, Braith, Feldman, Kallas, & Lowenthal, 2002b). Yet another study reported that *super slow movements* combined with fewer repetitions may increase muscle mass more than normal-speed movements (Ring-Dimitriou et al., 2009).

A good alternative exercise for increasing strength in older adults with painful arthritic joints is *isometrics*, the contraction of a muscle without movement at the joint. The typical way to engage in isometrics is to pull or push against a stationary object, usually against a wall or against another body part. Each contraction should be held for about 5 seconds, and repeated three times. Many exercise physiologists are reluctant to recommend isometric exercise for heart patients because of the increased likelihood of performing the *Valsalva maneuver* (i.e., holding one's breath). It is possible, however, to avoid this maneuver when doing isometrics.

Because there is no movement and no equipment, you can do isometrics any place, any time, and at no cost. The muscle that you select tightens but does not change length, thus there is no movement of the joint or the bone to which the muscle is attached. Isometrics, therefore, has the advantage of allowing you to build muscle at a fixed angle, avoiding those joint positions that may be affected by arthritic pain. On the other hand, unless you systematically alter the angle (about 20 degrees each time), you do not develop strength over the entire range of motion.

There are several problems to avoid with all strength-building techniques, but they can be especially problematic with isometrics. To avoid the unhealthy *Valsalva maneuver* (holding one's breath), for instance, focus on inhalation and exhalation. To improve range of motion, it is not only important to vary the isometric angle, but also to develop opposing muscle groups (e.g., quadriceps and hamstrings). Finally, the Borg scale for estimating appropriate aerobic intensity level can also be used with isometric exercise.

My favorite isometric exercise for older adults was one that I developed to avoid the common problem of knee pain. In a seated position, the adult places the palms of both hands on one leg, about 2 or 3 inches above the knee, pushing down with the hands and up with the knee. The angle of the knee is altered by raising it slightly off the ground, and then raising it slightly higher two more times (see Figure 4.4). Repeat with the other leg. This exercise targets the important quadriceps muscle, the largest muscle in the body. It is a good alternative to leg squats, which can exacerbate knee pain.

In addition to building strength and endurance, my resistance-training component included safety tips on how to lift objects and how to move one's body to avoid muscle strain, backaches, hernias, and the like. Injuries from weightlifting are not uncommon, and they increased by 300% from 1978 to 1998 for middle-aged women and men ("More People Lifting Weights," 2000). In weight rooms around the country you can frequently observe examples of incorrect techniques that lead to injury. Men (and I suppose some women, but I have not observed this) typically are hoisting too-heavy weights, arching their backs, holding their breath, swinging the weights or otherwise using momentum, and dropping the weights (in this case, both free weights and machine weights) when done.

Instead, manageable weights and proper technique should be used. Lift slowly and smoothly and return the weights under full control, maintain the natural curve of your back, exhale on exertion and inhale as you relax. If you break form, the weights are too heavy. Weightlifters who use correct form reduce injuries by strengthening joints and ligaments. Machine weights are safer than free weights because they help foster proper technique and prevent the weight from falling on you.

Sixty percent of weight lifters are males, down from 80% two decades ago. Women have learned that they need not fear building bulging muscles, because they have less

FIGURE 4.4   Isometric exercise for quadriceps that avoids knee pain.

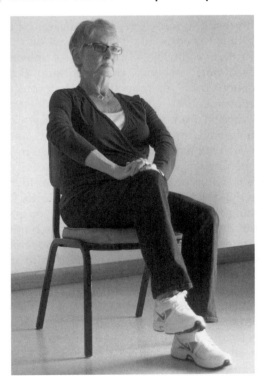

testosterone and fewer cells that make up muscle fiber. In addition to working toward a better appearance, female weightlifters enjoy the benefits of improving strength and balance and preventing or postponing osteoporosis.

Two research leaders who extol the benefits of resistance exercise (free weights, machines, isometrics, and rubber tubing), exercise physiologist William Evans and physician Maria Fiatarone, believe that strength building may be even more important for older adults than aerobic exercise. Although many physicians recommend walking because they think it is the safest activity, people who are weak have poor balance and are more subject to falling. Prescribing resistance exercise can give older adults the strength and confidence they need prior to beginning a systematic program of aerobic activity.

A joint effort by Tufts University and the CDC has produced an online interactive program entitled *Growing Stronger: Strength Training for Older Adults*. This online exercise program, and a booklet on strength training, are available free at www.go.tufts.edu/growing-stronger. Another resource on strength training is the website of Dr. Miriam Nelson, director of the John Hancock Center for Physical Activity and Nutrition, accessible at www.strongwomen.com.

The Flexibility and Balance Component

Different types of exercise activities for older adults result in different types of benefits. Programs emphasizing aerobics and strength building provide an array of benefits for older adults, but flexibility exercises are particularly well suited for improving the range of motion and reducing arthritic and other types of pain among older adults. It should be noted, though, that stretching as a method for preventing injury or soreness has not been supported by research (Thacker, Gilchrist, Stroup, & Kimsey, 2004).

Ballistic stretching, using quick and bouncy movements, works against the protective reflex contraction and can result in muscle tears, soreness, and injury. *Static stretching* is the type of stretching that I used in my exercise class and involves the slow and smooth advancement through a muscle's full range of movement until resistance or the beginning of discomfort was felt. The maximum position was then held 10 to 30 seconds, which allowed for the reduction of the protective reflex contraction and additional range of movement.

Stretching should always be preceded by a brief aerobic warm-up to increase heart rate, blood flow, and the temperature of the muscles, ligaments, and tendons. Conversely, stretching while muscles are cold may sprain or tear them. In my class, therefore, aerobics always preceded stretching.

A good way to develop different flexibility routines for older adults is to complete the Arthritis Foundation's 2-day PACE (People with Arthritis Can Exercise) training program to teach stretching to older adults. In addition, you receive the PACE manual, which includes a brief description of the purpose of each of the 72 movements, an illustration that demonstrates how to do each stretching movement, an explanation of the functional benefits of each movement, and the identification of special precautions— particularly for persons with arthritis or osteoporosis. There is also a separate section on teaching tips. To find out more information about the training program or the manual (the manual can be obtained separately), contact the local chapter of the Arthritis Foundation, or call the national office in Atlanta at 404-872-7100.

In each of my 10-week or 12-week classes, I attempted to bring in a *yoga* or *Tai Chi* instructor (preferably both) as an alternative activity in one or more of the stretching components of the class. The graceful movements and inner awareness of these techniques affect the mind as well as the body, and are popular with people of all ages, especially older adults. In several Chinese cities that I visited 35 years ago, I observed many outdoor groups of Tai Chi practitioners during my early-morning jogging, and noticed that a majority of the participants were older adults (Haber, 1979).

A meta-review of 35 systematic reviews of Tai Chi reported that there was no benefit of this type of exercise for treating cancer, Parkinson's disease, rheumatoid arthritis, or cardiovascular disease (Lee & Ernst, 2011). However, three of the four reviews for fall prevention demonstrated positive benefits, and four of the five reviews for psychological well-being demonstrated positive benefits. Most of these studies focused on older adults.

To demonstrate the popularity of yoga among older adults in the United States, I enjoyed sharing the story of Sadie Delany with the older students in my class. Sadie Delany reported in her book that she began her yoga practice in her 60s and continued it for 40 years, the last several of which she followed a yoga program on television (Delany, Delany, & Hearth, 1993). Sadie died in 1999 at the age of 109. She noted in her book that when her sister Bessie turned 80, she decided that Sadie looked better than she did, and Bessie then began doing yoga too. Bessie, however, probably started too late to reap the same longevity benefits as did Sadie. Her life ended prematurely in 1995, at the tender age of 104.

The most popular yoga activity is *hatha yoga*, a sequence of stretching, bending, and twisting movements that causes each joint to move slowly through its maximum range of motion, then is held for several seconds and repeated (see Figure 4.5). These practices improve body awareness, reduce stress, improve balance and coordination, and increase the maximum range of motion by expanding joint mobility.

FIGURE 4.5   **Shoulder roll.**

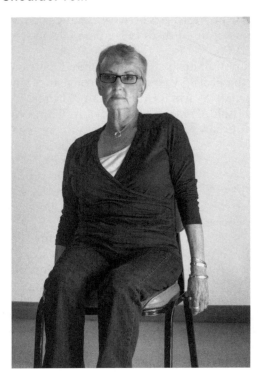

Hatha yoga and other types of stretching, twisting, and bending exercise programs possess two characteristics that make them highly desirable for older adults. They are well suited to all adults, even the very frail elderly (Haber, 1988a), and are exceptionally easy to incorporate into a daily routine. The movements of a stretching program, for instance, can be performed while one is watching television or talking on the telephone (not a good idea for yoga, though, where the attention should be on one's body and breath). Also, for people who engage in regular aerobic or strength-building activity, a brief flexibility routine can be added on at the end.

Performing yoga exercises in a group setting has become very popular with older adults. It was estimated that 18 million Americans were practicing yoga, a number that tripled during the 1990s ("Baby Boomers Turning to Yoga," 2000). For years I worked with older adults implementing yoga and related programs at senior centers (Haber & George, 1981–1982), congregate living facilities (Haber, 1986), nursing homes (Haber, 1988a), churches (Haber & Lacy, 1993), and other sites. Without exception, the programs were enthusiastically received and individual benefits were demonstrable.

One study by a group of researchers focused on yoga with stressed-out caregivers ranging in age from 45 to 91 years old. They reported that a daily yoga practice for 12 minutes, over 8 weeks, showed significantly lower levels of depressive symptoms and greater improvement in mental health and cognitive functioning, compared with a relaxation group (Lavretsky et al., 2012). The researchers also looked at the cellular level and found increased telomerase activity, which slowed ceullar aging.

For those interested in practicing yoga for therapeutic purposes, the International Association of Yoga Therapists (928-541-0004) will locate therapeutic yoga instructors in local areas. It should be noted though, that there is no regulatory body for yoga therapy and yoga instructors are unlicensed. There is no such thing as a certified or registered yoga instructor. It is particularly crucial that an individual, particularly a vulnerable older adult, choose his or her instructor carefully. Older adults may have to be guided into making changes in the moves that they are attempting.

For an interesting book on the ease with which many yoga participants have injured themselves, ranging from ruptured discs to leg paralysis to strokes, read *The Science of Yoga* by William Broad (2012).

Though not quite as popular as yoga in the United States, *Tai Chi* has increased in popularity as well over the past 15 years. Tai Chi consists of slow, graceful movements that are derived from a martial arts form in Asian cultures. It is gentle in nature and well suited to young and old. Persons of all ages in China can be observed practicing Tai Chi in groups in urban parks and in front of congregate housing. In addition to improving flexibility, Tai Chi is conducted with a lowered center of gravity (knees and hips held in flexion) and can contribute to lower-extremity strength building, body awareness, and balance control.

Question: What is the primary difference between flexibility exercises and yoga movements?

In terms of balance control, rigorously controlled studies—part of a 3-year exercise research project sponsored by the National Institutes on Aging and the National Institute for Nursing Research—supported the contention that Tai Chi has favorable effects upon the prevention of falls (Wolfson et al., 1996), and one Tai Chi group endured 48% longer than a comparison group before a first fall (Wolf et al., 1996). Older participants learn to stabilize their balance or regain it before they begin to fall. Other randomized controlled trials reported that Tai Chi improved sleep quality among older adults with moderate sleep complaints (Irwin, Olmstead, & Motivala, 2008) and augmented the immune response in older adults to fight off shingles (Irwin, Olmstead, & Oxman, 2007).

An alternative to yoga and Tai Chi that I have not tried in my exercise classes is the *tango*. In one study the tango produced the most positive effects on balance and movement control in persons with Parkinson's disease, followed by (believe it or not) the waltz and foxtrot. The treatment group in this randomized trial with 58 participants with mild to moderate Parkinson's disease improved significantly on the Berg Balance scale, 6-minute-walk distance, and backward stride length in comparison to a control group (Hackney & Earhart, 2009). Even if the effects of dance on balance and locomotion were not so promising, this would still be a fun option to insert into an exercise routine.

Balance issues emerge slowly and subtly over the life cycle, beginning in the mid-40s and becoming more obvious by the mid-60s. Loss of balance is a major contributor to falling, and each year about a third of persons 65 and older experience a fall, as do about half of persons over 80. Even the *fear* of losing one's balance can curtail activity, and this fear can be particularly counterproductive. Less activity leads to more weakness, and more weakness to more falls.

Regarding balance exercises, I included one or more of the following exercises at the tail end of some of my classes. All the exercisers stood next to a wall, chair, or something else that could be grabbed onto when needed.

1. Toe raise: Rise to tiptoes 10 times, reaching for support only if necessary. Repeat with eyes closed.
2. One-legged stand: Stand on one leg, flexing the other knee slightly. Balance on one foot for 10 seconds. Repeat with eyes closed.
3. Tandem walk: Walk across the floor, heel-to-toe, remaining next to a wall for support if necessary.
4. Sitting upside down (Figure 4.6): (Just kidding).

It is important to remind older adults that loss of balance can be caused by a number of conditions in addition to the physical losses that accumulate through a sedentary lifestyle. These conditions include problems with the inner ear, medications, poor posture resulting from arthritis or osteoporosis, poor vision, and muscle weakness. To rule out these problems, nothing takes the place of an evaluation by a health professional. Ideas to improve balance—such as vibrating insoles (Priplata et al., 2006) and cobblestone mat walking (Li, Fisher, & Harmer, 2005b)—appear on a regular basis.

The Health Education Component

One of the student instructors or one of the participating older adults facilitated the health education topic (with volunteers obtained at the end of the previous class) on a rotating basis. The health education topic for the class can be one of an endless number of subjects: describing an experience with a complementary medicine technique, providing a brief description of another health-promoting class in the community, sharing a healthy recipe, discussing fall-prevention ideas, sharing a list of sleep hygiene techniques, discussing tips for improving memory, and so forth. The topic may also be presented as a demonstration, rather than pedagogically, such as leading a stress management exercise like deep breathing or progressive muscle relaxation.

> **Question:** How would you improve upon my community-based exercise class?

FIGURE 4.6   A photograph of two fellows with pretty good balance, taken by the author in China.

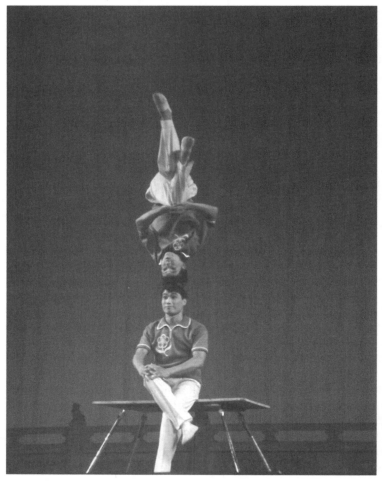

BOX 4.1   Best Practice for an Exercise Program With Older Adults

Leading exercise and aging specialists list five key practices in order for exercise programs to be effective with older adults (Cress et al., 2005). The key practices are: (1) Implement a multidimensional program that includes endurance, strength, balance, and flexibility training. (2) Utilize principles of behavior change, including social support, self-efficacy, active choices, health contracts, assurance of safety, and positive reinforcement. (3) Manage risk by beginning at a low intensity level and gradually increasing to a moderate intensity level. (4) Have an emergency procedure plan in place. (5) Monitor aerobic and strength-building intensity to ensure motivation and to encourage progression.

Chances are quite good that the exercise programs for older adults in your local community fall short of this model. Perhaps an alternative set of criteria can be useful: (1) Is it safe? (2) Is it fun? If yes to both, it may not be a "best practice," but it is certainly good enough for promoting health.

OTHER EXERCISES

Power yoga (an Americanized version of *astanga* yoga) is a blend of flexibility and strength building that has become popular mostly in New York and California. It was introduced into America by the aptly named Beryl *Bender* Birch (1995). Power yoga differs from traditional stretching programs, which encourage relaxation into a pose while stretching, in that proponents advocate for isometrically tensing specific muscles while relaxing the opposing muscles. *Vinyasakrama* is another yoga variant that blends flexibility with aerobics instead of strength building. Rather than holding postures for a long time, students do a series of yoga movements without pause, synchronized with deep yoga breathing.

According to Andrew Weil, there is also *disco yoga*, *tribal yoga* (to the beat of African drums), *aqua yoga*, and *iron yoga* (with light hand weights). As blasphemous as it may seem (or is), there are also *yoga competitions* in which participants are judged on the precision, appearance, and grace of their movements. Finally, there are hybrids like *Yogilates*, a blend of yoga and *Pilates*. Pilates (pronounced pi-LA-tees) is a technique that uses specially made exercise equipment with pulleys and springs to stretch and to strengthen your midsection. Trained instructors guide you through breathing exercises and a routine to help you move in a balanced way. To find a Pilates instructor in your city, call 800-474-5283.

The *Alexander technique* also attempts to promote balance and to retrain your body to carry itself properly, with particular attention to head, neck, and spine alignment. The technique combines good posture with simple movements to reduce muscle tension. To see if there is a program near you, call 800-473-0620. The *Feldenkrais method* is another alternative to train your body to move with efficiency and ease. A trained practitioner gently manipulates your muscles and joints to find the most comfortable ways to use your body. For more information, call 800-775-2118.

The following are two programs that emphasize muscle toning and stretching:

1. *The Sit and Be Fit program.* Developed by a registered nurse, Mary Ann Wilson, the program has been shown on public television for many years. If a program is not televised in your area, you can purchase a videotape for a general audience of older adults, or for persons with specific health problems—arthritis, stroke, osteoporosis, Parkinson's, multiple sclerosis, or COPD. Contact Ms. Wilson at 509-448-9438; or Sit and Be Fit, P.O. Box 8033, Spokane, WA, 99203-0033; or www.sitandbefit.org
2. *Body Recall program.* Dorothy Chrisman began her classes for persons age 50 and older more than 30 years ago. For more information about the program, the location of classes around the country, teacher certification, or the Body Recall manual, contact Ms. Chrisman at Body Recall, Box 412, Berea, KY 40403; or www.bodyrecall.org

Swimming may be a particularly relevant exercise for older adults, especially those with joint problems such as arthritis of the knee or hip. Swimming helps attain and preserve stamina and flexibility, as well as cardiac and respiratory function. There are more than 10 million residential pools and 300,000 public pools in the United States, but that does not necessarily mean they are conveniently located or affordable to every older adult.

One small study with 43 older persons reported that swimming three or four times a week lowered systolic blood pressure (Nualnim et al., 2012). Over a 3-month period, the swimmers reduced their systolic blood pressure 9 points on average in contrast to no change in the relaxation control group.

For those readers who have found no modality of exercise to their liking, there is always the promise of the work being done by Dr. Sanders Williams, dean of the Duke

University School of Medicine. Dr. Williams is working on chemical pathways that muscle cells use to build strength and endurance. This could lead to the development of a medication that will let people get the health benefits of regular exercise by just taking a pill! If you run out of patience waiting for this pill, try obtaining one of the products that received one of these patent numbers:

#6,024,678: *Vacuum cleaner leg exerciser.* This invention consists of shoes with bellows, so that when you walk around your house you create suction that pulls dirt into a cleaning wand and then into a tank strapped on your back.

#6,042,508: *Remote-control dumbbell.* This remote is built into a contoured weight that you lift up and down to switch television stations. It also calculates your pulse rate.

#5,984,841: *Shower step master.* This device makes you pedal in order to shower, with elastic bands that provide resistance. A side benefit is that you won't even know when you are sweating.

#7,037,243: *Cordless jump-rope.* A jump-rope minus the rope; all that's left is two handles (with moving weights inside that simulate the feel of a rope moving) and a pretend rope. The truly lazy can pretend to jump over the pretend rope.

Special thanks to WellnessLetter.com for alerting me about the first three of these patented gems. Regarding the cordless jump-rope, if you have your own silly idea to patent and want help, contact www.patentsilly.com.

Different Strokes for Different Folks

As the following chart of five exercise activities indicates, there is considerable variation in the types of benefits that can accrue, suggesting the importance of engaging in a balanced approach to exercise (Table 4.3). It should be noted that each of the exercises below can be performed in such a way as to improve its ranking in each of the three categories (e.g., power yoga increases strength, high-repetition weight lifting improves endurance, etc.).

THE ACTIVITY PYRAMID

Most people have heard of the USDA's food guide pyramid (see Chapter 5, "Nutrition and Weight Management"). Now several organizations have developed an *activity* version of a pyramid. Not having seen one that I like without modification, I offer my contribution in Figure 4.7.

Sedentary behaviors—like eating the junk food at the top of the food pyramid—should be done sparingly. It is acceptable to watch television and play computer games,

TABLE 4.3 Different Exercises and Benefits

EXERCISE	ENDURANCE	STRENGTH	FLEXIBILITY
Swimming	High	Low	Medium
Brisk walking/jogging	High	Low	Low
Yoga	Low	Low	High
Tai Chi	Medium	Medium	Medium
Weight lifting	Medium	High	Low

FIGURE 4.7   Activity pyramid.

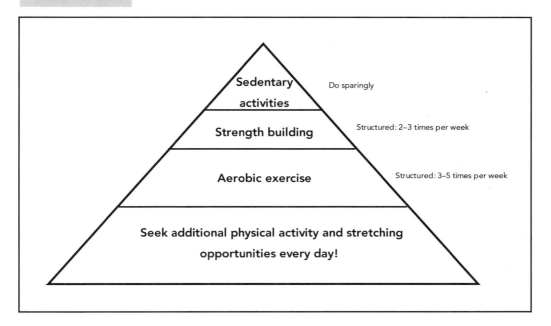

Sedentary activities — Do sparingly

Strength building — Structured: 2–3 times per week

Aerobic exercise — Structured: 3–5 times per week

Seek additional physical activity and stretching opportunities every day!

and even to eat junk food while doing it, but doing it to excess is dangerous to your health. On the other hand, slothfulness every now and then is an excellent antidote for wellness self-righteousness.

Two to three "servings" of structured strength-building exercises per week are recommended. Medium or vigorous aerobic intensity, such as jogging and some recreational activities, is recommended three or four times a week for those who have left the ranks of the sedentary far behind. Light to moderate exercise, such as brisk walking, stretching, and finding additional activity bouts in the course of the day, can be done *every* day.

Incorporating additional activity bouts into your everyday routine can be done in a variety of ways. Park your car farther away from the store, use stairs instead of escalators, walk the dog, work in your garden, and, perhaps most torturous of all, do not use the remote control when watching television—and change channels frequently.

People who are sedentary need to focus their attention on the base of the pyramid. The everyday activity at the base of the pyramid is different from the exercises above it. Activity can be defined as any body movement produced by skeletal muscles that results in energy expenditure. It is in the lower sector of the pyramid that we can emphasize the healthy pleasures of spontaneity and enjoyment. Activities can be enjoyable, for instance, when they are turned into social occasions with family and friends. Or you can take advantage of spontaneity in the lower sector of the pyramid by stepping up the intensity level of, say, vacuuming. You not only get your housecleaning done, but you also obtain a free bout of exercise in your home using your vacuum cleaner (or your duster, mop, or other household exercise tool).

Exercise, on the other hand, is planned, structured, and emphasizes repetitive body movement. It is in these upper sectors of the pyramid where maintaining a routine, rather than spontaneity, is desirable. Routine exercise can be enjoyable too, though for me, the highlight is when I am done with it and can savor the way my body feels for several hours afterward.

ARTHRITIS: A BARRIER TO EXERCISE AND ACTIVITY

This story, entitled "The Joys of Aging," has been circulating anonymously for years. It goes like this: "I have become quite a frivolous old gal. I'm seeing five gentlemen every day. As soon as I awake, Will Power helps me get out of bed. When he leaves, I go see John. Then Charley Horse comes along, and when he is here, he takes a lot of my attention. When he leaves, Arthur Ritis shows up and stays the rest of the day. He doesn't like to stay in one place very long, so he takes me from joint to joint. After such a busy day, I'm really tired and ready to go to bed with Ben Gay. What a day!"

One of the major barriers to performing resistance training, yoga, calisthenics, aerobics, and other types of exercise is arthritic stiffness and pain. The 2011 Profile of Older Americans reported that half of Americans over age 65 suffered from arthritis. The estimates of CDC and other government agencies are even higher I suppose, dependent on how you define "suffer from." The likelihood of arthritis rises with age.

Osteoarthritis (degenerative joint disease), the most common type found among older people, ranges in intensity from occasional stiffness and joint pain to disability. This disease is affected by genetics, obesity, injuries, and overuse of joint movement. Rheumatoid arthritis is less common, but can be more disabling. Although the cause is unknown, scientists believe it may result from a breakdown in the immune system.

Many people with arthritis think that any type of exercise will be uncomfortable—that is, cause joint or muscle pain or swelling of the extremities—or be downright harmful and lead to decreased functional abilities. These indicators of exercise intolerance, however, will typically not take place if exercise is performed properly. In fact, it is more likely that the joints will stiffen, the muscles will weaken, and the ability to function will decline if regular flexibility exercises are *not* performed.

To counteract arthritic stiffness, it may be necessary to briefly engage in flexibility exercises several times a day. It is also helpful to engage in strength-building exercise to strengthen the muscles that surround and support the joints and to force lubricating fluid into the cartilage that helps keep it nourished and healthy. The advice of a physical therapist, occupational therapist, or nurse can be especially helpful when developing an individualized exercise program that balances exercise and rest. One way to minimize aches and pains is to relax joints and muscles prior to exercise by applying heat (or soaking in a warm bath), or to gently massage muscles or apply ice packs. Weight control can also help keep unnecessary stress from joints.

Another technique for conquering the challenge of aches and pains in order to exercise is to choose a time of day when one is subject to the least amount of discomfort, stiffness, and fatigue. People who are on medication may find that their optimal time coincides with the period during which their medicine is having its maximum effect. Many persons with arthritis depend on anti-inflammatory drugs to alleviate aches and pains and to allow them to exercise.

Many others hold out hope for a miracle medication that will not only alleviate their arthritic pain, but also reverse the disease process. One prospect in this regard, discovered by the public more than 15 years ago, coincided with the publication of *The Arthritis Cure* (Theodosakis, 1997). The book touted two supplements, *glucosamine* and *chondroitin sulfate*, to stimulate the growth of cartilage and keep it from wearing down. Although many arthritis sufferers are already convinced of the benefit of these supplements, a multicenter, randomized controlled trial was equivocal, at best, on these two supplements.

Over 1,500 patients with symptomatic knee osteoarthritis were randomly assigned to glucosamine and chondroitin (individually and in combination) or to placebo, with no significant differences in the reduction of knee pain between groups (Clegg et al., 2006). A subgroup of patients with moderate to severe knee pain did receive benefit from the combination of supplements, but subgroup analysis is unreliable and can only be considered exploratory.

Another option for avoiding arthritic discomfort is finding a more appropriate exercise routine, such as *water aerobics*. An older adult who believes she is aggravating an arthritic knee during her walking program may find an aquatic program more desirable than a land-based exercise program. Water provides buoyancy, and can relieve some of the stress and strain of other exercise, where gravity and weight are greater influences. Body weight in water is less than 10% of its weight on the ground. Also, if the water is sufficiently warm it will allow greater range of motion since muscles stretch better when they are warm.

A free brochure from the Arthritis Foundation explains how to set safe exercise limits and includes tips for easing into exercises, such as taking a warm shower before engaging in exercise in order to loosen up. To obtain one, contact the foundation at 800-283-7800, or through its website, www.arthritis.org.

Other Barriers and Cautions

There are several *barriers to exercise* besides arthritis and the belief that exercise will be painful, unenjoyable, and perhaps even harmful. Some older adults engage in a level of exercise that is inadequate or that lacks the proper intensity to meet their needs, yet are under the mistaken belief that they are sufficiently active. Others have a problem with overexuberance, tackling an exercise program too strenuously and too quickly, and suffer the consequences of injury.

It is necessary to begin and end an exercise routine with adequate *warm-up* and *cool-down* periods consisting of gentle aerobics. It is important that the warm-up period begin with aerobics (walking, or a slow version of the exercise to be engaged in) and not stretching, as the latter can create damage to the muscles and joints if the body temperature is not warmed up first. The cool-down period prevents blood from pooling in lower muscles, which reduces blood flow to the heart and brain and can cause faintness or worse. Cooling down may also prevent muscle stiffness and soreness by restretching muscles that are shortened during exercise. One meta-analysis of randomized research trials, however, reported no significant effect of stretching on either muscle soreness or injury (Herbert & Gabriel, 2002).

Another inhibitor of activity is the *fear of falling*. More than one third of community-dwelling elderly persons fall each year. The potential for falling has been used as a justification for physical restraints in the nursing home. Fear of falling, reinforced by a caregiving spouse, may be a significant barrier to exercising. Some risk may have to be tolerated; however, the risk may be reduced by exercising in a seated or lying position or by a change in medication.

Medication usage can contribute to falling. Medications may require that exercise participants modify their exercise routine by decreasing the duration and intensity of an exercise, increasing fluid intake, or forgoing exercise for a period of time. One should be alert for dizziness, faintness, and fatigue that may result from a wide variety of medications, especially ones that belong in these categories: antiarthritic, psychotropic, antihypertensive, antiarrhythmic, antiparkinsonism, antihistamine, decongestant, and barbiturates.

To treat injury to a muscle or ligament in the form of a strain, sprain, or tear, and keep it from becoming worse, the most commonly recommended guideline is the acronym RICE, which stands for rest, ice, compression, and elevation. Rest the injured area immediately to cut down on blood circulation to that part of the body. Apply ice immediately, which shrinks blood vessels and reduces swelling. Compress the injured area with an elastic bandage or cloth to also help reduce swelling. Elevate the damaged part to a level higher than the heart.

Other barriers to exercise may include lack of transportation to an exercise facility, limited financial resources for joining a program, medical concerns, lack of access to consultation with a health professional, lethargy, inability to identify a pleasurable exercise that can sustain one's interest over time, and lack of time. Creative problem solving can overcome most barriers.

Some health professionals erroneously believe that older adults have considerably more discretionary time than younger adults. A perceived lack of time, however, is as likely to be a problem among older adults as among younger adults. In fact, a common response among older adults is that they lack the time for exercise because they provide care for a family member who is frail. Other older adults may also have a busy schedule that consists of sedentary hobbies, family events, and volunteer obligations.

In general, exercise is a safe activity. Research on exercise in the elderly rarely reports serious cardiovascular or musculoskeletal complications in any published trials. This is not to suggest that exercise is hazard-free. Walkers and joggers often share a path with persons on bicycles, and rare collisions do occur. Overexertion in hot weather can lead to heat exhaustion (with symptoms of dizziness and a rapid or weak pulse) or potentially fatal heat strokes. High humidity is dangerous because the air is saturated with moisture, which prevents heat from leaving the body through perspiration.

Occasionally, older persons with unsuspected heart problems embark on exercise programs. To avoid this problem, individuals may consider an *exercise stress test* prior to beginning an exercise program. This test—consisting of treadmills, cycle ergometers, and steps—is designed to identify individuals without symptoms who may be at high risk of suffering a medical complication during exercise because of undetected heart disease. A review of several studies on stress tests, however, found that they are expensive, of unproven benefit to low-risk adults without symptoms, and may serve as a deterrent to individuals who delay (perhaps permanently) exercise until they get one (Firestone, 2000).

The U.S. Preventive Services Task Force does not recommend stress testing in low-risk adults who do not have symptoms of heart disease. Individuals with known or suspected heart disease, however, should consider the test. Abnormal responses to a stress test may consist of a failure of the blood pressure level to increase as work intensity increases, a slow recovery of ventilation and heart rate, an excessive shortness of breath, chest pain, or electrocardiogram changes such as dysrhythmias. There are, however, an unusually high percentage of false positives (abnormal stress test results for people who can exercise) and false negatives (normal results for persons who should not exercise). False-positive tests can lead to additional psychological stress and invasive tests; false-negative tests can lead to delayed treatment.

SELECTED TOPICS

How to Respond to an Excuse

AARP's Staying Healthy After Fifty program (SHAF; now defunct) listed the most common excuses for not exercising: fatigue, fear of heart attack or hypertension, trouble catching breath, need to relax, too old, bad back, and arthritis. Each excuse was examined during the SHAF program and exposed as a myth or a general misunderstanding that can keep an older adult inactive.

Some examples of responses to these excuses are, respectively: improved strength makes daily tasks easier and less tiring; an exercised heart is stronger, works easier, and can lower blood pressure; heart, lungs, and muscles become more efficient through exercise and may make breathing easier; exercise can help relaxation; it is never too late to exercise—even nonagenarians benefit; bad backs are commonly caused by inadequate exercise, improper lifting, and poor posture; and exercise can alleviate the pain and stiffness of arthritis.

Benefits

A negative attitude also can be a barrier to exercise. When motivating someone to exercise, it is important to shift the emphasis from the negative—what will happen if you do not exercise—to the positive—how you will benefit if you do. The SHAF program listed benefits of exercise that are likely to motivate old and young alike: having fun; sleeping better; feeling more energetic; controlling body weight; feeling more relaxed; feeling stronger; increased joint flexibility; maintaining an independent lifestyle; improving heart, arteries, and lungs; new social contacts; improved morale and confidence; and enhanced agility and mobility.

> **Question:** Role play with a partner. Can you counter every excuse that your partner offers for not exercising by suggesting an idea that will encourage your partner to exercise?

If these benefits are not appealing, the humorist Erma Bombeck offered a particularly unique advantage to those who exercise: "The only reason I would take up jogging is so that I can hear heavy breathing again."

Health Club, Home, or Religious Setting

Membership in health clubs has risen steadily over the past two decades in the United States. About 25% of health club members are over age 55, with baby boomers the fastest-growing segment of the health club population. Bally Total Fitness centers and Gold's Gyms include older adults in their advertisements for new members. Curves, which targets middle-aged, female fitness novices, developed a 30-minute circuit workout that led to the launching of 8,000 health clubs worldwide.

There are many advantages to membership in a health club. Most clubs offer at least one free session from a qualified trainer as part of the membership fee. Weight machines are excellent for beginners because they are easy to use, and they reduce injury by controlling your form and preventing a weight from falling on you. Most health clubs arrange machines in a logical order to promote a balanced approach to strength building. Free weights are offered as an alternative; and though more likely to produce injury, they involve stabilizing muscles that help you progress faster. Finally, aerobic and yoga classes are commonly offered at health facilities.

The downside is that fees often range from $600 to $2,000 a year per individual. The more resources in the fitness facility and the greater your access to them, the higher the fee. Also, many older adults may feel shy or inadequate in a health club with a preponderance of young, fit participants. Finally, if motivation is marginal, sometimes all it takes is the prospect of a 15-minute drive, or longer, to the health facility to put you off.

Before joining a health club, it is wise to visit more than one, to go the same time of day that you intend to exercise, determine whether the classes are reasonable for your level of fitness, and find out whether a staff person is certified by a nationally recognized senior fitness organization to work with people who have age-related health issues. Additional questions for assessing whether the health club is age-friendly or suitable to beginners, are as follows:

1. If there is music, is it acceptable to you and set at a reasonable level?
2. Are the display panels on the equipment easy to read, change, and understand?
3. Do the treadmills start slowly, at 0.5 mph?
4. Are there recumbent bikes, and do they have comfortable seats?
5. Does the strength-building equipment have low starting resistance, no more than 5 pounds?

Exercising in the home setting, on the other hand, is as convenient as it gets. You do not have to worry about how you look, and you do not have to adapt to other people's musical tastes. The investment is a one-time expense consisting of weights, weight machine, treadmill, stair stepper, or other preferred equipment. If money is a barrier, an excellent exercise routine can be devised from using the floor, wall, chair, and your own body weight; or using household items as weights; or using a jump rope in a way that allows for a low- or medium-intensity level.

The downside is that you may be distracted by a ringing telephone, the television set, or a family member. You may also lack the peer support of an aerobics class or role models doing strength building. Home exercise equipment typically does not include the variety found in a health club.

If you are going to buy a piece of exercise equipment for your home, consider the low-tech treadmill. One study reported that the walking or jogging machine outperforms a rowing machine, a cross-country skiing simulator, a stationary bicycle, and a stair stepper when it comes to burning calories (Zeni, Hoffman, & Clifford, 1996). Regardless of the home exercise equipment you purchase, check a consumer magazine for recommendations; try out the equipment before you buy; and remember that flimsy, uncomfortable, or noisy equipment is likely to wind up as a clothes rack.

An interesting alternative to the health club or home setting is the faith-based fitness movement. Synagogues and churches are hosting a growing number of fitness programs. A fitness and nutrition program called *First Place* has been tried in 12,000 churches. Faith-based fitness is more likely to focus on fellowship and community, and less likely to be competitive or appearance-conscious. Sometimes an exercise session may end with a meditation or a prayer. Whether religious or not, however, two messages can easily apply to all exercisers regardless of setting: treat your body as your temple, and focus on both inner and outer health.

Two websites that relate to exercise and religious institutions are (1) www.beliefnet .com—which offers spiritually oriented information on fitness for many faiths; and (2) www.jcca.org which lists Jewish Community Centers that provide fitness programs and equipment.

Personal Trainer

Is it worth $85 an hour for a *personal trainer*? If you can afford it, the answer is probably yes, both in terms of expertise and motivation. Want to make sure that your instructor is certified? Ask about his or her certification and call to check on his or her credentials. Most qualified trainers have been certified by a national fitness organization, such as the following:

American College of Sports Medicine, 317-637-920
National Strength and Conditioning Association, 800-815-682
American Council on Exercise, 800-825-363
Aerobics and Fitness Association of America, 800-446-232
International Association of Fitness Professionals, 800-999-4332
Cooper Institute for Aerobics Research, 972-341-3200

Most exercise certifications are not specific for leading exercises with older adults. Make sure that the organization and instructors are experienced with working with older persons, and that the content of the training program addresses the needs and preferences of older adults.

There are also a number of online fitness trainers that match your personal health statistics and goals with a predesigned training program. Some sites send the user a daily e-mail prescribing that day's exercises; others display an exercise regimen on a personal monthly calendar that can be accessed by smart phone. Online sites produced by a single trainer tend to be less sophisticated and may merely consist of a training plan with illustrated exercises that are sent to you.

One study reported on older participants who received an instructional session and a hand-held computer that was programmed to monitor their physical activity levels twice per day, and provide them with daily and weekly individualized feedback, goal setting, and support. In comparison to a control group that received age-appropriate educational materials on physical activity, the treatment group of previously underactive adults reported significantly greater physical activity levels (King et al., 2008).

Wii-Hab for Degenerative Diseases

When Nintendo's Wii gaming system was released in November 2006, more than 19 million consoles were sold over the next 2 years in the United States alone. Unlike traditional video game systems controlled by a player's thumbs and fingers, Wii games respond to a player's whole body movement.

The Wii games—referred to by some therapists as *Wiihabilitation*—appeal to not only young and old alike but to therapists working with clients with Parkinson's disease and other degenerative diseases. Players wave a wireless controller that directs the actions of animated athletes on a screen. The Wii features simulated movements such as swinging a tennis racket, throwing a bowling ball, or engaging in golf, baseball, or boxing. Some of the movements are similar to traditional therapy exercises.

Significant improvements in rigidity, fine motor skills, energy level, endurance, reflexes, balance, and coordination have been recorded (Hinely, 2009). Although studies have focused on older adults in nursing homes, senior centers, and retirement communities, they tend to be clinical case studies rather than more rigorous random assignment to treatment or control group (Clark & Kraemer, 2009).

Eighteen months after the Wii gaming system was released, in May 2008, Nintendo followed up with the release of the Wii Fit system, with 40 exercise-oriented games such as yoga, ski-jumping, and hula hooping. Participants reported having a great deal of fun on their own or with others, as many of the games accommodate several players at a time. The Wii games are increasingly being located in both rehabilitation centers and in retirement communities.

Absence of the Health Educator in the Clinic Setting

The percentage of active older adults would likely increase if physicians were more inclined to recommend the health benefits of exercise to clients. A Harris poll reported that 85% of adult respondents believe a physician's recommendation would help motivate them to engage in regular exercise.

Yet over the past quarter century, physicians have not been so inclined. In 1983 less than half of the primary care physicians surveyed reported routinely asking patients about their exercise habits (Wechsler, Levine, Idelson, Rohman, & Taylor, 1983). A few years later, results from seven surveys of primary care physicians cited that an estimated 30% of all sedentary patients received counseling about exercise (Lewis, 1988). In 1999 a survey of 6,000 older adults 50 and older reported that only half of the respondents said their doctor asked about their level of physical activity or exercise during any of their medical checkups over the past year (Kruger et al., 2002). Perhaps due to lower expectations, physicians are even less likely to ask patients age 65 and over to change a health behavior than their younger patients (Centers for Disease Control and Prevention, 2002; Callahan et al., 2000).

The barriers to physicians counseling older patients include a lack of time, training, teaching materials, knowledge, reimbursement, and confidence in getting compliance from their patients. Perhaps some of these barriers can be avoided by using other health professionals in the office. There have been examples of nurses being effective with reaching out to patients and encouraging them to exercise. Nurses report that merely posting a sign by the office elevator giving directions to the nearest stairs is a good way to promote physical activity. Other nurses have been creative with implementing exercise programs for even the most physically and mentally compromised individuals (Colangelo, Stillman, Kessler-Fogil, & Kessler-Hartnett, 1997).

A trained receptionist can distribute exercise materials to patients, answer questions, and even follow up on whether patients are pursuing exercise goals and to answer additional questions and offer further encouragement. Perhaps the ideal solution for health promotion is for each clinic with a sufficient number of patients to hire a health educator, a cost that can be shared among providers (and justified by the goodwill and additional referrals this will generate). A more fiscally conservative approach would be to require patients who accept the services of a health educator to bear some or all of the costs involved.

A Farewell to Jack

Jack LaLanne, the father of the fitness movement, died at the age of 96 in 2011. He started working out with weights in 1936 when it was an oddity. Shortly thereafter, he opened the first fitness facility in an old office building in Oakland, California. He had limited business as people at the time thought there was a risk of heart attack with the use of weights. Things began to change with *The Jack LaLanne Show*, which made its debut in 1951 on television in the San Francisco area. His strength-building and aerobics routine quickly reached a national television audience that lasted almost 35 years, with over 3,000 shows.

Jack invented leg-extension and pulley devices, marketed juicers to blend vegetables and fruits, and sold exercise videos and fitness books long before Jane Fonda. At age 60 he swam from Alcatraz Island to Fisherman's Wharf, handcuffed and towing a 1,000-pound boat. At age 70, handcuffed again, he towed 70 boats and 70 people for a mile and a half.

Jack worked out 2 hours a day and his diet was equally rigorous. He maintained his health routine into his 90s, along with his 150-pound frame on his 5-foot-6 body.

I admired Jack LaLanne and his unbelievable fitness and eating routine, and appreciated the sentiment that he expressed: He hated to work out, but loved the results. I have to confess, though, when I saw him on television, he was a turn-off, a hectoring, badgering, guilt-inducing presence. Eventually, I learned for myself how to tolerate an exercise routine and loved the moment I stopped each day and could then start to feel good, a feeling that lasts the rest of the day.

It was Jack LaLanne, though, who got the ball rolling for the American fitness movement.

5

●●●●●○

NUTRITION AND WEIGHT MANAGEMENT

National Weight Control Registry   ten tips

body composition   diet drugs

diets   emotional distress

bariatric surgery   competitive eating

● ● ● ● Learning Objectives

- Evaluate the food guide pyramids, MyPlate, and the Nutrition Bull's-Eye
- Contrast nutrients and nutritionism
- Distinguish among fats
- Discuss the Mediterranean diet and its consequences
- Differentiate HDL, LDL, and the ratio of total cholesterol over HDL
- Evaluate the National Cholesterol Education Program guidelines
- Contrast complex and simple carbohydrates
- Explain the importance of fiber in the diet
- Analyze the consequences of added sugar to food and drink products
- Explain why socioeconomic status is related to obesity
- Examine the role of protein in the diet
- Explain the importance of hydration in older adults
- Identify the vitamins and minerals that have age-based recommendations
- Identify the clinical manifestations of nutritional deficiencies
- Analyze the influence of sodium on the blood pressure of older adults
- Examine calcium and vitamin D supplementation for older adults
- Summarize the federal legislation that regulates nutrition labels
- Describe the food rating systems
- Identify the risk factors for malnutrition
- Identify the relevance of boomers for organic food consumption
- Explain the consequences of fast food and junk food
- Identify nutritional consequences of sensory decline with aging
- Identify the signs of nutritional quackery
- List the advocacy accomplishments of the Center for Science in the Public Interest
- Analyze weight-gain trends in America over the past 40 years
- Examine weight gain over the life cycle
- Calculate body mass index and waist-to-hip ratio
- Examine the relationship between overweight and obesity, and morbidity and mortality
- Differentiate the contributions of genetics, lifestyle, and environment toward weight gain
- Identify environmental changes in response to obesity in America

- Critically evaluate whether we should gain weight with age
- Identify four measures of body composition
- Examine the influence of sex and aging on body composition
- Compare the effectiveness of a variety of weight-loss programs
- Describe bariatric surgery and its coverage by Medicare
- Summarize Medicare coverage for weight-loss counseling
- Identify and describe 10 tips for weight loss and maintenance
- Analyze the effectiveness of diet drugs
- Explain the impact of emotional distress and support on eating patterns
- Discuss competitive eating and its significance, if any

A dietitian was making a presentation to a group of older adults at a senior citizens center. She began her talk by asking, "Over the long term, what is the single worst food that you can eat?" Immediately, an older woman in the front of the audience stood up and declared, "Wedding cake!" She probably was not referring to the calories.

Older adults may have a sense of humor about their eating habits, but they most definitely take the topic seriously as well. National studies have reported that older people were more conscientious about managing their diets than were the middle-aged. A higher percentage of those over age 65 (approximately two thirds) than of those in their 40s (one half) reported trying "a lot" to limit sodium, fat, and sugar; eat enough fiber; lower cholesterol; and consume enough vitamins and minerals.

If older adults are paying more attention to their nutritional habits, one can only speculate that they may be motivated by more immediate feedback (heartburn, constipation, and so forth) or feelings of greater vulnerability (higher risk of impairment from disease and of loss of independence). The next cohort of older adults—today's baby boomers—bring more than motivation to the table. They also bring a higher level of formal education, including a strong interest in health education.

Advertisers are taking notice of the baby boomers reaching older ages. A series of clever television commercials targeted the Kellogg's Frosted Flakes that boomers used to eat when they were kids. Sales of this product increased appreciably as boomers combined their former love of this sugary cereal with appreciation for the statement on the cereal box that proclaimed "This product meets the American Heart Association's (AHA) food criteria for healthy people over age 2 when used as part of a balanced diet."

Apparently, the boomers and AHA are not paying as much attention to the high sugar content on the nutritional label. The criteria for the AHA's stamp of approval include limits on only fat, cholesterol, and sodium content. The AHA does have one more criterion: the willingness of the food manufacturer to pay them for their stamp of approval—$7,500 per product the first year, and $4,500 annually thereafter. Many healthy products made by small manufacturers do not get this stamp because their manufacturers are unwilling to pay the fee.

Middle-aged boomers and older adults are influenced not only by the AHA's stamp of approval, clever advertising, and an interest in reviving earlier eating habits, but also by nutritional content. Sometimes, however, it is difficult to ascertain the nutritional value of food. In 1993, for instance, newspaper headlines and television news announcers proclaimed the importance of bran in the diet, but then reversed those claims when the findings of a single research project with a small sample size indicated that the importance of bran was questionable.

Before the year was out, a new announcement declared, once again, that bran was an important component of the diet. By 1996 several controlled research studies supported the finding that bran and other forms of fiber reduced the risk of colon cancer and heart disease ("End of Debate," 1996). This was followed a few years later by impressive studies that used randomization and large sample populations, and concluded that a high-fiber diet did not reduce colon cancers (Alberts et al., 2000; Michels et al., 2000; Park et al., 2005; Schatzkin et al., 2000). Later studies, though, reported positive results with whole-grain intake and the reduction of cardiovascular disease, diabetes, and increased longevity (Jensen et al., 2006; Kaline, Bornstein, Bergmann, Hauner, & Schwarz, 2007; Sahyoun, Jacques, Zhang, Juan, & McKeown, 2006).

Although the relationship between fiber and colon cancer remains inconclusive, the evidence is strong that it lowers the risk of heart disease and diabetes (Liebman, 2008). As Liebman notes, "Fiber is back. Foods that never had any (yogurt, ice cream, juice) sometimes have some, and foods that always had some (cereal, bread, pasta) often have more" (p. 3). Though people may believe in fiber again and are seeking more of it, there is no research to support the effectiveness of the latest fad—inserting isolated fiber into food and drink.

The frequent controversies can be confusing and sometimes amusing, but they should not detract from the sensible advice that guides most educated adults. The best recipe for good health is moderation and balance; including ample fiber in the diet; and avoiding excessive fat, sugar, and sodium. (I should probably end this chapter here with this succinct summary statement; but no, I am going on.)

THE FOOD GUIDE PYRAMID AND VARIATIONS

In the spring of 1991, there were health-related headlines questioning whether the long-standing circle that depicted the four food groups should be changed to a pyramid. This was not merely a question of geometrical aesthetics. The equally divided circle implied that the four food groups—bread/cereal, vegetable/fruit, milk, and meat—were equal in value, whereas the pyramid better portrayed the desirable balance of foods we needed to eat, that is, greater space for complex carbohydrates, fruits, and vegetables on the bottom (and in our diet), and less space for fat and protein at the top. At the narrow apex, the sinful fats, oils, and sweets (see Figure 5.1).

However, after 11 years of study that finally led to the launching of the *Food Guide Pyramid* in 1991, the U.S. Department of Agriculture (USDA) quickly dropped the pyramid and returned to the circle. Many accused the agency of caving in to the dairy and meat industries. Supporters of the retraction denied the political pressure, though not very convincingly (Nestle, 2002). They claimed the pyramid concept overlooked the recent surge of low-fat dairy products and leaner meats that made these foods more acceptable. Also, because we still have to worry about anemia, malnutrition, and calcium deficiency, the claim was made that we should not cut back on milk and meat.

One year later, however, the pyramid concept overcame the dairy and meat industry lobbyists and became the accepted figure for good nutrition. Registered dietitians (RD) and nutritionists recommended more daily selections from the bread and cereal group (6 to 11 servings) and the vegetable and fruit group (5 to 9), and fewer daily selections from the milk (2 to 4) and meat (2 to 3) groups than they previously did.

Most Americans, however, fell short of achieving the recommended number of servings in the important bottom parts of the pyramid: grains, cereals, breads, rice, pasta, vegetables, and fruit. These deficiencies occurred despite the fact that it was not

FIGURE 5.1   Food Guide Pyramid.

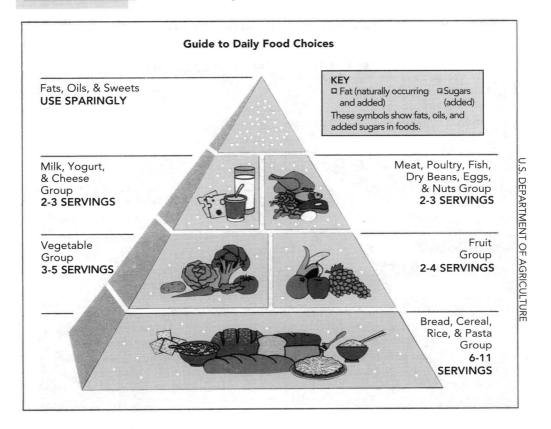

Guide to Daily Food Choices

Fats, Oils, & Sweets
USE SPARINGLY

KEY
◻ Fat (naturally occurring   ▨ Sugars
and added)   (added)
These symbols show fats, oils, and
added sugars in foods.

Milk, Yogurt,
& Cheese
Group
2-3 SERVINGS

Meat, Poultry, Fish,
Dry Beans, Eggs,
& Nuts Group
2-3 SERVINGS

Vegetable
Group
3-5 SERVINGS

Fruit
Group
2-4 SERVINGS

Bread, Cereal,
Rice, & Pasta
Group
**6-11
SERVINGS**

U.S. DEPARTMENT OF AGRICULTURE

as difficult to achieve the recommended number of servings as most adults thought. A pyramid serving is typically smaller than the "average helping." One slice of bread is one pyramid serving; as is one-half cup of cooked cereal, pasta, rice, most vegetables, and cut or canned fruit. The servings on your plate, therefore, often represent more than one serving within a food pyramid group.

Modified Food Guide Pyramids

Although the Food Guide Pyramid became the standard in 1992, appearing in classes in the public school systems and on shopping bags in supermarkets, less than a decade later it began to accumulate considerable criticism. The main problems were that the carbohydrates at the base of the pyramid did not differentiate between the complex and more refined food products; that the protein categories did not differentiate among products that had high saturated fat content, such as red meat, and other products like fish, beans, and nuts; and that the fat category at the top of the pyramid did not differentiate among monounsaturated, polyunsaturated, saturated, and partially hydrogenated fats.

Another line of criticism had to do with not targeting the Food Guide Pyramid to different age groups, particularly to older adults who have been lumped together into the 50+ category by nutritionists for many decades. The first change in the *Modified Food Pyramid for Mature (70+) Adults* (Russell, Rasmussen, & Lichtenstein, 1999) was to add a new foundation to the pyramid—eight 8-ounce glasses of water. Older adults have a reduced thirst mechanism and must consciously think of hydration in order to avoid cardiovascular and kidney complications, as well as constipation. Also, a flag at the top of the pyramid served as a reminder to older adults that many of them were not able to get adequate amounts of calcium, vitamin D, and vitamin B_{12}, and that supplements in these areas may be necessary.

Yet this modified pyramid was clearly not sufficiently revised; in fact, the modifications only occurred at the top and bottom of the Food Guide Pyramid. Instead, the bottom of both the original and modified pyramids should have been exclusively complex carbohydrates, and the refined carbohydrates should have been placed near the top of the pyramid and eaten more sparingly. In the protein categories and at the apex of the pyramid there needs to have been a differentiation among fats, with saturated and partially hydrogenated fats at the top and eaten sparingly, and monounsaturated and polyunsaturated *omega-3* fats lower down. In other words, fish, beans, nuts, vegetable oils, and similar products should be consumed in greater amounts than red meat, butter, refined carbohydrates, and sweets. A pyramid that incorporated some of these changes was the *New Healthy Eating Pyramid* (Willett, 2005).

MyPyramid

The federal government's 2005 Dietary Guidelines for Americans—the guidelines are redrafted every 5 years by the USDA and the Department of Health and Human Services (DHHS)—produced not only a 70-page blueprint for nutritional policy, but a revised Food Guide Pyramid, dubbed *MyPyramid*, and a website, www.mypyramid.gov. The Food Guide Pyramid had not been updated for 13 years, and the website was a new initiative. The entire update had been billed as an interactive food guidance system rather than a one-size-fits-all initiative.

The Food Guide MyPyramid update engendered a whole host of positive and negative reactions; we will start with the positive. The content of the dietary guidelines appears to reflect more of the thinking of the scientific community than in the past, and the industry-representing USDA and its food-industry lobbyists appear to have had less influence than in years past. The guidelines basically encouraged Americans to eat fruits, vegetables, whole grains, and low-fat or fat-free dairy products, and there was much more detail on the consumption of these foods than was provided by previous guidelines.

Fruits and vegetables were increased; salt guidelines were made specific for the first time, limiting it to 1 level teaspoon a day; trans fat was identified, and the advice was to keep it as low as possible; saturated fat limitations were specific, keeping it to 10% of calories or less; cholesterol level was to be less than 300 milligrams; added sugars or sweeteners were discouraged for the first time, particularly in drinks; whole grains were differentiated from the broad category of carbohydrates, and the recommendation was that half the grains should be whole grains.

The old pyramid used ambiguous serving sizes, whereas the new one switched to cups, ounces, and other (allegedly) easier-to-grasp household measures. The old pyramid ignored exercise, whereas the new one advised a half hour a day. School lunches and programs that provided meals to seniors had to follow the guidelines, so these constituencies should receive more whole grains, fruits, and vegetables, and less salty foods and sugary drinks.

Finally, on the good side of the ledger, the website lets people assess their diet and exercise habits. Depending on a person's age, gender, and activity level, the new pyramid comes in 12 versions. The user will get specific dietary recommendations on grain, vegetable, fruit, milk, meat/beans, total fat, saturated fat, cholesterol, sodium, oils, and fats/sugars. Types and duration of each physical activity are assessed as well, with specific recommendations. The website is interesting and informative.

Now for the dark side. There was no budget for mass-media or other educational initiatives, so the overall effort can be considered a token one. While the website is very good, only the most motivated and educated—those least likely to need guidance— are likely to access it. The new pyramid symbol, which many Americans did see, was awful. Perhaps no symbol can adequately capture and disseminate useful information, but this one was confusing. The symbol was a triangle with six colorful vertical stripes of differing widths representing general food groups and a stair-climbing stick figure on its side.

The new pyramid image was cryptic in telling you what to eat. There was no text attached to the pyramid, and you had only a vague idea about what the symbol meant. It was not surprising that the new graphic was created by a public relations firm rather than one with an educational mission.

Bottom line: This 4-year, $2.5 million initiative was a bust and did not last long. Perhaps any effort is doomed to failure, because much of the salt, fat, and sugar that are in processed and prepared foods do not penetrate the consciousness of the consumer, and the food and drink industry spends billions of dollars in advertisements to promote these products.

> **Question:** Review the website, www.mypyramid.gov. What did you learn from it?

MyPlate

Perhaps this time! After two decades of various USDA food pyramid diagrams, on June 2, 2011, the *plate* took over. The MyPlate icon (see www.choosemyplate.gov) depicts a place setting with a plate divided into four food groups unequally divided (See Figure 5.2). The plate is approximately 30% grains, 30% vegetables, 20% fruits, and 20% protein. This is accompanied by a smaller circle representing dairy, such as a glass of low-fat milk or yogurt cup.

If the latest icon does not work, we can at least share the blame with the United Kingdom, Australia, and the American Diabetes Association, which also use plate

FIGURE 5.2   MyPlate.

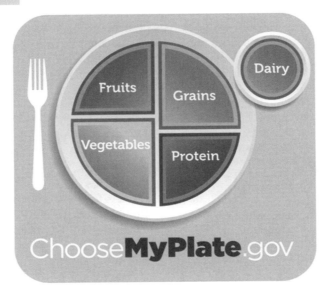

diagrams. A stated improvement are associated slogans that are easy to visualize. For example: "Make half your plate fruits and vegetables." "Make at least half your grains whole." This is easier to follow through on than attempting to measure individual items in ounces or cups.

But guess what? The new icon is also being criticized! Who could have guessed? I suppose anyone who thinks icons are too simplistic to differentiate saturated fats from monounsaturated and polyunsaturated omega-3 fats; beans and fish from red meat; complex carbohydrates from simple carbohydrates … would not be a fan.

Which brings us to an icon that I prefer.

The Personalized Nutrition Bull's-Eye

Nutritionist Covert Bailey may have been the first to develop a replacement for the Food Guide Pyramid, calling it the *nutrition bull's-eye* (Bailey, 1996). The goal of the bull's-eye is for people to consume the nutritious foods that are listed in the center of it. These foods are low in saturated fat, sugar, and sodium, and high in fiber. They include skim milk, nonfat yogurt, most fruits and vegetables, whole grains, beans and legumes, and water-packed tuna. As you move to the foods listed in the rings farther away from the bull's-eye, you eat more saturated fat, sugar, sodium, and low-fiber foods. In the outer ring of the bull's-eye, therefore, are most cheeses, ice cream, butter, whole milk, beef, cake, cookies, potato chips, and mayonnaise.

Unlike the Food Guide Pyramid, Bailey's bull's-eye makes important distinctions *within* food categories. Whole-wheat products, for instance, are in the bull's-eye, whereas products from refined white flour and/or with added sugar are placed in the outer circles. Fresh fruits and vegetables are in the bull's-eye, but juiced vegetables and fruit that lose fiber and/or concentrate sugars are placed in a ring just outside of the bull's-eye. Skim and low-fat milk, nonfat cottage cheese, and part-skim mozzarella are in the center ring, whereas whole milk and most cheeses are in the outer circles of the target.

When used in a one-to-one setting and focused on the specific foods and drinks that an individual consumes, I have found this technique helpful. I offer my own personalized version of a nutrition bull's-eye. In this version, you begin with a blank bull's-eye, and then add food and drink products that you usually consume to each of the rings. The foods and drinks in the bull's-eye (see Figure 5.3) are clearly superior; the second ring is not quite as nutrient dense or lists neutral products that are not particularly harmful or helpful; and the outer ring includes the least nutritious foods and drinks that should be consumed sparingly.

If it provides additional motivation, you can add a scoring system to this technique. One system might consist of the following: Give yourself 10 points for each food or drink you consume in the bull's-eye, 0 points for items in the second ring, and minus 50 points for items in the outer ring.

Question: Create your own nutrition bull's-eye, filling in the foods and drinks that you consume or might consider consuming. Use it for a week to guide your eating choices. Take a list of the food products listed in the center of your bull's-eye to the supermarket with you. Did you find this technique to be helpful?

Add up your points, which I call pennies (real ones), and at the end of each month, if your point count is on the minus side, send that amount of money to the Center for Science in the Public Interest (CSPI, P.O. Box 9661, Washington, DC 20077; www.cspinet. org), an advocacy organization that has had a substantial impact on improving

FIGURE 5.3   The personalized nutrition bull's-eye.

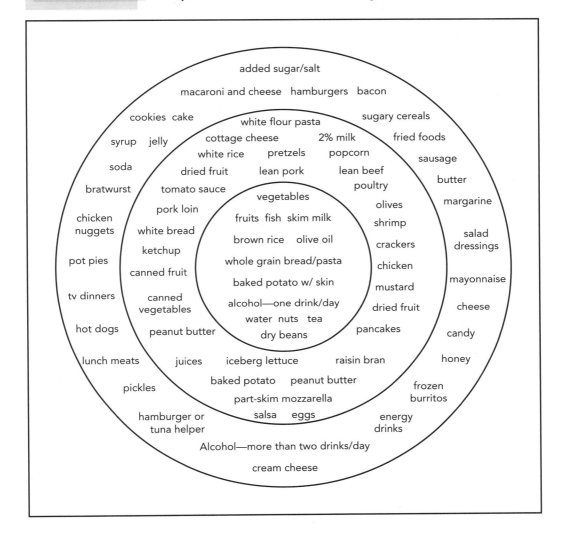

nutrition in America. Because I have not coordinated this effort with the center itself, do not be surprised to find that if your point count is on the plus side, you are unlikely to receive a check from them.

GOOD NUTRITIONAL HABITS

The principles of moderation, selectivity, variety, and balance are widely believed to be the keys to healthy eating. Reduce the size of portions; consume less sugar, saturated fats, and salt; and consume more fiber, including a balance of vegetables, fruits, and whole-grain breads and cereals. Interestingly, these recommendations are not too different from what the USDA first proposed by way of dietary recommendations in 1917 (Nestle, 2002)!

Although educated Americans believe good nutrition is based on these principles, they find them easier to endorse than to practice. The good news is that some progress has been made. The USDA reported that Americans consumed less fat over the past decade. The bad news is that during this time period, people consumed more calories.

Diet is only one component in the development and exacerbation of disease (heredity, environment, medical care, social circumstances, and other lifestyle risk factors also play a part), but eating and drinking habits have been implicated in five of the leading causes of death—heart disease, cancer, stroke, diabetes, and liver disease—as well as in several debilitating disorders like osteoporosis and diverticulosis.

Basic Nutrients

Nutrients are substances in food that build and maintain body tissues and are necessary for bodily function. Nutrition education helps us learn how to provide our bodies with the more than 40 nutrients they need. Good dietary habits help us feel energetic and avoid obesity and other health problems; whereas poor nutrition contributes to feelings of fatigue and weakness, and contributes to health problems.

The basic categories of nutrients are carbohydrates, fats, proteins, fiber, water, vitamins, and minerals. Carbohydrates—sugars (simple carbohydrates) and starches (complex carbohydrates)—are our main source of energy. Fats provide a reserve of energy. Proteins are needed for the growth and repair of tissues. Fiber aids in the regulation of bowel function. Water—the main ingredient in the body—provides the proper environment for the body's processes, which vitamins and minerals help to control and regulate. Large quantities of fats, carbohydrates, protein, fiber, and water, and small quantities of vitamins and minerals, are needed by the body.

Nutritionism Versus Food

One caution needs to be observed before each nutrient is separated and discussed. In his book *In Defense of Food*, Michael Pollan (2008) argues that we have been seduced by *nutritionism*, the belief that what matters most is not the food but the nutrient. This reductionism began several decades ago when members of Congress criticized certain foods, such as meat and whole milk, and the food manufacturers made sure that the culprits were not reelected. Nutrients, however, were allowed to be criticized by congressmen and other government representatives with impunity, just as long as specific foods were not identified. The industry was more agreeable with allowing the consumer to be cautioned about eating less desirable nutrients such as fats and simple carbohydrates in moderation.

Pollan's advice? Let's get back to talking about food and less about nutrients, and in particular let us differentiate between whole fresh foods and processed food products. The former consist primarily of fruits and vegetables, which are even better if they are homegrown or from a nearby farmer's market. The latter have ingredients that are unfamiliar and unpronounceable, and these edible *food like* products have taken over the supermarket, often proudly proclaiming some aspect of nutritionism: This product is low in fat, or has healthier fat, or is high in antioxidants, or is low in carbs, and so forth. Pollan's "Eater's Manifesto" is stated in the first line of his book: *Eat food. Not too much. Mostly plants.*

FAT

Between 1981 and 2000, heart disease and stroke death rates fell by one third for those age 65 and over. Public education was given much of the credit for this decline; Americans not only became more knowledgeable about the risk factors for heart disease—smoking, inactivity, and diet—but also began to do something about them.

The American public became particularly well informed about fats. In 1984, 8% of Americans considered fats their greatest dietary concern; by 1992, 48% designated it their major concern. Many Americans shifted their beliefs from cholesterol being the chief health problem in their diet (when only 20% of the population is very sensitive to cholesterol-rich diets), to fats, which have been implicated in heart disease and other diseases and conditions.

Fat is an essential part of our diet and a major source of energy. It is the most concentrated energy source, with each gram of fat supplying 9 calories to the body. Most Americans consume too much of it. According to data from the USDA's food consumption surveys, the average consumption of fat has always been high, reaching 40% in the 1970s, and declining in 1994 to 33% of total calories, still above the recommended limit of 30%. In recent years, however, fat consumption has leveled off, although the recommendation for daily fat intake has declined among some nutritionists to 25% or even 20%.

Does lowering fat in our diet improve our health? The low-fat-diet trial of the Women's Health Initiative involved a sample of 49,000 women and produced controversial results. Women joined one of two groups: (1) the group that reduced their fat intake to 20% of daily calories, and increased their vegetable and fruit intake to five servings per day and their intake of grains to six servings per day, or (2) the group that continued to eat their normal diet. The healthier diet produced *no* benefit to the hearts of postmenopausal women, did *not* lower the risk of colorectal cancer, and did *not* protect postmenopausal women against breast cancer.

The low-fat diet, however, proved to be difficult for the average woman to follow. The women in the experimental group, despite ongoing support from *nutritional counseling*, were unable to reach the dietary goal of 20% of calories from fat; and, in fact, as the study progressed, their fat intake rose to 29%, not too different from the average diet. Moreover, lowering fat intake, as flawed as the attempt was, did lower breast cancer by 8%, though this was lower than a statistically significant result. Finally, the study measured overall fat, and current research is leaning more toward the replacement of saturated and trans fats with monosaturated and polyunsaturated omega-3 fats as a means for improving health. So, the jury is still out.

Another long-standing, but less controversial, fat issue has been partially hydrogenated fats or trans fatty acids, which for years managed to escape detection on nutritional food labels. Many processed foods contained trans fatty acids, such as crackers, cookies, pastries, deep-fried products, candy, cakes, and TV dinners. The only way to have determined whether this kind of fat was in a food product prior to 2006 was through a chemist in a laboratory. *Trans fats* are solid fats that are created by chemically adding hydrogen atoms to a liquid oil. This hydrogenation process makes the fats artificially hard at room temperature, and helps products last longer on store shelves. It also, however, appears to raise blood cholesterol about as much as saturated fats.

Margarine was considered for a number of years to be a healthy alternative to butter. This belief was compromised, however, when it was discovered that margarine relied heavily on trans fatty acids that made it as least as unhealthy as the saturated fat in butter. The only margarine exception is products such as Promise, which are made without trans fat.

As far back as 1993, the CSPI and other advocacy agencies called for the Food and Drug Administration (FDA) to expose trans fat and add it to the nutrition label. In 2006, 13 years after the CSPI petitioned the FDA to require trans fat on nutrition labels, the FDA finally required it. Just before trans fat had to be listed on the food label in 2006, many food manufacturers chose to eliminate it from their products.

After an initial unsuccessful effort in 2006 by the New York City Board of Health to persuade restaurants to eliminate trans fat voluntarily, the board voted to ban artificial trans fats from all restaurant foods on July 1, 2008. That same month California became the first state to ban trans fats from restaurant food. This type of ban is not without precedent, as Denmark has successfully banned trans fat in restaurant food, and all restaurants—including McDonald's—have complied in that country.

To end on a humorous note (though I recognize that written humor is in the eye of the beholder), the Indiana State Fair banned the sale of products with trans fats in the summer of 2007, though this didn't exactly turn standard state fair cuisine into health food. In fact, added on to the battered Snickers bar, Oreo cookie, and Reese's Peanut Butter Cup was frying oil that was trans-fat free. And in celebration of the trans fats ban was a new product at the Indiana State Fair—deep-fried Pepsi. This new item consisted of Pepsi-based dough, dipped in a batter made with Pepsi and deep-fried for 90 seconds. Outside the booth of this Pepsi concoction was a proudly posted sign (I swear, I saw it with my own eyes): Trans-fat free!

Not All Fats Are Created Equal

The *Mediterranean diet* became popular in America in 1997, as we discovered that the countries along the Mediterranean had among the lowest rates of coronary heart disease and many common cancers found in the Western world. This near-vegetarian diet was high on unrefined grains, potatoes, fruit, vegetables, fish, wine, and olive oil, and low on meat, cheese, refined sugar or flour, butter, and margarine. Although the Mediterranean diet is more expensive than most Western diets (Lopez et al., 2009), research reports that it lowers overall mortality (Knoops et al., 2004; Trichopoulou et al., 2005) and slows cognitive decline (Feart et al., 2009).

A decade later, though, the Mediterranean diet was in full retreat in Greece and other countries along the Mediterranean (Rosenthal, 2008). Two thirds of the children were overweight, and longevity was likely to be reduced in comparison to their parents. The increasing percentage of working mothers and the spread of supermarkets and convenience foods may have accounted for this change. Ironically, while the diet was shrinking in terms of the number of adherents abroad, it was still expanding in the United States. In a large study of Americans, those who followed the Mediterranean diet had significantly lower all-cause mortality rates, especially from heart disease and cancer deaths (Mitrou et al., 2007).

Surprisingly, the diet is not low in fat, with more than 35% of calories coming from it—primarily from olive oil, which consists mostly of monounsaturated fat. Thus, Americans began to extol the virtues of olive oil and other monounsaturated and polyunsaturated fats like canola, safflower, sunflower, corn, sesame, soybean, and peanut oils.

Monounsaturated fats are the best type of fat because they appear to slightly lower low-density lipoprotein (LDL) but leave the high-density lipoprotein (HDL) intact or may even raise it a little (Curb et al., 2000). *Polyunsaturated fats*, such as sunflower, corn, and soybean oils, appear to lower LDL, but may be less desirable because they may slightly lower HDL as well. Not all polyunsaturated fats are created equal.

Omega-6 is abundant in vegetable oils, particularly sunflower, corn, and soybean oils, and is less healthy than *omega-3*, which is found in fish like salmon, and in nuts, green leafy vegetables, tofu, flaxseeds, and canola oil. Unfortunately, more than 90% of the polyunsaturated fats we consume are omega-6 (Dietary fat, 2001).

Saturated fats, solid at room temperature and contained in butter, cheese, and meats, are more damaging than the liquid fats. Saturated fat is converted into LDL, the cholesterol that clogs arteries. It should be noted, however, that *all* fats are a mix of saturated, monounsaturated, and polyunsaturated fatty acids, so even the best fats contain some saturated fat.

Most nutritional experts fall short of suggesting that total fat content is now irrelevant, provided we obtain most of it from monounsaturated and polyunsaturated omega-3 fats. They point out that the Mediterranean-style cooking is healthy not just because it limits saturated fats, but because it relies heavily on vegetables, grains, and beans (de Lorgeril et al., 1999; Trichopoulou et al., 1999). Moreover, the people in the Mediterranean countries have traditionally benefited from being more active than Americans, and more successful at burning off excess fat (Brody, 1998).

CHOLESTEROL

Cholesterol is a lipid—a waxy, white, fatty substance that is manufactured by the liver and supplemented through the diet. Excess cholesterol can cling to the interior walls of the arteries and restrict the flow of blood to the heart; over time, it can narrow the passage enough to cause a heart attack.

Two types of proteins, called lipoproteins, carry cholesterol: LDL and HDL. Researchers believe that LDL carries cholesterol toward the body cells, leading to plaque buildup, and that HDL carries cholesterol away from the cells to the liver, to be further processed and excreted. Saturated fat in the diet increases the LDL lipids in the blood. Exercise and smoking cessation will increase the HDL lipids in the blood. The AHA recommends a total cholesterol level of less than 200 mg, and an HDL of 40 mg or higher in men and 50 mg or higher in women. The recommended ratio between the two is 4.2 or less for middle-aged and older persons.

The implications of the research findings on cholesterol level in *older* adults are still debated due to insufficient evidence determining whether data on middle-age men can be extrapolated to older persons, who have been studied less extensively. Some experts, like P. J. Palumbo, director of clinical nutrition at the Mayo Clinic in Minnesota, endorsed the popular belief of many health professionals that older persons can tolerate a higher level of cholesterol than the general adult population. Other experts, like William Castelli, director of the Framingham Heart Study in Massachusetts, believed that older adults may be even more vulnerable than others to the effects of a high cholesterol level, and the standards should be more, not less, stringent.

The research evidence tilts toward managing cholesterol levels in older adults, and the use of cholesterol-lowering medication for high-risk groups independent of age (Aronow, 2005). It should be noted, though, that few patients in these types of studies were 80 years of age or older (Wilson, 2005).

National Cholesterol Education Program Guidelines

The National Heart, Lung, and Blood Institute launched the *National Cholesterol Education Guidelines* (NCEP) in 1985 and last updated in 2004. Over these two decades the guidelines have become increasingly stringent, with the number of Americans recommended for cholesterol-lowering drugs increasing from 13 million designated under the 1993 guideline update, to 36 million under the 2001 update, to 43 million under the 2004 update.

This tripling of persons recommended for lipid-lowering drugs will help many people avoid heart disease, stroke, and other major vascular events. But it will also financially challenge individual American consumers, even those with insurance, as costs go up as medication usage rises.

The last NCEP guidelines are not only more aggressive, but more complicated as well (see Table 5.1). The guidelines state that *high-risk* patients should aim for a LDL goal of below 100 mg/dL, with an optional goal of below 70 for patients at *very high risk*. *Moderate-risk* patients should aim for below 130 mg/dL, and *lower-risk* patients below 160 mg/dL.

The *major risk factors* are cigarette smoking, hypertension, HDL below 40 mg/dL, family history of premature coronary heart disease, and age (men over 45 and women over 55). Having an HDL score above 60 mg/dL, however, removes one risk factor from the total count. Low risk is zero to one risk factor; moderate risk is two or more risk factors; and high risk is defined as coronary heart disease or its risk equivalent, such as diabetes.

Although exercise and dietary interventions are noted in the revised guidelines, they are dismissed as not having been effectively introduced into the lifestyle of most Americans. Nonetheless, recommendations are made: the reduction of saturated fat below 7% of total calories, cholesterol below 200 mg per day, increased fiber to 10 to 25 g/day, weight reduction, and increased physical activity. A review of the NCEP report, however, revealed limited attention to the lifestyle approach, and when it did focus on lifestyle it provided unrealistic recommendations, such as a daily limit on dietary cholesterol to less than the amount in the yolk of a single large egg. There appears to be a clear bias toward the use of statins and other drugs as the best way to reduce cholesterol levels.

> **Question:** The author expresses several benefits of, and reservations toward, the latest NCEP Guidelines. What is your opinion of the overall value of these guidelines?

A health promotion policy advocate, however, might suggest that part of the estimated $50 billion that is recommended to be spent annually on cholesterol-lowering drugs to an expanding number of people could be better spent on a large-scale research initiative to examine how clinicians can more effectively counsel patients to improve nutrition and exercise habits. Moreover, long-term use of good nutrition and exercise habits do not have adverse side effects, but the same cannot be said of using cholesterol-lowering drugs at earlier and earlier ages, because we do not have research data on adverse effects of long-term usage.

TABLE 5.1 LDL Cholesterol Targets

<100	Optimal for *high-risk* patients
100–129	Optimal for *moderate-risk* patients
130–159	Optimal for *low-risk* patients
160–189	High for all patients
>189	Very high for all patients

CARBOHYDRATES AND FIBER

Carbohydrates are the starches (complex carbohydrates), sugars (simple carbohydrates), and fiber in our diet. Complex carbohydrates are found most commonly in breads, dry beans, potatoes, grains, pasta, carrots, peas, and corn. Many older adults have subscribed for years to the myth that all carbohydrates, especially bread and pasta, are fattening. In fact, when carbohydrates are whole grain, they are moderate in calories and rich in fiber and nutrients.

Grains are the seed-bearing fruits of edible grasses. Each kernel of grain has a nutritionally dense "germ" or seed at its core, and a layer of bran that surrounds the kernel itself. When grains are refined into white flour, white rice, and so forth, a process that began in the 1940s, the bran and germ of the whole-wheat kernel are removed through the milling process, losing fiber, vitamins, and minerals, but not fat content.

The term *whole grain* means that the kernels are unrefined, still containing the germ and the protective bran coating. The germ provides fiber, B vitamins, and vitamin E; the bran contains fiber. The most familiar whole grains are wheat, barley, oats, rye, rice, and corn, and the uncooked grains can be added to boiling water or simmering soup. When whole grains are a regular part of the diet, the risk for heart disease and adult-onset diabetes declines.

However, when grains are ingested exclusively in the form of mashed potatoes, white rice, and other processed foods that have little of their fiber left, the starch converts quickly to sugar. Thus, it is important to pay attention to the nutritional bull's-eye. Just as all fats are not created equal, the same holds true for carbohydrates and other nutrients.

Vegetables and fruits are complex carbohydrates that are low in fat and high in fiber, vitamins, and minerals. The exceptions are items like olives, avocados, salads with high-fat dressing, and vegetables that are fried or seasoned with margarine or butter. Unfortunately, the most popular vegetable is the fried potato, that is, French fries. Not counting the dubious French fry, Americans of all ages tend to eat less than half of the recommended amount of fruits and vegetables. A diet rich in fruits and vegetables protects against cardiovascular disease, cancers, and other morbidities.

Fiber is the indigestible residue of food (e.g., the husk, seeds, skin, stems, and cell walls) that passes through the bowel and is eliminated in the stool. It appears to have a positive effect on cholesterol reduction, though scientists do not know exactly how this works. Fiber is a natural laxative that promotes regularity, adds bulk to stool, absorbs water, and reduces the amount of time that stool is in the bowels. A diet that is high in fiber is especially important in later years, when constipation is likely to be a problem. Among persons age 65 and older, a diet high in fiber will lower the risk of cardiovascular disease. However, only about 5% of American adults follow the National Cancer Institute's recommendation to eat at least 20 grams of fiber a day.

Fiber supplements like Metamucil do not contain the essential nutrients found in high-fiber foods, and their nutritional benefits are questionable. Some older adults rely on laxatives that are costly and, in the long run, self-defeating because they create a "lazy bowel." Although laxatives and supplements are not effective complements to fiber, fluid intake is. In fact, fiber needs fluid to be effective, and about 64 ounces of water daily is recommended.

About half of the American diet consists of carbohydrates, and many nutritionists recommend that this be increased to 55% to 60%. The key, of course, is to focus on complex carbohydrates.

SUGAR

Sugars (also referred to as fructose, glucose, dextrose, maltose, lactose, honey, syrup, molasses, etc.) are carbohydrates. Some are naturally present in nutritious foods, such as fruit and milk, but a good many are added to foods. Added sugar provides calories that have no nutritional value (i.e., empty calories) while increasing the likelihood of dental caries. Natural sugar in fruit, vegetables, and dairy products differs from added sugar in that it is accompanied by vitamins, minerals, and fiber.

Much of the sugar we ingest is hidden: almost one third of Heinz tomato ketchup and Wish-Bone Russian salad dressing is sugar. Sugar also makes up two thirds of Coffee-mate nondairy creamer; one half of Shake 'n Bake; and a high percentage of processed soups, spaghetti sauces, frozen dinners, yogurts, and breads.

The American population consumes more than double the recommended amount of sugar, and the amount of sugar consumed by the public has steadily increased over the past 25 years. The movement toward low-fat foods worsened the trend, as many of the products used sweeteners to make up for the lost fat flavor. Many low-fat foods, therefore, result in only a small caloric reduction—or no caloric reduction—from their full-fat counterparts.

The CSPI petitioned the FDA to change nutrition labels so that sugar can also be included in the percentage of the daily value it represents. At the present time, however, it is listed in grams as a subset of carbohydrates, but it is exempted from the percentage-of-daily-value category, which would be more useful to consumers. A nutritionally sound diet should probably derive no more than 10% of its calories from added sugar, a percentage that is almost half of what is consumed by the average American.

Recommendations for added sugar range from 8% of calories by the CSPI, to up to 25% of calories by the Institute of Medicine (IOM) as part of their September 5, 2002, report (www.iom.edu). The high end of the IOM's more liberal recommendation is obviously not meant for the average American, given that the panel was especially concerned about the rapidly rising number of people who are overweight or obese.

PROTEIN

Proteins form antibodies, which help the body resist disease and enable the growth and repair of body cells—organs, muscles, skin, bones, blood, and hair. Amino acids, the units from which proteins are constructed, are the end products of protein digestion. Complete protein foods contain, in proper amounts for adults, eight essential amino acids that must be available for the body to properly synthesize protein. Fish, dairy products, and eggs—complete protein foods— contain all the essential amino acids.

Proteins obtained from vegetables are low in some of the essential amino acids. Previously, it was believed that protein complementing needed to occur within a *single* vegetarian meal, but that theory has been discredited. Moreover, proteins obtained from vegetable intake may have the added benefit of decreasing bone loss and the risk of hip fracture more than proteins obtained from meat and cheese (Sellmeyer, Stone, Sebastian, & Cummings, 2001). The theory behind this research is that, unlike plant protein, animal protein produces an overflow of sulfuric acid into the bloodstream, and in order for the body to neutralize this excess it must leech calcium from bones.

Protein should account for an estimated 12% to 20% of the total calories in the diet, and Americans tend to get at least that much. Older adults who are ill, however, are the most likely segment of society to experience protein deficiency. They suffer loss of appetite and often eat very little if any meat because of the cost, denture problems, lack of ability or desire to cook, or philosophy. Protein deficiency in older adults can result in a lack of vigor or stamina, depression, poor resistance to infection, impaired healing of wounds, and slow recovery from disease.

| BOX 5.1 | The Low Cost of Eating Poorly |

We get five to nine times the amount of calories for the buck when we choose energy-dense (junk) foods rather than nutrient-dense foods (Monsivais & Drewnowski, 2007). Why is that? The $75-billion-a-year Farm Bill subsidizes crops like corn and soy, which are used for added sugar and fats in our food (Pollan, 2007), but not fruits and vegetables. Given the perverse incentives, farmers produce ever-increasing amounts of corn and soy; and the price of soda, for example (which has plenty of liquid corn), stays low, whereas the cost of fresh produce continues to rise.

If you eat on a budget, the most rational *economic* strategy to get sufficient calories is to eat junk food. This helps explain why a much higher percentage of poor people are overweight or obese than those who are economically better off. And obesity among low-income Americans has been costly in terms of Medicaid expenditures and emergency room utilization.

Nonetheless, the Farm Bill does not generate a health debate in America, just an economic one—and this mostly occurs between congressmen and lobbyists. These two groups value agribusiness profits over the quality of food accessible to all socioeconomic levels. What do you value, and what can be done about it?

WATER

Although we can get by without most nutrients for several *weeks* at a stretch, we cannot survive without water for several *days*. Water is the medium in which all the reactions in cells take place. Water lubricates joints; transports nutrients and salts throughout the body; hydrates the skin; promotes adequate blood volume; moistens the eyes, nose, and mouth; carries waste; and regulates body temperature. Nevertheless, older adults tend to drink only about three cups a day, less than what they need. This is due in part to reduced thirst perception with age.

Inadequate hydration can have many deleterious effects, beginning with constipation and fatigue and moving on to hypotension, hyperthermia, dizziness, breathing difficulties, and irregular heartbeats. Prolonged dehydration can lead to a variety of diseases. It is important, therefore, that older adults with inadequate fluid intake build up gradually to eight cups of fluids per day (including that which is found in food), regardless of thirst. It should be noted, though, that researchers have been unable to find a single study that supports the need for the widely circulated recommendation to drink an additional eight glasses of water a day (Valtin, 2008). Much of the water we need exists in the food we eat, and the additional amount of water that any one individual needs is not particularly challenging to achieve, with the exception of older adults and their declining thirst mechanism. For most Americans, "schlepping water bottles around all day long" is unnecessary (Negoianu & Goldfarb, 2008).

Dehydration in the elderly is responsible for a substantial number of additional days of hospital care, at a significant cost to Medicare. The American Medical Association (AMA)'s Council of Scientific Affairs recommended that undergraduate, graduate, and continuing-education programs for nurses, allied health professionals, and physicians include the importance of hydration in older adults.

Water, juice, and milk meet hydration needs. More than 80% of many fruits and vegetables, about 50% of meat, and about one third of bread consists of water. Alcohol, caffeinated tea and coffee, and soft drinks raise the fluid level more modestly because of their diuretic effect. One study, however, reported that caffeinated drinks do not dehydrate the body more than noncaffeinated drinks (Grandjean, Reimers, Bannick, & Haven, 2000). Alcohol consumption is not effective for hydration purposes. However, moderate alcohol consumption of one to two drinks per day may lower cardiovascular risk (Mukamal et al., 2003), dementia risk (Ruitenberg et al., 2002), and the all-cause mortality rate (Lee, Ayers, & Kronenfeld, 2009).

VITAMINS AND MINERALS

Vitamins in the right amounts are needed for normal growth, digestion, mental alertness, and resistance to infection. The body also needs 15 *minerals* that help regulate cell function and provide structure for cells. Since 1941 the Food and Nutrition Board of the National Academy of Sciences has published the Recommended Dietary Allowance (RDA) for the majority of vitamins, minerals, and protein that we require, and have updated these recommendations every few years based on research findings. The RDA is the average daily dietary intake level that is sufficient to meet the nutrient requirement of nearly all healthy individuals (97% to 98%) in a particular life stage and sex category.

In 1998, Dietary Reference Intakes were developed that added additional guidelines, such as Tolerable Upper Intake Level (highest safe intake level) to warn against the potential for adverse effects. Although the surplus *water-soluble* vitamins—C and eight of the B vitamins—are excreted in urine, adverse effects can still result from exceeding the upper-level recommendations. The surplus *fat-soluble* vitamins—A, D, E, and K—are stored in body tissue, and excessive amounts can become toxic.

RDAs (see Table 5.2) have been difficult to establish, especially for older adults who have been broadly, and inadequately, defined for the past several decades as persons age 51 and over. Although we know that increasing age alters nutritional requirements, the Food and Nutrition Board had delayed for many years the establishment of separate categories for adults over 50, based on insufficient research data. The insufficient data has been caused by such research problems as inadequate numbers of older adults in

TABLE 5.2 Age-Related Recommended Dietary Allowances (RDA) by the National Academy of Sciences

		RDA	UPPER LEVEL	FOOD/DRINK SOURCES
Vitamin B$_6$	Women 50+	1.5 mg	100 mg	Meat, poultry, seafood, liver, and fortified foods
	Men 50+	1.7 mg	100 mg	
Vitamin D	Ages 51–70	600 IU	4,000 IU	Sunlight, fatty fish, and fortified foods
	Ages 70+	800 IU		
Calcium	Ages 50+	1,200 mg	2,000 mg– 3,000 mg	Dairy, fortified foods, leafy green vegetables, canned fish
Iron	Women 50+	8 mg	45 mg	Red meat, poultry, seafood, and whole-grain flour
	Men	8 mg	45 mg	

studies, higher nonresponse rates from older adults, and the confounding influence of selective mortality. In addition, vitamin, mineral, and protein requirements for older adults in particular are complicated by diversity in physiological changes, living arrangements, transportation access, and disability (Wakimoto & Block, 2001).

As the research base has improved over the past decade, RDAs are being expanded into a broader range of categories. The most important change regarding older adults has been to create a separate category for people age 50+ (vitamin B_6, calcium, iron) and to differentiate adults age 51 to 70 versus adults older than age 70 (vitamin D).

A meta-analysis of studies focused on nutrition and age reported that nutritional intake declines with age (Wakimoto & Block, 2001). This is not surprising, as energy output and muscle mass decline with age as well. Along with nutritional-intake decline, though, potentially important declines in protein, zinc, calcium, folate, thiamine, riboflavin, and vitamins D, E, B_6, and B_{12} were observed (see Table 5.3). This raises two questions that need further research: Which nutrient intakes should decline with age, given that energy output declines as well? Which should increase with age, given that absorption and utilization efficiency decrease with age?

On the positive side, fruit and vegetable consumption appears to increase with age, especially among older women, along with vitamin A, vitamin C, and potassium intake. Older persons—again, particularly women—are more likely to consume vitamin supplements (Wakimoto & Block, 2001). To improve the intake of important nutrients, Table 5.4 identifies some of the best food group sources for older adults.

TABLE 5.3 Nutrients and Clinical Manifestation of Deficiency in Older Adults

Protein	Inability to cope with metabolic stress like infection or broken bone
Zinc	Impaired immune function, delayed wound healing, lethargy
Calcium	Increased risk of fracture
Folate	Increased risk of stroke, anemia, appetite loss, fatigue
Thiamine	Compromised nervous system, weight loss, fatigue, decreased reflexes
Riboflavin	Problems with lips and tongue
Vitamin D	Bone pain, fatigue, gait disturbances
Vitamin E	Uncertain, perhaps reduction of antioxidant effect
Vitamin B_6	Nausea, dizziness, confusion, depression, fatigue
Vitamin B_{12}	Nausea, fatigue, depression, memory problems, anemia, neurological disease

TABLE 5.4 Good Sources of Nutrition for Older Adults

TO INCREASE SOURCE OF	EAT MORE
Protein, iron, niacin, vitamin B_{12}	Meats
Calcium, riboflavin, protein	Milk products
B vitamins	Breads and cereals
Vitamins C and A, potassium	Fruits and vegetables
Vitamin D	Fatty fish

Two minerals of particular nutritional importance for the aging body are sodium chloride (salt) and calcium. Typically, we consume too much of the former and too little of the latter.

SODIUM AND HIGH BLOOD PRESSURE

Sodium keeps muscles and nerves working properly and attracts water, thereby helping us retain the proper amount of body fluid. Too much sodium in the system, however, causes the body to retain excess water, increase the blood pressure level, and make the heart work harder.

Americans consume more than twice the recommended amount of sodium for adults at high risk, which includes older adults—3,500 mg versus 1,500 mg. The latter figure is low, to be understated about it, about a half-teaspoon of salt. That would pretty much preclude eating at restaurants, and eating anything processed. Processed and restaurant food rely heavily on salt as a cheap way to enhance flavor and texture and preserve food.

To help approach the 1,500 mg level, at its 2006 meeting the AMA urged the food industry to cut the amount of salt in restaurants and in processed foods by 50% within the decade. The AMA also urged the government to require high-salt foods to be labeled, and to revoke salt's G.R.A.S. ("generally recognized as safe") status granted by the FDA.

Because many foods already contain high levels of sodium (such as potato chips, processed meats, frozen dinners, ketchup, most sauces, and canned foods) and it is hidden in a wide variety of other foods, it is quite a challenge for individuals to limit salt (40% sodium and 60% chlorine) sufficiently, even if it is not added to food, which it often is. About half the women who prepared food at home used salt when preparing it, and about one third used salt at the table.

The amount of salt used in cooking should be reduced for most people, and the salt shaker removed from the table. Some foods that contain large amounts of salt, such as canned soup or processed lunch meat, should be avoided altogether. Labels should be read for sodium content, and people should be made aware that sodium may be indicated by complex names (e.g., monosodium glutamate).

Most Americans associate sodium intake with high blood pressure, yet the percentage of Americans whose high blood pressure can be attributed to salt sensitivity is unknown. In the absence of definitive research findings, many registered dieticians (RD) recommend that sodium reduction be practiced widely. Others suggest a more targeted approach through an informal test for determining salt sensitivity. An individual can alternately restrict salt and then remove salt restrictions for specified periods of time, and assess the impact on the person's blood pressure levels.

Salt restriction is recommended for older adults and for people with an elevated blood pressure level. One study reported that salt restriction may be more effective than daily walking in lowering blood pressure among postmenopausal women (Seals et al., 2001). Salt restriction is also recommended by the U.S. Public Health Service for people with a family history of high blood pressure, and for African Americans, who are more likely to be highly sensitive to excess sodium.

In 1995 two leading medical journals, the *British Medical Journal* (*BMJ*) and the *Journal of the American Medical Association* (*JAMA*), published articles that offered contradictory conclusions—conclusions that are still controversial today! The *BMJ* article concluded that the traditional association between salt intake and blood pressure was accurate, and monitoring salt intake was still important. Moreover, the relationship appears to be stronger in middle-aged persons than in young adults.

The *JAMA* article, however, concluded that low-salt diets had virtually no effect on people with normal blood pressure, making low-salt diets irrelevant to the majority of the population. Moreover, a subsequent research study reported that a low-sodium diet was associated with higher readmission rates for congestive heart failure patients, perhaps due to detrimental renal and neurohormonal effects (Paterna, Gaspare, Fasullo, Sarullo, & Di Pasquale, 2008). The study has been criticized for under-representing high-risk groups like older adults and Blacks, and not controlling adequately for medication usage.

The controversy is not easy to sum up. Norman Hollenberg (2006) of Harvard Medical School recognized that reduced salt intake could make a substantial contribution to reducing hypertension, particularly among older adults, the obese, Blacks, and those with diabetes and hypertension, but also believed it was premature to invoke mandatory reductions in salt content that affected all people.

Conversely, the AMA has stuck to its position of salt reduction on a general basis, and has advocated that American food makers and restaurants reduce salt content. I agree with the AMA on this policy position, but I should warn the reader that the AMA has not had a good track record when it comes to health policies. It supported the tobacco industry for years after research warned against smoking, and it did not favor the passage of Medicare.

In January 2010 New York City set voluntary guidelines recommending maximum amounts of salt for a variety of restaurant and store-bought foods, with the goal of reducing salt levels in food by an average of 25% over 5 years. Restaurants and food manufacturers were encouraged to lower salt content gradually so consumers do not notice. This innovative project, called the *National Salt Reduction Initiative*, has attracted the endorsements of 25 other city and state health agencies; 17 national health organizations; and 28 national food companies, retailers, and supermarket chains. The suggested salt reductions in products range from a 20% drop in peanut butter to a 40% decline in canned vegetables. Food industry representatives have reacted cautiously so far, stating they will take this initiative under consideration.

CALCIUM AND OSTEOPOROSIS

Calcium is essential for maintaining bone strength. If the amount of calcium contained in the diets of older adults is inadequate, the body takes calcium from the bones and uses it for other purposes. When people lose calcium from their bones, or their body's ability to absorb calcium is reduced (a process associated with age and exacerbated by the excess use of such products as mineral-oil laxatives, caffeine, and alcohol), bones become more brittle and fragile.

This condition, known as osteoporosis, is characterized by low bone mass and an increase in the risk of fracture from ordinary skeletal stress. Over the years, the bones of a person with osteoporosis gradually thin, until some break, causing pain and disability. Almost half of women age 50 and older have osteoporosis or the condition leading up to it—osteopenia (Siris et al., 2001). Approximately 1.5 million fractures attributable to osteoporosis occur each year, located most often in the vertebra (700,000), hip (300,000), or wrist (300,000).

Older adult women consume about 500 mg/day of dietary calcium, considerably less than the 1,200 mg/day recommended for postadolescent females, or the 1,500 mg/day recommended by the National Institute on Aging. The most common sources of calcium are dairy products, fortified foods, and dark green leafy vegetables (kale and broccoli, but not spinach). Regarding calcium supplementation, though, there is concern that cardiovascular health could be compromised and the risk of kidney stones elevated at lower levels of calcium supplementation than previously thought. Regarding vitamin D, which helps to absorb calcium, most older adults fall far short of the 400 IU (ages 51–70) to 600 IU (ages 70 and above) recommended. We will further examine the importance of vitamin D and calcium in Chapter 6, "Complementary and Alternative Medicine."

Weight-bearing exercise helps to maintain strong bones by increasing bone mineral density and reducing calcium loss. The positive effect of exercise on bone strength, however, appears to be lost within a relatively short period of time if the exercise program is discontinued. Hormone replacement therapy (not a good option) and bisphosphonates can reduce or reverse bone loss.

> **Question:** Can you give three examples in which changing dietary habits might be an acceptable alternative to taking a medication for a health problem?

For information and resource materials on osteoporosis, contact the National Osteoporosis Foundation, 1232 22nd St. NW, Washington, DC 20037; 202-223-2226 (www.nof.org).

NUTRITION LABELS

The Nutrition Labeling and Education Act passed by Congress in 1990, but not fully implemented until 1994, required the FDA to enforce food labels that were more educational and less confusing. The initial confrontation pitted consumer advocates against the food industry, which only wanted amounts on the label, rather than explain that an amount contained 25% of the total fat that you should consume in a single day. After substantial debate and controversy, consumers won out over the food industry.

The content of this legislation was broad. Terms like *light, low-fat*, and *reduced-calorie* had to be based on federal definitions. Many food labels had implied positive characteristics that were, in fact, meaningless, such as *light, natural*, or *pure*. *Light* now had to mean a 50% reduction from that which existed in the original product; *low-fat*, 3 grams or less of fat per serving; and *low-calorie*, 40 calories or less per serving. Similar definitions applied to *lean, sugar, sodium, high-fiber, healthy*, and so forth.

Health or medical claims must be backed by solid research. All packaged foods must have a standard nutrient chart, with standardized portions to make nutritional and caloric data meaningful. The chart must include information on calories, calories from fat, the amount of fat, saturated fat (and, since 2006, trans fat), cholesterol, carbohydrates, protein, and sodium.

In 1995, 1 year after the *nutrition labels* debuted, 56% of consumers used the new labels often. Unfortunately, the public fixated on fat content rather than on nutrients or total calories. As a consequence, from 1995 to 1998 more than 6,500 reduced-fat foods were introduced to the public ("Counting on Food Labels," 2000), many of which were low in fat but not low in calories, and obesity continued to rise. Although the interest in nutrition labels rose to nearly 80% of Americans in 2006, according to a national AP-Ipsos poll, 44% of the people who looked at nutrition labels admitted that they didn't let the label, regardless of content, dissuade them from buying the product.

The nutrition labeling law had other defects. Ground beef, for example, accounts for about half of the meat sold in the United States, and added more saturated fat to the average American's diet than any other single food. Yet a package of ground beef, which can provide 14 grams of fat in a single serving, can have an "85% *lean*" label on it.

The latest refinements of labeling are *food rating systems*, in which numerical ratings, star ratings, or letter grades are posted on the shelf next to each product in a grocery store. The problem is that assigning value to foods requires considerable judgment. How many points should be earned for whole grains, fiber, vitamins, and minerals? How many points should be deducted for saturated fat, trans fat, cholesterol, and added sugars or sodium? Without federal guidelines, nine large U.S. food manufacturers (with the input of academic nutrition professors—shame on them) developed the Smart Choices Food Labeling Program in 2009. This rating system allowed for processed foods high in sugar, such as Froot Loops cereal and Cracker Jack snack food, to be rated as "smart choices." After several months of bad publicity, it was terminated by federal regulators because it was deemed misleading.

Shoppers and well-respected nutritional leaders want a food rating system, but a few questionable rating systems could diminish the value of all of them. Nonetheless, the use of rating systems is likely to spread, and could be legitimized by a government-sanctioned national standard.

Fast-food restaurants have long resisted legislation that mandates calorie labeling on menus and menu boards, because these restaurants typically serve high-calorie food. Over the past four decades, consumers have doubled the percentage of their food dollars spent at restaurants—to about 46%—most of which takes place at fast-food restaurants. Not surprisingly, overweight and obesity has doubled in America during this time as well.

New York City is the leader in advocating for transparent caloric content of food in restaurants. After a series of courtroom battles, the New York City Board of Health required in July 2008 that all NYC restaurant chains having at least 15 outlets across the country must post the calories in each of their offerings in large type and in readily visible areas, such as the menu, menu board, or near cash registers. This legislation affected more than 10% of the 23,000 licensed restaurants in New York City.

As part of the Affordable Care Act (see Chapter 12, "Public Health Policy"), all restaurants with more than 20 locations will have to post calorie counts on their menus, though the timetable for compliance was not established as of this writing. In anticipation of this mandate, McDonald's, with its 14,000 locations in the United States, began to post calorie counts on its menus near the end of 2012.

Nationwide, the 10% of restaurants that are chains serve almost two thirds of restaurant traffic. One national survey reported that 83% of restaurant diners wanted nutritional information posted. Studies show, however, that when given this type of information, only 10% to 20% of diners would choose lower-calorie options (Rabin, 2007). Nonetheless, nutritionists argue that with additional education and publicity, labels can play an important role in helping diners eat fewer calories.

MALNUTRITION

Americans are no longer dying of pellagra, rickets, beriberi, or scurvy—caused by deficiencies in niacin, vitamin D, thiamine, and vitamin C—thanks largely to the fortification and enrichment of our foods. Nonetheless, *malnutrition* remains a serious problem. Between 16% and 30% of older Americans are malnourished or at high risk of it, with higher percentages among older hospital patients and nursing-home residents (Beers & Berkow, 2000). These malnourished older adults take 40% longer to recover from illness, have two to three times as many complications, and have hospital stays that are 90% longer.

There are many risk factors for malnourishment in older adults (Table 5.5). The link between malnutrition and social isolation is particularly strong, and suggests that encouraging participation in clubs and the sharing of meals with friends or neighbors may be far more effective in improving dietary intake than providing nutrition education. Men living alone consume fewer fruits and vegetables and have a much greater

TABLE 5.5 Risk Factors for Malnourishment in Older Adults

Inappropriate food	Loss of appetite	Decreased thirst	Dental problems
Social isolation	Poverty	Dementing illness	Medical disease
Physical condition	Alcoholism	Endurance problems	Balance problems
Depression	Medication usage	Medication withdrawal	

propensity for selecting easy-to-prepare foods, which are high in fat and low in complex carbohydrates, than do those who have companions. Loneliness, bereavement, and social isolation are associated with poor dietary intake in later life. An increasing percentage of older adults report difficulty in preparing meals, particularly after age 85.

Many elderly individuals depend on meals prepared at a congregate nutrition site or meals-on-wheels program. As the demand for services of this type increases along with the number of very old, frail adults, the likelihood that the supply of such services will meet the need is unlikely based on funding trends. Malnutrition is therefore likely to increase.

Nutrition screenings examine characteristics known to be associated with dietary and nutritional problems, in order to identify high-risk individuals. One such screening initiative, a collaborative project by the American Academy of Family Physicians, the American Dietetic Association, and the National Council on Aging, resulted in the production of a manual that begins with a checklist, "Determine Your Nutritional Health," shown in Figures 5.4A and 5.4B. The manual includes a variety of screening tools on nutrition and related topics, including *body mass index* (BMI), eating habits, functional status, cognitive status, and depression. To order copies, contact *Nutrition Screening Manual for Professionals Caring for Older Americans*, Nutrition Screening Initiative, 1010 Wisconsin Ave. NW, #800, Washington, DC 20007; or access www.aafp.org.

When older clients lose their appetites, the following is recommended: eat smaller and more frequent meals; take advantage of when you feel good and are hungry, regardless of the time; eat higher-calorie foods or consider taking a nutritional supplement; postpone beverages toward the end of a meal; create a pleasant eating atmosphere, and find company to enjoy the meal with; and see a physician to either change a medication that is affecting appetite, or add a medication that may relieve nausea, heartburn, or other symptoms that occur when you eat.

SELECTED NUTRITION TOPICS

Organic Foods

As Whole Foods Market, Trader Joe's, and other chains that cater to consumers interested in *organic* foods expand throughout the country, their marketing executives have noticed that their typical customer is increasingly becoming a well-educated female baby boomer. This sentiment has been shared by the Organic Trade Association, which believes that the buying trend of the past decade has been led by the health-conscious baby boomers. One of these boomers is first lady Michelle Obama (she just made it—born in 1964), who seized upon an opportunity in 2009 to organically grow vegetables and assorted herbs on the White House grounds.

Boomers will have to be educated advocates to preserve the integrity of the organic movement. (Organic does not necessarily mean healthy, as organic donuts and organic chips are just as high in fat and calories as the conventional kind.) The national standards will have to be preserved regarding pesticides, hormones,

FIGURE 5.4A   Determine your nutritional health.

The Warning Signs of poor nutritional health are often overlooked. Use this checklist to find out if you or someone you know is at nutritional risk.

DETERMINE YOUR NUTRITIONAL HEALTH

Read the statements below. Circle the number in the yes column for those that apply to you or someone you know. For each yes answer, score the number in the box. Total your nutritional score.

	YES
I have an illness or condition that made me change the kind and/or amount of food I eat.	2
I eat fewer than 2 meals per day.	3
I eat few fruits or vegetables, or milk products.	2
I have 3 or more drinks of beer, liquor or wine almost every day.	2
I have tooth or mouth problems that make it hard for me to eat.	2
I don't always have enough money to buy the food I need.	4
I eat alone most of the time.	1
I take 3 or more different prescribed or over-the-counter drugs a day.	1
Without wanting to, I have lost or gained 10 pounds in the last 6 months.	2
I am not always physically able to shop, cook and/or feed myself.	2
TOTAL	

Total Your Nutritional Score. If it's —

0-2   **Good!** Recheck your nutritional score in 6 months.

3-5   **You are at moderate nutritional risk.** See what can be done to improve your eating habits and lifestyle. Your office on aging, senior nutrition program, senior citizens center or health department can help. Recheck your nutritional score in 3 months.

6 or more   **You are at high nutritional risk.** Bring this checklist the next time you see your doctor, dietitian or other qualified health or social service professional. Talk with them about any problems you may have. Ask for help to improve your nutritional health.

These materials developed and distributed by the Nutrition Screening Initiative, a project of:

 AMERICAN ACADEMY OF FAMILY PHYSICIANS

 THE AMERICAN DIETETIC ASSOCIATION

 NATIONAL COUNCIL ON THE AGING, INC.

Remember that warning signs suggest risk, but do not represent diagnosis of any condition. Turn the page to learn more about the Warning Signs of poor nutritional health.

FIGURE 5.4B Determine your nutritional health.

The Nutrition Checklist is based on the Warning Signs described below. Use the word DETERMINE to remind you of the Warning Signs.

DISEASE

Any disease, illness or chronic condition which causes you to change the way you eat, or makes it hard for you to eat, puts your nutritional health at risk. Four out of five adults have chronic diseases that are affected by diet. Confusion or memory loss that keeps getting worse is estimated to affect one out of five or more of older adults. This can make it hard to remember what, when or if you've eaten. Feeling sad or depressed, which happens to about one in eight older adults, can cause big changes in appetite, digestion, energy level, weight and well-being.

EATING POORLY

Eating too little and eating too much both lead to poor health. Eating the same foods day after day or not eating fruit, vegetables, and milk products daily will also cause poor nutritional health. One in five adults skip meals daily. Only 13% of adults eat the minimum amount of fruit and vegetables needed. One in four older adults drink too much alcohol. Many health problems become worse if you drink more than one or two alcoholic beverages per day.

TOOTH LOSS/ MOUTH PAIN

A healthy mouth, teeth and gums are needed to eat. Missing, loose or rotten teeth or dentures which don't fit well or cause mouth sores make it hard to eat.

ECONOMIC HARDSHIP

As many as 40% of older Americans have incomes of less than $6,000 per year. Having less--or choosing to spend less--than $25-30 per week for food makes it very hard to get the foods you need to stay healthy.

REDUCED SOCIAL CONTACT

One-third of all older people live alone. Being with people daily has a positive effect on morale, well-being and eating.

MULTIPLE MEDICINES

Many older Americans must take medicines for health problems. Almost half of older Americans take multiple medicines daily. Growing old may change the way we respond to drugs. The more medicines you take, the greater the chance for side effects such as increased or decreased appetite, change in taste, constipation, weakness, drowsiness, diarrhea, nausea, and others. Vitamins or minerals when taken in large doses act like drugs and can cause harm. Alert your doctor to everything you take.

INVOLUNTARY WEIGHT LOSS/GAIN

Losing or gaining a lot of weight when you are not trying to do so is an important warning sign that must not be ignored. Being overweight or underweight also increases your chance of poor health.

NEEDS ASSISTANCE IN SELF CARE

Although most older people are able to eat, one of every five have trouble walking, shopping, buying and cooking food, especially as they get older.

ELDER YEARS ABOVE AGE 80

Most older people lead full and productive lives. But as age increases, risk of frailty and health problems increase. Checking your nutritional health regularly makes good sense.

The Nutrition Screening Initiative, 2626 Pennsylvania Avenue, NW, Suite 301, Washington, DC 20037
© The Nutrition Screening Initiative is funded in part by a grant from Ross Laboratories, a division of Abbott Laboratories.

chemical fertilizers, antibiotics, irradiation, bioengineering, artificial preservatives, flavors, synthetic ingredients, conservation of soil and water, and humanely treatment of animals.

Walmart has begun to offer organic foods in its nearly 4,000 stores, and the consequences may be far-reaching. In the Walmart tradition, cost is a factor, and they have vowed to keep costs to only 10% over conventional food, instead of the additional 25% or more charged elsewhere. The good news is that many more people will be able to afford organic food.

There is more possible good news. Critics were concerned that Walmart would look for large-scale producers to keep prices low and begin the decline of local organic farming. Instead, Walmart announced an initiative to double, to 9%, the amount of locally grown fruits and vegetables it sells. The shorter travel distances would help to reduce air pollution. Now let's see if Walmart follows through, and launches more green initiatives.

Junk Food and Fast Food

Junk food—also known as *energy-dense and nutrient-poor foods* in the nutrition business—provides about one third of the daily calorie intake of American adults. Younger adults slightly prefer salty snacks, candy, and soft drinks; whereas older adults slightly prefer fats and desserts (Kant, 2000). In 2001, Americans ate about 6.5 billion pounds of snacks, with potato chips and tortilla chips leading the way.

Fast foods, which also tend to be energy-dense and nutrient-poor, are on the rise as well. In 1970, Americans spent about $6 billion annually on fast food; in 2000, over $110 billion. One of the newer wrinkles in fast food is called dashboard dining. The automobile driver can drink 13 varieties of soup in heat-and-sip cups. Yogurt can be consumed through squeeze tubes. Cookies can be eaten from cans that fit neatly in car cup holders. Frozen peanut butter and jelly sandwiches—crustless for the kids—can also be taken along for the ride.

Older adults at home often opt for the convenience of prepared, frozen microwaveable meals. These foods, unfortunately, are typically high in fat, sodium, and cholesterol. Healthier options were made available to consumers after ConAgra's former CEO Mike Harper suffered a heart attack, and shortly thereafter created Healthy Choice Dinners. Other companies followed suit.

What are the dietary habits of future cohorts of older adults likely to be? McDonald's, Pizza Hut, Domino's, and other fast-food outlets are located in about 30% of public high schools in the United States (Schlosser, 2001). Ronald McDonald is second only to Santa Claus in familiarity among children ("How McNuggets," 2001). In 1955 Americans spent 19% of their food dollars on restaurants; today, that figure has increased to 41%. The average American eats out more than four times a week, and more than half the time at a fast-food restaurant. Restaurant meals contain 20% more fat than home-cooked meals and are less desirable in terms of sodium, cholesterol, calcium, and fiber content.

Coffee

Coffee has been cast as either a vice or a virtue for centuries. For instance, a few monarchs destroyed coffeehouses around 1600, believing that coffee incited gossip and rebellion; about that same time, a pope found it so delicious that he baptized it. The latest research leans more toward virtue, and it may even promote longevity.

Researchers analyzed the coffee-drinking habits of 400,000 people ages 50 to 71. Whether caffeinated or not, they found that controlling for risk factors (smoking, diet, exercise, etc.), the more coffee a person consumed, the less likely he or she was to die from a number of health problems, including diabetes, heart disease, respiratory disease, stroke, and injuries or accidents (Freedman, Park, Abnet, Hollenbeck, & Sinha, 2012).

Researchers have also found that those who consumed up to six cups of coffee a day were almost 20% less likely to develop prostate cancer over two decades than those who drank none, and 60% less likely to develop a lethal form of the disease (Wilson et al., 2011). Other researchers believe that coffee is a major source of dietary antioxidants, and that coffee consumption is associated with reduced risk of death from inflammatory and cardiovascular diseases (Andersen, Jacobs, Carlsen, & Blomhoff, 2006), diabetes (Salazar-Martinez et al., 2004), and cirrhosis (Klatsky, Morton, Udaltsova, & Friedman, 2006). Up to six cups a day can be counted toward one's recommended liquid intake as it is, contrary to popular belief, no more of a diuretic than water.

Sensory Decline

An age-related decline in the sense of smell—rather than taste—directly affects a person's ability to taste or enjoy food. About 30% of persons between the ages of 70 and 80, and 65% of persons over age 80, experience problems with their sense of smell. Older persons have more trouble identifying pureed foods, for instance, than do younger persons. If younger persons held their noses while eating, their ability to identify foods would drop to the level of older adults.

Because individuals try to compensate for the loss of smell and taste, they may add too much sugar or salt to make food taste better, which can affect heart disease, stroke, diabetes, and other diseases. To enhance food aromas for older adults, herbs and spices are encouraged. Adding flavors and sweeteners also can enhance taste. Another technique for stimulating appetite is a combination of different textures—for example, adding granola to yogurt.

Quackery

Dietitians and nutritionists individualize a nutrition plan and make sure that fat, salt, and sugar are limited and complex carbohydrates and fiber are emphasized. They encourage lifelong eating guidelines, regular exercise, ongoing behavior management techniques, and identifying sources of emotional support to help clients sustain changes in their eating habits. They advocate for the consumption of a wide variety of foods, and suggest supplements primarily when needs cannot be met through diet. They do not promise cures, and they do consult with physicians. They are also more likely to have earned a degree from a 4-year accredited college or university, or to be RD, which requires passing a national exam.

Quacks, on the other hand, rely on testimonials, are not shy about promising to cure a disease, typically foresee quick results, often emphasize one or two food groups, frequently encourage megadoses of vitamins, and repeatedly denigrate other people's ideas, even those based on scientific evidence.

Want a qualified nutritionist to design a healthy eating plan? Call the Nutrition Information Line of the American Dietetic Association, at 800-366-1655, to find an adviser in your area.

Socioeconomic and Cultural Sensitivity

In addition to the physiological changes that occur with age, health professionals need to be sensitive to the *socioeconomic* and *cultural* factors that influence their clients. For example, health professionals ought not to try to increase the protein consumption of low-income clients by recommending diets that contain expensive lean meat, fish, or poultry. Nor should health professionals recommend diets that completely ignore the food preferences of members of particular ethnic groups. Ethnic foods are a source of pride, identity, and fond memories. Every effort should be made to incorporate food preferences in nutritional planning.

Food Films

My first date with my wife was to see the movie *Like Water for Chocolate*. This great Mexican—and date—film is about how a young woman transfers her feelings of forbidden love into her cooking. Her passion is channeled into her food preparation, and those who subsequently dine on her creations experience her emotions as well.

There are other films in which people pour their love into the preparation of food. *Babette's Feast* is about a group of quarreling people who become transformed by a magnificent feast and end the meal by forgiving and blessing one another. *Eat Drink Man Woman* is about a famous Chinese chef concerned about his daughters, but only able to communicate through loving meal preparations. *Big Night* is about two Italian brothers trying to save their restaurant through the feast of a lifetime. In all these films the food is fresh and delicious, and prepared slowly and lovingly. (Interested in the slow food movement? Visit www.slowfood.com.)

At the other end of the continuum is the movie about fast food, called *Super Size Me*. Morgan Spurlock is a healthy young man who became fascinated by two young people who sued McDonald's for making them fat. Spurlock then decided to make a movie about eating at McDonald's for three meals a day, 30 straight days. Spurlock at first found the meals to be tasty, but eventually he sustained liver damage, stomach pains, vomiting, weight gain, depression, and impaired sexuality (though perhaps the attitude of his girlfriend—a vegan chef—toward his project contributed to the last problem).

Just before *Super Size Me* began appearing in movie theaters in 2004, McDonald's (they claimed coincidentally) eliminated their super size option, and also announced the introduction of a new, healthier menu. Spurlock's film had less of an influence on me. I took my wife to see it and discovered that it wasn't nearly as good a date film as *Like Water for Chocolate*.

Advocacy

The CSPI is an educational and advocacy organization. Its educational component consists of the *Nutrition Action Health Letter*, published monthly, which informs more than 800,000 subscribers, including this author. The organization is best known, however, for its advocacy accomplishments, under the leadership of its executive director and cofounder (in 1971), Michael Jacobson.

Jacobson and CSPI staff, for example, have led the fight for nutrition labels on food items in the supermarket; for exposing the hidden fat in Chinese, Mexican, Italian, and delicatessen food; for pressuring movie theaters to stop cooking popcorn in artery-clogging coconut oil; for warning labels on Procter & Gamble's fake fat, Olean, which may interfere with the absorption of nutrients and cause loose stools and cramping; for more accurate labeling of ground beef in supermarkets; and for the listing of trans fat on nutrition labels.

For more information, contact the Center for Science in the Public Interest, 1875 Connecticut Avenue NW, Suite 300, Washington, DC 20009; or visit their website, www.cspinet.org.

Nutrition Newsletters

To obtain a newsletter on nutritional topics, contact one of the following:

Nutrition Action Health Letter, Center for Science in the Public Interest, 1875 Connecticut Avenue NW, Suite 300, Washington, DC 20009; www.cspinet.org

Environmental Nutrition: The Professional Newsletter of Diet, Nutrition and Health, 2112 Broadway, New York, NY 10023; 800-829-5384

Mayo Clinic Nutrition Letter, Mayo Foundation for Medical Education and Research, 200 1st Street SW, Rochester, MN 55905

Diet, Nutrition and Cancer Prevention, National Cancer Institute, Building 31, Room 10A24, Bethesda, MD 20892; 800-4-CANCER

National Center for Nutrition and Dietetics, 216 W. Jackson Boulevard, Suite 800, Chicago, IL 60606-6995

Tufts University Diet & Nutrition Letter, P.O. Box 57857, Boulder, CO 80322-7857; 800-274-7581

University of California Berkeley Wellness Newsletter, P.O. Box 420148, Palm Coast, FL 32142; 800-829-9170

Nutrition Websites

Center for Nutrition Policy and Promotion (www.usda.gov/cnpp): The USDA's online Interactive Healthy Eating Index helps you assess the quality of your daily diet.

American Dietetic Association (www.eatright.org): For information on nutrition and health, call 800-366-1655.

Cyberdiet (www.cyberdiet.com): Commercial site that provides nutritional information and support for a better diet and healthier lifestyle.

I WISH I HAD KNOWN

In the 1973 science fiction comedy movie *Sleeper,* a character played by Woody Allen is frozen in time and comes back to life centuries in the future. There he finds that deep-fried fat, hot-fudge sundaes, and steaks are the real health foods. Products like wheat germ and organic honey have long been exposed as worthless.

TRENDS IN WEIGHT GAIN

The U.S. Preventive Services Task Force (USPSTF) recommends that clinicians screen all adults for *obesity* (BMI of 30 or above) and offer intensive behavioral counseling to obese adults. This decision seems to be based not so much on the effectiveness of clinician counsel, which is questionable, but rather on the evidence that overweight and obesity have become epidemic in America.

In 1960, when weight was relatively stable in America, women ages 40 to 49 averaged about 140 pounds. By 2000, the average weight of women in that age group had jumped to 169 pounds (Kessler, 2009). This is not even the heaviest age group, that distinction goes to adults ages 50 to 69, followed by those age 70 to 79. In 2010, according to the U.S. Federal Interagency Forum on Aging-Related Statistics, 38% of people aged 65 and older were obese; an increase of 16% in only two decades. Overall, 68% of adults are overweight and 34% are obese today.

This epidemic has escalated despite the fact that Americans spend about $40 billion a year on diet products and programs; that excess weight is widely known to be a risk factor for disease and death; that obesity is a social stigma in our society and continues to offend most people's personal vanity; and that a health revolution had supposedly occurred in America.

It does appear that a limited health revolution occurred in America during the past 40 years. Cigarette smoking declined significantly during this time; alcohol abuse was identified as a common risk factor and steps were taken to curtail it, especially among automobile drivers; seatbelt use had risen steadily; brisk walking, jogging, aerobic dancing, and other exercises had attracted millions of new participants; and the use of low-fat food alternatives had proliferated. How could the nation have grown fat while all of this was happening?

Some health analysts believe that the fitness revolution was limited to only a segment of the population, perhaps 20%, with the majority of Americans still sedentary and consuming more calories than ever. Others theorize that significant numbers of Americans have been responding to the computer age by relying on their computers rather than physical activities for entertainment as well as work. Another theory is that many people in this highly stressful era have been using food as a coping device to combat the anxiety and depression caused by violence, job reductions, divorce, and so forth. It has also been suggested that although many Americans have been preoccupied with fat reduction, they were not as vigilant with calorie reduction. Yet another theory is that legions of ex-smokers have turned to overeating.

Each of these ideas contains some element of truth, but perhaps none more than the fact that our society is aging. As noted in Chapter 1, "Introduction," the familiar population pyramid, with a few old people at its top and many young people at its base, is fast becoming a rectangle. This population rectangle, which has been taking shape over the past 40 years, will complete its metamorphosis over the next two decades. In 1980, nearly three times as many persons were under age 18 as were over age 65 (28% vs. 11%). By 2030, the percentages will be equivalent (20%).

As we age, our *metabolism*—the chemical processes that build and destroy tissue— gradually slows. When it comes to eating, our fat oxidation, or fat-burning rate, slows by about 30% with age. The metabolism that breaks down food components releases them in the form of energy and heat more slowly. Thus, the number of calories that were required to maintain our weight when we were young no longer maintains our weight, but increases it. Also, chronic conditions—most notably arthritis—that accompany the aging process can place limitations on our ability to stay active. Activity is a crucial factor in long-term weight management.

According to the Harris poll and the National Health and Nutrition Examination Survey, obesity reaches a peak among people in their 50s. More specifically, obesity peaks between the ages of 45 and 55 for men, and between 55 and 65 for women. Between the ages of 25 and 55 the average American gains 30 pounds of weight, about a pound a year. Moreover, during this time period most Americans are sedentary and *lose* about 15 pounds of muscle mass, so the 30-pound weight gain actually translates into a 45-pound *fat* gain.

After age 75 there begins to be a tendency to lose weight. Unfortunately, this weight-loss is due more to loss of muscle than loss of fat, so older persons not only become thinner, but weaker and less functional as well.

Obesity is most prevalent among low-income minority women. Regarding *income*, 25% of women above the poverty level are obese, whereas 37% of women with incomes below the poverty level are obese. Regarding *sex and ethnicity*, Mexican American women are 40% obese, compared to 29% for Mexican American men; African American women are 50% obese compared to 28% for African American men (Flegal, Carroll, Ogden, & Johnson, 2002; Squires, 2002). Using the less rigorous criterion of being overweight, more than 80% of African American women 40 or older are overweight (Flegal et al., 2002).

OVERWEIGHT AND OBESITY

The BMI has been the standard gauge of weight status. It provides a simple and roughly accurate method for determining population (but not individual) overweight and obesity. BMI can be calculated by multiplying weight in pounds by 700, divided by height in inches, and then dividing by height again; or if you have a pocket calculator, divide body weight (kg) by height squared (m²). People who have a BMI between 25 and 29.9 are overweight, between 30 and 39.9 are obese, and 40 or over are extremely (or morbidly) obese. According to these criteria, about two thirds of adult Americans are overweight, one third are obese, and 5% of the obese are morbidly, or extremely, obese.

The BMI is a useful, and sufficiently accurate, tool for screening the *general* population; but, similar to height/weight charts, it fails to differentiate fat from lean body mass in individuals. Also, centrally obese apple-shaped bodies are more of a heart risk factor than pear-shaped bodies. The two shortcomings of this tool that are associated with age are:

1. Excess body fat in older adults may be underestimated by a BMI score because it is counteracted by a loss of muscle mass with age. The net result can be a BMI under 25 for an older person, despite the excess body fat.
2. It is not uncommon for older adults to lose about two to three inches in height as they age, and there is no consensus on whether to use the new or old height (or an in-between height) in determining BMI.

A *waist-to-hip ratio* is a better predictor of heart attack than BMI (Yusuf et al., 2005). This ratio refers to waist measurement divided by hip measurement. A score above .85 in women, or .9 in men, shows a risk for heart disease. The higher the ratio, the greater the risk of a heart attack. This association is not as strong using the BMI measurement. The BMI measurement, however, is a lot easier to calculate, and serves research well when used on large data sets.

Morbidity and Mortality

One study reported that even being modestly overweight increases the chances of developing heart failure. This study of almost 6,000 adults reported that although the risk of heart failure is double in obese people, it is still a substantial 34% higher in those who are only overweight (Kenchaiah et al., 2002). For each increment of one unit on the BMI scale, the risk increased 5% for men and 7% for women.

Obesity, however, is the major risk factor. It is associated not only with heart disease, but also with diabetes (Pereira et al., 2005); cancers of the breast, colon, and prostate (Calle, Thun, Petrelli, Rodriguez, & Heath, 1999; Feigelson et al., 2006; Renehan, Tyson, Egger, Heller, & Zwahlen, 2008); osteoarthritis of the weight-bearing joints (Leveille, Wee, & Iezzoni, 2005); dementia (Kivipelto et al., 2005; Whitmer, Gunderson, Barrett-Connor, Quesenberry, & Yaffe, 2005); metabolic syndrome (Maison, Byrne, Hales, Day, & Wareham, 2001); gallbladder disease (Dittrick, Thompson, Campos, Bremers, & Sudan, 2005); and premature mortality (Peeters et al., 2003).

Moreover, obesity appears to be a cause of heart disease, even beyond its association with cardiac risk factors like hypertension, diabetes, and hyperlipidemia (Kenchaiah et al., 2002). A follow-up of the Framingham Heart Study reported that obesity decreased life expectancy by 6 to 7 years, and the difference in life expectancy between obese and normal-weight adults is similar to that between smokers and nonsmokers (Peeters et al., 2003).

Surprisingly, a national survey of seriously overweight persons reported that 70% did not view their excess pounds as a health concern ("Most Patients," 1999). Although most respondents were not in denial about being overweight or about the stigma associated with their appearance, they were in denial about the health consequences of their excess weight.

> **Question:** Some people argue that, despite the amount of obesity in old age, the bigger geriatric concern is malnutrition. What is your opinion on this? Why?

Costs

Obesity is associated not only with a wide range of diseases, but also with increased expenses—Medicare costs accrue with these diseases. Obese Medicare recipients accumulate $170,000 more in Medicare charges than normal-weight patients (Raebel et al., 2004). The heavier people were in middle age, the more they accumulated in annual Medicare charges later on. Health economists have calculated that nearly 10% of health spending in 2008—$147 billion—was related to obesity, nearly double the total of a decade ago (Finkelstein, Trogdon, Cohen, & Dietz, 2009).

The incremental cost of obesity far exceeds that of smoking. A 7-year study reported that smokers do not live as long as the obese because the latter are being kept alive with drugs for heart disease, diabetes, and other fat-related diseases (Moriarity, 2012). The extra costs for these prescriptions as well as additional hospitalizations adds up over time.

GENETICS, LIFESTYLE, AND ENVIRONMENT

Genetics

Although genes do not destine you to become fat, a family history of obesity increases your chances of becoming obese by about 25% to 30%. Moreover, if you are genetically inclined to carry the extra weight primarily around your waist (apple shaped), you are at higher risk for heart disease, hypertension, stroke, and diabetes than the noncentrally obese (pear shaped).

There may also be a genetic thermostat for body fat. *Set-point theory* states that a genetic thermostat for body fat maintains a fairly constant weight. If body weight decreases through dieting, the set-point either triggers appetite or makes the body conserve energy—lowers the basal metabolic rate—to maintain the fat cells and a set weight. The body burns calories more slowly than normal when weight is lost. This was a useful compensation when sources of food were unpredictable or possibly scarce.

Lifestyle

Although genetics is a contributor to the development of obesity, a more important (in terms of being able to do something about it) reason that an individual becomes overweight or obese is related to lifestyle. By limiting the types and quantity of food and increasing daily energy expenditure through physical activity and exercise, one has the ability to make a significant impact on body weight.

The *National Weight Control Registry* is a landmark study of 800 persons, average age 45, who have shed at least 30 pounds and kept the weight off for at least 5 years (Klem, Wing, McGuire, Seagle, & Hill, 1997). Weight loss was confirmed in a variety of ways, including documentation from physicians, interviews with family members or friends, and photographs. The researchers concluded that persistence was one of the most important components of successful weight loss. The average person failed half a dozen times before success was obtained.

Moreover, there was no single magical way to achieve success, unless you count modifying eating and exercise habits as magical. About 44% limited their food portions, 40% counted calories, 33% limited fat intake, 25% kept track of fat grams, and 4% relied on diet drugs.

Most of the registry's participants had been overweight since childhood, nearly half had at least one overweight parent, and more than a quarter had two overweight parents. Genes may predispose some toward obesity, but apparently lifestyle changes can initiate and sustain weight loss. On average, the participants reduced their body weight by 29% and successfully moved into the normal weight range.

A similar study with a smaller sample size (*n* =160) was conducted earlier by Anne Fletcher (1994), an RD, and reported in her book *Thin for Life*. Fletcher distilled her strategies for success from persons who kept off at least 20 pounds (average weight loss was 63 pounds) for a minimum of 3 years (most more than 5 years). The successful strategies employed by this sample of adults included the following:

1. Focus on what you can eat, not on what you cannot eat.
2. Do not deny yourself your favorite foods and do not worry about periodic slip-ups.
3. Identify and then avoid high-risk situations and emotional eating.
4. Find a way to incorporate exercise into your weekly routine.
5. Identify when you need to seek outside help.

Environment

Perhaps it is not our genes or our lack of will power. Perhaps our environment is a major contributing factor. Our society produces an abundance of food: food that is high in fat, sugar, and salt—much of it processed and packaged for our convenience; food that is advertised with costs of tens of billions of dollars per year; and food that is available everywhere—gas stations, drugstores, food courts in shopping malls, and vending machines located just about everywhere, including in 98% of our high schools.

> **Question:** Regarding weight management, which do you believe is more important: lifestyle counseling or environmental change? Explain your answer.

Also, during the last 30 years Americans have doubled the frequency with which they eat at restaurants; and when they eat out, they eat more. In a busy society, consumers seek the convenience that restaurants provide. Consumers also have been seeking greater value at restaurants. Profit-seeking restaurant owners have come to the realization that the food itself is the least costly ingredient of a food product, compared to the costs of labor, packaging, and marketing. Thus, restaurant owners are providing ever-larger portion sizes, with little increase in cost.

Food is low cost and overproduced in the United States. According to Marion Nestle, an endowed professor in nutrition and health at New York University, there are 3,800 calories produced per person, per day in the United States, and we only need about half of that (Nestle, 2002). Food is abundant, ubiquitous, cheap, and fattening, and it is promoted everywhere, all the time.

Environmental Change to Accommodate Obese Americans

Given how difficult it has been for people to lose weight, it is not surprising that businesses are focused on a complementary challenge: adjusting the environment for bigger people. Restaurants provide larger chairs for obese customers or switch to armless chairs and reinforced seats. Airlines have allowed—and charged for—obese customers to take up two adjoining seats. Some obese customers request seatbelt extenders.

Slacks labeled "regular" are now "slim cut." Larger sizes are "easy fit," "loose fit," or "baggy fit." Larger-sized women's clothing now has smaller-sized numbers: what used to be a size 12 is now labeled a size 8. The petite health writer Jane Brody, who believes she is at best a size 4, was thrilled to find a pair of size 0 slacks that fit perfectly.

Hospitals use larger beds and bigger wheelchairs. To avoid the embarrassment of taking a patient down to the loading dock for the use of a scale, human scales have been developed to accommodate up to 1,000 pounds. Rear ends are so large that extra-length needles are necessary for the injection to pass through the fat and reach the buttocks muscles. Medical clinics add loveseats to the waiting room. Open MRI machines are not just for claustrophobic patients, but for obese ones as well. Blood pressure cuffs, body fat calipers, and patient gowns are super-sized.

Exam tables have been anchored into the floor to prevent obese patients from flipping them as they sit on the end. Floor-mounted commodes prevent them from being pulled out of the wall. Doorways have been widened from 36 to 52 inches. Portable hoists are placed by bedsides to prevent worker injuries. Hospital suppliers have developed more than 1,000 items specifically for obese patients, including a wider body bag—which leads to a final comment: Funeral homes now offer extra-large coffins that accommodate up to 700 pounds. They are selling briskly.

SHOULD WE GAIN WEIGHT WITH AGE?

Many argue that gaining a few extra pounds with age may be not only common in America, but healthy. Dr. Reubin Andres, former clinical director of the National Institute on Aging, conducted a series of long-term studies and found that people in their 60s who were somewhat overweight (according to the Metropolitan Life Insurance charts), but not grossly obese, had a better chance of living into their 80s and 90s than those whose weight was normal. Thus, he created age-specific weight tables that generally have upper weight limits that are 10 to 20 pounds higher than the insurance-based tables.

A study by the Cooper Institute for Aerobics Research (Lee, Blair, & Jackson, 1999) appeared to support Andres's contention that we need to be more lenient with recommended weight ranges, especially among persons who maintain their fitness. Men who gained significant amounts of weight over time but remained moderately or very fit had lower death rates than men who were in the average weight rate for their group but were unfit.

The chief opponent of Dr. Andres's theory was Dr. Roy Walford of the UCLA School of Medicine, who died at age 79, 41 years short of his goal to live to 120. Dr. Walford practiced what he preached, which was to maintain reduced caloric intake, and placed himself on a life-long diet in adulthood of 1,500 calories a day. His animal research had shown that underfed rats lived one third longer than well-fed rats. Other studies have reported that a caloric intake decreased by 30% in young or middle-aged laboratory animals prolonged longevity (Colman et al., 2009; Masoro, 2005).

Critics of Dr. Walford's research, however, were concerned not only with his extrapolation from rodents to humans, but also with whether longer life on an "eat less" diet, even among the rats being studied, is associated with stunted growth, lower energy levels, and greater irritability. Comedians are also critical of Dr. Walford's diet, lamenting that eating less may not really lengthen life; it may just make life *seem* longer.

For those willing to risk lowered energy levels, increased irritability, malnutrition, and reduced interest in sex, there is the California-based *Calorie Restriction Society*. The 900 members have cut their calories by about 30% in hopes of living longer lives. For more information, visit www.calorierestriction.org.

Before you join, though, consider a 25-year study funded by the National Institute on Aging. Rhesus monkeys (N = 121) fed a calorie-restricted diet (30% reduction in calories) lived no longer than monkeys fed a normal-calorie diet (Mattison et al., 2012). The response to this study, conducted by well-respected researchers, some of whom were calorie-restrictors themselves, was surprise and disappointment.

Dr. Andres's extra-weight theory also generated studies that both supported and refuted his ideas. Critics noted that Andres's sample was biased toward the affluent elderly who could pass life-insurance medical examinations, and that he ignored health problems like diabetes, hypertension, and hyperlipidemia that were often unfavorably influenced by weight gain.

The Nurses' Health Study also suggested that the increasingly permissive weight guidelines may be unjustified. The researchers tracked the health status of 115,000 female nurses for 16 years and discovered a direct correlation between weight and susceptibility to stroke (Rexrode et al., 1997). Women whose BMI score rose into the 27 to 31 range during the 16-year period were 1.7 times more at risk for stroke; women who rose to a BMI of at least 32, more than doubled their risk.

The controversy was further muddled, however, by the results of a large and rigorous study conducted by researchers at the Centers for Disease Control (CDC) and the National Cancer Institute. They concluded that people who were overweight had a *lower* death risk than people of normal weight (Flegal, Graubard, Williamson, & Gail, 2005). Many critics applauded the rigor of the study's methodology; others argued that if overweight led to hypertension, heart disease, diabetes, hyperlipidemia, and sleep apnea, the results of the study appeared to be biologically implausible.

Despite the seemingly contradictory findings, there are studies that help to make sense of the controversy (e.g., Corrada, Kawas, Mozaffar, & Paganini-Hill, 2006; Dahl et al., 2010; Lenz, Richter, & Mühlhauser, 2009; Reynolds, Saito, & Crimmins, 2005). Being overweight in midlife increases morbidity and physical and mental decline in late life, but it may have no effect on longevity, or it may even extend longevity. This may be due to improved medications that are able to reduce mortality, the extra weight lowering the risk of hip and other types of fractures, and the cushion against weight loss that accompanies some major diseases. Obesity, though, may increase death rates by 20%, and extreme obesity by 200%. Obesity increases the likelihood of coronary heart disease, which not only affects morbidity and disability, but mortality as well.

BODY COMPOSITION

Body composition is a better measure of health and fitness than body weight. Improving your fat-to-muscle ratio helps protect you from serious ailments and improves your fitness. No one, however, has been able to evaluate the ideal percentage of body weight that should be fat versus lean tissue. Researchers have attempted, though, to develop broad guidelines for body fat ranges for men and women. Table 5.6 was derived from data provided in an article by Gallagher and associates (2000).

Notice that the relationship between age and body fat is less strong, and more susceptible to lifestyle intervention, than the relationship between sex and body fat. One study reported that middle-aged and older men with more than 24% body fat, and women with more than 31%, are at increased risk for heart disease, stroke, various cancers, high blood pressure, diabetes, and degenerative joint disease (Howley & Franks, 1997).

There are several ways to measure body fat. The gold standard is *hydrodensitometry*, or underwater weighing; it is based on the principle that fat is less dense than water and that overweight individuals weigh less in water. *Skin-fold caliper* is quick and reasonably accurate. Fat is pinched and measured in several areas, including the triceps, suprailium, and thigh for women; and chest, abdomen, and thigh for men. This technique, though, came into use in the 1950s, when people were leaner. Now, nearly 25% of women in their 50s have too much body fat to be measured with the traditional two-inch calipers, and they were being excluded from research samples (Himes, 2001).

Bioelectrical impedance is another way to measure body fat. One electrode is attached to an individual's foot and another to the hand, and a weak electrical current (that is safe and painless) is sent from one electrode to the other. The technique is based on the premise that the signal will travel faster through muscle than fat, because water conducts electricity and muscle is 70% water. Fat, on the other hand, is about 9% water.

Another technique is the *Bod Pod*, which works on the premise that a muscular body is denser and takes up less space than one that has more fat. The pod has a built-in computer that uses your weight and how much space you take up, and then converts it into a percentage of your body that is fat.

TABLE 5.6 Age and Recommended Body Fat Ranges

AGE	MEN	WOMEN
18–39	9%–19%	22%–32%
40–59	12%–21%	24%–33%
60–79	14%–24%	25%–35%

DIETS

Americans spend over $40 billion a year on diets and related attempts to lose weight. Despite this investment, 95% of people who lose weight regain the weight in 5 years, and the percentage of overweight American adults continues to increase. Diets tend to reduce weight in the short run—primarily due to loss of water and high short-term motivation—but invariably prove ineffective in the long run. But they still do not lose their popularity, because along comes another one that this time "really works!"

The *low-carbohydrate, high-protein* diet has been around since the early 1970s, and resurfaced years later as the *Dr. Atkins' New Diet Revolution* (1992). Variations of this diet have been developed by Barry Sears, *Entering the Zone* and *Mastering the Zone* (1995, 1997); H. Leighton Steward and colleagues, *Sugar Busters* (1998); Arthur Agatston, *South Beach Diet* (2003); and others. This diet is unique in its longevity and in the number of research studies that support it—much to the surprise of many experts. It may work, however, for reasons other than the one offered by its proponents.

If carbohydrates are restricted, so the theory goes, blood sugar levels will be restricted and the pancreas will produce less insulin. With less insulin, the body is forced to burn fat reserves for energy. Opponents of this theory say dieters eat fewer calories, both by consuming fewer carbohydrates and by eating a monotonously high-protein diet that curbs their appetite. Despite the bacon and other high-fat foods that are permitted on this diet, the typical Atkins dieter amasses only 1,500 calories a day (or about 1,700 with the Zone diet).

The differences between these two low-carbohydrate, high-protein diets and the recommendations of the AHA are summarized in Table 5.7. (I provide the average of two different estimates of Dr. Atkins's plan, from the *Nutrition Action Healthletter*, March 20, 2000, issue, page 6; and *Health* magazine, the January/February 2001 issue, page 94.) Protein and fat are doubled in the Atkins diet compared to the AHA recommendations, and carbohydrates are drastically reduced. The Zone and other low-carbohydrate, high-protein disciples—like Sugar Busters—are less extreme.

The Atkins diet, compared to a conventional low-fat, low-calorie diet, produced favorable results after 6 months or a year. Not only did participants lose considerably more weight than the low-fat, low-calorie diet, but there were also improvements in HDL and triglycerides (Foster et al., 2001; Gardner et al., 2007a; Yancy et al., 2001). Also, a more rigorous test was conducted over a 2-year period with random assignment, and favored a low-carbohydrate diet over a Mediterranean diet or a low-fat diet (Shai et al., 2008). The results of greater weight loss and greater reduction in lipids was consistent with a meta-analysis comparing these same diets for geriatric patients (Watson, Chandrasekran, & Steinle, 2012).

Dr. Jules Hirsch, an emeritus professor and physician in chief at Rockefeller University who has been researching obesity for nearly 60 years, cautions dieters about low-carbohydrate and high-protein diets by noting: "When carbohydrate levels are low in a diet and fat content is high, people lose water" (Kolata, 2012). I suspect most people prefer to lose fat rather than water.

High-fat foods and protein do promote satiety. In order to satisfy hunger, though, one need not encourage an Atkins or similar diet program, but just greater consumption of high-fiber complex carbohydrates, lean protein, monounsaturated fats and polyunsaturated omega-3 fats.

Low-fat diets also have a huge constituency. The Women's Health Initiative study randomized nearly 49,000 postmenopausal women to a low-fat diet or their regular

TABLE 5.7 Low-Carbohydrate and High-Protein Diets

WEIGHT-LOSS PLAN	PROTEIN	FAT	CARBOHYDRATE
American Heart Association	15%	30%	55%
Dr. Atkins	27%	61%	12%
The Zone	30%	30%	40%

diet and found, to the surprise of many, no significant difference in weight loss (Howard et al., 2006). Moreover, diets that limit fat to no more than 10% of their daily caloric intake, such as the Pritikin (1984) and Ornish (2001) diets, may be deficient in essential fatty acids and fat-soluble vitamins such as A, D, and E. Thus, the last word on this diet must be given to the Irish dramatist George Bernard Shaw: No diet will attempt to remove all the fat from your body, because the brain is entirely fat; without a brain, you might still look good, but all you could do is run for public office.

Christian weight-loss programs began in 1957 when Presbyterian minister Charles Shedd urged his readers to pray their weight away. During the 1990s, Christian diet books and church-based weight-loss programs began to proliferate, combining evangelical theology, psychology, and nutrition education. Critics have expressed concern about the accuracy of the nutritional advice and the questionable association between losing weight and gaining God's approval.

One of the more successful Christian diet books was Gwen Shamblin's (1997) *The Weigh Down Diet*. This book sold more than a million copies and was followed up with a second book, *Rise Above* (Shamblin, 2000). One concern with her advice is that despite her background as an RD, Shamblin advocated that even people with serious weight problems should turn to God rather than to medical professionals. "Trust God, not exercise. The only exercise you need is getting down on your knees to pray."

BOX 5.2   **You Need Divine Intervention to Choose Among Religion-Based Diet Programs**

The religion-based diet programs are, to state the obvious, mostly unscientific, and some are a bit eccentric as well. The Hallelujah Diet by Rev. George Malkmus was inspired by the Bible's Book of Genesis, chapter 1, verse 29: "And God said, 'Behold, I have given you every plant yielding seed which is upon the face of all the earth, and every tree with seed in its fruit; you shall have them for food.'" Therefore, this vegan diet basically consists of fruits and vegetables, and 80% of what is eaten must be raw.

The Maker's Diet was created by Jordan Rubin, a Messianic Jew, who drew his inspiration from the book of Leviticus, and discourages readers away from the vegan regimen of the Hallelujah Diet. Instead, it promotes organic meat and non-pasteurized dairy products. Another program called Bod4God relies on God and low carbohydrates. Pastor Steve Reynolds leads this program in Baptist churches across America; and he has his work cut out for him, as Baptists have the highest rates of obesity among several denominations studied (Salmon, 2007).

It is unclear whether incorporating any type of religious ideology into a weight-loss or weight-management program is helpful to participants in terms of guidance, motivation, or other factors. Regardless of the ideological content, however, program participants in synagogues and churches that follow nutritiously sound diets—a major qualifier—can take advantage of the fellowship, trust, and support that typifies these settings.

Do you know older adults who are open to change in their own eating patterns? Do you think the persons you have in mind would be more or less motivated to attend a program located in their religious institution? Would they be more or less motivated to attend if there were dietary practices linked to religious ideology compatible with their own beliefs?

Weight Watchers encourages participation in a weekly support group meeting and a nutritional strategy that assigns a point value based on calories, fat, and fiber content. The dieter is allocated a preferred number of total points each day, which can be spent anyway one likes. Adding exercise to one's daily routine allows for additional points to be spent. This commercial weight-loss

> **Question:** If you had developed your own weight-loss program and you wanted to pilot-test this program with older adults in your community, which of these three sites would you choose: a physician's office, a religious institution, or a shopping mall? Why?

program has done well in a few controlled studies that compared it to other strategies (Heshka et al., 2003; Tsai & Wadden, 2005).

Volumetrics is a diet based on portion size and energy density. Dr. Barbara Rolls and colleagues at Pennsylvania State University found that people tend to eat about the same weight of food each day, but the number of calories packed into a given amount of food determines weight gain or loss. Low-caloric, that is, low-energy, low-density foods such as fruits, vegetables, low-fat dairy products, and whole-grain breads and cereals have a positive association with weight loss and weight maintenance (Ledikwe et al., 2006). Foods with high water and fiber content result in a low density score and are encouraged. Fiber not only adds noncaloric volume to foods, but also holds water, which slows the absorption of food and may lead to a quicker feeling of satiety.

Another option, chosen by about 4,000 overweight individuals each year, is to undertake a pilgrimage to Durham, North Carolina, in order to participate in weight-loss and nutrition programs, as well as to transfer $51 million into the city's economy. These programs are effective, with one caveat. When you return home, the weight returns as well. The programs provide group support, a supportive culture, personal attention, and medical care associated with weight problems—none of which are brought back home.

The most unique weight-loss program (appealing to my eccentric personality) is "fidgeting," or what researchers so eloquently refer to as *nonexercise activity thermogenesis* (Levine et al., 2005). Spontaneous fidgeting can make a significant contribution to daily energy expenditure, whereas nonfidgeters may experience a 10% additional weight gain. Fidgeting is likely to be genetically based, however, and it is unlikely that patients can be successfully counseled to fidget more.

Along this same vein was a purported study (no reference provided) in *Health* magazine that reported on gum chewing. Chomping for an hour on a big wad of sugarless gum raises the metabolic rate 19% and burns 11 extra calories. The researchers alleged that chewing gum every waking hour can knock off 10 pounds a year. It would seem to me that chewing gum every waking hour and missing three meals a day would result in a weight loss of more than 10 pounds a *week*—until there was no more you. (See Figure 5.5 for a similar fanciful diet.)

The *Imaginary Diet* was reported on in the prestigious journal *Science* (Morewedge, Huh, & Vosgerau, 2010). People who first imagined themselves eating several pieces of a specific food, became less likely to gorge on that specific food afterward. The imagining habituates you to the real thing and lessens your desire to eat as much of it. The best part of this diet is the—imaginary for the time being—cookbook. It would be all pictures, the first diet flip book.

Perhaps the most preposterous diet is practiced by the *Breatharians*, who allegedly live off the air and the energy from sunlight. This fasting to the extreme has led to several recruits dying of starvation or dehydration, as well as lawsuits (Lagesse, 2002). This suggests that the last word on diets should be given to the late comedian and quasi-nutritionist Art Buchwald who said the word *diet* comes from the verb *to die*.

| FIGURE 5.5 | The 10-calorie diet. |

MONDAY	Breakfast:	Weak tea
	Lunch:	1 Bouillon cube in ½ cup of diluted water
	Dinner:	1 Pigeon thigh and 30 oz. of prune juice (gargle only)
TUESDAY	Breakfast:	Crumbs scraped from burned toast
	Lunch:	½ dozen Doughnut holes
	Dinner:	2 Jellyfish skins
WEDNESDAY	Breakfast:	Boiled out tablecloth stains
	Lunch:	½ dozen Poppy seeds
	Dinner:	Bee knees and mosquito sautéed in vinegar
THURSDAY	Breakfast:	Shredded eggshell skin
	Lunch:	Belly buttons from navel oranges
	Dinner:	2 Eyes from Irish potatoes
FRIDAY	Breakfast:	2 Lobster antennas
	Lunch:	1 Guppy fin
	Dinner:	1 Filet of softshell crab claw
SATURDAY	Breakfast:	4 Chopped banana seeds
	Lunch:	Broiled butterfly liver
	Dinner:	Jellyfish vertebrae
SUNDAY	Breakfast:	Pickled hummingbird tongue
	Lunch:	Prime rib tadpoles
	Dinner:	Aroma of empty custard pie plate, tossed paprika and 1 cloverleaf

The first week you lose 50 pounds, the second week you lose another 50 pounds, and the third week we lose you.

Happy Holiday!

The good news is that many Americans gain only four fifths of a pound during the mid-November to mid-January holiday period. The bad news is that this gain may not be reversed during the rest of the year, and this translates to a 24-pound weight gain over 30 years of celebrating the end-of-year holidays (Yanovski et al., 2000).

BARIATRIC SURGERY

Bariatric surgery is the modification of the gastrointestinal tract for the purpose of initiating substantial weight loss. The most common bariatric procedure uses surgical staples to close much of the stomach so that it can only hold a small amount of food, as well as shortening the intestines. Due to the incidence of complications, subsequent dietary restrictions, and expense ($30,000 for the surgery and 6 months of follow-up care), this technique is often reserved for clients with extreme obesity—those with a BMI of 40 or more—who have attempted nonsurgical weight loss without success.

In 2002 the Internal Revenue Service designated obesity as a disease, allowing eligible taxpayers who spend over 7.5% of adjusted gross income on medical care because of obesity to deduct expenses for bariatric surgery (as well as weight-loss drugs and nutritional counseling). Two years later, the Centers for Medicare and Medicaid Services reversed a long-standing policy and also recognized obesity as a disease, opening the door for Medicare reimbursement of bariatric surgery. Medicare coverage had always been limited to treatments for illness and injury based on the 1965 law that created it.

In 2006 the Centers for Medicare and Medicaid Services began to cover bariatric surgery for seniors (along with previously covered disabled persons), provided they had a BMI of 35 or more, had at least one obesity-related condition, and had unsuccessfully attempted weight loss without surgery. Just prior to this Medicare policy change, bariatric surgeries rose from 47,000 in 2001 to an almost fourfold increase in 4 years—to 170,000 in 2005. Given that 14 million seniors are estimated to be obese, the number of bariatric surgeries is expected to increase substantially in the coming years.

A major concern with bariatric surgery is complications. An unpublished study by the Agency for Healthcare Research and Quality reported that 40% of 2,522 patients who underwent weight-loss operations in 2001 and 2002 had complications develop within 6 months. These complications increased costs by 20% and, for those whose complications required readmission to a hospital, the costs increased more than 100%. The most common complications range from the relatively common vomiting and diarrhea to the more serious abdominal hernias, infections, pneumonia, respiratory failure, and the leaking of gastric juices caused by imperfect surgical connections.

Since that time, surgical techniques and the quality of care has improved, and some hospitals that specialize in the procedure have been designated as "centers of excellence." To be covered by Medicare, bariatric surgeries must be performed at these centers, where it is believed that older patients do as well as younger ones. One study, though, reported that the risk of complications increased slightly for each additional year over age 60 (O'Rourke et al., 2006). After the Medicare rule change, however, the number of bariatric surgeries at certified centers increased, and length of stay and overall complication rates decreased (Nguyen et al., 2010)

The good news is that the death rate for bariatric surgery is a relatively low two per thousand patients, and that laparoscopic surgery, which requires only small incisions, has a lower complication rate. As laparoscopy becomes an increasingly favored mode of treatment, complications should be reduced.

Even more good news is that type II diabetes completely resolves itself in about 80% of individuals who undergo gastric bypass surgery (Saliba, Wattacheril, & Abumrad, 2009). Surprisingly, the immediate effects on glycemic control *precede* the substantial weight loss that is typically associated with these changes. One possible explanation relates to changes in hormonal effects accompanying the surgery. The Medicare program is considering covering bariatric surgery for diabetes alone.

MEDICARE COVERAGE FOR WEIGHT LOSS COUNSELING

If you have a BMI of 30 or higher, Medicare will pay for one counseling session a week for the first month, then five more monthly sessions. If you have lost at least 6.6 pounds by the end of the 6th month, you can get 6 more monthly sessions. If you have not, you must wait 6 more months before Medicare will cover another weight loss attempt. Weight-loss sessions are covered under Medicare Part B, with no copayment or deductible if they are conducted by a qualified practitioner in a primary care setting.

TEN TIPS FOR WEIGHT LOSS OR MAINTENANCE

Applying the *10 Tips* model from Chapter 3, "Health Educators: Collaboration, Communication, and Behavior Change," to weight loss or weight maintenance produces the following list of suggestions:

1. *Motivation.* Two general categories of motivation when it comes to behavior change are improved function and disease prevention. Is the client motivated by functioning better, that is, more energy, better mood, and so forth? Or is she or he motivated by avoiding, or alleviating the impact of heart disease, arthritis, and so forth? With the topic of weight loss or weight maintenance, though, there is another motivational source: appearance. Does the client want to look good, fit into his or her clothes, and garner the approval of others? The challenge is to find out which motivation works best for the client, and then encourage him or her to be conscious of this motivation on a daily basis, perhaps through strategically placed written reminders.

2. *Modest.* Clearly a loss of 1 pound of weight each week is more achievable than a 40-pound weight-loss goal with no particular time frame in mind. An even more modest goal is to avoid a focus on poundage and to focus instead on improved nutrition and exercise. That is, establish a goal to eat one additional fruit and vegetable each day, to substitute one whole-grain product for a refined one each day, or to walk briskly an additional time or two each week.

3. *Measurable.* Make sure that the client's goal is measurable, and that it is also for a measurable and modest period of time, perhaps a week or a month. What will clients accomplish at least 4 days during the upcoming week: one additional vegetable serving on each of the targeted days? Do clients' measurable goals modestly allow them to have days during the week when they do not have to be met?

4. *Memory.* Can clients place a subtle, or not-so-subtle, sign on the refrigerator? Can a list be prepared before going food shopping, and complied with during shopping? Do clients need a friend to call regularly to remind and motivate them? Do clients need to associate a brisk walk with an existing habit that they will rarely miss, such as dinner, and then decide to walk just before or after it?

5. *Positive thoughts.* It is hard to nurture positive thoughts when it takes the average person several failed attempts before s/he succeeds at weight loss. Hard, but not impossible. Encourage clients to be persistent, until positive thoughts finally match positive deeds.

6. *Reinforcement.* Losing weight or maintaining a desired weight tends to be reinforcing in its own right. If clients need additional external reinforcement, just about any reinforcement not involving food will do.

7. *Environmental Support.* If at all possible, keep junk food out of the house. Have a jar of healthy snacks handy. Keep another jar of water in a prominent place in the refrigerator, and make sure it is always stocked with carrots or celery. Place health magazines around the house. Keep enjoyable activities (crossword puzzle, letter writing, organizing a photo album) at strategic locations in the house, as a substitute activity for snacking.

8. *Stress Management.* This is particularly important with weight loss or weight maintenance, because emotional disturbances can lead to poor eating habits. One of the best stress managers is also the best technique for long-term maintenance of weight loss—exercise. For most people, timing exercise before meals decreases appetite; or timing it between meals, when you are most likely to snack, can take your mind off eating. Other techniques, such as deep breathing or progressive muscle relaxation, may also work.

9. *Social Support.* Someone who used to be overweight and has kept the weight off makes for a particularly effective social support person. But just about any person who genuinely cares for the person will do. Multiple sources of support are preferable to reliance on a single person.

10. *Problem Solve.* The typical person can examine several failed previous attempts at achieving a desired weight, or anticipate new problems likely to emerge in the future. Another problem-solving strategy is to keep a record of what is eaten, where it is eaten, and who it is eaten with, and try to reduce unhealthy eating patterns triggered by emotions (see Table 3.2, Food-Behavior Diary, in Chapter 3, "Health Educators: Collaboration, Communication, and Behavior Change").

SELECTED WEIGHT-MANAGEMENT TOPICS

Diet Drugs

In the 1960s and 1970s the drug of choice for desperate dieters was amphetamines, or speed, which promoted weight loss by boosting metabolism. Unfortunately, the drugs caused more problems than they solved, not the least of which were addiction and serious side effects.

In the 1990s, a new drug was introduced to Americans: *fen-phen* (fenfluramine and phentermine). With one third of Americans obese, and a majority of them unsuccessfully attempting to reduce to a healthier and more socially acceptable weight, it was not surprising that fen-phen became a best-selling diet drug. New prescriptions for fen-phen increased by 6,390% in the 4 years before it was taken off the market in 1997. The drug worked by curbing people's appetites, and studies reported the average weight-loss to be about 20 pounds in a year's time. The drug, however, was linked to heart valve abnormalities, pulmonary hypertension, and brain cell damage.

Defenders of diet drugs proclaim that the hazards from serious obesity are a far greater risk, resulting in 300,000 deaths a year from heart disease, diabetes, kidney disease, and stroke. Many people who had taken the diet drugs, however, were not getting the results they wanted; some were not even obese and were getting the drugs from commercial weight-loss clinics without a physician's supervision.

The next generation of anti obesity drugs activated different weight-loss mechanisms. *Meridia* came on the market in 1998; it acted on the brain to reduce hunger and enhance satiety and, therefore, helped to reduce portion size and snacking. Dieters using this drug lost about 10 pounds more than non-drug-taking dieters. After a dozen years, the medication was taken off the market in 2010 because it increased the risk of heart attack and stroke in patients with a history of heart disease.

Xenical was approved by the FDA in 1999. It interfered with the enzyme that digests fat and reduced by a third the amount of dietary fat a person absorbs. Trial results indicated that those taking Xenical lost 14 pounds during the first year, whereas those taking a placebo lost 8 pounds. For a 6-pound weight loss, though, the consumer paid $6 a day, took a multivitamin pill to compensate for the fat-soluble vitamins blocked by the drug, and may have experienced unpleasant gastrointestinal side effects. Also, weight loss occurred during the first 8 months; after that, subjects started to regain weight (New diet pill, 2000).

Nonetheless, in 2006 the FDA recommended that the weight-loss pill, Xenical, be sold over the counter. The drug took a new name, *Alli*, and consumers received with it a weight-loss and exercise guide and a free online behavioral support program. Along with the convenience of obtaining the over-the-counter Alli and its supplementary material, however, one also acquires its side effects, such as diarrhea and oily stools.

The next pill, *Acomplia,* not only helped clients to lose weight, but allegedly helped them to quit smoking, lower alcohol and drug abuse, and reduce risk factors for heart disease and diabetes. The trial study resulted in greater weight loss and fewer side effects than Xenical/Alli or Meridia, though one side effect that was particularly disturbing was the 8.5% of patients reporting psychiatric disturbances, compared to 3% on placebo.

In the last several years, herbs have grown popular for promoting weight loss. St. John's wort, taken for years in Germany to lift sagging spirits, has been used for weight loss in America. Repackaged with names similar to the unavailable fen-phen, like Herbal Phen Fuel and Diet Phen, this herb has not been tested for weight loss.

An herbal mixture used at Nutrisystem weight-loss centers was called *Herbal Phen-Fen,* a combination of St. John's wort and ephedra. *Ephedra,* an herb that is also known as ma huang, is a major constituent in many herbal weight-loss products and appeared to work in the short run. Ephedra was also the likely culprit in approximately 800 health problems reported to the FDA, including more than 40 deaths.

In 2004 the FDA banned the sale of dietary supplements containing *ephedra*—the first time the FDA had banned a dietary supplement since the Dietary Supplement Health and Education Act (to be examined in Chapter 6, "Complementary and Alternative Medicine") had been passed in 1994. In 2005, though, the ban was partially overturned to permit low-ephedra products, with fewer than 10 milligrams, to be sold.

And now we've come full circle. *Belviq* won approval from the FDA in 2012 even though it worked like the fen-phen combination that was withdrawn from the market in 1997 because it damaged heart valves. The good news? Medicare Part D does not pay for weight-loss drugs and other insurers tend to follow suit, including private insurers and 40 of the 50 state Medicaid programs.

Emotional Distress

One of the few studies of overweight older adults that focused on *emotional distress* reported that those individuals ($n = 183$) who exhibited the most effective dieting behaviors needed to avoid the emotional distress of having desired foods removed from their diet (Rosendahl & Kirschenbaum, 1992). Dieting may be especially difficult for older adults who have to deal with both the deprivation of favorite foods, and the inevitably slow progress that results from their slower metabolic rates.

A program called *The Solution Method* encouraged older dieters to add aerobic exercise and social support to the changes undertaken in their eating patterns, and to focus attention on counteracting a tendency to seek love and comfort from food or drink. These interventions may help to offset the emotional distress and discouragement that can result from dieting (Mellin, Croughan-Minihane, & Dickey, 1997). Aerobic exercise may also be an effective component of a weight-loss program. It may not only enhance the ability to achieve dieting goals, but may also improve mood, reduce depression, decrease somatic symptoms, and reduce muscle tension.

A social support component of weight-loss programs may be especially important to older dieters who are vulnerable to emotional distress while dieting. Social support may be provided by sharing experiences with peers or by seeking support from a spouse or health professional. In one study, two thirds of people who received strong support from friends, both within and outside of a weekly weight-loss meeting, sustained their weight loss for at least 10 months, compared with just one fourth of those who attended the meetings without such support (Wing & Jeffery, 1999).

Another intervention for keeping off extra weight is yoga, despite the fact that it doesn't burn off much in the way of calories. Researchers found that people in their 50s who regularly practiced yoga lost about 5 pounds over 10 years; whereas a comparison group, controlled for physical activity and diet and that didn't practice yoga, gained more than 13 pounds (Kristal, Littman, Benitez, & White, 2005). The researchers believed that yoga helped people cultivate awareness—particularly toward stress, sadness, and other emotions—making them less likely to overeat.

Competitive Eating and Implications for Advocacy

Given America's fixation on food and on competitive events, it was not surprising to find out that there is an International Federation of Competitive Eating, and most of the events take place in America. The most popular *competitive eating* event takes place in Coney Island, New York, on July 4 each year, and is hosted by Nathan's, known for its hot dogs. Nathan's has sponsored this annual event almost every year since 1916.

The dominant gurgitator (competitive eater) had been a relatively slender Japanese man named Takeru Kobayashi, who won the contest every year from 2001 to 2006, capping it off with his record-breaking 53.75 dogs in 12 minutes on July 4, 2006. Kobayashi's technique is to separate the bun, dip it in water to condense it (yum!), and eat it separately from the hot dog. Apparently this technique takes you only so far, as the American Joey Chestnut has beaten Kobayashi each July 4 after 2006.

Although Steve "the Terminator" Keiner ate only 20 hot dogs at one of Nathan's Annual Hot Dog Eating Contests, he was quite proud of his very American strategy—a pile-driver approach, keeping hot dog and bun together as he rammed them down his throat. When explaining his eating philosophy, the Terminator said he combines the American pile-driving strategy with a Zen philosophy: "I went down a path that the hot dog was one with me and I was one with the universe."

Aside from the fact that these competitions are too disgusting for most of us to watch, there is something sad and funny about this anecdote. Sad, because many Americans have an unhealthy relationship with food. Besides the excess weight, gorging on food can pose immediate health dangers. Funny, because Americans are a diverse and tolerant lot, and perhaps we do not need to get the Wellness Police to shut down a New York tradition into its ninth decade. (In the interest of reportorial candor, I should note that Nathan's hot dogs were one of my favorite foods as a child in Brooklyn about 6 decades ago.)

There is a similar conflict in attitude regarding obesity. Most persons would argue that obesity is unhealthy and we need to do as much as possible to reduce this epidemic. Yet a growing number of health promoters advocate a more laissez-faire approach, because some overweight Americans are fit and should be left alone, and others are not helped by the stigma and rejection that add to their burden.

A more laissez-faire approach toward overweight *individuals*, however, does not necessarily mean a do-nothing approach. The food industry spends $30 billion on marketing food each year, and the government spends only a tiny fraction of that amount on nutrition education. What should be done to address this imbalance?

Should we tax junk food to subsidize nutrition education? Should all restaurants be required to provide nutritional and caloric content of their food servings in a conspicuous place? Should breakfast cereals that have as much sugar as candy bars be required to display labels that they are breakfast candy rather than cereal? Should "lean" beef be redefined so that the beef is actually lean?

The general issue of health advocacy, including advocating for better nutritional habits in this country, is discussed in more detail in Chapter 12, "Public Health Policy."

Surfing for Slimness

Here are three computer-related strategies for losing weight:

1. www.eDiets.com: This website claimed that its 800,000 registered members had lost a total of 1,744 tons. That sounds like a lot of tons, but it actually turns out to be a modest 4.36 pounds per person.
2. www.HealthandAge.com: This website does not make claims for weight loss, but it does provide interesting articles. It also provides its older web surfers with a choice of normal, large, or extra-large font size for their reading pleasure.
3. The last strategy for losing weight is, ironically, to spend less time in front of your computer screen.

The End of Overeating

In his book *The End of Overeating*, David Kessler (2009), former commissioner of the FDA, pointed out that the average weight of Americans grew by three quarters of a pound each and every year between 1960 and 2000. Something happened beyond the decline of individual willpower that instigated this 40-year obesity revolution. Kessler argued that food manufacturers have learned how to combine fat with sugar or salt in order to stimulate dopamine in the brain, for an effect similar to drugs like cocaine or amphetamines. Then the manufacturers added on the emotional gloss of advertising, eating tasty foods with friends, having a good time, and food products became addictive.

What to do about it? Kessler argues that we should limit the advertising of foods that have excessive combinations of fat, sugar, and salt, and increase the number of messages about the consequences of unhealthy foods. Also, practice these six tips:

1. Determine ahead of time what you will eat for meals and snacks.
2. Figure out how much food you need, and put it on your plate. No seconds.
3. Select foods that satisfy, rather than stimulate, such as whole grain, fruits, and vegetables, and combine them with lean protein and a small amount of fat.
4. Anticipate what to do when you encounter stimulating food, and rehearse your response.
5. Recognize emotions like sadness and anxiety that stimulate overeating.
6. Remove the image of a trigger food in your mind before you start to debate whether or not to eat it.

I find Kessler's ideas preferable to Jack LaLanne's well-known dictum: "If it tastes good, spit it out."

6

COMPLEMENTARY AND ALTERNATIVE MEDICINE

Key Terms

National Center for Complementary and Alternative Medicine

mind–body medicine

manipulative body-based therapy

energy therapy

dietary supplement

biomedical model

naturopathy

Dietary Supplement Health and Education Act

vitamins and minerals

antioxidants

herbs

hormone supplements

nutritional drinks

ConsumerLab.com

Dietary Supplement Verification Program

nutraceuticals

Learning Objectives

- Define complementary and alternative medicine
- Review the history of the National Center for Complementary and Alternative Medicine (NCCAM)
- Summarize the accomplishments of the NCCAM
- Contrast CAM and the biomedical model
- Review the usage of CAM among Americans of different ages
- Differentiate the categories of CAM
- Describe popular types of CAM

- Apply a CAM technique with an individual or small group
- Define naturopathy
- List CAM techniques covered by medical insurance
- Assess the accomplishments of Andrew Weil and Deepak Chopra
- Define dietary supplement
- Critically evaluate the Dietary Supplement Health and Education Act
- Evaluate the effectiveness of dietary supplements
- Describe the strengths and weaknesses of ConsumerLab.com and the Dietary Supplement Verification Program
- Define *nutraceuticals*

NATIONAL CENTER FOR COMPLEMENTARY AND ALTERNATIVE MEDICINE

The Office of Alternative Medicine existed between 1992 and 1998 as the newest and smallest institute of the National Institutes of Health (NIH). In 1998 it was renamed the *National Center for Complementary and Alternative Medicine* (www.nccam.nih.gov) and given a budget increase to $50 million, up from an initial budget of $2 million. A decade later, in 2008, the budget had increased to $122 million. This 61-fold increase in the budget for complementary and alternative medicine over a 16-year period confirmed the growing significance that the U.S. Congress had attached to this movement.

The change in name in 1998 was not arbitrary. *Alternative medicine,* as used in the original name of the office, was considered to be too adversarial, as if the consumer must choose between it and more conventional medicine. *Complementary medicine,* another popular term, suggested that these types of activities are used only in conjunction with traditional allopathic medicine. The compromise term—complementary and alternative medicine—and its acronym CAM reflect that consumers use it sometimes as an alternative to mainstream medicine and sometimes along with it. Hence, the National Center for Complementary and Alternative Medicine (NCCAM).

Two other labels that were often used were *integrative medicine* and *holistic health care.* However, CAM became the most popular term once the U.S. Congress gave it its blessing with the renaming of the national center.

The purpose of the National Center for Complementary and Alternative Medicine is to sponsor research on nontraditional topics such as *mind–body medicine, manipulative and body-based therapy, energy therapy, dietary supplements,* and other modalities that are off the beaten research path. The primary goal of the NCCAM is to begin to separate research fact from practitioner and consumer fancy, and to answer the question: Do these therapies work?

The question of effectiveness is not unique to CAM, as the parallel movement toward more evidence-based medicine in mainstream medicine attests. Nor is the safety of CAM services necessarily an issue more than it is for traditional allopathic medicine. The Institute of Medicine (IOM) reported more than 100,000 deaths from medical mistakes in 2009, even greater than a decade earlier when IOM declared a call to action to lower these deaths. The IOM also reported that drug errors injure at minimum 1.5 million Americans annually.

What is unique about CAM, though, is that despite the consistently unimpressive research findings, it remains a rapidly growing field of business, reaching $34 billion-a-year (Offit, 2012).

| BOX 6.1 | Complementary, Alternative, and Unimpressive? |

After spending a total of $1.6 billion over the years, the National Center for Complementary and Alternative Medicine (NCCAM) and its predecessors have very little to show for their investment. Large-scale, rigorous government studies have produced few positive findings. Distance prayer heals heart disease? Not a chance. Echinacea cures colds? No. Ginkgo biloba improves memory? Well, it worked for me, but I can't remember anything about the research findings. (Remember, humor is an important health promotion tool; the reader, however, may be better at using it than I am.) In summary, almost two decades of increasingly funded complementary and alternative medicine (CAM) research has produced no big wins.

Proponents of CAM suggest that its content areas are hard to research. For example, there are multiple manufacturers of the same herb using different techniques for production, and producing different versions of the same product. Would the results be better if another manufacturer, technique, or version of the product was used? There are plants, such as echinacea, that have nine different species, most of which have not yet been tested. One herbal brand might contain a plant's flowers, another its seeds, and another its stems and leaves, and in varying amounts. There are also natural sources versus synthetic forms of some vitamins. Finally, although the government's outlay on CAM research has been growing, it is still a tiny overall investment relative to past and current spending on conventional medications and interventions.

Opponents argue that CAM techniques and products are running far ahead of the science, resulting in true-believer/advocates who pressure funding agencies for more research dollars. Some of the studies seem downright foolish from a scientific perspective—for example, distant healing by anonymous prayer (supported by $1.5 million in NCCAM research funds), acupuncture results explained by body meridians, coffee enemas to treat pancreatic cancer, magnets to improve a whole host of bodily problems, lemon or lavender scents to improve arthritis—none of which are based on biological prinicples.

Where do you stand on this topic? Over the next few years would you favor giving more, less, or the same funding to the NCCAM? Would you fund CAM studies even if they are not based on a scientific foundation? Would you require multiple successful pilot studies before approving a large-scale CAM grant?

See whether your opinion is strengthened or changed after you read this chapter.

PREVALENCE OF COMPLEMENTARY AND ALTERNATIVE MEDICINE

In 2008 the National Center for Health Statistics reported that almost 40% of American adults used some type of complementary or alternative care. This is not surprising, given the more attractive set of characteristics that describe CAM than allopathic medicine (i.e., the *biomedical model*) (see Table 6.1). The number of visits to providers of CAM exceeded the number of visits to all U.S. primary care physicians by 37 million, despite the fact that only 25% of the cost of CAM is covered by health insurance.

The highest period of CAM usage is between the ages 50 and 59, followed by ages 60 to 69 and then ages 40 to 49. These decades include all individuals in the baby boom cohort (see Figure 6.1), making the topic particularly relevant to a book on aging. This should not be surprising, given that these techniques are primarily utilized for chronic conditions—conditions that begin to increase in number and severity during the boomer years.

TABLE 6.1 Characteristics of Complementary and Alternative Medicine and the Biomedical Model

COMPLEMENTARY AND ALTERNATIVE MEDICINE	BIOMEDICAL MODEL
Patient responsibility	Health professional responsibility
Mind/body/spirit	Body and mind separate
Healer serves as guide	Physician in charge
Holistic	Specialized
Promoting health	Fighting disease

FIGURE 6.1   Complementary and alternative medicine use among adults and children: United States, 2007.

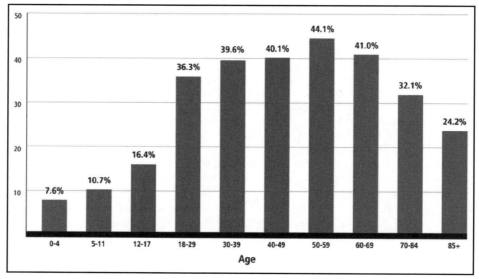

Source: Barnes, Bloom, and Nahin (2008).

Among all age groups there is a failure among clients of CAM to notify their physicians about their treatments. Surveys consistently report that more than half of the participants in CAM therapies neglect to communicate with their physicians. For instance, among older adults, 52% of White Americans and 58% of African Americans failed to communicate their CAM use with their physician (Flaherty et al., 2001). Among Medicare recipients in another study, 58% did not discuss CAM use with their physicians (Astin, Pelletier, Marie, & Haskell, 2000). Regarding dietary supplement use, one study examined the medical charts of 182 older adults; only 35% of self-reported dietary supplements were documented in the medical charts (Cohen et al., 2002a).

There are several reasons CAM users may not want to communicate such participation with their physicians. They may believe that their physicians do not approve of their activities, do not understand their motivations, or do not have the expertise to contribute to their own CAM knowledge. The consequences of this lack of communication, however, can be serious. For instance, over-the-counter herbal therapy—plant-derived preparations to improve function, prevent illness, or counteract pain—can diminish or alter the effects of prescription drugs.

TYPES OF CAM

Exactly what constitutes CAM has never been clearly established. Reinforcing this assertion, the NIH provided a definition of CAM that described what it is not, rather than what it is: "Those treatments and health care practices not taught widely in medical schools, not generally used in hospitals, and not usually reimbursed by medical insurance companies."

Despite the imprecision, some practices have been consistently associated with CAM. Herbal medicine and other dietary supplements fit into the CAM bailiwick, for instance, and will be given considerable space in this chapter. Some CAM techniques are hard to categorize, such as *homeopathy* (treatment with highly diluted substances that have little or no active chemical content, but that leave an "energy signal"), and *chelation therapy* (intravenous infusion of ethylenediamine tetra-acetic acid to bind heavy metals in the bloodstream), and are of dubious benefit.

Most others fall into one of three categories. A collection of techniques referred to as *mind–body medicine* falls within CAM and might include such modalities as meditation, visualization, prayer, humor, Tai Chi, yoga, and support groups. Another set of techniques associated with CAM, often referred to as *manipulative and body-based therapies*, includes chiropractic, massage therapy, postural restructuring, acupuncture, and osteopathic medicine. *Energy therapies* refer to yet another group of CAM methods that include healing touch, Reiki, magnetic field therapy, and laying on of hands.

There are also activities involving nutrition education and exercise that are sometimes included in CAM. Nutrition and exercise, however, are claimed by many different types of practitioners as part of their purview, including the practitioners of allopathic medicine. Often in mainstream medicine, however, they are only included as add-on strategies and superficially presented to a patient.

POPULAR CAM TECHNIQUES

Diaphragmatic Breathing

One symptom of stress is shallow and rapid breathing. A way to counteract this symptom is through diaphragmatic breathing, also called belly breathing, deep breathing, or yoga breathing. This technique is simple, convenient, and has face validity for most adherents. In other words, people feel better quickly. From a research perspective, the technique's short- or long-term effect on stress management is largely untested, and the results with disease management are mixed (Cahalin, Braga, Matsuo, & Hernandez, 2002; DeGuire, Gevirtz, Hawkinson, & Dixon, 1996). However, one study on slow breathing, that is, slowing respiration to 6 breaths per minute, reported a decrease in blood pressure in hypertensives (Joseph et al., 2005).

This technique is not easy for many older adults to learn (based on my personal experience teaching it). The imagery I use to facilitate learning is to visualize your stomach and chest as a pitcher to be filled with air. Place one hand on your stomach and the other on your chest, and inhale for about 6 seconds through the nose (this warms and moistens the air and screens impurities). Raise the lower hand (by expanding your stomach) as the air fills up the bottom of the pitcher, then the upper hand as the top of the pitcher is filled. Exhale for about 8 seconds, with the upper hand moving in first as the top of the pitcher is emptied; then draw in the abdomen as the bottom of the pitcher is emptied last and the lower hand moves in. The placement of the hands on the stomach helps to clarify this breathing procedure (see Figure 6.2).

Because most persons are shallow chest breathers, light-headedness may occur. To reduce or avoid light-headedness, decrease the length of the inhalation and exhalation. After sufficient practice, this exercise can be extended in time and repeated multiple times over the course of the day.

FIGURE 6.2   **Belly breath.**

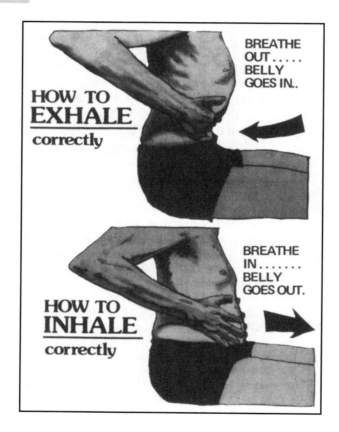

BREATHE OUT . . . . . BELLY GOES IN . .

HOW TO **EXHALE** correctly

BREATHE IN . . . . BELLY GOES OUT.

HOW TO **INHALE** correctly

Progressive Muscle Relaxation

Another symptom of stress is muscle tension. Edmund Jacobson began his work on reducing muscle tension through progressive muscle relaxation in 1908. Jacobson believed that tension can manifest itself in any muscle in the body, and in order to relax you must learn to differentiate between muscle tension and relaxation. There has been little scientific inquiry to produce evidence in support or refutation of this technique.

This may not be the ideal relaxation technique for older people with painful arthritis or a heart condition. Clients with these conditions need to consult with their physician and may choose to eliminate or just to imagine the tension phase of the technique, or clients can focus exclusively on visualization, which tends to follow this technique.

One way to determine which sequence of muscle groups to tense and relax is to start from your head or your feet, and continue up or down your body. For each part of your body, hold your breath and the tension for 3 or 4 seconds, and then relax. When relaxing, exhale slowly and steadily. After exhalation, spend a few seconds paying attention to the way you feel, and then move on to the next part of your body:

1. Tense your forehead by raising your eyebrows.
2. Wrinkle your nose and press your lips together.
3. Tense your whole face, squeezing it in like a prune.
4. Shrug your shoulders.
5. Tense your left arm, then your right arm.
6. Tense your left fist, then your right fist.
7. Tense your shoulders toward the back, slightly arch your back, and lift your head up.
8. Squeeze your abdomen tight.
9. Squeeze your buttocks together.
10. Tense your left leg, then your right leg.
11. Bend your left toes, cock your left ankle, then your right toes, then your right ankle.

After some practice at this technique you may begin to recognize and locate tension that consistently collects in a specific part of your body. You can then use a mini-version of this procedure at any time to let go of tension in that area.

Visualization

Relaxation can be further facilitated by following progressive muscle relaxation with 10 minutes of visualization or imagery. One popular image is to recall the warmth of the sun, the sensation of a gentle breeze, the sound and smell of the ocean, and the sight of a swaying palm tree. Just visualize and relax.

Or, if you like wellness guru Donald Ardell's offbeat sense of humor (I do, please don't hold it against me), try the imagery that he suggests:

> Picture yourself near a stream. Birds are singing in the crisp, cool mountain air. Nothing can bother you here. No one knows this secret place. You are in total seclusion. There is the soothing sound of a gentle waterfall, and the cool water is fresh and clear. And, without any effort, you can make out the face of the person whose head you are holding under the water.

Interactive guided imagery is a component of visualization that involves guidance by a trained therapist. The therapist may focus on relaxation and visualization and then direct your attention to an ailing part of your body (including internal organs) and ask you to focus healing thoughts on it. One study using guided health imagery with former smokers found that after 24 months, abstinence rates were double for the guided-imagery group versus the placebo-control group (Wynd, 2005).

Relaxation Response and Meditation

The relaxation response is based on the technique of meditation, but without the Eastern spiritual overtones. It operates on the premise that the repetition of a sound or word (like *one* or *peace*) is equivalent to the repetition of an Eastern philosophy-derived mantra, a one- or two-syllable sound that is part of a meditation technique. (For more information on the relaxation response technique and theory, see Herbert Benson's [1984] landmark book, *The Relaxation Response*.) The repetition of either a Western word or an Eastern philosophy-derived sound produces the same effect: deep relaxation.

Researchers at the Maharishi University in Fairfield, Iowa, have reported in academic journals that the technique of transcendental meditation—first brought to the United States in the 1950s by Indian guru Maharishi Mahesh Yogi and later popularized by the Beatles—is an effective option for lowering high blood pressure. Through randomized and controlled, single-blind trials, the researchers report that meditation lowers blood pressure as effectively as hypertension drugs but without the side effects (Castillo-Richmond et al., 2000; Paul-Labrador et al., 2006), and may decrease mortality in older persons (Schneider, Zaslavsky, & Epstein, 2005).

Meditation may also be associated with changes in the brain's physical structure. The prefrontal cortical area—an area of the brain associated with attention—was thicker in meditation participants than in matched controls (Lazar et al., 2005). Differences were especially notable in older persons, suggesting that meditation may help reduce the cortical thinning that occurs with age.

Both the relaxation response and meditation are based on the technique of letting thoughts drift away from the mind as they arise. This generally is referred to as emptying one's mind, but in actuality the technique is better described as allowing thoughts to pass through the mind as they arise, while the participant keeps returning to the chosen repetitive sound. The meditation may be performed in the following way:

1. Find a comfortable position. Most individuals prefer to be seated, though some choose to lie down. (People complain that they are likely to nap when they lie down; it is unclear whether, or by how much, a short nap is less effective at revitalizing the body and mind.)
2. Sit quietly with eyes closed; perhaps run through a quick version of progressive muscle relaxation.
3. Begin to repeat to yourself, softly, your word or sound (choose one that is pleasing to you and that you are not likely to forget).
4. Continue for 15 to 20 minutes, opening an eye to check the time if you like, or set a timer in another room so you will hear it as a soft auditory reminder.
5. Practice once, preferably twice, a day, before a meal, when digestive processes are not too distracting, and at a consistent time of the day (e.g., before breakfast and dinner) in order to establish a habit.
6. Most important, do not evaluate each session, even if you believe (and undoubtedly you will) that your thoughts have dominated your attention and prevented you from repeating your word or sound very often. Instead, choose a trial period (perhaps 1 month) and determine whether the sessions as a whole are having a beneficial impact.

Although repeating a sound or word is the most popular meditative device, some people prefer to visually focus on the center of a yantra (a geometric form) or to imagine a peaceful scene (such as the beach or the woods), or to pay attention to their inhalation and exhalation patterns.

Stress management techniques such as meditation are deceptively simple. As a one-time meditator for 20 years (I switched to deep-breathing techniques), this technique is easy to learn but difficult to sustain. To help develop a stress management habit, it is important to establish a consistent routine and it is helpful to have a partner to reinforce your practice.

One form of meditation, although some argue it is the opposite of meditation, is *mindfulness*, defined as paying attention to one's immediate experience, approaching it with curiosity, openness, and acceptance. One researcher argues that this technique is particularly relevant to older adults attempting to cope with chronic disease, pain, and disability (Rejeski, 2008).

Acupuncture

One major source of stress is coping with chronic physical pain. In November 1997 a committee of independent physicians and scientists at the NIH reviewed a wide range of research findings and concluded that acupuncture treatment—the 2,500-year-old Chinese needle therapy that has been on the fringe of American medicine for years—is effective for pain control and nausea, and has the promise to be beneficial in other areas as well.

The NIH committee encouraged insurers, both public and private, to cover acupuncture services for nausea caused by anesthesia, chemotherapy, and pregnancy, as well as for postoperative dental pain (National Institutes of Health Consensus Development Panel on Acupuncture, 1998). Only 19% of health plans provide acupuncture benefits, however, and Medicare is not one of them.

The Chinese theory behind acupuncture—that the body is made up of channels of energy flow called qi (pronounced *chee*) and that inserting needles into specific points on the body relieves energy blockages along these channels—has not received support from Western science. Research does support the idea, though, that acupuncture needles inserted into specific nerve junction points on the body and rotated or electrically stimulated will increase the production of the body's own natural painkilling chemicals.

In 2009, 41 states and the District of Columbia licensed or regulated the practice of acupuncture by nonphysicians and provided training standards for certification. In addition, the Food and Drug Administration (FDA) regulates the needles as part of its medical device authority. The number of acupuncturists in the United States has grown to 11,000, including 3,000 physicians who are members of the American Academy of Medical Acupuncture. To find a licensed or certified specialist, contact the National Certification Commission for Acupuncture and Oriental Medicine (www.nccaom.org) or the American Academy of Medical Acupuncturists (www.medicalacupuncture.org).

Research on the effects of acupuncture on cocaine addiction, rheumatoid arthritis, low back pain, asthma, emesis, menopausal symptoms, and myocardial disease has been mostly negative (Berman et al., 2004; Margolin et al., 2002; Shen et al., 2000; Vickers et al., 2004; Witt et al., 2005). Interestingly, the placebo effect—sham acupuncture, which consists of needles placed superficially at nonacupuncture sites—can have a positive impact on participants (Melchart et al., 2005; Witt et al., 2005).

To find information about *acupressure*—pressure applied by hands rather than needles—consult the American Organization for Bodywork Therapies of Asia, at www.aobta.org. One randomized, double-blind study with patients in six dementia units in Taiwan reported that acupressure applied to older residents with dementia decreased agitation and aggressive behaviors in comparison to a control group (Lin et al., 2009).

Therapeutic Massage

Chances are you will feel better after a good massage. In addition, there are studies to suggest that a therapeutic massage has a greater impact on lower back pain than does acupuncture (Cherkin et al., 2001), and produces migraine relief as well (Hernandez-Reif, 2001; Hernandez-Reif, Field, Krasnegor, & Theakston, 2001). For a listing of licensed professionals in your area contact the American Massage Therapy Association (www.amtamassage.org).

Chiropractic

Chiropractors focus on spinal and extremity manipulation, physical medicine modalities, rehabilitation, and nutrition. They are licensed in all 50 states and can become board certified in such subspecialties as orthopedics, sports medicine, and nutrition. Patients seek chiropractic doctors for musculoskeletal disorders, with low back pain being the most likely referral. Several studies report that, compared with medical treatment for low back pain, manipulation by chiropractors provided as much or more pain relief, higher activity levels, and greater patient satisfaction (Hurwitz et al., 2002; Sierpina, 2001).

One study reported that chiropractors spent more time with their patients than physicians, explaining their treatment for low back pain and advising them about self-care once they get home (Hertzman-Miller et al., 2002). Consequently, chiropractic patients were more satisfied with their care. Differences in satisfaction disappeared, however, when equal time was spent by the two types of professionals on explanations and advice about self-care.

It should also be noted that chiropractic manipulation is not without risk. If you want additional information on this practice or referral information, contact the American Chiropractic Association, 1701 Clarendon Blvd., Arlington, VA 22209; 703-276-8800; www.acatoday.com.

Hypnosis

A committee of independent physicians and scientists at the NIH reported that hypnosis may be effective for treating some types of pain. Hypnosis is a deep state of relaxation, accompanied by inertia, passivity, and a narrowing of consciousness. This technique has considerable potential for reducing anxiety and has been used with patients undergoing coronary angioplasty (Kanji, White, & Ernst, 2004). Guides are available to help clients learn self-hypnosis (Davis, Eshelman, & McKay, 2000), and there is a professional society that focuses on hypnosis research (Society for Clinical and Experimental Hypnosis, www.sceh.us).

Biofeedback

The NIH committee recommended biofeedback for tension headaches. Biofeedback uses a machine to make you aware of bodily processes that you do not ordinarily notice (muscle tension, skin surface temperature, brain wave activity, skin conductivity or moisture, blood pressure, and heart rate) so that you can bring them under voluntary control. A directory of certified biofeedback practitioners by local area is published by the Biofeedback Certification Institute of America, 10200 W. 44th Ave., Suite 310, Wheatridge, CO 80033-2840; 303-420-2902; www.bcia.org.

Magnet Therapy

A few poorly controlled studies that generated substantial publicity following positive results led to $200 million in sales in 1999 for magnets manufactured for healing purposes. When studies began to use control groups and participants proved unsure who was wearing real versus sham magnets ("Attracted to Magnets?" 2000; Collacott, Zimmerman, White, & Rindone, 2000) or ionized versus placebo bracelets (Bratton et al., 2002), no differences in pain relief were found.

One magnet study utilizing a treatment and a control group was able to report differences in self-rated pain and physical function. The use of a single-blind sample was probably offset by the fact that the magnet pad attracted metal objects (Hinman, Ford, & Heyl, 2002). Although only 10% of treatment participants admitted to detecting this, others may have noticed an attraction and experienced a placebo effect from the discovery.

Aromatherapy

Aromatherapy may have been in use since 3000 B.C. It is based on the practice of treating patients with essential oils extracted from plants. There is speculation that beyond the effects of the treatment's pleasant smell, the oils may affect certain parts of the body when inhaled or absorbed by the skin. One study found that 60% of severely demented patients who had lemon balm rubbed into their faces and arms twice a day for 4 weeks reported a significant reduction in their symptoms of agitation, compared to only 14% of those treated with a placebo lotion (Ballard, O'Brien, Reichelt, & Perry, 2002). Other small studies have utilized the lavender plant for easing anxiety.

Laughter

There are organizations that certify people as laughter leaders, and there are laughter clubs. There is also an International Laughter Day each year on May 6—mark your calendar! One study reported an inverse relationship between laughter and heart disease (Clark, Seidler, & Miller, 2001). But does laughter ward off heart problems, or are people with heart disease just less likely to laugh? It doesn't matter; go ahead and laugh. For information on training and speakers, access the Association for Applied and Therapeutic Humor (www.aath.org).

CAM AND MEDICAL EDUCATION

Most medical schools and residency programs in the United States were teaching CAM content or practices in one or more required or elective courses, usually in a department of family practice or internal medicine. This interest in CAM in medical education, however, does not necessarily amount to an endorsement of it.

Some medical schools and residency programs offer CAM courses and lectures in order to better inform physicians and students about what patients are doing. One large midwestern medical school reported that most first-year medical students (84%) were interested in learning about CAM because they believed this knowledge will be important to them when they become physicians and discover that some of their patients are using it (Greiner, Murray, & Kallail, 2000).

NATUROPATHIC MEDICAL COLLEGES

Naturopathy emphasizes the healing power of nature, and practitioners attempt to support the body's own healing capacity with natural therapies. There are seven naturopathic medical colleges in the United States and Canada, and in 15 states and the District of Columbia licensed naturopaths can legally practice medicine as primary care physicians. Between 4,000 and 5,000 naturopaths have graduated from 4-year accredited programs.

The state of Washington leads the country in naturopathic medicine. Seattle is the home of Bastyr University, the largest naturopathic school in the country, and in 1996 Washington became the first state to require insurance companies to cover complementary and alternative therapies in their benefit plans. The first publicly funded natural medicine clinic—staffed with naturopaths, other alternative therapists, and conventional health professionals—opened shortly thereafter in the Seattle area.

Naturopaths complete 4 years in a medical college and take national licensing exams. These physicians receive training similar in many ways to that of traditional physicians, plus they receive excellent training in the areas of nutrition (comparable to that of registered dietitians) and herbal medicine. These practitioners use herbal medicine, massage, and acupuncture; take X-rays, and blood and urine tests; and in some states perform minor surgery and prescribe antibiotics.

> **Question:** Can you imagine any medical problems that you might develop in the future for which you would consider enlisting the paid services of a licensed naturopath? Why or why not?

Naturopaths are more inclined than medical doctors, however, to try alternative treatments that have little or no credible scientific backing, such as *homeopathy*—prescribing infinitesimal doses of herbs and minerals that in larger amounts would produce an ailment's symptoms, in order to stimulate the body's curative powers; color therapy—wearing purple to lower blood pressure and yellow to prevent stroke; and colonic irrigation—a powerful, machine-delivered enema. The Liaison Committee on Medical Education, the accrediting body for U.S. medical schools, does not recognize naturopathic medical colleges.

To acquire more information, contact the American Association of Naturopathic Physicians (www.naturopathic.org), or call 866-538-2267 (toll-free).

SELECTED CAM TOPICS AND RESOURCES

CAM Insurance

About two thirds of health maintenance organizations (HMOs) offer coverage for at least one form of CAM, usually chiropractic (65%) or acupuncture treatments (19%), followed in single-digit percentages by massage therapy, biofeedback, and homeopathy ("Getting a Boost," 1999). Coverage of chiropractic treatment is mandated by 42 states, acupuncture by seven states, and massage therapy by two states. The state of Washington requires that insurers cover all categories of providers, including acupuncturists, massage therapists, and naturopaths.

Chiropractic coverage is endorsed by some insurers because there are studies reporting that this type of treatment is as successful at treating patients with chronic low back pain as allopathic care although costing substantially less. One study, however, reported that chiropractic care is more expensive than medical care for the treatment of low back pain (Kominski, Heslin, Morgenstern, Hurwitz, & Harber, 2005).

CAM coverage is endorsed by some insurers in the hope of attracting better-educated consumers with higher incomes and above-average health. In general, though, CAM coverage is quite limited, with insurers waiting for research results on clinical efficacy and cost-effectiveness. When insurers do cover a CAM therapy, it must be deemed medically necessary, visits are limited, and deductibles and copayments are high.

Oxford Health Plans in Connecticut became the first major U.S. health care plan to offer comprehensive coverage for a wide range of CAM services. Its network of 2,000 alternative providers include licensed practitioners of acupuncture, chiropractic, naturopathy, massage therapy, nutrition, and other specialties such as yoga and Tai Chi. These services are available for an additional premium.

In 2006 Medicare made a breakthrough by approving participation in two prevention programs developed by physicians Dean Ornish and Herbert Benson, though the first patients did not begin until May 2011. These comprehensive health promotion programs—nutrition education, exercise, cognitive restructuring, and others—also include CAM activities such as yoga, meditation, deep breathing, and support groups. Ornish's program is offered at eight sites in Pennsylvania and at five medical centers in West Virginia; Benson's program is available in Indiana, Rhode Island, Tennessee, Washington, and Virginia.

This marked the first time that the federal government had reimbursed Medicare beneficiaries for lifestyle intervention programs. These two programs have prompted a shift from an exclusive focus on the biomedical model to a regimen also including complementary medicine. Coverage is for 36 sessions within an 18-week period, with a possible extension to 72 sessions in 36 weeks. Medicare eligibility is limited to those with cardiovascular conditions and it has approved these programs for intensive cardiac rehabilitation. Typically, once Medicare establishes a reimbursement policy, most private insurance companies follow Medicare's lead.

> **Question:** What CAM services or dietary supplements would you like to see generally covered by health insurance? Why?

Weil and Chopra

Andrew Weil is on the medical school faculty at the University of Arizona in Tucson, where he developed a 2-year residency program that integrates traditional medicine and other disciplines, such as meditation, nutrition, herbal medicine, acupuncture, and osteopathic manipulation. He has published several books, such as *Spontaneous Healing, Eight Weeks to Optimum Health*, and *Healthy Aging*, and he reports receiving thousands of questions a week online at www.drweil.com.

Dr. Weil is without question the best-known and most influential purveyor of CAM. His opinions have become more mainstream over the years, and he has regularly appeared on the covers of national magazines and on television shows. His ideas on exercise, nutrition, and stress management are sensible and sciencebased. His views on dietary supplements, however, are way ahead of the research, in my opinion. Dr. Weil appears to take the generally more supportive and less rigorously conducted European studies on dietary supplements at face value and, as a consequence, prematurely recommends an astonishingly broad array of supplements.

Deepak Chopra's ideas lie more in the mystical realm. He writes books and a monthly newsletter; records spiritual lyrics and poetry; delivers lectures and seminars; sells tapes, herbs, and aromatic oils; and has plans—yet unrealized—for a nationwide chain of healing centers. The Chopra Center for Wellbeing in Carlsbad, California (www.chopra.com), dispenses a wide range of CAM along with conventional medicine.

Dr. Chopra's popularity may be waning, the same fate that befell prior charismatic health and spiritual gurus. To the extent that they advocate critical thinking and provide a more balanced view toward the medical mainstream, they serve a useful purpose for expanding our strategies for improving health. To the extent that they are interested in being seen as gurus and raking in every last buck from a gullible public, they are expanding their bank accounts more than our health care options.

CAM Organizations

The *American Holistic Medical Association*, 23366 Commerce Park, #101B, Beachwood, OH 44122; 216-292-6644; www.holisticmedicine.org.

The *American Holistic Nurses Association*, 323 N. San Francisco St. #210, Flagstaff, AZ 86001; 800-278-2462; www.ahna.org

The *Center for Mind-Body Medicine*, 5225 Connecticut Ave. NW, Suite 414, Washington, DC 20015: 202-966-7338, www.cmbm.org

Commonweal (cancer patients and health professionals who treat them), Commonweal, P.O. Box 316, Bolinas, CA 94924; 415-868-0970; www.commonweal.org

Ayuredic Institute (medicine of India), 11311 Menaul Blvd. NE, Albuquerque, NM, 505-291-9698. www.ayureda.com

Herb Research Foundation, www.herbs.org

The *National Wellness Institute* hosts an annual summer conference at Stevens Point, Wisconsin, P.O. Box 827, Stevens Point, WI 54481; 800-243-8694; www.nationalwellness.org

The *Complementary & Alternative Medicine Program* at Stanford is the only university-based research center focused on CAM and aging adults, Stanford Prevention Research Center, Hoover Pavilion, 211 Quarry Rd. N229, Stanford, CA 94305; 650-723-8628; http://camps.stanford.edu

CAM Journals

Alternative Therapies in Health and Medicine, www.alternative-therapies.com
Holistic Nursing Practice, http://journals.lww.com/hnpjourn
Journal of Alternative and Complementary Medicine, www.liebertpub.com/acm
Alternative Medicine Review, http://altmedrev.com
Positive Health, www.positivehealth.com

DIETARY SUPPLEMENTS

For many years the conventional wisdom in the nutritional sciences has been that a balanced diet is sufficient to achieve all nutritional goals. More than two decades ago, Horwath (1991) reported that purchasing healthy foods within the context of a balanced diet is more effective and less costly than purchasing supplements. She also noted that the presumed value of any particular dietary supplement is subject to change with each new research finding. Horwath concluded that it is best to rely on the variety of good foods provided by nature.

Over the following two decades, however, an increasing number of researchers have found evidence of the need for specific dietary supplements. For example, the research supporting folate as a supplement was so persuasive that the FDA required manufacturers of breads, cereals, pasta, and other grain products to fortify their products with it. The American public, however, has gone one giant step further, finding the need to buy a *wide range* of dietary supplements, nutritional or food supplements containing vitamins, minerals, herbs, or other ingredients. This perceived need is so strong that one study reported that 71% of regular patrons of dietary supplements would continue to use them even if research proved them to be ineffective (Blendon, DesRoches, Benson, Brodie, & Altman, 2001)!

Cautions

There are good reasons to be more cautious in taking dietary supplements than the general public appears to be. It is not clear, for example, if dietary supplements are adequate substitutes for the nutrients in foods. Most dietary supplements are narrowly targeted, whereas the nutrients in foods work in synergy.

Phytochemicals are illustrative of this distinction. These chemical compounds are found in abundance in fruits and vegetables, and seem to exert a powerful synergistic effect in cancer prevention. These compounds, however, are impossible to replicate in pill form. Adults who eat a poor diet and try to compensate with a variety of specific supplements will not derive the same benefits they would from healthy eating because of the inability to replicate synergistic chemical compounds in pill form.

Another caution with taking supplements is that they can be dangerous. An overdose of vitamin A can cause headaches, nausea, diarrhea, liver problems, and hip fracture. Excessive vitamin D intake can cause appetite loss, fatigue, nausea, and constipation; can lead to abnormal calcium deposits in the body; and can adversely affect the kidneys. An overdose of bran can lead to seriously reduced calcium absorption. Excess vitamin B_6 can cause numbness, vitamin E can cause bleeding, and niacin can lead to gastric problems and liver damage.

In addition, people on medication need to be careful about taking dietary supplements. For instance, a person taking coumadin, a blood-thinning medication, should avoid vitamin K, which can negate the effect of this medication, and also avoid several herbs (including ginkgo biloba) that can unsafely exacerbate the effects of blood-thinning medication.

Finally, people need to be cautious about the proclaimed benefits of dietary supplements, which are often exaggerated. If consumers acquire a false sense of security regarding supplements, it may contribute to failure to pay sufficient attention to the nutritive value of the foods they eat.

Dietary Supplement Health and Education Act

In 1994 the federal government passed the *Dietary Supplement Health and Education Act*, which eliminated premarket safety evaluations for a wide variety of dietary supplements, including many herbs, vitamins, minerals, and hormones. The FDA can now intervene only after consumers complain about illnesses from supplements, and even then the FDA can restrict the product only if it can be proven that the specific supplement caused the harm. This is difficult to accomplish because it is hard to separate out people who did not take the supplement as directed, or who exceeded the recommended dose, or who took different types of supplements simultaneously, or who engaged in some other confounding practice.

Before 1994 the FDA regulated nutritional supplements through premarket safety evaluations, similar to the procedure required for foods and drugs. Most herbs and all vitamins that were sold in dosages exceeding 150% of the recommended daily allowance were considered to be prescription drugs in 1993.

Though the lay public remained bullish on the prospects of dietary supplements, after the 1994 legislation passed, the FDA quickly logged more than 2,500 reports of side effects associated with dietary supplements, including 79 deaths (Neergaard, 1998). Because the government decided to take a caveat emptor, or "buyer beware," approach to regulating supplements, there has been insufficient consumer guidance about what works, what does not work, and what the potential side effects are.

The 1994 legislation also allowed advertisers to make unproven claims for their products—for instance, that their product reverses aging—as long as the product is not being sold at the same time (i.e., the advertisements are physically separated from the items being promoted). Even the placement of false claims on product labels, which is illegal, is not being punished because government agencies lack the resources for enforcement. Moreover, the unprotected consumer has to contend with the lack of regulation over product purity, as well as over the amount of active ingredient in a supplement. Two packages of the same product may contain vastly dissimilar amounts of the active ingredient(s).

With no safeguards against grandiose advertisement claims, it is not surprising that dietary supplements became a booming business after the legislation was passed. Dietary supplement sales in the United States went from $9 billion in 1995, to $16 billion in 2000, to $21 billion in 2005, to $23 billion in 2009. A corresponding amount of money was spent on *functional foods*, foods "enhanced" by supplements.

In 2000, 52% of Americans used dietary supplements on a sometime (32%) or regular (20%) basis (Blendon et al., 2001). A survey of Americans age 50 and older reported that 59% used dietary supplements at least once a month, with 52% taking them daily (Eskin, 2001).

Utilizing herbs, vitamins, minerals, hormones, enzymes, and many other "natural" products, Americans have attempted to improve mood, ease achy joints, enhance memory, strengthen immune function, increase intelligence, boost stamina, improve sleep, relieve stress, prevent wrinkles, or reverse the aging process. All such claims are being allowed on the labels of dietary supplements without evidence to support them, thanks to the Dietary Supplement Health and Education Act.

It took a whole decade for this legislative Act to ban even a single supplement—ephedra—and even then the ban was partially rescinded to allow small amounts of this product. Ephedra products claimed to promote weight loss and increase energy, but they also drove up blood pressure and were linked to many cases of heart attack and stroke. The FDA finally banned sales of most ephedra products in 2004, after more than 18,000 adverse events and an estimated 100 deaths had been tied to this weight-loss product, which contains an amphetamine-like herb.

Fourteen years after the passage of the Dietary Supplement Health and Education Act, in 2008, things had gotten so out of hand under the "get the government off our backs" political climate, that even the dietary supplement industry backed federal legislation enacted that year requiring supplement manufacturers to report to the FDA serious adverse events linked to their products. Typically, in previous occurrences, such as with ephedra, it would eventually come to light that a manufacturer had been sitting on a large number of adverse-event reports it had received over the years, as it was not obligated to pass them on to the FDA. Even though that is no longer allowed, it may not be enough to correct the problem. The decisions whether to test and how to test a new product are left up to the manufacturers. And with more than 40,000 products on the market, the FDA has limited resources to ensure compliance.

> **Question:** How would you change the Dietary Supplement Health and Education Act so that it provides as much consumer freedom as possible while protecting the safety of the public?

Given the widespread public use and limited government regulation of these products, it is important to encourage research on dietary supplements. Unfortunately, research studies in the United States have been limited. Many dietary supplements are naturally occurring substances that cannot be patented, which reduces the incentive for manufacturers to invest money in research. Research on dietary supplements has been a more common practice outside the United States, but the methodologies have been less rigorously designed.

VITAMIN AND MINERAL SUPPLEMENTS

Multivitamin Preparations

Half of American adults are taking multivitamins and minerals. In an earlier edition of this book, the evidence appeared to support this practice. Since then, this recommendation has become more controversial. Let's start with the positive side.

The late Robert Butler, Pulitzer Prize-winning author and former chair of the Department of Geriatrics and Adult Development at New York's Mount Sinai Medical Center, supported the practice of routine multivitamin use. Butler once considered vitamin and mineral supplements a rip-off, but his concern about the methods of food production and processing led him to recommend that older adults consume an inexpensive multiple-vitamin supplement on a daily basis.

In an essay in the *Journal of the American Medical Association*, Ranjit Chandra (1997)—a physician twice nominated for the Nobel Prize in medicine—reported that deficiencies in vitamins and trace elements have been observed in almost onethird of sampled older adults. He further observed that because it was expensive and impractical to analyze the blood levels of various nutrients in individuals on a periodic basis, all older adults should take a multivitamin containing modest amounts of *vitamins and minerals* as good preventive medicine practice.

A review of studies that were published between 1966 and 2002 concluded that all adults, and especially older adults, should take a daily multivitamin (Fletcher & Fairfield, 2002). A review of nutritional interventions involving older adults in clinical trials found that nutritional supplements boost immunity among older adults (High, 2001). Dr. Chandra (2001) conducted a placebo-controlled, double-blind study with 86 older adults and concluded that those who took a multivitamin supplement showed significant improvement in short-term memory, problem-solving ability, abstract thinking, and attention, and a decline in infection-related illnesses. No improvement in cognition or immune response was found in those who took the placebo.

What has happened since then? The research of the internationally recognized Dr. Chandra on the strengthened immune response of older adults who took daily multivitamins has been discredited. Independent statisticians concluded that his methods and statistical findings were so dubious that it was unlikely that the studies had even been done. An independent panel convened by Dr. Chandra's university concluded that he had pretended to recruit participants and then fabricated results. When asked for his raw data, Dr. Chandra reported that they had mysteriously disappeared. The editor of *Nutrition* wrote an editorial acknowledging serious statistical flaws in an article of his that the journal had published, regretting that their peer-review process had failed to identify them before publication of the article.

Dr. Chandra's research, from the time he contributed to *Lancet* in 1992 to the printing of the *Nutrition* article in 2001, had been lauded as a landmark contribution to the fields of nutrition and immunity. During that time, Dr. Chandra formulated and then patented a supplement based on his "findings" and licensed the rights to his daughter, who founded a company that sold the multivitamin, called Javaan 50. Experts denounced not only the validity of Dr. Chandra's findings, but also the linking of his research results to the selling of this profitable dietary supplement. According to a statement in Dr. Chandra's divorce proceedings, he is now living off of $2 million (Canadian) held in 120 bank accounts around the world and spends most of his time in Switzerland and his native India.

A study released since then reported that regular use of commonly available multivitamin and multimineral supplements is *not* likely to reduce infections or associated use of health services for people living at home (Avenell et al., 2005). A panel of nutritionists, biostatisticians, and epidemiologists met at the NIH in May 2006 and concluded that there was no evidence to support the regular use of multivitamins. Moreover, given that 65% of Americans consume fortified foods or beverages, they may be unknowingly exceeding the upper safe limits of some vitamins. After an 8-year follow-up period in the Women's Health Initiative clinical trials, multivitamin use was found to have little or no influence on the risk of cancer, heart disease, or total mortality in postmenopausal women (Neuhouser et al., 2009).

Case closed? Not so fast. In a randomized trial that included nearly 15,000 male physicians age 50 and older, long-term daily multivitamin use resulted in a statistically significant reduction in cancer—but not heart disease—after more than a decade of treatment and evaluation (Gaziano et al., 2012; Sesso et al., 2012).

Vitamin D and Calcium

For the past few years vitamin D has been the "in" supplement, with allegedly far-ranging benefits. Studies trumpeted this supplement's role in strengthening bones, and reducing the risk of cancer, heart disease, and diabetes. However, new dietary guidelines, based on more rigorous studies, have deflated this balloon. Moreover, too much of either vitamin D or calcium may be detrimental to one's health.

The IOM panel in 2010 recommended 600 IU of vitamin D for people age 51 to age 70, and 800 IU beyond age 70. Although this was an increase over the prior recommendations (400 IU and 600 IU), it was quite a bit below a wide range of recommendations recently proferred. The safe upper limit was raised from 2,000 IU to 4,000 IU, again below recent recommendations. The latest round of evidence regarding the impact of vitamin D on cardiovacular disease, diabetes, cancer, and other diseases was inconclusive.

Calcium supplementation was, with caution, recommended up to 1,200 mg daily for women age 51 and older, 1,000 mg for men age 51 to 70, and 1,200 mg for men over age 70. The upper safe limit was between 2,000 and 3,000 mg. Given that vitamin D enhances the absorption of calcium, recommendations for calcium could be adjusted downward, but the Institute did not state anything specific in this regard.

The U.S. Preventive Services Task Force was even more deflating by stating that vitamin D and calcium supplementation did not prevent fractures in most older women (Kuehn, 2012). Regarding vitamin D, there was no benefit of vitamin D supplementation at low doses, that is, at 400 IU, but there was no clear evidence about taking higher doses of vitamin D to make a recommendation one way or the other. Regarding calcium, there was concern that cardiovascular health could be compromised and the risk of kidney stones elevated at lower levels of calcium supplementation than previously thought (Zarowitz & Hauersperger, 2012).

Routine supplementation is no longer recommended for vitamin D (Sareh, Sourwine, Rochester, Steinle, & Steinle, 2011) or calcium (Bolland et al., 2011), and the new recommendation is that providers assess individual levels in older patients and use supplements when necessary to correct insufficient levels.

It should be noted, though, that vitamin D, although found in fatty fish and eggs and added to dairy products and some cereals and breads, can be difficult to get in sufficient amounts from food and drink among older adults. Moreover, many older adults have digestive issues that can cause their bodies to absorb less vitamin D than younger adults.

Therefore, some researchers recommend that vitamin D supplementation at 800 IU or greater *is* a good idea for fracture prevention. One team of researchers pooled 31,000 subjects, mean age 76, from 11 double-blind, randomized, controlled studies and reported that supplementation at 800 IU or greater would lower the risk of hip fracture and nonvertebral fractures among older adults (Bischoff-Ferrari et al., 2012). The researchers also noted that high levels of calcium supplementation (more than 1,000 mg) can *reduce* vitamin D's benefit.

Once again . . . stay tuned! This is an active area of research.

Vitamin E

Many areas of nutritional research involve a pendulum effect. At first there were a number of promising observational studies that associated high intakes of vitamin E with protection against cancer and heart disease. Studies of older adults taking vitamin E supplements of 200 IU/d (significantly higher than the 30 IU/d currently recommended) reported improvements in T-cell function and other immune functions (Meydani et al., 1997). As we age we produce fewer T-cells and antibodies that help us attack viruses and cancers and fight infection.

Vitamin E also appeared to be important in reducing the risk of heart disease. It seemed to be a potent antioxidant that attaches directly to low-density lipoprotein (LDL) cholesterol to prevent damage from free radicals. A study (Stephens et al., 1996) reported that adults who were given 400 or 800 IU of vitamin E a day for 18 months had a 77% lower risk of heart attacks. Vitamin E supplementation appeared to reduce prostate cancer incidence and mortality in male smokers in Finland and provided some protection against colorectal and lung cancer among persons of this ethnic background (Heinonen et al., 1998). Yet another study reported that 1,000 IU of vitamin E twice a day slowed the progression of Alzheimer's disease, though it did not stop or reverse it (Sano et al., 1997).

The next generation of research studies was more rigorously conducted, however, and the results were *not* positive. The effects of long-term vitamin E supplementation were not significant in comparison to a placebo, in terms of cancer incidence, cancer deaths, myocardial infarction, stroke, or cardiovascular deaths (HOPE Trial, 2005; Lee et al., 2005). In fact, the risk of heart failure was *higher* in the vitamin E group than in the placebo group (HOPE Trial, 2005). A meta-analysis of 19 randomized, placebo-controlled trials reported that vitamin E *increased* the risk of all-cause mortality, and this dose-dependent increase began at the 150 IU/day level of supplementation (Miller et al., 2005). Yet another study reported that vitamin E supplement was significantly correlated with increased risk for prostate cancer in men (Klein et al., 2011).

A study of 9,500 patients at high risk for cardiovascular events reported that treatment with vitamin E for 4.5 years had no apparent effect on cardiovascular outcome in comparison to a randomly assigned control group (Heart Outcomes Prevention Evaluation Study Investigators, 2000). Another study reported that vitamin E supplements did not reduce the risk of cardiovascular disease over a 3-year period (Hodis et al., 2002). Yet another study reported that vitamin E provided no benefit for age-related cataracts (Christen, Glynn, Chew, & Buring, 2008).

What *was* promising? Food intake. One study reported that vitamin E in food (green, leafy vegetables, corn, whole grains, nuts, olives, and vegetable oils) slowed decline in mental function among older adults, whereas a vitamin E supplement did not (Morris, Evans, Bienias, Tangney, & Wilson, 2002). Another study conducted with 5,395 residents in the Netherlands, age 55 and older, reported vitamin E intake from food may reduce the risk of developing Alzheimer's disease, whereas vitamin E from supplements may not (Engelhart et al., 2002). A study in the *New England Journal of Medicine* (Kushi et al., 1996) reported that older women who eat more foods rich in vitamin E reduce their chance of getting heart disease by almost twothirds.

Because most of the studies that supported vitamin E supplementation were observational as opposed to more rigorous clinical trials (for an examination of potential problems with observational research, see the discussion of hormone replacement therapy in Chapter 2, "Clinical Preventive Services"), two additional explanations emerge: (a) Persons taking vitamin E supplements may also have had a diet richer in vitamin E, and this may have accounted for the early positive results. (b) Persons taking vitamin E supplements may also have been more likely to include healthier lifestyle practices in their daily routines.

When the more recent wave of studies reported that daily vitamin E doses of 400 IU or more can increase the risk of heart failure, and even 150 to 400 IU/day may have a detrimental effect, U.S. sales of vitamin E supplements declined 25% in 2005. For those who choose to continue to take a vitamin E supplement although the research remains inconclusive at best, it is not clear what the recommended amount should be—though

150 IU/day or less seems prudent. Also, vitamin E supplementation is not recommended for individuals on anticoagulant therapy, as vitamin E is itself an anticoagulant.

Vitamin C

For almost 30 years, millions of people followed the lead of Nobel laureate Linus Pauling and consumed vitamin C pills to fight the common cold and cancer. The late Pauling earned his laurels for work in molecular structure, however, not vitamin C research, and most scientists rejected his theory that vitamin C is an antioxidant that fights disease-causing free radicals. One study reported that vitamin C supplementation failed to reduce the incidence of the common cold in the population, with the possible exception of people who are exposed to brief periods of severe physical stress (Douglas, Hemilä, Chalker, & Treacy, 2007).

Nonetheless, studies on the positive effects of vitamin C still appear from time to time. The most promising of these studies suggest that vitamin C supplementation may prevent cataracts. Cataracts are thought to result from the oxidation of lens protein, and vitamin C may prevent this oxidation. One study found that long-term vitamin C supplement use among 492 nondiabetic women over a 15-year period was associated with a 60% reduction in the risk of cataracts, compared with no supplement use (A. Taylor et al., 2002).

Most nutritionists argue that the recommended five daily servings of vitamin C–rich fruits and vegetables would easily meet the minimum daily recommendation for vitamin C. Unfortunately, only 9% of Americans eat the recommended minimum of five daily servings of fruits and vegetables.

Antioxidant Cocktail

The antioxidant vitamins are vitamin E, vitamin C, and beta-carotene. Many advocates of antioxidant vitamins recommended a cocktail of all three.

Antioxidants stabilize free radicals, which are unstable forms of oxygen. Oxygen is used during metabolism to change carbohydrates and fats into energy. During this process, oxygen is converted into stable forms of water and carbon dioxide, but some oxygen (i.e., free radicals) ends up in an unstable form with a normal proton nucleus but a single unpaired electron. The unpaired electron seeks to steal a second electron from a stable molecule, and in so doing it damages proteins and lipids in a process that likely contributes to heart disease, cancer, and other diseases. This chain reaction among unpaired electrons continues until antioxidants become available to help stabilize the free radicals so they will not be so reactive.

Antioxidants are found in foods, especially fruits and vegetables. As mentioned, though, few Americans get adequate servings of fruits and vegetables in their daily diets. Thus, nutritionists have recommended the *antioxidant cocktail* (Cooper, 1994; "Is This the Right Way," 1995). The typical cocktail guidelines ranged from 250 to 1,000 mg of vitamin C, 200 to 800 IU of vitamin E, and 10,000 to 25,000 IU of beta-carotene.

Based on later research, many nutritional leaders no longer recommend the cocktail. Antioxidant supplements do not delay mortality. A meta-analysis of 67 randomized clinical trials with a total of 230,000 participants reported no evidence that antioxidant supplements decrease mortality; in fact, some studies report that vitamin A, beta-carotene, or vitamin E may increase mortality (Bjelakovic, Nikolova, Gluud, Simonetti, & Gluud, 2008).

One ray of hope for the antioxidant cocktail lies with macular degeneration. A modified version of the original cocktail—400 mg of vitamin E, 500 mg of vitamin C, but only 15 mg of beta-carotene—plus 80 mg of zinc and 2 mg of copper—provided the first effective treatment for this leading cause of vision loss among older adults. Among persons with macular degeneration who have not yet lost the central portion of their vision to the disease, the cocktail reduced the risk of vision loss by 20% in one study (Jampol et al., 2001) and by 35% in another (van Leeuwen et al., 2005).

Vitamin B$_{12}$

The prevalence of vitamin B$_{12}$ (cobalamin) deficiency is age dependent, and older adults are the most susceptible, especially those who take antacids or multiple medications, or have gastrointestinal problems (Ionica, Sourwine, Steinle, & Rochester, 2012). Vitamin B$_{12}$ helps maintain red blood cells and nerve cells and is needed to make DNA. It is found naturally in animal foods such as meat, poultry, fish, eggs, and dairy products. Up to 20% of older Americans have marginal vitamin B$_{12}$ status (Ionica, Sourwine, Steinle, & Rochester, 2012).

A deficiency in B$_{12}$ can lead to fatigue, memory loss, balance problems, constipation, and depression. Close to 80% of older adults with a B$_{12}$ deficiency do not know it, according to Dr. David Spence, a neurologist at the Robarts Research Institute in London, Ontario, and are in danger of acquiring permanent neurological damage.

The National Academy of Sciences, which advises the federal government on nutrition, urged people over age 50 to take a vitamin B$_{12}$ supplement or to eat cereals fortified with B$_{12}$. The academy reviewed several research studies and concluded that up to 30% of persons over age 50 cannot absorb B$_{12}$ in foods, primarily due to the onset of atrophic gastritis—a reduction in the ability to secrete stomach acid that allows us to separate vitamin B$_{12}$ from the protein in food and thereby utilize it.

The Framingham Offspring Study reported that 39% of their national sample had low B$_{12}$ levels. Some participants had a primarily vegetarian diet and failed to get enough of the vitamin in their foods. Others did get sufficient amounts of meat, poultry, and fish but had difficulty with absorption. The authors speculated that an increased use of antacids may contribute to the absorption problem (Tucker et al., 2000).

Researchers are beginning to suggest that persons over age 50 consider increasing the recommended daily allowance of vitamin B$_{12}$ in their diets from 6 µg to 25 µg. Though most multivitamin supplements have only 6 µg, Centrum Silver and other supplements designed for older adults typically have 25 µg. An option to dietary supplementation that is nearly as effective is to eat B$_{12}$-fortified cereals and dairy products five or more times a week (Tucker et al., 2000). Some researchers argue that B$_{12}$ is water-soluble, likely safe even in large doses, and should be added to flour as is now done with another B vitamin, folate. Others maintain that vitamin B$_{12}$ has not been adequately tested in randomized clinical trials, and even if safe it is likely to be insufficient as a supplement in flour to correct even a mild deficiency.

HERBS

The medicinal benefits of plants are undeniable. *Herbs* are the basis for aspirin, morphine, digitalis, and other medicines. Most of the millions of dollars that consumers spend on herbal remedies do not produce beneficial outcomes, however, and a not-insignificant number create health risks. Even among those products that appear to be helpful, the consistency of ingredients is unregulated and uncertain.

The regulation of herbs in Europe, where they are treated almost like drugs, sharply contrasts with the situation in America. In Europe herbal labels warn people with diseases or conditions that might leave them susceptible to bad outcomes. Germany's Commission E of the Federal Department of Health has tested hundreds of herbs, approving those with absolute proof of safety and some proof of efficacy (though nowhere near the research standard for efficacy that is used in the United States). These clearly labeled herbal medicines outsell prescription drugs in most European countries.

In contrast, Americans can access herbs over the counter, but they must rely on books for safety and efficacy information—or they need to contact the nonprofit educational and research organization the American Botanical Council at www.herbalgram. org (512-926-4900).

Ginkgo Biloba

Ginkgo biloba is the best-studied and most popular herbal medicine in Europe. It is also the most popular herb used by older adults in the United States and is believed to be a memory enhancer. Numerous well-controlled studies show that an extract from the leaves of the ginkgo biloba tree dilates blood vessels and can improve blood flow in the brain and the extremities.

A placebo-controlled, double-blind randomized trial in the United States reported that ginkgo biloba was safe and appeared capable of stabilizing, and in some cases improving, the cognitive performance and the social functioning of demented patients for 6 months to a year (Le Bars et al., 1997). This study, however, was limited by a high dropout rate and small differences between treatment and control groups. A team of Dutch researchers employed the same ginkgo preparation as did the U.S. study and did not find significant differences between ginkgo recipients and placebo recipients (Van Dongen, van Rossum, Kessels, Sielhorst, & Knipschild, 2000). Although both trials appeared to be methodologically sound, the Dutch trial had a lower dropout rate.

Another randomized controlled trial with 230 people over age 60 with no signs of memory impairment found that the ginkgo biloba supplement worked no better than a placebo on learning, memory, attention, concentration, naming, and verbal fluency outcomes (Solomon, Adams, Silver, Zimmer, & DeVeaux, 2002). Finally, researchers at six universities across the United States studied more than 3,000 adults aged 72 to 96 over an 8-year period with normal mental functioning or mild cognitive impairment. Compared with a placebo, the use of ginkgo biloba did not result in less cognitive decline (Snitz et al., 2009). Given the plethora of well-controlled studies that refute the claim that ginkgo biloba improves memory and related cognitive function, sales, which had been steadily increasing in the United States through 2007, went down 8% in 2008.

The Other G's

In addition to ginkgo biloba, there are other popular herbs that begin with the letter *g*: ginseng, garlic, and ginger. These are anticoagulants and can increase the risk of bleeding problems, especially when taken with aspirin, warfarin (Coumadin), and other over-the-counter and prescription blood-thinning medications.

Ginseng products are used as energy boosters and to cure a wide range of ills. The few well-designed studies of ginseng do not bear out the claims that it boosts energy (Engels & Wirth, 1997) or enhances psychological well-being (Cardinal & Engels, 2001) when compared with a placebo-control group. Another problem is that authentic ginseng in standardized doses is difficult to find. *Consumer Reports* tested 10 ginseng products and found that one contained almost none of the active ingredient and the remainder varied by 1,000%.

The typical claim for garlic is that it lowers the cholesterol level and improves cardiovascular health. A panel of experts reviewed 1,800 studies on the potential health benefits of garlic and found little evidence that it lowers cholesterol, blood pressure, or blood sugar, or that it prevents heart attacks, cancer, or blood clots ("Garlic: Case

Unclosed," 2000). Commission E, the agency that advises the German public and health professionals on herbal medicines, no longer recommends garlic for cholesterol reduction. The small reductions in cholesterol in some of the short-term studies were no longer evident at 6 months or longer. A randomized clinical trial found garlic had no significant effects on LDL, high-density lipoprotein (HDL), triglycerides, or total cholesterol level (Gardner et al., 2007b).

Ginger is typically taken to relieve nausea associated with seasickness, motion sickness, and anesthesia. Studies of ginger extract and its effect on the lowering of cholesterol have been promising, but have focused on mice (Fuhrman, Rosenblat, Hayek, Coleman, & Aviram, 2000). Ginger, like the other "g" herbs, can exacerbate internal bleeding.

St. John's Wort

St. John's wort is a weed native to the western United States and parts of Europe. This weed is named for St. John the Baptist, whose birthday is celebrated on June 24, about the time the plant puts forth its yellow blooms.

St. John's wort is the second most popular herbal medicine (after ginkgo biloba) in the United States, but it is the most popular antidepressant in Germany, where it outsells Prozac 4 to 1. St. John's wort was not effective in the treatment of moderate or severe depression in two separate studies (Hypericum Depression Trial Study Group, 2002; Shelton et al., 2001), but there was evidence that it was effective with milder depression in comparison to a prescription antidepressant (Philipp, Kohnen, & Hiller, 1999; Woelk et al., 2000). The studies of milder depression, however, have been criticized for the lack of rigor in their design (Kupfer & Frank, 2002; Spira, 2001).

Prozac costs on average eight times more than a regimen of St. John's wort. Researchers warn, however, that the German studies supporting the efficacy of St. John's wort involved small numbers of patients, brief trial periods, nonstandardized diagnoses of depression, and varied potency and dosages.

St. John's wort can interfere with drugs for depression, cancer, heart disease, asthma, and AIDS, as well as with antibiotics. Clinicians warn about the adverse effects of stopping prescribed antidepressants on one's own or taking St. John's wort while taking prescription antidepressants such as Prozac. Older adults are particularly susceptible to the hazards of combining the herb with prescription antidepressants and are likely to experience dizziness, confusion, headaches, and anxiety.

Finally, several organizations have analyzed dozens of brands of St. John's wort and found serious deficiencies in a majority of the products ("St. John's Worts and All," 2000).

Saw Palmetto

Extracts of the berries of saw palmetto, a small palm tree native to the southeastern United States, are used widely to improve urinary flow in men with noncancerous enlarged prostate, or benign prostatic hypertrophy (BPH). A review of 18 randomized controlled trials examining saw palmetto extracts for the treatment of BPH was generally positive (Wilt et al., 1998). The United States Pharmacopeia (USP), a quasi-governmental agency that sets manufacturing standards for drugs and advises health professionals, reported in April 2000 that there is moderate evidence of effectiveness for saw palmetto in men with BPH (Schardt, 2000b).

In contradiction to these findings, an exceptionally well-designed government study found that men randomly assigned to a saw palmetto-taking group did not differ in symptoms, prostate size, urinary flow, or quality of life from placebo takers

(Bent et al., 2006). This study lasted 1 year and was carefully blinded: the placebo had a similarly strong taste and smell as saw palmetto, perhaps revealing a weakness in blinding in prior studies. The study also used an extract recommended by alternative medicine experts.

The potential market for saw palmetto extracts is huge, with half of all men over the age of 50 having enlarged prostates. Moreover, prescription prostate drugs have substantial side effects. Saw palmetto is definitely not a substitute for conventional medical prostate treatment. In fact, it does not actually shrink the prostate but may relieve the symptoms of enlargement, such as the frequent urge to urinate. Saw palmetto is not effective when the dried berry or extract is made into a tea.

Echinacea

Extracts of the plant echinacea, a purple coneflower, are widely used in the United States and some European countries for the treatment or prevention of common colds (upper respiratory tract infections). A review of 16 randomized and quasi-randomized trials with 3,396 participants suggested that a few echinacea preparations may be better than placebo (Melchart, Linde, Fischer, & Kaesmayr, 2000). Subsequent studies, however, have not been supportive of this herb's effectiveness. Compared with a placebo, echinacea provided no detectable benefit in more rigorous randomized trials (Barrett et al., 2002; Sperber, Shah, Gilbert, Ritchey, & Monto, 2004; Turner, Bauer, Woelkart, Hulsey, & Gangemi, 2005). Despite a growing list of negative clinical studies, however, echinacea retains its popularity.

Black Cohosh and Other Herbs for Menopausal Symptoms

After the publication of the results of the Women's Health Initiative on the risks of hormone replacement therapy, many women sought alternatives for the treatment of menopausal symptoms. As noted by one reviewer, though, dietary supplements for the relief of menopausal symptoms receive little scientific support for their efficacy despite their popularity (Albertazzi, 2006).

Most studies report that black cohosh, soy supplements, ginkgo biloba, ginseng, St. John's wort, and combination herbal remedies are *no* more effective than placebos for alleviating symptoms, though they all may be perceived as effective by up to 40% of women (comparable to placebos). Not surprisingly, twothirds of current users of these supplements believe they are effective in relieving symptoms, whereas 70% of former users believe they did not help (Ma, Drieling, & Stafford, 2006).

In the general absence of support for dietary supplements, women who are no longer willing to take hormone replacements may want to consider exercise, relaxation techniques, improved sleep hygiene, and nutritional changes. The common side effect of these interventions is good health, and no additional money has to be spent.

For those who persist in using black cohosh, which is the most popular supplement for menopausal symptoms, there are three caveats: (1) One study examined 11 black cohosh products in stores and reported that three contained no black cohosh at all, and most of the remaining products substituted cheaper versions of the herb (Jiang, Kronenberg, Nuntanakorn, Qiu, & Kennelly, 2006). (2) When a black cohosh product is legitimate, it has not shown to be more effective than placebo (Newton et al., 2006). (3) Only about half of the women using dietary supplements for alleviation of menopausal symptoms tell their doctors, despite the fact that some of these products have adverse interactions with prescribed medications (Ma et al., 2006).

HORMONE SUPPLEMENTS

Human Growth Hormone

Human growth hormone (HGH) is secreted by the brain's pituitary gland and helps regulate growth during childhood and metabolism during adulthood. HGH levels begin declining by age 30 along with the body's muscle mass. By age 70, hormone levels are only 25% of the peak reached by most people between the ages of 18 and 30. An estimated 20,000 to 30,000 American adults take a synthetic version of HGH. Injecting growth hormone appears to boost lean body mass and improve physical function, and HGH is promoted as an antiaging remedy. It allegedly improves strength, energy, and immunity and has been used as a treatment for heart disease, cancer, impotence, and Alzheimer's disease.

Although there is limited or no evidence for some of these claims, there is more evidence that this hormone supplement is more harmful than beneficial. It can lead to carpal tunnel syndrome, edema, joint and muscle pain, high blood pressure, congestive heart failure, and tumor growth, and it can worsen the effects of arthritis and diabetes. Two studies have associated HGH with increased mortality rates (Demling, 1999; Maison et al., 1998). HGH does not yet translate into improved function for older adults, and the risk of adverse effects is substantial (Cassel, 2002). Researchers conclude that the participation of older persons in this therapy should be confined to controlled studies (Blackman et al., 2002). Moreover, buying pills or getting shots that can cost up to $15,000 a year and are not covered by insurance is a poor financial investment (Boling, 2000).

Nonetheless there is a strong and growing black market demand for HGH, for both older and younger persons. For the former, the antiaging movement and, in particular, the *American Academy of Anti-Aging Medicine* tout HGH as a way to stop or reverse the aging process. Its appeal has been particularly strong among people aged 40 to 60. Perhaps the lucky ones are only wasting their money. A recent analysis by ConsumerLab.com of products for oral use that claim to contain or release HGH reports that only a minuscule amount of this substance can be found in the supplements sold at health food stores or on the Internet.

The appeal of HGH to young athletes was revealed in 2006 when Arizona Diamondbacks pitcher Jason Grimsley was caught using it and then disclosed that many other major league baseball players were using it as well. The ballplayers were acquiring HGH on the black market, and it was considerably more potent than the brands available to the average consumer through commercial outlets. Baseball's drug testing for steroids began in 2003, but it did not include a test for detecting HGH until 2012. Unfortunately, the test is administered only once annually, prior to the baseball season, and HGH stays in the system only a short while, making it easy to avoid detection as the testing system is currently set up.

Testosterone

Testosterone is also a hormone, popular with men for gaining muscle strength. Experience with testosterone therapy to restore vitality in aging has been disappointing. Testosterone therapy appears to be beneficial only to those with an original deficit in the hormone, regardless of age (Snyder, 2001). From the perspective of the young athlete, however, testosterone is believed to be a performance booster. Floyd Landis, briefly the winner of the 2006 Tour de France, tested positive for a level of testosterone too high to have been naturally produced.

Supplemental testosterone replacement may be as risky for men as hormone replacement therapy has been shown to be for women (see Chapter 2, "Clinical Preventive

Services"). There have been concerns that this therapy increases the risk for stroke and prostate cancer (Rhoden & Morgentaler, 2004). The National Institute on Aging (NIA) formed a task force to evaluate the benefits and risks of testosterone therapy (for more information, go to www.nia.hih.gov). In 2010 NIA embarked on a study of the potential mental and physical benefits of testosterone therapy with 800 older men at 12 facilities nationwide. This 6-year, $45 million study will present preliminary results in 2015.

DHEA (dehydroepiandrosterone) is made by our adrenal glands and is converted into testosterone and estrogen in our cells. Studies report that there were no differences after 2 years between those who took DHEA and those who were given a placebo, in terms of muscle mass and strength, exercise capacity, and quality of life.

Despite the likely health risks and the lack of research support for the benefits of testosterone therapy, prescriptions for testosterone soared in 2011, to $1.6 billion, almost triple the amount spent in 2006, primarily due to television advertising and websites promoting its use. In addition, Solvay Pharmaceuticals, the makers of the best-selling synthetic testosterone, AndroGel, has been accused by the Federal Trade Commission (FTC) of paying off two firms to terminate their production of generic versions of this product in exchange for financial payoffs. This would prevent AndroGel, with its $300 monthly cost, from having to compete with a $45 per month generic version.

Melatonin

Melatonin is a hormone produced in the brain by the pineal gland, and it is believed to set the body's sleep cycle. It was the first best-selling hormone supplement, with 20 million new users in 1995 in the United States. Adults also use melatonin to reduce the effects of jet lag.

These uses of melatonin have not received much research support. Scientists are not convinced that there is an age-related decline in melatonin levels, or that sleep problems typical of older people occur because of a deficit in this hormone (Duffy et al., 2002). A meta-analysis reviewed 25 controlled trials that tested melatonin against placebos for various kinds of sleep disorders. The review did not provide much support for the use of melatonin for sleep disorders (Buscemi et al., 2006). Melatonin might not be an effective jet lag antidote either. Traveling physicians randomly assigned to a melatonin treatment group or a placebo- control group did not report differences in jet lag symptoms after a trip from Norway to New York (Spitzer et al., 1999).

For free fact sheets on melatonin, DHEA, HGH, estrogen, and testosterone, call the NIA at 800-222-2225.

OTHER DIETARY SUPPLEMENTS

Glucosamine and Chondroitin

Glucosamine and chondroitin in the human body are used to make cartilage and have been touted as a way to reverse the effects of arthritis since the publication of the best-selling book *The Arthritis Cure* (Theodosakis, 1997). In supplement form, these compounds come from crab shells, cow tracheae, and shark cartilage and appeared to ease arthritic aches and slow the loss of cartilage.

In one study, persons with mild to moderate knee arthritis who took 1,500 mg of purified, standardized glucosamine once a day for 3 years had 20% to 25% less pain and disability than those taking a placebo pill. Also, X-ray examinations showed that arthritis progressed slowly or not at all in the treatment group, whereas the placebo group continued to lose cartilage at the expected rate (Reginster et al., 2001).

There was also evidence to suggest that chondroitin was effective in the treatment of osteoarthritis (Leeb, Schweitzer, Montag, & Smolen, 2000; Mazieres, Combe, Phan Van, Tondut, & Grynfeltt, 2001). One meta-analysis of 15 clinical trials of glucosamine and chondroitin found a moderate treatment effect for glucosamine and a large effect for chondroitin (McAlindon, LaValley, Gulin, & Felson, 2000). Conversely, another meta-analysis on the efficacy of chondroitin in relieving pain from osteoarthritis reported that the supplement was not effective (Reichenbach et al., 2007).

Chondroitin is a more expensive supplement than glucosamine, and it is difficult to make. Twelve of 14 glucosamine samples had at least 90% of the ingredient amount listed on the label, but only 5 of 32 chondroitin samples contained the listed amount (Schardt, 2000a).

In a long-awaited NIH-supported multicenter trial, researchers examined the dietary supplements glucosamine (1,500 mg) and chondroitin (1,200 mg) in 1,583 patients with knee arthritis. Sixty percent of the patients who received the placebo reported at least a 20% reduction in pain, compared to 65% of patients taking one or the other supplement, or both together (Clegg et al., 2006). The 5% difference, however, was not statistically significant. Only Celebrex (which was found to double the risk of heart attack and was taken off the market in 2004), which led to pain relief in 70% of patients, was statistically significant in its percentage difference from the placebo.

When researchers examined people with moderate to severe knee pain (eliminating those with mild pain), 79% taking the supplement combination reported pain relief, a significantly higher percentage than those taking a placebo (54%) or Celebrex (69%). Subgroup analysis can be notoriously unreliable, though, and often is not confirmed in follow-up research. Such was the case with these two supplements in a 2-year follow-up to the 2006 NIH study. A double-blind, placebo-controlled study at nine sites reported that nothing worked better than the placebo to slow the progress of arthritis and its discomfort (Sawitzke et al., 2008).

In 2008 there were worldwide sales of $1.9 billion for glucosamine and chondroitin—up 60% from 2003—with half that amount spent in the United States. This sixth-top-selling dietary supplement in the United States typically costs individuals between $30 and $50 a month.

Nutritional Drinks

Ensure, Sustacal, Nutrastart, and Boost are liquid meal supplements touted as energy increasers. The supplements were designed for elderly persons who have debilitating health conditions that make it difficult for them to eat or keep food down. Advertisers are also promoting the products to baby boomers and the young-old who are still in good health but are seeking more vitality, for whom these supplements may be expensive and ineffective. Sometimes the nutrients in these supplements are not fully absorbed by the body and provide only a third of the calories (about 240 versus 750) of a meal if used as a substitute.

There are also many protein drinks on the market, some advertised as energy boosters and others as meal replacements. These drinks are twothirds protein and are useful for the few adults who have a protein deficiency. But they lack some of the vitamins, minerals, fiber, phytonutrients, fat, and carbohydrates found in whole foods. Protein bars are likely to be less healthy than the drinks, as they tend to be high in saturated fat. Based on tests by ConsumerLab.com, 60% of 30 protein bar products tested failed to meet their labeling claims.

CONSUMERLAB.COM AND THE DIETARY SUPPLEMENT VERIFICIATION PROGRAM

Unlike drugs, dietary supplements are not required to undergo premarket safety testing, which means that a brand may not contain the ingredients claimed on the label. The ingredients may also be unsafe, perhaps due to contamination or to amounts that exceed safe limits. In response to this situation, *ConsumerLab.com* subjects different brands of dietary supplements to laboratory analysis and posts the results on the Internet (available to subscribers for a fee). Results appear every 4 to 6 weeks, and it is not uncommon to find that 25% or more of products studied fail to contain the labeled ingredients in the amounts described, or fail related tests of disintegration and impurity levels. Three studies, for example, reported that 25% of ginkgo biloba product labels were inaccurate, 32% of multivitamins, and 37% of saw palmetto product labels.

Typically, when a product fails to contain the designated amount of a labeled ingredient, the amount is inadequate—sometimes even nonexistent. However, a review of B vitamin supplements (complexes and single B vitamins) found that 9 of 21 products *exceeded* the established Tolerable Upper Intake Levels for adults, above which there is increased risk of side effects with regular use. Also, Centrum Chewables had 173% of the vitamin A listed on the label, which can be toxic to one's liver. ConsumerLab found almost no connection between the price of the product and its quality.

The ConsumerLab.com website has its detractors. It sometimes does not publish the names of failing products. It samples only one batch of a product, and herbal products are notorious for being inconsistent from batch to batch because of the nature of the plants and the processing technique. It does not test for bioavailability, that is, whether the substance will be absorbed and actually utilized by the body. And finally, even if the label is accurate, the site does not evaluate the benefit of the product.

The USP launched a *Dietary Supplement Verification Program* in 2002. The USP mark, which states "Dietary Supplement Verified," refers to the presence, quantity, and purity of a supplement's ingredient. If a bottle of ginseng pills bears the USP seal, it means that the product contains the amount of ginseng listed on the label and that the ingredient is free from contamination.

The USP seal does not verify safety or possible benefits. The bottle of ginseng pills that bears the USP seal, for example, does not verify that ginseng provides additional energy or that it is safe. Neither the USP seal nor the accompanying explanation makes that distinction clear.

These are at least steps in the right direction, and other organizations, including Consumers Union (www.consumersunion.org), are joining in. Unfortunately, efforts to regulate dietary supplements remain woefully inadequate overall, and caveat emptor—buyer beware—is an inadequate descriptor of the state of events in dietary supplements. Perhaps the situation was best described by the *UC Berkeley Wellness Letter* ("Is This the Right Way," 2000): "Not since the early 1900s, when unregulated patent medicines were sold from circus wagons, has there been such a free-for-all."

NUTRACEUTICALS, OR FUNCTIONAL FOODS AND DRINKS

Americans have been eating fortified foods since 1924, when manufacturers added iodine to salt to prevent goiters. Since then we have had vitamin D-fortified milk, calcium-fortified orange juice, flour enriched with B vitamins and iron, and other useful products.

Nutraceuticals represent a new pathway in the field of functional foods: exploiting nutritionally weak foods and marketing them as health products. Waffles with refined flour and orange drinks with sugar and water are now calcium fortified. Corn chips have kava to promote relaxation. Donuts are vitamin fortified and portrayed as healthy. A chocolate-chip cookie is laced with 500 mg of calcium and called Calci-cookie. Tortilla chips contain St. John's wort to boost your mood. And potato rings have ginkgo biloba to increase memory and alertness. The function of most functional foods and drinks is to make a profit for the manufacturer. Sales reached $16 billion in 2000 and then almost doubled, to $31 billion, in 2008.

Not all fortified products are soft drinks, breakfast cereals, and snack chips. Two margarines, Benecol and Take Control, are functional foods with probable benefit. These products, as part of a low-fat diet, can reduce the LDL cholesterol level up to 10%. The FDA allows the manufacturers of these products to claim that these margarines may reduce the risk of heart disease. It is unclear, however, whether there is an unhealthy effect on the body from the unprocessed oils that are also in these products.

Some foods are merely getting image makeovers. Ketchup is now more than a mere condiment; it is the richest dietary source of lycopene, which may ward off prostate cancer (though the evidence is questionable). So squirt a little ketchup on a super-sized order of French fries and avoid cancer. Milk (calcium), tea (flavonoids), grapes (phenols), carrots (beta-carotene), broccoli (sulforaphane), and beef (linoleic acid) have also undergone image makeovers (Haney, 1999).

Some of these products may turn out to be useful, but manufacturers are unwilling to wait for the research to be completed. As previously mentioned, glucosamine and chondroitin are dietary supplements that may or may not have promise in the area of reduc-

> **Question:** Do you think there is too much skepticism in America about CAM? Why or why not?

ing pain from arthritis. Rather than wait for definitive and consistent research results, though, Coca-Cola formed a partnership with Procter & Gamble to market the drink Elations, which has 1,500 mg of glucosamine and 1,200 mg of chondroitin added to it. The advertisers brazenly proclaim that you will receive joint comfort in 6 days, and significant improvement in only 3 days. Their motto: "The drink that brings 'Joy for Joints.'"

The good news is that the herbal supplements added to most functional foods are in amounts so minuscule that they are quite safe. The bad news is that you are wasting your money. The additional bad news is that junk foods and drinks with a supplement added are still junk. The bad news on top of that is that manufacturers could start adding unsafe dosages of herbs without premarket safety testing. Then it will be up to a sufficient number of sick consumers to demonstrate that it was the functional food and not some other factor that caused their health problem.

7

●●●●●●

SELECTED HEALTH EDUCATION TOPICS

●●● Learning Objectives

- Describe the history of smoking prevalence in the United States
- Review the diseases associated with smoking
- Cite the smoking quit ratio

- Examine age, gender, and educational differences in smoking
- Compare smoking cessation interventions
- Examine the impact of taxes on smoking
- Review the history of secondhand tobacco smoke and the tobacco industry settlement
- Review the history of smoking bans in public places
- Summarize the Family Smoking Prevention and Tobacco Control Act
- Describe Medicare smoking cessation coverage
- Define alcoholism and describe types of alcoholism
- Review alcohol assessment tools
- Examine alcohol prevalence among older adults
- Review diseases and problems associated with alcoholism
- Describe the positive effects of alcohol
- Examine medication usage in the United States
- List medication problems that are patient versus physician initiated
- Explain the consequences of television advertising of prescription drugs
- Review medication safety resources
- Examine the prevalence of falls
- Review fall prevention strategies and resources
- Examine motor vehicle safety issues and interventions for older drivers
- Review whether older drivers are required to have their licenses renewed more frequently
- Analyze the consequences of older adults' quitting driving
- Examine pedestrian safety issues
- List resources for driving safety
- Examine sexuality and intimacy with age
- Describe changes in sleep as we age
- Review medical sleep disorders and sleep hygiene issues
- Contrast behavioral interventions with the use of medications for sleep disorders
- Cite sleep interventions and resources

Health professionals and older adults need to be informed about a great many health education topics. In this chapter, we will explore a few of these topics: smoking, alcohol, medication usage, injury prevention (fall prevention and motor vehicle/pedestrian safety), sexuality and intimacy, and sleep.

SMOKING

Although most health providers proclaim the leading causes of death to be heart disease, cancer, and stroke, health educators view these diseases as pathological diagnoses rather than as causes. The latter group cite the leading causes of death as smoking, diet, inactivity, and alcohol. From the perspective of these analysts, the number 1 cause of death is smoking tobacco, and the Americans who are most likely to die as a result of smoking are over the age of 65.

Prevalence

The prevalence of smoking in the United States declined between 1965 and 1990, from 44% of American adults to 25.5%, and then leveled off over the next decade. It then decreased again, to 19.8% in 2007. This is the lowest smoking rate since just after World War I. This recent decline in smoking has been attributed to three factors: increasing smoking bans in public places, higher cigarette taxes, and more options to help people quit.

Tobacco is a worldwide problem and, unlike the case in the United States, it has been steadily increasing not only over the past half century, but in the past few years as well. An estimated 1.25 billion people currently smoke cigarettes and more than half of them will die from the habit.

The future worldwide looks bleak. The *Tobacco Atlas*, released in 2009 by the American Cancer Society and World Lung Foundation, predicted that tobacco alone will kill a billion people in the 21st century, 10 times the toll it took in the 20th century.

Smoking is a leading cause of premature death in all developed countries, but it is growing even faster in developing countries. The *Tobacco Atlas* estimates that 70% of the deaths from cigarette smoking in the coming century will occur in developing countries. Since 1960, tobacco production has increased threefold in low- and middle-income countries, but in richer countries production has been cut in half.

Associated Diseases

In May 2004 the 941-page Surgeon General's report was published, titled *The Health Consequences of Smoking*. It was based on a review of 1,600 research articles and produced by a team of 20 scientists at the Centers for Disease Control and Prevention (CDC). This panel of scientists concluded that the list of diseases linked to smoking had grown considerably.

These diseases included cancers of the lung, larynx, bladder, kidney, esophagus, cervix, pancreas, stomach, and mouth; leukemia; chronic obstructive pulmonary disease (COPD); pneumonia and other respiratory diseases; cardiovascular disease; cerebrovascular disease; osteoporosis; peptic ulcers; reproductive diseases; cataracts; periodontitis; cognitive decline; and abdominal aortic aneurysms. (Plus, the U.S. Preventive Services Task Force recommended a one-time ultrasound screening for abdominal aortic aneurysms for all 65- to 75-year-old males who have ever smoked.) If that is not enough damage, evidence is still being considered for associations between smoking and colorectal cancer, liver cancer, prostate cancer, and erectile dysfunction.

Cigarette smoke irritates and inflames lungs and air passages and produces excess mucus. Over time, these effects lead to or exacerbate a variety of lung diseases, including cancer and COPD. More deaths occur from lung cancer than from any other type of cancer; yet lung cancer is rare among those who have never smoked. Smokers with a habit of two packs or more per day have lung cancer rates about 20 times greater than those who have never smoked.

Cigarette smoking accounts for more than 60,000 of the 80,000 deaths each year that are due to COPD. Moreover, death from COPD usually is preceded by an extended period of disability due, in most cases, to chronic bronchitis or emphysema. In addition, smokers are about three times more vulnerable than nonsmokers to the incidence of coronary heart disease and to the risk of sudden death.

Among the estimated 440,000 people who die from smoking-related diseases each year, about 300,000 of those deaths are people age 65 and older.

Quit Ratio and Benefit

I phoned my dad to tell him I had stopped smoking. He called me a quitter.

—Steven Pearl

It's not that difficult to quit. I did it a thousand times.

—Mark Twain

In 2007 the United States had about 43 million smokers, but also an equal number of people who had quit smoking. Difficult to quit? Yes! Impossible? Not by a long shot! In 2010, 53% of older men age 65 and over previously smoked cigarettes, whereas 29% of older women were former smokers.

About 57% of smokers age 65 and older report a desire to quit, and about 10% of them stop smoking each year. Seniors who try to quit smoking are more likely to succeed than younger age groups, and their relapse rate is lower than for younger adults. Older participants in one study were more likely to quit smoking after receiving a serious health diagnosis (Whitson, Heflin, & Burchett, 2006). Many seniors now realize that they can reduce their risk of death from heart disease to that of nonsmokers within 2 or 3 years after quitting.

Researchers who conducted a meta-analysis of former smokers reported that *smoking cessation* benefits were evident through the highest ages of their sample—even people aged 80 and older (Gellert, Schöttker, & Brenner, 2012)! There was an 83% increased mortality for current smokers versus a 34% increased mortality for former smokers, and relative mortality of former smokers continued to decrease with time since cessation, regardless of age.

Age

The percentage of older adults who smoke (9% in 2008) is less than half that of the adult population (21%) in general. Part of that is due to mortality. Smoking is linked to a higher mortality rate, shortening lives up to 13 years, and preventing some people from reaching old age.

Older smokers have a personal history of more unsuccessful quit attempts than do younger smokers. They contend with a longer smoking history, the tendency to be thoroughly addicted due to a heavy smoking habit, the likelihood of not being exposed to the nonsmoking norms and influences in the modern workplace, less knowledge than younger adults have about the physical effects of smoking, and less likelihood of being told by their physician to quit than for younger smokers. Nonetheless, the number of failed attempts in their earlier years appears to be unrelated to success in quitting at a specific point in their later years.

Two stereotypical attitudes about smokers who survive into old age are (1) they must be resistant to the health hazards of smoking, and (2) because of their advanced age, they no longer have time to benefit from a reduction in risk by quitting. In fact, smokers who continue to smoke as older adults continue to increase their risk of morbidity and mortality. Conversely, even 65-year-old men who quit smoking gained 2 additional years of life, and 65-year-old women gained almost 4 years (Taylor, Hasselblad, Henley, Thun, & Sloan, 2002). Those who quit smoking, even late in life, can improve their physical function and overall health in comparison to those who continue smoking.

A presentation by Virginia Reichert of the Center for Tobacco Control at the 2007 American College of Chest Physicians conference stated that smokers over age 65 reported—most frequently—that their motivations for quitting smoking were physician pressure and stress due to a major health problem. In contrast, younger smokers reported cigarette costs and tobacco odor as prime motivations for quitting.

Gender

Although the prevalence of smoking among adults in general declined between 1980 and 2000, the decline was considerably lower among females. In fact, there was even a slight rise among female smokers who were age 65 and over. By 2000 the prevalence of older women smokers equaled that of men. The American Cancer Society predicted that women's deaths from smoking-related disease will exceed men's in about 2020.

Lung cancer death rates are estimated to climb rapidly about 20 to 30 years after a large increase in the incidence of smoking. Men began smoking in large numbers after the turn of the century, and their death rate from smoking peaked during the first half of the century. Women's rapid rise in smoking began in the 1950s, and by 1986 lung cancer had surpassed breast cancer as the leading cause of cancer death among women.

Forty-five percent of women who have ever smoked have quit, versus 52% of men. Researchers believe that it is more difficult for women to quit smoking because many depend on cigarettes to control their weight. A nationwide survey of adults over age 35 revealed that gaining weight is a more ardent concern for women smokers, and women who gave up smoking gained an average of 11 pounds and men 10 pounds (Flegal, Troiano, Pamuk, Kuczmarski, & Campbell, 1995). Although from a health perspective a modest weight gain is much more desirable than continued cigarette smoking, it is a difficult trade-off for many female American smokers to make because of the perceived stigma associated with additional weight. One study, though, reported that women who exercise while trying to quit smoking are twice as likely to quit—and only gain half as much weight—as those who did not exercise (Marcus et al., 1999).

The good news for women is that a study of 17,000 smokers reported that they have a lower rate of fatal outcomes from lung cancer compared to men. The bad news is that women smokers have twice the likelihood of developing lung cancer than men (Henschke, International Early Lung Cancer Action Program Investigators, Yip, & Miettinen, 2006). They appear to have increased susceptibility to tobacco carcinogens, though not as prematurely fatal as it is for men.

Education

Among Americans in 2007 who never graduated high school, 25% smoked. Of those with undergraduate degrees, 11% smoked; and of those with graduate degrees, 6% smoked. You would not think it would take a college degree to understand that this increasingly expensive habit kills 443,000 people annually (from smoking and second-hand smoke) through cancer, lung disease, heart disease, and other causes, but there is a strong correlation between smoking rates and formal educational achievement.

Smoking Cessation Interventions

About 70% of all adult smokers visit a physician each year, and the American Cancer Society reports that almost 80% of the heavy smokers claim they would stop smoking if their doctors urged them to do so. Only half of all smokers, however, report having heard an antitobacco admonition from their physician. One problem is with the training of physicians. A majority of U.S. medical school graduates are not adequately trained to treat tobacco dependence.

Even when physicians give patients a prescription for nicotine replacement therapy, the physicians provide very low levels of any form of smoking cessation assistance beyond how to use the replacement therapy (Solberg, Asche, Boyle, Boucher, & Pronk, 2005).

Fewer than a quarter of the more than 1,000 patients surveyed reported that their physician followed up on their smoking cessation therapy.

When client readiness is combined with the authority of the physician, even *brief* smoking cessation counseling by primary care physicians—especially when reinforced by follow-up visits or telephone calls during the first 4 to 8 weeks—is effective in getting clients to quit (Kottke et al., 2000). An attempt to quit is at least twice as likely to occur among smokers who receive nonsmoking advice from their physicians compared with those who are not advised to quit (Milch, Edmunson, Beshansky, Griffith, & Selker, 2004).

Physicians either overestimate the percentage of smoking patients whom they counsel to stop smoking on a regular basis, or their patients do not hear them do so. In several studies, a much higher percentage of physicians reported that they counseled smokers compared with the percentage of smokers reporting that they received counseling from a physician. Physicians are more likely to communicate effectively with smoking clients if they are well prepared for the task.

One simple but effective smoking cessation intervention consists of asking whether patients smoke, motivating those who do to quit, setting a date, providing a written reminder or prescription, and using either a nicotine patch or gum as a supplement. These principles have been incorporated into the *Doctors Helping Smokers* (DHS) system, which was developed by Minnesota physicians Thomas Kottke, a cardiologist, and Leif Solberg, a family practitioner. The system was implemented in 31 Minnesota clinics and reimbursed through Blue Plus, a health maintenance organization.

DHS is based on the four A's—which, in 2000, expanded to five: *A*sk if patients smoke. *A*dvise them that smoking is harmful. *A*ssess their readiness to quit. *A*ssist them by providing self-help guides, education, and counseling. *A*rrange for a follow-up visit, mailing, or telephone call as the proposed quit date nears. Nurses and receptionists assist the physician in counseling and follow-up duties. In addition, follow-up audits allow the team to devise ways to improve the system.

Nursing interventions for smoking cessation appear to be effective, based on a meta-analysis of 16 studies. There were significant increases in patients' quitting rates due to nursing intervention compared to a control group or usual care (Rice & Stead, 2002). Moreover, there was no evidence that interventions classified as intensive had a larger effect on patients than less intensive ones, such as the offering of brief advice. If the latter finding even partially holds up, it could make it less challenging to incorporate smoking cessation interventions by nurses as part of the standard practice in hospitals, clinics, and other settings.

Since the nation's 3 million nurses represent the largest group of clinicians in the country, and they can be effective in helping people stop smoking, the government has developed a free guide titled *Helping Smokers Quit: A Guide for Nurses*. The government replaced this guide in 2009 with *Helping Smokers Quit: A Guide for Clinicians*, and it can be accessed through ahrq.gov/about/nursing/hlpsmksqt.htm.

Telephone counseling services that offer smoking cessation counseling (i.e., "quitlines") appear to be effective. More than 3,000 smokers were given self-help materials and randomized either to a treatment group that received up to seven telephone counseling sessions or to a control group that did not. Abstinence rates doubled over a 1-year period for those who received the counseling (Zhu et al., 2002). Thirty-three states have established quitlines for smokers, including 10 quitlines that the American Cancer Society coordinates from Austin, Texas. To access one in your area, call 800-ACS-2345.

It should be noted that more than 90% of successful quitters do not participate in organized smoking cessation programs. Nevertheless, some evidence suggests that those who smoke more heavily and more addicted smokers may be the best candidates for formal smoking cessation programs (Fiore et al., 1990). If every primary care provider offered a cessation intervention to smokers, it is estimated that an additional 1 million would quit each year.

Nicotine Replacement

It is estimated that more than 95% of smokers relapse after their first attempt to quit (NIH State-of-the-Science Panel, 2006). Withdrawal symptoms, such as irritability, anxiety, restlessness, and a craving for nicotine, are the major cause of relapse. Nicotine is the psychoactive drug that is primarily responsible for the addictive nature of tobacco use.

The transdermal nicotine delivery system, commonly referred to as the nicotine patch, was developed to combat withdrawal symptoms. The patch, along with related nicotine replacement strategies, has grown from a $129 million market in 1991 (when the patch was first approved) to an $800 million market in 2007.

The patch is placed on a different non hairy part of the upper body each day, and it delivers nicotine at a relatively steady rate. In 1991 the Food and Drug Administration (FDA) approved three nicotine patches: Nicoderm, Habitrol, and ProStep. Nicoderm has become the best-selling patch and employs a weaning process that releases 21 mg of nicotine a day, then drops to 14 mg, followed by 7 mg over an 8- (for light smokers) or 10-week (for heavy smokers) period. In 1996 Nicoderm became available over the counter as NicoDerm CQ, and soon thereafter its sales increased to about one-half of the smoking cessation aids market.

Nicorette nicotine gum—which the FDA approved even earlier, in 1984, as the first nicotine replacement aid—controls 40% of the market. Nicotine gum is systematically chewed, 12 to 15 pieces of gum per day, using a continuous "chew and park" technique. Nicotrol, available first as a patch, then as an inhaler or nasal spray, captured 10% of the market. The inhaler consists of a mouthpiece and a cartridge that allows you to puff in, rather than inhale, 10 mL of nicotine. The nicotine nasal spray delivers nicotine the most rapidly, but can lead to abuse, and nasal or throat irritation. There is also a lozenge that should not be chewed but allowed to dissolve slowly in the mouth.

The manufacturers of these nicotine replacement therapies highly recommend that their aids be used as a component of a behavior modification and support group program. These educational programs typically include self-monitoring of daily living habits to determine which habits need to be changed to support a lifestyle without cigarette use. Other program components include a combination of breathing and other stress management exercises, nutrition education, assertiveness training, exercise, peer support, and tips for relapse prevention.

It may take a combination of strategies for smoking cessation to work (Jolicoeur et al., 2009). A patch followed by a nasal spray was more effective than a patch alone, and the antidepressant Zyban combined with a patch was more effective than a patch alone. One randomized clinical trial reported that a nicotine patch plus lozenge produced a 6-month abstinence rate of 40%, compared with the 22% rate of the placebo group (Piper et al., 2008). Given the risk of nicotine overdosing, the combined strategies require a physician's supervision and careful monitoring of blood pressure.

However, the patch as well as other nicotine replacement strategies may be more efficacious (successful in controlled and short-term clinical trials) than effective (successful over the long term in everyday practice). One study reported that 75% of nicotine patch users relapsed over an 8-year period (Yudkin et al., 2003). Other studies have also concluded that nicotine replacement therapy helps people to quit, but is not enough to prevent relapse in the longer run (Carey, 2012). What may help more than nicotine replacement techniques are support from family and friends, increased tobacco taxes, and the tightening of smoking bans.

Other Interventions

In addition to nicotine replacement therapies, there is *Zyban* (also known as Wellbutrin), which was initially marketed exclusively as an antidepressant. In 2006 a nicotine-free antismoking pill, *Chantix*, which blocks nicotine receptors, was FDA approved after 22% of successful users remained smoke-free after 1 year of a clinical trial (Klesges, Johnson, & Somes, 2006). By 2008 Chantix sales reached $846 million. Chantix is taken twice a day and has the effect of making smoking unpleasant while reducing withdrawal symptoms.

A problem with consuming either Chantix or Zyban is that in 2009 the FDA required these two smoking cessation drugs to carry the strongest "black box" warning. This warning was based on a substantial number of people who reported feelings of depression, suicidal thoughts, or other unwanted changes in behavior.

One study reported that supportive text messages on cellphones helped smokers quit (Free et al., 2011). Participants who received motivational texts were twice as likely to be smoke-free as those who did not. Five texts were sent each day for the first 5 weeks and three a week for 26 weeks thereafter. Smokers could also text for help during cravings or relapses.

Another innovation is the *electronic cigarette*, a battery-powered device that can be bought online. It can deliver an odorless dose of nicotine and flavoring without tar or additives, and produces a vapor mist nearly identical to tobacco smoke. Because "e-cigarettes" produce no smoke they can be used in the workplace and any public facility, prompting one distributor to name its product Smoking Everywhere. The downside is that it is unapproved by the government—which has halted shipments of electronic cigarettes at the U.S. border, and one FDA study reported that two leading e-cigarette makers had products with several toxic chemicals. There is pending legislation and ongoing debate about the safety of e-cigarettes.

They cost between $100 and $500 for a starter kit with battery-powered cigarette and replaceable cartridges that typically contain nicotine but can be purchased without. Some kits just include flavoring such as tobacco, menthol, and cherry, and propylene glycol, which produces the smoke-like mist. One study, financed by an electronic cigarette company, reported that users receive 10% to 18% of the nicotine delivered by a tobacco cigarette and produced no carcinogens.

Taxes

In 1988 the California Tobacco Control Program was initiated, increasing cigarette taxes by 25 cents a pack and requiring that 20% of the tax money be used for smoking cessation programs, especially for an antismoking television campaign. Subsequently, there was a 14% decrease in lung cancer in that state over the following decade, compared to only 2.7% in the rest of the country ("Tough Anti-Tobacco Effort," 2000), and a lower rate of death from heart disease during this same time period (Fichtenberg & Glantz, 2000).

Smokers will do what it takes, though, to minimize economic disincentives. A study of the effects of taxes on cigarette consumption from 1955 through 1994 reported that state taxes are less effective than federal taxes because smokers will bootleg cigarettes across state lines to avoid state taxes (Meier & Licari, 1997). Children, however, have had fewer options in this regard. California raised its excise tax on cigarettes by 50 cents on January 1, 1999, and sales went down 29% over the next 6 months—particularly among children—compared with the previous year (California cigarette sales, 1999).

In New York City, where the price of cigarettes escalated to $8 a pack and to $65 a carton, the percentage of public high school students who smoked dropped to 11% in

2006, compared to 23% in 1999. The biggest decline in youth smoking occurred among Black and Hispanic students, who had smoked at a higher rate (29%) and were considerably poorer than White students.

Many states struggling with budget deficits raised their cigarette taxes substantially, mostly for the purpose of raising revenue. As a consequence of the steep price increases, smokers became a lot more creative at dodging them. Popular strategies included buying on American Indian reservations, in low-tax states like Virginia and Kentucky, from illegal sources, and over the Internet. To fight the avoidance of state taxes through online cigarette purchases, states have attempted to outlaw these purchases, or they have obtained the customer lists of Internet cigarette vendors and sent tax bills to residents who purchased online. The black market in contraband cigarettes appears to be more robust than it was after the 50-cent cigarette tax increase in California resulted in only 5% of cigarette buyers turning to low-tax or no-tax sources.

> **Question:** Do you think raising cigarette taxes in *your* state next year would lead to lower consumption rates? Why or why not?

Secondhand Smoke and Attacking the Tobacco Industry

In January 1993 an Environmental Protection Agency (EPA) report that was widely publicized in the media declared that passive tobacco smoke is a human carcinogen responsible for 3,000 lung cancer deaths annually among U.S. *non*smokers and that there was an increased risk of cancer, lower respiratory tract infection, and severe asthma symptoms among children. Subsequent research has also documented the link between *secondhand smoke* and lung cancer (Kreuzer, Krauss, Kreienbrock, Jöckel, & Wichmann, 2000), heart disease (Kawachi et al., 1997), stroke (Bonita, Duncan, Truelsen, Jackson, & Beaglehole, 1999), and respiratory symptoms (Janson et al., 2001). Mortality is about 15% higher among nonsmokers who are exposed to smoke at home than among those not exposed (Hill, Blakely, Kawachi, & Woodward, 2004).

With the accompanying media attention of the 1993 report and the subsequent alarming research findings, restaurants and other public places imposed restrictions in response to the fear of legal action by patrons and employees. Excise taxes on tobacco were raised to fund educational programs for the public, especially ones targeted toward the dangers of secondhand tobacco smoke.

About the same time, Michael T. Lewis, a personal injury lawyer from Clarksdale, Mississippi, developed a strategy for attacking the tobacco industry on the basis of secondhand tobacco smoke and tobacco-related illnesses. Realizing that smokers as plaintiffs had had little success winning conventional lawsuits (after all, the argument goes, it is a free country to do what you want), this small-town lawyer convinced the Mississippi attorney general to sue the tobacco companies to recover money the state spent in *Medicaid bills* for cigarette-*related* illness. By April 1997, 25 states had filed copycat suits against the tobacco industry.

Also, the FDA commissioner David Kessler became convinced that the smoking industry deliberately relied on nicotine to hook smokers and also that they intentionally marketed to minors. In 1996, in fact, daily smoking among 12th graders had reached its highest level (21.6%) since 1979. Dr. Kessler unveiled a proposal to restrict the sale and marketing of cigarettes to minors, and in 1996 President Clinton, realizing that smoking curbs on young persons were politically viable, allowed the FDA to enforce it.

In 1998 California became the first state to extend a smoking ban to bars, casinos, and even private clubs. The main motivator was not a clamor from the public, but the state's legal liability to waitstaff and bartenders who were forced to inhale secondhand smoke during the workday. After the ban took place, the respiratory health of bartenders improved dramatically with the establishment of smoke-free environments. Respiratory irritations to eyes, nose, and throat decreased from 77% to 19% among bartenders; and coughing, wheezing, shortness of breath, and phlegm symptoms decreased from 74% to 32% (Eisner, Smith, & Blanc, 1998).

Attacked on economic, legal, and political fronts, the tobacco industry in 1998 began to pay out a $246 billion legal settlement for the Medicaid expenses associated with smoking-related illnesses. Other features of the legal settlement included regulation of nicotine content, advertising and labeling restrictions especially as they relate to minors, and financial penalties if youth smoking rates did not decrease. In exchange, the tobacco industry received immunity from lawsuits for punitive damage that their products cause and a cap on other damages.

In turn, the tobacco companies raised the price of cigarettes 44% over the next 2 years and increased their marketing budget by 33% in 2000. They also shifted more attention to exporting tobacco products to overseas markets. Finally, they surreptitiously increased the addictive nicotine content of cigarettes by 10% between 1998 and 2004, according to a Massachusetts Department of Public Health report. In response, the FDA tried on its own to regulate nicotine as a drug, but a conservative Supreme Court struck down that effort. Cigarette content remained less regulated than cosmetics or pet food.

In addition, only 5% of the $246 billion tobacco settlement money was spent by state governments on smoking control. (States are not required to spend settlement monies on antismoking programs.) North Carolina spent 75% of its tobacco settlement money to provide assistance to tobacco producers, including a tobacco auction house and a video history of tobacco cultivation. Michigan, which spent no money on tobacco prevention or cessation, used its settlement monies on general education. New York used some of its money to buy golf carts. In 2009 antismoking programs accounted for only 2.3% of the more than $25 billion that states collected from tobacco taxes and payouts from the 1998 tobacco settlement money.

On June 27, 2006, the surgeon general issued a report on secondhand smoke, titled *The Health Consequences of Involuntary Exposure to Tobacco Smoke*, which can be accessed at www.surgeongeneral.gov/library/secondhandsmoke. The report states that second-hand smoke is not a mere annoyance but a serious health hazard. Surgeon General Richard Carmona declared that smoking sections with the best ventilation systems were still not safe, and advocated for completely smoke-free buildings and public places throughout the United States.

The 670-page study reports that there is "overwhelming scientific evidence that secondhand smoke causes heart disease, lung cancer, and many other illnesses." The report helped to accelerate an already growing movement toward statewide smoking bans in public spaces. (It also accelerated the "retirement" of Surgeon General Richard Carmona by the Bush administration, which viewed the report as too antibusiness.)

Smoking Bans

There have been a growing number of statewide bans on smoking in all enclosed public places, including restaurants and bars. In fact, North Carolina, which produces nearly half of the nation's tobacco, and Virginia, the second-leading state producer of tobacco, became the 25th and 26th states in January 2010 to ban smoking in enclosed public places. Seven states have less comprehensive public *smoking bans*, such as allowing bars to permit smoking if they choose. Conversely, 13 states have not enacted a single state-wide ban on any space that is not government-owned.

There have been several workplace or public smoking bans that have demonstrated effectiveness. One such ban on all workplace smoking sites in Pueblo, Colorado, led to a 41% reduction in the rate of heart attacks requiring hospitalization over a 3-year period. There was no such drop in two neighboring areas that did not enact this ban (www.msnbc.msn.com/id/28450513/). A review of 13 studies of public and workspace smoking bans revealed a 36% reduction in heart attacks over a 3-year period in communities in the United States, Canada, and Europe (Lightwood & Glantz, 2009). According to the authors of this meta-analysis, the data add to the already strong evidence that secondhand smoke causes heart attacks, and that passing 100% smoke-free laws in all workplaces and public places will produce substantial health benefits.

A smoking ban was taken one step further by the city of Calabasas in California. Their smoking ordinance prohibits smoking in all public places, indoors *and* outdoors. The ban includes outdoor cafes, bus stops, soccer fields, condominium pool decks, parks, and sidewalks. If you are going to smoke in your car in Calabasas, you need to close the windows if anyone is nearby. California has always been in the vanguard when it comes to ratcheting up smoking bans, beginning with the first statewide ban on smoking in restaurants, workplaces, and many public venues in 1995. In 2000, smoking was prohibited on most southern California beaches and piers. In 2006 California officially declared secondhand smoke a toxic air pollutant.

Whole countries are now banning indoor smoking. Ireland began the trend in 2004, followed by Norway, New Zealand, England, Scotland, Puerto Rico, and others. In 2006 Latin Americans joined in when Uruguay banned smoking in the workplace, shopping malls, and many other public spaces. The president of Uruguay, who promoted the ban, also happened to be a practicing oncologist. In Cuba you cannot even smoke a legendary Cuban cigar in most public places. In cigarette-friendly France, a ban on smoking in schools, offices, and other public buildings took effect in 2007, and was followed up in 2008 by including restaurants, dance clubs, and some bars.

In China, however, there is resistance. Two thirds of Chinese men are smokers, including 60% of physicians. Smoking takes place in hospitals, and hospital shops sell cigarettes. There are 360 million smokers in China, and thanks to China's becoming a member of the World Trade Organization, Western tobacco companies are eagerly attempting to break into this lucrative market.

What is happening in China? There is a state-owned tobacco monopoly that provides 60 million jobs and 10% of national tax revenue. The official website of the tobacco monopoly advertises cigarettes as a miracle drug: it prevents ulcers, reduces the risk of Parkinson's disease, relieves schizophrenia, boosts brain cells, speeds up thinking, improves reaction time, eliminates loneliness and depression, and increases work efficiency.

A 2005 survey reported that 90% of the Chinese population believed that smoking had little effect on their health, or that it was good for them. By 2011, though, the worldwide trend had an impact on the government. Indoor smoking bans were legislated throughout China; but enforcement, so far, has been patchy at best.

The Family Smoking Prevention and Tobacco Control Act

The *Family Smoking Prevention and Tobacco Control Act* (FSPTC) is a landmark piece of legislation passed in 2009 that gives federal officials for the first time the power to regulate cigarettes and other forms of tobacco. The law gives the FDA power to set standards that could reduce nicotine content and regulate the chemicals in cigarette smoke. The law also bans most tobacco flavorings (granting an unfortunate waiver to menthol). The law tightens restrictions on the marketing and advertising of tobacco products, replacing colorful advertisements and store displays with black-and-white-only text. All outdoor advertising of tobacco within 1,000 feet of schools and playgrounds is illegal. Terms such as "light" and "low tar" are banned, and large, graphic health warnings were to be placed on cigarette packages by 2012 (no such luck, see next section). Finally, tobacco companies had to submit lists of all their product ingredients to the government and disclose research results about their health effects.

As if that weren't enough, cigarette companies must pay the fees for the creation and administration of a new FDA tobacco oversight department, which could add another 6 cents to a pack of cigarettes and further discourage smoking. The Congressional Budget Office has estimated that the new law will reduce youth smoking by 11% and adult smoking by 2% within the next decade.

Bloody Mouths

When it comes to truth in advertising, American tobacco companies thought they had it bad in the mid-1960s when they had to make space on cigarette packs for a warning that cigarette smoking is a health hazard. In 2001 the Canadian government went one giant step further: Over 50% of each cigarette pack had to be adorned by a graphic warning of what those health hazards look like. Among the 16 designs they chose from were bloody mouths in acute periodontal distress, cancerous lungs, stroke-clotted brains, and damaged hearts.

In 2011, Canada strengthened its tobacco warning labels to cover 75% of each cigarette package and increased the number of designs to 20. In 2012, Australia one-upped them. All logos, including distinctive colors and brand designs, must be stripped from cigarette packs and replaced by a drab and uniform shade of olive, and feature graphic health warnings and images such as cancer-riddled mouths, blinded eyeballs, and sickly children.

Ireland and Belgium are joining in, and other countries of the European Union are considering it, because smokers constitute one third of the population in Europe. Among their pictures are a grisly photograph of a man with a cancerous growth on his neck and a picture of a drooping cigarette meant to represent impotency. It remains to be seen if this strategy will be more effective than the U.S.'s warning on cigarette packs, which appears to have slipped out of the consciousness of most American smokers.

The FSPTC attempted to escalate warnings to American smokers by requiring graphic health warnings on cigarette packages by 2012. But that year a U.S. judge sided with the tobacco companies and ruled that reglations requiring large graphic designs on cigarette packaging and advertising violate free-speech rights under the first amendement of the U.S. Constitution.

Medicare Smoking Cessation Coverage

Initially, in 2005, Medicare offered coverage for smoking cessation counseling only for beneficiaries who had tobacco-related diseases (e.g., cardiovascular, cancer, respiratory, gastrointestinal, osteoporosis, cataracts, blood clots) or who were on drug regimens that were adversely affected by smoking (e.g., insulin, hypertensive medications, treatments for blood clots or depression). Thanks to the Affordable Care Act (see Chapter 12, "Public Health Policy") and its emphasis on prevention, however, help was expanded to all Medicare-eligible people who want to quit smoking. The Centers for Medicare and Medicaid Services (CMMS) estimates that 4 million seniors fit this profile.

Two quit attempts are covered per year, each consisting of up to four counseling sessions. Smoking counseling must be prescribed by a doctor, as well as provided by a qualified doctor or a Medicare-recognized practitioner. CMMS, however, does not provide guidelines when it comes to qualifications, and encourages clinicians to become appropriately trained until a consensus on national credentialing emerges. Medicare does not cover the cost of over-the-counter nicotine patches, gum, or other products. There is, however, a national quitline available to smokers at 800-QUITNOW, and a national network of smoking cessation quitlines accessed through www.smokefree.gov.

Additional Programs and Materials

Fresh Start is a group smoking cessation program that is offered by many local chapters of the American Cancer Society. To locate your local chapter or to obtain free publications on smoking cessation, contact the American Cancer Society, 1599 Clifton Road, Atlanta, GA 30329; 800-227-2345 (information service); www.cancer.org.

Two booklets, *Clearing the Air—A Guide to Quitting Smoking* and *Guide to Quit Smoking for Your Health and Your Family* (the latter available in Spanish as well), offer strategies and suggestions for quitting and staying a nonsmoker. These booklets (up to 200 copies free) are available from the Office of Cancer Communications, National Cancer Institute, Building 31, Room 10A24, Bethesda, MD 20892; 800-422-6237; www.cancer.gov.

Freedom from Smoking is offered by local affiliates of the American Lung Association. To locate your local chapter or to obtain manuals, audiotapes, videotapes, films, posters, or buttons, contact the American Lung Association, 1720 Broadway, New York, NY 10019-4374; 800-586-4872; www.lungusa.org.

The *Smoking and Health Bulletin*, a free guide entitled *Out of the Ashes: Choosing a Method to Quit Smoking*, a free bibliography on smoking and health, and materials on smoking cessation techniques are available from the Office on Smoking and Health, Park Building, Room 1-16, 5600 Fishers Lane, Rockville, MD 20857. Smoking cessation kits are available from the American Academy of Family Physicians at 800-944-0000 (www.aafp.org).

Also available are *Smoking Cessation Resources from the National Library of Medicine*, www.americanheart.org, and www.nlm.nih.gov/medlineplus/smokingcessation.html; *Smoking Cessation: You Can Quit Smoking Now*, www.surgeongeneral.gov/tobacco; and *How to Quit: Resources to Quit Smoking*, www.cdc.gov/tobacco/how2quit.htm.

ALCOHOL

Definition

No consensus exists among alcohol researchers and other experts regarding what constitutes moderate drinking and what constitutes *alcoholism*. The Department of Agriculture somewhat arbitrarily defined moderate drinking as no more than two drinks a day for men and one drink a day for women, with a drink defined as approximately 12 ounces of beer, 5 ounces of wine, or 1.5 ounces of spirits. Some researchers conclude, however, that given the substantial increase in the proportion of body fat with aging and the concomitant decrease in volume of total body water, a maximum of one drink a day may be advised for both older women and men.

It may be best when attempting to define alcoholism to avoid associating it with a specific number of drinks. The National Council on Alcoholism and Drug Dependence define it as impaired control over drinking, preoccupation with the drug alcohol, use of alcohol despite adverse consequences, and distortion in thinking.

The diagnostic criteria for alcohol dependence used in the *Diagnostic and Statistical Manual of Mental Disorders* (American Psychiatric Association, 2000) is the persistence for a month or more of three or more of the following nine criteria:

1. Drinking more or over a longer period than previously.
2. Persistent desire or unsuccessful efforts to cut down or control use.
3. Considerable time spent in obtaining, drinking, or recovering from the effects of alcohol.
4. Intoxication or withdrawal when expected to fulfill major obligations.
5. Important activities given up or reduced because of drinking.
6. Continued use despite knowledge of having persistent or recurrent psychological or physical problems related to alcohol.
7. Marked tolerance.
8. Withdrawal symptoms.
9. Drinking to relieve or avoid withdrawal symptoms.

Types

About one third of elderly alcoholics are late-onset, reactive problem drinkers. *Late-onset* alcoholics are likely to be the product of a life cycle crisis, such as the death of a spouse or the loss of a physical function. Once the precipitating event is identified and therapy is pursued, the condition may be reversible. A return to moderate drinking may be viable for late-onset alcoholics. *Early-onset* drinkers have had a drinking problem for many years and have either avoided or undergone unsuccessful treatment. Although the prognosis for successful treatment of chronic, lifelong problem drinkers is poor, it is not impossible to treat.

Assessment

The U.S. Preventive Services Task Force recommends that all adults be screened for alcohol misuse, with referral for counseling if necessary. During the early stages of alcoholism, though, no physical signs or symptoms signal the shift from health to disease. Often, behavioral problems such as repetitive accidents or injuries, or ongoing work and family problems, accompany alcohol misuse.

It may be especially difficult to detect alcohol problems among retired persons, who have fewer opportunities to experience problems in the work or community setting. It appears to be particularly difficult for physicians to detect. When presented with early symptoms of alcoholism, only 6% of 462 physicians mentioned substance abuse as a possible diagnosis (Schmidt, 2000). It is estimated that physicians make the correct diagnosis of alcoholism in older adults in only about one third of actual cases seen in emergency departments or during hospitalizations.

Even when alcoholism is recognized, the physician is less likely to initiate or recommend treatment for older clients than for younger clients. Some physicians believe it is too late in their older patients' lives to do anything about the problems of alcoholism (Butler, Lewis, & Sunderland, 1998). Other physicians believe it is too difficult and time-consuming to accurately assess. One qualitative study of 14 primary care physicians at a Veterans Affairs General Internal Medicine Clinic revealed that providers often did not pursue disclosures from older patients about alcohol problems, or provided advice that was typically vague and tentative—particularly in contrast to smoking-related advice given to younger patients (McCormick et al., 2006).

One of the most popular assessment tools for busy health professionals and one that has been tested with older clients is the CAGE questionnaire. It has good sensitivity and specificity for alcohol abuse in general, though is less sensitive to early problem or heavy drinking (U.S. Preventive Services Task Force, 1996). The four questions in the CAGE are

Have you ever:

Thought about	Cutting down?
Felt	Annoyed when others criticize your drinking?
Felt	Guilty about drinking?
Used alcohol as an	Eye opener?

Two or more affirmative responses to the above questions suggest an alcohol problem.

Although the CAGE instrument is practical for the busy health care professional, more sensitivity and specificity can be obtained with longer questionnaires, especially the 25-item Michigan Alcohol Screening Test (MAST), which has been tested with older adults. The MAST, however, is too lengthy for routine screening. There is a 10-item version of the MAST targeted toward older adults that is used in outpatient settings, called the Short Michigan Alcoholism Screening Test–Geriatric Version (Naegle, 2008). It appears to capture different aspects of unsafe drinking, however, and perhaps both it and the CAGE instrument need to be used (Moore, Seeman, Morgenstern, Beck, & Reuben, 2002).

A third commonly used assessment tool is the Alcohol Use Disorders Identification Test (AUDIT). The value of the AUDIT is that it incorporates questions about quantity, frequency, and binge behavior. The AUDIT focuses on drinking during the previous year and is less sensitive for past drinking problems that can help the clinician distinguish between late-onset versus long-term drinking problems.

Question: Do you have any ideas on how we can better detect problems with alcohol among older adults?

Another assessment option is a biochemical test for diagnosing alcohol abuse. The carbohydrate-deficient transferrin test, approved by the FDA, improved upon the specificity and sensitivity of previous biochemical tests and could help break through the denial and rationalization of a patient.

Prevalence

Estimates of the percentage of Americans who are problem drinkers vary widely, from 2% to more than 10%, with men having three times the rate of alcoholism as women. A national survey of Medicare beneficiaries, though, reported that 9% exceed recommended drinking limits, with a prevalence of 16% for men and 4% for women (Merrick et al., 2008). About 10% of patients who go to an emergency room with an alcohol-related problem are over age 60, although the prevalence of alcohol-related hospitalizations declines with age for both men and women.

It is not easy to estimate the scope of problem drinking in late life because much of it may take place out of the glare of work and community life. It is easier to predict that alcohol abuse and dependence are likely to increase in the coming decades, due to baby boomers having a history of greater alcohol consumption than the current cohort of older adults.

Associated Diseases and Problems

Although problem drinking in late life is less common than for younger adults, the risks of alcohol abuse for older drinkers are elevated in terms of falls and accidents, dementias, medical problems, reaction time, memory, and interactions with prescription and over-the-counter drugs. Nutritional deficiencies, particularly vitamin and protein deficiencies, are more common among older alcohol drinkers as well because of the increased inhibition of the absorption of many nutrients.

With age, the body absorbs a higher percentage of the alcohol consumed. This occurs because alcohol is more soluble in water than in fat; and as we age, the water content in our body declines. Lean body mass that is high in water content decreases, and body fat that is low in water content increases. Thus, alcohol reaches a higher concentration in the blood of an older person. Also, as we age there is a decline in a stomach enzyme—alcohol dehydrogenase—that can break down alcohol before it reaches the bloodstream. This further increases the blood alcohol level and places an extra burden on the liver, where most alcohol metabolism takes place.

Moreover, as we age, blood flow through the liver declines, as does kidney function, which means that alcohol is eliminated more slowly from the blood. Consuming the same amount of alcohol as a younger person, the older person will have a blood alcohol level that is 30% to 40% higher.

Although alcohol adds calories to the diet, it adds almost no nutrients; therefore, malnutrition becomes a problem as well. Other problems of excess alcohol consumption are an increased risk of injury or accident, especially when driving and, along with excess caffeine and medications, an adverse affect on sleep.

At least 100 of the most commonly prescribed medications interact negatively with alcohol. This interaction effect, along with the increased vulnerability of older adults to alcohol abuse, accounts for the fact that older adults are hospitalized as often for alcohol-related problems as for heart attacks.

Intervention and Referral

Most patients with suspected drinking problems receive no counseling from primary care physicians. Although physicians report having counseled patients on alcohol abuse, it is much less likely to appear on patients' medical records when they are examined. One study of patient records revealed that only 18% of patients were counseled by physicians. When physicians do offer problem drinkers advice and additional workbook materials, problem drinking may be reduced and maintained for at least a year (Fleming et al., 2000). One study reported that physician referral to a specialist—regardless of whether it was implemented—was associated with less drinking (Crawford et al., 2004).

Older adults often drink in response to depression and loneliness, whereas younger adults are likely to use multiple substances to assuage their anger, frustration, tension, interpersonal conflicts, and social pressure. If interventions are to be effective, most older adults with alcohol abuse problems will need to be referred by their health professionals to groups or specialists who recognize the different needs of older versus younger persons. Only 18% of 13,749 substance abuse programs nationwide, however, offered specialized treatment for elders.

Some evidence indicates that persons referred to age-specific support groups remain in treatment longer and complete treatment more often than those in age-mixed groups. Problems such as widowhood and retirement, which are not of universal concern, may be particularly difficult for older people to share in support groups of mixed ages. Older adults tend to grapple with different health issues, want a more peaceful environment in which to share, and expect a different pace of verbal interaction than younger adults (Gross, 2008).

About a third of those who attend Alcoholics Anonymous (AA) meetings are over age 50, and many communities launch groups specifically for older adults. The geriatrician Robert Butler suggests: "Because of the magnitude of drinking problems among older people, it would be useful to have AA programs set up especially for them" (Butler, Lewis, & Sunderland, 1998, p. 178).

AA employs a strategy that encourages public confession, intense social support, contrition, and a spiritual or philosophical awakening. Founded in the 1930s, AA expanded to about 90,000 groups around the world, and close to 2 million members. Companion organizations have been set up for spouses (Al-Anon), teenage children of alcoholics (Alateen), and adult children of alcoholics (ACOA).

The anonymous nature of membership in AA makes it difficult to evaluate this type of intervention. Even if researchers could randomly assign alcoholics to an AA group or an alternative intervention, that research design would eliminate one of the most important elements of joining a group, namely, the ability to seek the intervention voluntarily. Older alcoholics may raise a unique set of research questions when evaluating the effectiveness of AA groups. Are older adults prepared for the openness that characterizes these types of support groups? Do older adults have access to a support group with other older alcoholics to whom they can relate?

Professionally led programs should be viewed as complementary to AA and other peer support groups, rather than as in competition with them. Professionally run treatment programs may be more effective than AA groups for some older individuals, but they have disadvantages as well. They are typically costly and time-bound, in comparison to support groups that can and do meet frequently (some several times a week) and that are ongoing.

The self-management strategies and vulnerability to relapse discussed for smoking cessation are applicable to alcohol addiction as well. Behavior management techniques may need to be reapplied on multiple occasions.

Positive Effects

Individuals who consume moderate amounts of alcohol reduce their risk of heart failure; and if a heart attack occurs, these individuals are more likely to survive it in comparison to teetotalers or heavy drinkers (Abramson, Williams, Krumholz, & Vaccarino, 2001; Mukamal, Maclure, Muller, Sherwood, & Mittleman, 2001). Moderate alcohol consumption also appears to have a protective effect against ischemic stroke (Sacco et al., 1999). People who drank only one or two drinks daily had a 45% lower risk of stroke caused by insufficient blood flow to the brain.

It is not clear why moderate drinking appears to have a positive effect on health, but it may act to lower blood pressure, as well as raise protective HDL cholesterol or reduce the likelihood of blood clots. Interestingly, if the alcohol is removed from red wine, that is, dealcoholized, blood pressure reductions more than doubled in one study (Chiva-Blanch et al., 2012). The polyphenols in alcohol may weaken the antihypertensive effect, but as they are not present in dealcoholized red wine, the benefits increase.

A survey of 490,000 adults, ranging in age from 30 to 104, concluded that taking one alcoholic drink a day provides a slight edge in longevity over nondrinkers (Thun et al., 1997). People who drank a small amount of alcohol on a daily basis reduced their incidence of heart disease and stroke, which modestly outweighed the increased risks associated with regular drinking, that is, death from cancer (especially breast cancer) and accidents. The study authors were not touting alcohol as the preventive therapy of choice because limiting oneself to one serving of alcohol daily is not the drinking pattern of many Americans.

"Reasonably small and controlled alcohol intake may be of benefit to the elderly, as it may stimulate appetite, increase socialization, and may play a 'protective' role against coronary artery disease" (Lamy, 1988). Nursing homes may be one type of facility where the introduction of controlled alcohol intake can be an effective preventive therapy. Unpublished research reports indicate that moderate alcohol drinking in nursing home institutions improves mental health and physical functioning, although the effects of an increased opportunity for socialization and increased personal control may be contributing to the positive outcomes as well.

Resources

For written material and other resources on alcohol abuse, contact:

Alcoholics Anonymous, 475 Riverside Drive, 11th Floor, New York, NY 10115 (www .aa.org); or the local chapter of Alcoholics Anonymous, Al-Anon, and Adult Children of Alcoholics, listed in the phone book or at www.al-anon-alateen.org

National Clearinghouse for Alcohol and Drug Abuse Information, P.O. Box 2345, Rockville, MD 20852; 800-729-6686; www.health.org

Hazelden's brochure, *How to Talk to an Older Person Who Has a Problem with Alcohol or Medications*, and other materials, 800-257-7810; www.hazelden.org

Smart Recovery, online and other types of support groups for abstaining from alcohol addictive behavior, 7504 Mentor Avenue, Suite F, Mentor, Ohio 44060; 866-951-5357 (toll-free); www.smartrecovery.org

National Institute on Alcohol Abuse and Alcoholism, at www.niaaa.nih.gov

---

BOX 7.1	Gerontologizing Smoking Cessation and Alcohol Counseling

Among the health education topics discussed in this chapter, tobacco and alcohol are two problems likely to be associated with interventions that focus primarily on younger adults. Suppose, however, that an alcohol abuse specialist and a smoking cessation specialist, both of whom have had practices almost exclusively with young adults, are being confronted for the first time with older clients. What advice would you give to each of them to help them become more responsive to the needs and interests of older clients? Think about topics that are unique to older adults, such as motivation for behavior change in late life, perceived stigma toward drinking or smoking, polypharmacy or comorbidity issues, responsiveness to group facilitation strategies, and so forth.

Alcohol and smoking abuse programs can be run by professionals who have had training with more of a clinical bent, such as nurses, clinical psychologists, or social workers, or by professionals with more of a health education perspective, such as graduates of health education departments or gerontology programs. The relative effectiveness of these professionals for health behavior change has yet to be studied, and it is hard to draw a distinct line between offering health education and providing counseling. Either way, an awareness of the issues impacting on older adults is paramount.

MEDICATION USAGE

More than 10,000 prescription drugs are currently available to Americans, and over a billion prescriptions are dispensed per year. There are also 300,000 over-the-counter medications, including 600 that would have required a prescription just a few years ago. It is not unreasonable to suggest that most Americans consider taking medications a normal part of life. In fact, Americans buy much more medicine per person than do citizens of any other country.

Because vulnerability to chronic disease increases over time, medication usage becomes more typical with age. More than half of all insured Americans are taking prescription medicines regularly for chronic health problems. Although adults aged 65 and over comprise only 13% of the population, they account for 34% of outpatient prescription medications and a similar percentage of those purchased over the counter. Among seniors, 28% of women and 22% of men take five or more medicines regularly.

Many diseases that used to be fatal, including some cancers and AIDS, have now turned into chronic conditions. Older persons rely on drugs to survive, to alleviate pain and discomfort, and to give them a sense of security and control in sometimes frightening health situations. Drugs, however, can make matters worse as well as better. The potential for serious adverse drug reactions is great.

Misuse

About 50% of prescriptions are not taken properly, and according to the National Council on Patient Information and Education, an estimated 125,000 Americans die each year from prescription drug misuse. In fact, there are more deaths from prescription medication than from accidents, pneumonia, or diabetes.

On an outpatient basis about 5% of Medicare patients are made ill by their medications during the course of a year, leading to as many as 1.9 million drug-related injuries (Gurwitz et al., 2003). More than half of these adverse drug events are preventable, ranging from mistakes made by physicians to failure of patients to adhere to medication instructions.

In 2012 the Institute of Medicine reported that drug errors injured about 1.3 million Americans yearly, an estimate that is much lower than others. This conservative figure included only drug errors in hospitals, nursing homes, and among Medicare outpatients. It did not include mistakes in physician offices or those made by patients themselves. The Institute recommended two strategies for lowering its estimate, (1) that electronic prescriptions become the standard, and (2) that patients be strongly encouraged to carry complete listings of their prescriptions to every doctor's visit.

About 11% of hospital, nursing home, and emergency department admissions of older adults are the result of adverse drug reactions (Hohl, Dankoff, Colacone, & Afilalo, 2001; Vik, Maxwell, & Hogan, 2004). This percentage is probably underestimated because medical personnel are not enthusiastic about filing the additional reports required by the FDA. Adverse drug reactions probably affect older adults three times as often as they do the general population.

To avoid adverse drug reactions, patients need to comply with their medication regimen, report unexpected side effects, and exercise caution with over-the-counter medications. They also need to know more about their medications. Only 15% of elderly patients who visited an emergency department were able to accurately report on their medications, dosages, frequencies, and indications—even with patients who were disoriented or medically unstable excluded from this study (Chung & Barfield, 2002). Audiotaped office visits from 185 outpatient encounters revealed that physicians addressed adverse effects of new medications, and how long to take them, only one third of the time with patients (Tarn et al., 2006).

Physicians need to take a good drug history, carefully assess dosage, communicate the rationale for the drug treatment and the expected response and common side effects, and monitor patient reactions. The aging process complicates this course of action because it affects the absorption, distribution, metabolism, and excretion of medications.

Physicians also need to know which medications are inappropriate for older persons. About 1 million older patients were prescribed 1 of 11 medicines that a panel of geriatric medicine and pharmacy experts agreed should always be avoided by older adults (Zhan et al., 2001). Five percent of older HMO (health maintenance organizations) members received at least 1 of these 11 drugs, and 13% received a medication classified as rarely appropriate (Simon et al., 2005). In one study of 162,000 elderly outpatients, 21% filled a prescription for a drug that should be avoided by older persons (Curtis et al., 2004).

Overprescribing is common as well. Even when nonpharmacological treatments are suitable for a given condition, physicians often prescribe medications, sometimes encouraged by their patients. Predictably, the greater the number of drugs prescribed, the greater the risk of inadvertent or intentional misuse of drugs by the patient or caregiver.

Polypharmacy is the use of more medications than are clinically indicated. Older adults are particularly vulnerable to polypharmacy because most of the chronic conditions associated with aging are potentially responsive to medications. This leads to the increased risk of multiple drug use among older adults, complicated by the fact that many older patients see more than one health care provider. With more than one provider, prescription and over-the-counter drug usage may not be coordinated, and older clients are vulnerable to potential interactions—drug–drug, drug–allergy, drug–food, drug–drink, and drug–disease—and therapeutic duplication.

This challenge has been met to some extent by the fact that almost all pharmacies in this country are now using computers. Nonetheless, many pharmacies do not have complete computer records of all the medication usage of their clients.

On the basis of an article by Montamat and Cusack (1992), 10 patient-related and physician-related factors may contribute to polypharmacy and other types of drug misuse:

Patient-Related Drug Misuse Factors

1. Expectation for physician to prescribe medication for a problem.
2. Inadequate reporting of current medications being taken.
3. Failure to complain about medication-related symptoms.
4. Use of multiple, automatic refills without visiting a physician.
5. Hoarding and using prior medications.
6. Use of multiple pharmacies or multiple physicians.
7. Borrowing medications from family members or friends.
8. Self-medication with over-the-counter drugs.
9. Impaired cognition or vision.
10. Underuse of medications due to side effects or cost considerations.

Physician-Related Drug Misuse Factors

1. Presuming that patients expect a prescription to be written.
2. Treatment of symptoms with drugs without sufficient clinical evaluation.
3. Treatment of conditions without setting therapy goals.
4. Communicating instructions in an unclear, complex, or incomplete manner.

5. Failure to review medications and their possible adverse effects at regular intervals.
6. Use of automatic refills without adequate follow-up.
7. Lack of knowledge of geriatric clinical pharmacology, leading to inappropriate prescribing practices.
8. Failure to caution about medication interactions.
9. Failure to simplify drug regimens as often as possible.
10. Failure to identify and adequately communicate the equivalency of cost-effective generics.

Finally, we can anticipate greater use of illicit drugs among older adults as baby boomers enter their ranks. A survey conducted by the Substance Abuse and Mental Health Services Administration reported that 8% of adults between the ages of 50 and 59 admitted to taking an illicit drug in 2010. The most common illicit drug was marijuana, followed by unprescribed drugs, most often painkillers. Also, 2.4 million people ages 50 to 59 reported that they abused prescription or illegal drugs within the past month—almost three times as many people as reported that behavior in 2002.

Prevention

One of the most effective prevention strategies is to avoid unnecessary medication. Many Americans unthinkingly take pills to alleviate constipation, insomnia, indigestion, headache, and other types of pain or discomfort. Diet, exercise, and stress management, however, may be effective alternatives that avoid the danger of medication side effects. Elderly clients with high blood pressure, for instance, are susceptible to severe adverse drug reactions. Treating some patients with mild to modestly high blood pressure with nonpharmacological alternatives, therefore, may be appropriate. Many older adults can be responsive to a reduction in sodium intake, or to exercise that positively affects blood pressure levels.

Physicians and patients must have an understanding of the degree to which the other favors chemical versus psychological and behavioral coping strategies. Many patients, and some physicians, believe that a productive medical encounter requires the writing of a prescription. In support of this assertion, about 75% of all physician visits result in the prescription of a drug. If prescriptions do become the treatment of choice, patients may be willing to participate actively in choosing among medication alternatives (type, dosage, and schedules) in order to enhance their adherence.

Advice From Pharmacists

Pharmacists are required to give Medicaid patients advice about their prescription drugs. When the (former) Health Care Financing Administration implemented these rules, some state boards of pharmacies expanded them to cover all patients.

In addition to informing patients verbally and in writing, pharmacies must maintain files of patient information (including a list of the medicines and health care devices being used by the patient). The pharmacist must provide specific information about each medication and its common side effects, potential interactions, contraindications, and must instruct patients on how to monitor their responses, explain what to do if a dose is missed, and inform patients on how to store the medicine. Pharmacies are required to provide an area suitable for confidential patient counseling. Over the years, these regulations have been increasingly adhered to.

The consumer who is most disadvantaged, especially in the way of monitoring potential interaction effects, is the one who pharmacy-hops for either financial purposes or convenience. It is not unusual for a patient to obtain prescription drugs from multiple sources, such as a community pharmacy, a hospital pharmacy, a mail-order pharmacy, and directly through samples from the physician. To offset this inconsistency, it would be useful to implement a credit card system to enable patients to carry prescription records with them wherever they go.

A Physician's Experience

"Recently, I spoke to a group of older people. I told them that as a young doctor I had spent most of my time putting patients on drugs. But now that I'm an old doctor, I spend a lot of my time taking patients off drugs. I thought the remark might elicit a few smiles or chuckles. Instead, they rose as a body, cheering and clapping" (Morgan, 1993). Although it is true that many new medications have been miraculous for the functioning of older adults, many older adults clearly have suffered the consequences of drugs as well.

Advertising

Only the United States and New Zealand permit advertising of prescription medicines to consumers. As the number of advertisements continues to rise, along with consumer spending on advertised prescription medications, this practice has become increasingly controversial. The 50 most advertised prescription medicines in 2000 contributed an additional $10 billion in spending on medications. The television messages are almost irresistible: after taking a medication, people with allergies are now able to romp happily in an open field, or those with painful heartburn are able to scarf down a pepperoni pizza.

In 2000 Merck & Company spent $161 million on advertising Vioxx, an arthritis drug, and sales of that one drug alone increased more than $1 billion. (Vioxx was voluntarily withdrawn from the market in 2004 because of its association with increased risk for heart attacks and stroke.) The amount spent on advertising for Vioxx that year was more than PepsiCo spent to advertise Pepsi or Budweiser spent to advertise beer. Besides prescription arthritis drugs, the most heavily advertised medications were cholesterol-lowering drugs, antidepressants, allergy medicine, and heartburn medicine (Petersen, 2001). By 2007 drug advertising had reached $5 billion, generating untold billions of additional dollars spent on medications. The good news is that from 2008 to 2011 drug advertising declined steadily. The reason was the increasing competition from generic drugs, which compete on their lower price rather than with advertising dollars.

Greater exposure to prescription drug advertising was significantly associated with a higher probability of patient requests for advertised drugs. Among older adults who were exposed to direct-to-consumer advertisements, 31% in one sample requested a prescription drug from their physician (Datti & Carter, 2006). Physicians grant about 75% of these requests for advertised drugs, and about half of these transactions result in drug prescriptions that physicians would not choose for a similar patient with the same condition (Mintzes et al., 2003).

Does television advertising increase overall awareness of drugs that might otherwise be underprescribed, or does it stimulate patient demand for unnecessary medication? You decide. My opinion, though, is in line with that of geriatrician John Morley: "Nancy Reagan's 'Just say no to drugs' campaign may have been more effective if it had been aimed at adults rather than teenagers" (2002).

Resources

Many readily available booklets on medication are good sources of consumer safety advice for today's cohort of older adults. These booklets list important questions to ask physicians and pharmacists, offer ideas to improve daily compliance with prescription indications, identify generic equivalents, note commonly reported side effects of medications, and include blank charts for listing prescription and over-the-counter medications prior to an appointment with a physician.

Consumers who are particularly vulnerable to psychological and emotional appeals that may influence their use of medications can obtain free copies of a booklet titled *So Many Pills and I Still Don't Feel Good: Suggestions for Preventing Problems with Medications*. The booklet helps individuals recognize times when they may be at risk for misuse of medications, suggests ways to manage medications, lists questions to ask the doctor or pharmacist about medications, and suggests things to do if there is a problem with medication usage. Up to 50 free copies can be ordered from AARP (formerly the American Association of Retired Persons) Fulfillment, 601 E St. NW, Washington, DC 20049; order no. PF 4767(1091)-D14581 (no telephone orders).

Two other booklets are provided free by AARP: *The Smart Consumer's Guide to Prescription Drugs* [PF 4297(389)-D13579] and *Using Your Medicines Wisely: A Guide for the Elderly* [PF 1436(1185)-D317]. Contact AARP Publications, Program Resources, 601 E St. NW, Washington, DC 20049.

For answers to questions about the drug approval process, drug reactions, and new and approved medications, contact the FDA, Center for Drug Evaluation and Research, CDER Executive Secretariat (HFD-8), 5600 Fishers Lane, Rockville, MD 29857; 301-827-4570; or go to the FDA website at www.fda.gov.

AARP's mail-order pharmacy is for members of AARP (who must be age 50 or older and pay a small annual membership fee). This network of regional pharmacies provides information on common prescription drugs, their side effects, and cost differences between brand names and generic drugs: AARP Pharmacy Services, 500 Montgomery Street, Alexandria, VA 22314, 800-456-2277.

> **Question:** If you wanted to reduce polypharmacy and drug misuse through a grant proposal and could focus on only one group—older persons, physicians, or pharmacists—which one would it be? Why? What strategies would you recommend?

Additional sources of free information on older persons and medications are the *Elder Health Program*, School of Pharmacy, University of Maryland at Baltimore, 20 N. Pine St., Baltimore, MD 21201, 410-706-2434; the National Institutes on Aging, P.O. Box 8057, Gaithersburg, MD 20898-8057, 800-222 2225; and for prescription safety guidelines, go to www.prescriptionfor-safety.com.

Finally, contact the *National Council on Patient Information and Education* for free booklets and other information on prescriptions, at 4915 Saint Elmo Ave. #505, Bethesda, MD 20814-6082; www.talkaboutrx.org. For the free booklet *Prescription Medicines and You*, call 800-358-9295. To find out about nonprescription products, go to www.bemedwise.org.

INJURY PREVENTION

Unintentional injuries were the fifth leading cause of death in the United States in 2009, accounting for 118,000 deaths. While the percentage of deaths from unintentional injuries was lower among persons age 65 and older, the mortality rate from injuries for older adults was more than twice that of other age groups.

Although hip fracture hospitalization rates vary from year to year among older adults, problems related to this injury consistently exceeded the Healthy People initiative's target rates. Women, in fact, had problems numbering almost three times above the 2010 target rate, and nearly double the number for men. Hip fracture was the most serious type of fall-related fracture and is a major contributor to death and disability among older adults.

Two of the most common antecedents of injuries are falls and motor vehicle accidents. A number of physical and environmental factors contribute to the greater frequency and severity of injuries from both falls and vehicle accidents among older adults: diminished vision and hearing, poor coordination and balance, slower reaction time, and arthritis and neurological disease. In addition, medication use, which increases with age, can produce drowsiness, confusion, and depression, increasing the likelihood of accidents.

Certain factors are extrinsic to the increased incidence of falls among older people. Homes age along with people; uneven floor surfaces and the absence of safety equipment, such as grab bars for bathtubs and showers, in older homes contribute to accidents. Other culprits in the home are throw rugs, inadequate lighting, steep stairs, and lack of handrails on stairs.

Accidents can also result when road repairs and improvements and law enforcement fail to keep pace with the increased demands of automobile traffic. Transportation systems and cars are not designed with older people's capacities in mind. And few cities acknowledge the need to extend the duration of walk signals at crosswalks to accommodate older pedestrians.

Fall Prevention

According to a 2009 updated report from the CDC (www.cdc.gov/HomeandRecreational Safety/Falls/adultfalls.html), more than one third of older adults fall each year in the United States. Falls are the leading cause of death due to injury among older adults, and fall-related deaths among older adults have risen significantly over the past decade. Falls are also the most common cause of nonfatal injuries and basis for hospital admissions.

About 25% of older adults who fall suffer moderate to severe injuries that make it hard for them to get around or live independently. A majority of older adults who suffer a serious hip fracture—the most common fall-related fracture—never regain their previous function. Falls result not only in decreased physical functioning, but also in decreased confidence and a heightened fear of falling. This fear can lead to a cycle of social isolation, further functional decline, and depression.

The older the person, the greater the fall risk. The rate of fall injuries for adults age 85 and older is four to five times that of adults age 65 to 74. Nearly 85% of deaths from falls occur among people age 75 and older. People age 75 and older who fall are four to five times more likely to be admitted to a long-term care facility for a year or longer.

Many fall risk factors are preventable. Tai Chi, for instance, improves balance and reduces falls (Wolf et al., 1996; Wolfson et al., 1996). Weight-bearing and other types of exercise reduce the risk of hip fracture and falls (Robertson et al., 2001). Persons with osteoporosis—which can lead to falls—can be helped by treatment with medications that increase bone density. Footwear is important, with sneakers associated with the lowest risk of a fall, and going barefoot or in stocking feet associated with the highest risk (Koepsell et al., 2004). Environmental changes, such as adding night lights, adjusting placement of objects and furniture, removal of tripping hazards, use of nonslip floor mats, and installation of grab bars in the bathroom, can lead to a reduced incidence of falls by older adults.

An innovative exercise program combining balance training and strength training was incorporated into daily life activity, and led to a significant reduction in falls in older adults compared to those who participated in a more structured exercise program

(Clemson et al., 2012). Participants in the (Lifestyle Integrated Functional Exercise) LIFE program sought opportunities to exercise, such as standing on one leg while working at the kitchen counter or doing a squat to close a draw, rather than adhere to a prescribed exercise routine. By doing this exercise opportunistically in the course of daily life, the participants not only increased their frequency of exercise compared to a more traditional exercise program, but had one third fewer falls over a 12-month period.

Up to 40% of older adults living in the community fall each year, and 75% of these falls occur within the home. It behooves the health professional, therefore, to recommend a home assessment to identify conditions that increase the risk for falling, to suggest environmental changes, and to educate clients to help reduce the risks.

An environmental assessment of the homes of 1,000 persons age 72 and older was conducted in Connecticut, and the prevalence of environmental hazards was high. Two or more hazards were found in 59% of the bathrooms and in 23% to 42% of the remaining rooms (Gill, Robison, Williams, & Tinetti, 1999).

Two thirds of all deaths due to falls in the home are preventable. The following is a list of 10 simple precautions that can reduce the risk of falls within the home:

1. Provide proper illumination and convenient light switches—by the bed, at the end of the hall, and at the top and bottom of stairs. Older persons generally need two to three times as much illumination as younger persons do.
2. Install handrails and place nonslip treads in strategic locations.
3. Tack down or remove loose throw rugs, and repair or replace torn carpet.
4. Install grab bars and place adhesive strips in shower and bath. Only about 6% of dwelling units of older persons have grab bars in their bathrooms.
5. Eliminate such hazards as trailing electrical cords, sharp corners, slippery floors, and household items that require a step stool to reach.
6. Lower bed height for ease in getting in and out.
7. Wear footwear that provides adequate traction, such as supportive rubber-soled, low-heeled shoes.
8. Exercise to improve balance, flexibility, strength, and coordination.
9. Avoid the misuse of medications and alcohol.
10. Limit fluids after dinner, which can reduce the need for nighttime trips to the bathroom.

Several health conditions, listed in Table 7.1, place older individuals at increased risk for falling. A multidisciplinary geriatric assessment can identify those at risk and help to prevent serious injuries from falls. An increasing number of departments of internal medicine and family medicine at university medical schools, as well as private practitioners, provide multidisciplinary geriatric assessments. Teams invariably include a physician and nurse, and those with enhanced benefit to consumers also include several of the following health professionals: occupational therapist, physical therapist, counselor, social worker, health educator, and pharmacist.

In 2011, the American Geriatrics Society and the British Geriatrics Society issued updated guidelines for health professionals on preventing falls in older persons. Health professionals should determine whether their older patients are at risk of falling by asking: "Have you fallen recently? Are you unsteady walking?" If yes to either question, patients should be assessed for muscle weakness, poor balance, orthostatic changes in blood pressure, foot problems and footwear, and other factors.

About the same time, the United States Preventive Services Task Force also came out with recommendations for older adults who are at high risk of falls. They should be encouraged to see a physical therapist, to exercise, and to consider a supplement of

TABLE 7.1 Primary Risk Factors for Falling

Balance abnormalities	Muscular weakness
Visual disorders	Gait abnormalities
Cardiovascular disease	Osteoporosis
Cognitive impairment	Alcohol
Antihypertensive and sedating psychotropic drugs	Environmental hazards

800 IU of vitamin D (Leipzig et al., 2010). The benefits from these three interventions would reduce the risk of falling by 13% to 17%.

Several strategies are available to protect older adults at risk of falls. A telephone emergency alert system, for instance, uses a signaling device that is worn around the neck or on the belt of an older adult who has a tendency to fall. Anatomically designed external hip protectors reduced the risk of hip fracture among frail elderly adults in one study (Kannus et al., 2000), but not, however, in another (Kiel et al., 2007). Regardless, hip protectors are a difficult sell to older women.

Universal design is an architectural philosophy for new homes, or the modification of existing ones, to make them safer for older persons and those with disabilities. Universally designed homes may include grab bars that look like towel racks, counters with stripes around the edge to enhance definition for people with poor vision, showers with pull-down seats, entrances with no steps, doorways that are wider to accommodate wheelchairs, and bedrooms and bathrooms on the same level as the main entrance so that stairs will not hinder access.

A guide that includes summaries of innovative programs to prevent falls, short descriptions of research findings on the topic, a home safety/fall prevention assessment tool, and educational strategies is provided by AARP. For a copy of *The Perfect Fit: Creative Ideas for a Safe and Livable Home* or *Fall Prevention Guide*, contact AARP/Program Resources, 601 E St. NW, Washington, DC 20049.

> **Question:** Think about your classroom space, your neighborhood, or your home. What steps can you take to reduce the chances that an older person will have an accident in one of these locations?

Falls Free is an electronic newsletter intended to enhance communication among individuals interested in fall prevention. This bimonthly newsletter provides the latest literature on fall prevention, tools and resources, highlights from model programs, and funding opportunities. For a free subscription, contact the National Council on Aging Center for Healthy Aging (www.healthyagingprograms.org).

Motor Vehicle Safety

On July 16, 2003, an 86-year-old driver killed 10 people and injured 60 more when he plowed into a crowded farmer's market in Santa Monica, California. Despite widely publicized tragedies like this one, older drivers kill fewer motorists and pedestrians than any other age group and have the lowest crash rate per licensed driver (Swoboda, 2001). Experts attribute this to self-imposed limitations, such as driving fewer miles, and avoiding driving at night, in bad weather, and during rush hour.

As older drivers increase in number, however—there were 34 million registered drivers over age 65 in 2012, with a sharp increase expected in the next two decades as more baby boomers enter the ranks of the older adult—they will account for an increasing share of motor vehicle accidents each year. Once a person reaches age 75 and beyond, collision risk is nearly equal to that for drivers age 16 to 24. For older adults in a collision, however, the risk of serious injury and death is much higher.

A number of physiological changes affect the driving of older adults. Arthritis makes it difficult to turn one's head and directly observe cars coming up from behind. Slower reflexes make emergencies more dangerous to contend with. Susceptibility to the blinding effects of glare, poor adaptation to the dark, and the need for additional light make night driving riskier. Cognitive impairment rises with age and has been linked to higher motor vehicle crash rates in elderly individuals.

Driving in late life is not necessarily an all-or-nothing proposition, however. Older adults who find driving an automobile increasingly difficult can restrict their driving to areas with little traffic, avoid rush hours and driving at night, and drive primarily or exclusively on familiar routes. In addition, older adults may need to be vigilant about restricting their driving to those periods when their medications are not slowing their reaction time or compromising their vision.

A 2012 national survey by the Automobile Association of America (AAA) auto club reported that many drivers age 65 and older self-police, with 61% not driving in bad weather, 50% avoiding night driving, and 42% not driving in heavy traffic. Eighty-eight percent of respondents said the inability to drive a car altogether would be a problem.

Some additional measures to prevent motor vehicle accidents among older drivers follow:

1. Enroll in a driver safety class designed for midlife and older motorists, such as a course available through AARP 55-Alive or the state motor vehicle department.
2. Adjust to hearing and vision losses: keep the radio, air conditioner, and heater noise low; crack windows to help you hear warning signals; wear good-quality sunglasses; and keep windows clean inside and out.
3. Stop frequently to stretch muscles and rest eyes.
4. Use seat belts all the time, even on short trips and in cars with airbags in order to prevent injury from side collision.
5. Keep the car in good working condition.
6. Avoid drinking before driving.
7. Lobby for state policies that are more responsive to the functional abilities of older drivers.
8. Lobby for state policies that require physicians to report motorists who have health problems that could affect their driving ability.

In regard to advocating for more responsive state policies (measure 7), selected states have begun to make the following traffic improvements: wider highway lanes, larger road signs with bigger letters and numbers, more reflective pavement markers to better illuminate roads at night, and street names displayed well in advance of intersections.

In regard to advocating for more responsible physician reporting (measure 8), six states—California, Delaware, Nevada, New Jersey, Oregon, and Pennsylvania—require physicians to report motorists who have health problems that could affect their driving ability. In the District of Columbia, physician certification of physical and mental driving competency, a vision test, and sometimes a reaction test are required for the person renewing a driver's license at age 75 or older.

In one study, using a convenience sample of older patients at a medical clinic in Hawaii, 24% of older adults who had been diagnosed with poor brain function reported that they currently drove. Poor cognitive performance was often unrecognized by physicians. Doctors identified mental problems in only 5% of the older adults with intermediate impairment and 11% of older adults with poor mental performance (Valcour, Masaki, & Blanchette, 2002). One study reported that many people with early Alzheimer's disease or mild dementia may initially be able to drive safely, but their driving skills predictably decline over a 1- to 2-year period to a level that often precludes safe driving (Ott et al., 2008). The researcher highlighted the need for valid screening tests of cognition and driving skill that can identify at-risk drivers in a timely fashion.

There is no consensus on whether, or at what age, older drivers should be required to be screened more frequently. The earliest age for accelerated renewal is 61, in Colorado, and the latest is 81, in Illinois. Illinois, however, has a frequent renewal cycle: every 2 years between ages 81 and 86, and every year for age 87 and older. Iowa drivers over age 70 can only receive driver licenses for 2 years before renewal is required. Overall, 18 states have adopted an accelerated renewal cycle for older drivers, six require that older drivers renew their licenses in person, nine require additional vision tests for older drivers, and two require additional road tests for older drivers.

Illinois and New Hampshire are the two states that mandate road tests for drivers age 75 and over (and, as previously noted, Illinois requires an annual driving exam once a driver turns 87). Some advocates, including AARP, argue that this is age discrimination. The Tennessee legislature seems to agree, as it has legislated that licenses issued to drivers over age 65 do not expire and no renewal is necessary.

Opponents of AARP's position, like myself, can argue, "You're right! This *is* age discrimination." But in the driving arena it is appropriate to discriminate by age, based not on age prejudice but on the physical and mental decline associated with aging. One study of older drivers in British Columbia reported that restricted licenses, limited to daylight driving only plus a speed maximum, led to a lower crash risk among the restricted older drivers than among the unrestricted drivers (Nasvadi & Wister, 2009). Another study reported that states that mandate in-person license renewal for older adults had a 17% lower death rate among drivers 85 years and older compared with those states without such laws (Grabowski, Campbell, & Morrisey, 2004).

Research results, though, can be complicated. For instance, a Florida law that was enacted in 2001 required drivers age 80 and older to have their vision tested. Over the next 5 years, the fatality rate in that age group declined by 17%, whereas the overall rate in Florida increased 6% (McGwin, Sarrels, Griffin, Owsley, & Rue, 2008). Researchers believed that some drivers were not allowed to renew their licenses because of poor vision, some did not bother to seek a renewal because they did not think they would pass a test, and some took steps to correct their vision. However, lending support to the idea that few things in life are simple, the researchers also concluded that there was little evidence overall indicating that poor vision had played a role in car crashes.

The topic of age discrimination, important though it may be, is likely to take a back seat to financial concerns in tough economic times. Extra costs are a deterrent to states' legislating additional driver screenings for older age groups. Even the legislator most supportive of additional driver testing with age is likely to be roadblocked by state budgetary concerns.

Those Who Quit Driving

The stakes are high for those who give up driving (about 600,000 people age 70 or older each year) and do not find effective transportation alternatives. One study reported that older adults who give up driving are more likely to enter an assisted living facility or a nursing home (Freeman, Gange, Muñoz, & West, 2006). For those who remain in their homes, a researcher reported that older adults will live about 10 years more after they stop driving. During this time they will need to rely on other forms of transportation. Many older adults find negotiating bus schedules and multiple transfers confusing.

The 2011 Florida Aging Road User Survey asked older driver respondents about their plans for the day when they are no longer able to drive safely. Eighty-three percent reported that they had no postdriving plan. Many responded they had never thought about it, and a few said they would die before they needed to stop driving.

An innovative response to the challenge for older adults who give up driving is the *Independent Transportation Network*. If an older adult agrees to stop driving and trades in the car, its value is booked into an account from which the person can draw to receive rides. About $8 is deducted for each car ride given by a paid driver, and less when a ride is scheduled in advance or shared.

The Independent Transportation Network program was started by Katherine Freund, whose 3-year-old son was hit by an elderly driver in Portland, Maine. (Her son recovered and eventually attended the University of Oregon.) Pilot programs are being started in several cities. For more information, contact www.itnportland.org.

To prepare professionals, family members, and concerned community members to engage in effective conversations about driver safety and community transportation issues with older adults, including alternatives to driving, there is a 2009 publication titled *Driving Transitions Education: Tools, Scripts, and Practice Exercises*. It was developed by the American Society on Aging and the National Highway Traffic Safety Administration, and can be obtained free on the web at www.nhtsa.dot.gov, or toll-free at 888-327-4236. For more information, visit www.asaging.org/drivewell.

Question: Think of an older adult you know who has given up or will eventually give up driving, and what you can do to reduce this person's chances of becoming isolated and depressed. What ideas can you suggest to enhance this person's ability to remain connected to the world?

For a booklet on how to talk to an older family member who may need to consider giving up the driving privilege, contact The Hartford, *Family Conversations With Older Drivers*, 200 Executive Blvd., Southington, CT 06489.

In the same way that people prepare for retirement, older adults will also need to plan ahead for the resources they will need after they stop driving. If adequate attention is not paid to this challenge, social isolation and depression may result.

Motorcycle Safety

An interesting *motor vehicle safety* issue for the future is motorcycle riding, a popular hobby for baby boomers. In 2006, 41% of motorcyclists killed in the United States were between the ages of 40 and 60, according to the National Highway Traffic Safety Administration. The median age of motorcycle owners has been going up each year, reaching age 43 in 2008. Some boomers do not realize that their skill levels and reflexes are not as good as they once were, and that today's motorcycles are heftier and more powerful (see Figure 7.1).

Other boomers have begun to recognize their limitations, such as slowing reflexes, bad knees, and aching joints, and have started to "trike" it. Trikes are three-wheeled motorcycles and are not only popular with boomer men, but women as well. Sales of trikes increased 45% in 2011. Three-wheelers do not require boomer riders to lean into curves or hold them steady at stoplights.

Pedestrian Safety

On February 15, 2006, Mayvis Coyle, age 82, was given a $114 ticket for taking too long to cross a Los Angeles street. Ms. Coyle, who used a cane, was unable to make it to the other side of the street before the light turned green for oncoming traffic. While Ms. Coyle

FIGURE 7.1   **Motorcycle riding is not just for young adults and boomers. Motorcycle rider, Hazel Poole.**

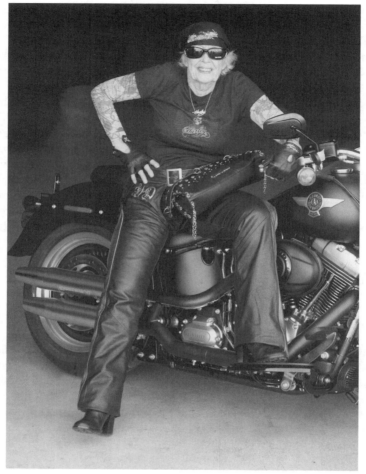

Source: The Star Press, Muncie, IN. Photographer, Jeri Reichanadter.

was fighting city hall for receiving what she deemed to be an outrageous ticket, city council members acknowledged the error of their ways and voted to lengthen the walk light time at that intersection. They also waived her fine.

A pedestrian is killed in traffic every 110 minutes, and one is injured every 9 minutes, according to the National Highway Traffic Safety Administration. Older adults are more likely than members of any other age group to be injured by motor vehicles while crossing a street and experience the highest death rate from pedestrian accidents. A study of 1,249 residents age 72 or older from New Haven, Connecticut, revealed that less than 1% of these pedestrians had a normal walking speed sufficient to cross the street in the time typically allotted at signalized intersections (Langlois et al., 1997).

Crosswalk markings at sites with no traffic signal or stop sign are particularly hazardous to older pedestrians (Koepsell et al., 2002). Motor vehicles struck and killed 48,000 pedestrians in the United States during the prior decade (2000–2009), with older pedestrians at especially high risk. People age 70 and older accounted for nearly 20% of all pedestrian deaths, nearly double what would be expected on the basis of age-related pedestrian statistics. AARP and the Institute of Transportation Engineers are identifying trouble spots in cities by doing pedestrian safety audits. To find out how you can make your neighborhood safer, go to www.aarp.org/communityexchange.

Some other measures to prevent pedestrian accidents follow:

1. Wear highly visible clothing, preferably of light-colored or even fluorescent material.
2. Do not assume that drivers in moving vehicles see pedestrians.
3. Do not return to the curb if the "don't walk" sign begins to flash. Continue to walk at maximum comfortable speed, moving your arms to be more visible.
4. Lobby local officials to install properly timed pedestrian traffic signals.

Resources

AARP's 55 Alive/Mature Driving Program was launched 30 years ago and is now available all around the country. It is an 8-hour, classroom-based (no actual driving) driver education refresher course for persons 50 and older, and it is taught by instructors who are also 50 and older. Almost 600,000 older drivers enrolled in AARP's classes in 2000, an increase of 60% over the 1990 figure. In some states, drivers who complete the course are eligible for a discount on automobile insurance. For more information, contact AARP toll-free at 888-227-7669.

The *AARP Driver Safety Online Course* is an 8-hour class that can be taken at one's own pace for $15.95. The content focuses on compensating for age-related changes; reducing traffic violations, crashes, and injuries; and updating one's knowledge of the rules of the road. In some states, the online graduate of this course is eligible for an insurance discount. For more information, visit www.aarp.org/drive/online.

A CD-ROM titled *Roadwise Review: A Tool to Help Seniors Drive Safely Longer* is available at AAA branches. This assessment tool measures physical and mental abilities that predict crash risk, such as leg strength and mobility, neck flexibility, high- and low-contrast visual acuity, and working memory. This CD-ROM is available at Community Safety Services, AAA Michigan, 1 Auto Club Dr., Dearborn, MI 48126.

For tips on driving safety for older adults, the AAA Foundation launched a traffic safety website, www.seniordrivers.org. Other useful websites are those of the National Highway Traffic Safety Administration, at www.nhtsa.gov, and the Insurance Institute for Highway Safety, at www.highwaysafety.org. For a free comprehensive guide, *Assessing and Counseling Older Drivers*, contact Catherine Kosinski, Older Drivers Project, American Medical Association, 312-464-4179; www.amaassn.org/go/olderdrivers. For the free guide *Alzheimer's Disease, Dementia & Driving*, contact www.thehartford.com/alzheimers.

SEXUALITY AND INTIMACY

Older adults can share intimate support in many ways. Some older adults, for instance, cherish playing with grandchildren, watching a sunset with a companion, feeding ducks with children by a pond, walking with a friend in the woods, and enjoying sexual intimacy. Playing, watching, feeding, and walking are not problematic for most older adults; *sexual* intimacy, however, may present more of a challenge.

A national survey of Americans aged 57 to 85 reported that the majority of older couples remain sexually active, but sexual practices decline with age. Seventy-three percent of Americans between ages 57 and 64 had sex, 53% between ages 65 and 75, and 26% for those aged 85 and over (Lindau et al., 2007). Sexual problems are common among older adults but are rarely discussed with physicians. Men are more likely than women to have a partner, more likely to be sexually active with that partner, and to have more positive and permissive attitudes toward sex (Waite, Laumann, Das, & Schumm, 2009).

Although these surveys may be reassuring in that they report that sexual practices continue into late life, they ignore the more important topic of intimacy, and the warmth, sharing, touching, and intimate communication that is maintained in good relationships. As consumers of research, we might find it useful to pay more attention to the studies that give primacy to intimacy over intercourse.

We also need to pay attention to samples of aging Americans that are not limited (see Chapter 11, "Diversity") to heterosexual activities, to Caucasians, and to healthy older adults. Sexual function and aging vary by race and ethnicity (Huang et al., 2009) and by sexual orientation (Jackson, Johnson, & Roberts, 2008). Also, patient–provider communication about sexual health among unmarried middle-aged and older women can be problematic when providers make assumptions about marital status and sexual orientation, and when patients view questions and discussion as judgmental (Politi, 2009).

The sexual expression of aging Americans can get waylaid by psychological factors, such as depression, guilt, monotony, performance anxiety, and anger. Young and old alike can be hampered by negative attitudes that reveal hostility or disgust toward the expression of sexuality in late life. Physical limitations are yet another cause of sexual dysfunction. Arthritic pains, cardiovascular disorders, respiratory conditions, hormonal imbalances, and neurological disorders can interfere not only with sexual performance, but also with intimacy. In addition, various medications can lead to a loss of interest in sexuality.

The most significant cause of sexual inactivity or lack of intimacy, particularly among women, is widowhood or lack of opportunity. This problem is exacerbated in older adults who are not accepting of alternative intimacy practices. Family members might try to expand the options of an older adult by arranging to have a respected health professional prescribe the reading of a book that was way ahead of its time in open-mindedness, *The Joy of Sex* (Comfort, 1972), in which the physician-author, Dr. Alex Comfort, presented a wide variety of ideas on sex and intimacy. Older women who have a problem with their sexuality, though, are less likely than men to consult a physician or other health professional (22% versus 38%; Lindau et al., 2007).

When talking about sex and aging it would be remiss to ignore the CDC data that indicate that the topics of gerontology and HIV/AIDS are beginning to converge. Along with the aging of the boomers has been an increase in the number of adults age 50+ with HIV/AIDS. Such cases rose from 65,000 in 2001 to 104,000 in 2004, an increase of 59% in 3 years! Yet very little HIV prevention education was targeted toward boomers or older adults. In fact, the CDC recommendation to test everyone for HIV/AIDS between the ages of 14 and 64, reinforces an implied irrelevancy of testing and prevention education for adults age 65 and over.

Intimacy for older adults is often as simple as touching. The importance of touching was clearly demonstrated to me when a yoga class, which had been enthusiastically received by older adults at senior centers and congregate living facilities (Haber, 1983a, 1986), was presented at 10 nursing homes (Haber, 1988a). After unsuccessful attempts to engage these nursing home residents were made during the first three classes, we decided to begin each class with massage—mostly instructor-

Question: The anecdote on the importance of touch should probably have included a cautionary note. What would that be?

to-resident massage (with help from student assistants), but also resident-to-resident and self-massage (see Figure 7.2).

FIGURE 7.2   Massage.

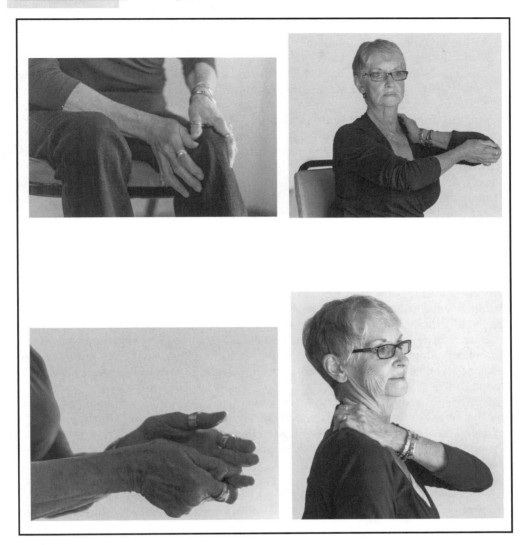

As a consequence of this innovation we witnessed a dramatic increase in—there are no other words that come to mind—*fun* and *intimacy*. The nursing home residents enthusiastically awaited the remaining classes.

This demonstration of the need for touch and intimacy brought to mind a passage from a book by Ebersole and Hess (1990): "When a group of Boy Scouts completed their performance for (a group of nursing home) residents, (an old woman) beckoned to the scout leader and said, 'Do you suppose I could hug one of those little boys?'"

SLEEP

Normal aging is accompanied by lessened quality and quantity of sleep. There appears to be a measurable decrease in the ability of the healthy older adult to initiate and maintain sleep, accompanied by a decrease in the proportion of the deeper, more restorative sleep (Espiritu, 2008). But does this mean that most older adults have *insomnia*, defined as difficulty in initiating or maintaining sleep? People require different amounts of sleep, so it is hard to give a definitive answer. Based on self-reports, though, chronic, primary insomnia in older adults is estimated at 10%, with about 50% of older adults complaining about sleep problems from time to time.

Significant sleep disturbance is likely to impact quality of life. Insomniacs are 2.5 times more likely to have accidents than other drivers; are more likely to be anxious, depressed, or forgetful; and may recover more slowly from an illness. Inadequate sleep has also been associated with hypertension (Gangwisch, Malaspina, Boden-Albala, & Heymsfield, 2006) and weight gain (Gangwisch, Malaspina, Boden-Albala, & Heymsfield, 2005).

A national survey conducted by the National Sleep Foundation reported that 56% of Americans experienced one or more symptoms of insomnia (though not full-fledged insomnia), including difficulty falling asleep, waking up during the night, waking up too early, and waking up feeling fatigued. Forty percent of the adults in this survey reported being so sleepy some days that it interfered with their daily activities. Yet only 4% were seeing a health care provider for advice or treatment.

Sleep Changes With Age

There are four *stages of sleep*, three non rapid eye movement (REM) sleep phases and one REM or dreaming sleep phase. Stage 1 sleep is light and constitutes about 5% of sleep time. Stage 2 is also considered light sleep and takes up about 50% of sleep time. Older adults tend to spend more time in the lighter stages of sleep and to have more awakenings. Stage 3 is deep sleep and is defined by the presence of low-frequency, high-voltage electroencephalographic (EEG) waves called delta or slow waves. We are least easily awakened in stage 3 sleep. As we grow older we tend to lose time spent in deep sleep (Vorona, 2009).

REM sleep is defined by rapid eye movements and intense dreaming. With the exception of our eye muscles and the principal muscle of respiration, the diaphragm, we are paralyzed during REM sleep, perhaps to keep us from acting out our dreams. REM sleep occupies about 20% to 25% of sleep time and there is disagreement on whether it tends to decline with age.

Sleep efficiency is the proportion of time spent in bed asleep. As we age, sleep efficiency declines from 90% to 70%. Does this mean that the *typical* older adult has sleep problems? Most experts do not think so. Too much sleep or too little sleep, however, is a problem. Studies suggest that the lowest mortality rate in adults is associated with approximately 7 hours of sleep a night, and that 5 or less and 9 or more hours of sleep are associated with higher mortality (Gangwisch et al., 2008).

Sleep-Related Medical Disorders

Restless legs syndrome (RLS) is defined as intense discomfort in the legs during periods of inactivity, particularly at night. Movement alleviates the unpleasant symptoms but disrupts sleep, and RLS can reoccur when the legs are again at rest. About 10% of the population in the United States is afflicted with RLS, and most are over the age of 50 (Vorona, 2009). Patients are instructed to minimize caffeine and alcohol and to avoid antihistamines. Some are asked to take warm baths, to get massages, or to exercise. There are also medications, vitamins, and minerals that may be effective.

Obstructive sleep apnea syndrome (OSAS) is the repeated complete or near complete occlusion of the upper airway during sleep. Often found in obese people, it is marked by cycles of loud snoring, obstruction, and gasping for breath. This is the most common sleep disorder and is age related, peaking after age 65. It is considered to be a secondary cause of hypertension and is associated with heart problems, stroke, cognitive impairment, and dementia (Yaffe et al., 2011). Patients are often instructed to lose weight and to reduce or avoid alcohol. Keeping the airway open with continuous positive airway pressure, using mouth guards, and undergoing surgery are recommended for some.

There are a host of other sleep-related diseases and disorders to consider as well, such as gastroesophageal reflux disease, heart problems, dementia, depression, and renal disease (affecting urinary frequency), to name a few.

Interventions

Identifying the cause of sleeplessness can be rather complicated, but it is necessary for identifying effective interventions. Potential causes of insomnia can be far-ranging, as can interventions to alleviate the condition (see Table 7.2). Most sleep specialists recommend the application of behavioral interventions for nonmedical sleep disorder problems rather than the long-term use of sleep medications.

Regarding exercise, older adults with moderate sleep complaints slept almost an hour longer and reduced by half the amount of time it took to fall asleep as a consequence of participating in a low-impact aerobics program (King et al., 1997). Even a sample of healthy older adult caregivers with no reported sleep complaints saw improvements in sleep quality after completing a moderate-intensity exercise program (King et al., 2002).

Another effective exercise may be Tai Chi. Older adults with moderate sleep complaints improved self-rated sleep quality with a 6-month low- to moderate-intensity Tai Chi program (Li et al., 2004). One hundred and twelve persons aged 59 to 86 with moderate sleep complaints were randomized into a Tai Chi group or a health education class. A significantly higher percentage of the former group moved from the poor sleeping range into the good sleeping range compared with the latter group (Irwin et al., 2008). The researchers concluded that Tai Chi was a useful nonpharmacological approach to improving sleep quality in older adults with moderate complaints.

As for therapy, after 8 weeks of an insomnia study, behavioral therapy was slightly more effective than drug therapy. Follow-up assessments up to 14 months later, however,

TABLE 7.2 Causes of, and Interventions for, Sleep Disorders

CAUSES		
Arthritis	Hyperactive thyroid	Sleep apnea
Restless legs syndrome	Anxiety	Too much caffeine
Poor circulation	Inadequate sleep hygiene	Inactivity
INTERVENTIONS		
Restricting caffeine	Keeping a regular bedtime schedule	Using relaxation techniques
Managing daytime napping	Avoiding reading and watching television in the bedroom	Limiting drinking, particularly alcohol, after dinner
Avoiding heavy meals at night		Monitoring medications
Cognitive/behavioral therapies	Medical interventions	
	More exercise	

indicated that *only* behavioral therapy led to sustained benefits (Morin, Colecchi, Stone, Sood, & Brink, 1999). Sleeping medication may be almost as effective as behavioral therapy in the short run, but in the long run individuals build up tolerance, the dosage must be raised, and the risks for memory impairment, hypertension, and more frequent accidents are increased. Another study reported similar results: Older patients with insomnia who implemented cognitive-behavioral therapy had greater improvement in their sleep than did patients who received the sleep medication zopiclone (Sivertsen et al., 2006).

Another study reported that two different behavior programs significantly improved sleep patterns among older adults with chronic illnesses who had trouble sleeping. The cognitive-behavioral program consisted of group education sessions. The home audio relaxation treatment consisted of audiotapes that instructed listeners in muscle, breathing, and cognitive relaxation techniques similar to the ones taught in the cognitive-behavioral program. Fifty-four percent of participants in the cognitive-behavioral program, 39% of persons in the home audio relaxation treatment, and 6% of the members in the control group significantly improved their sleep efficiency, the time awake after sleep onset, and total time in bed (Rybarczyk, Lopez, Benson, Alsten, & Stepanski, 2002). The authors concluded that older adults with chronic illness are able to make substantial improvements in their sleep patterns without resorting to medication. This is particularly important among older persons who take other drugs for existing chronic medical conditions.

Seventy-five patients (mean age 55) with persistent primary sleep disorder for an average of 13 years were randomly assigned to cognitive-behavioral therapy (changes in attitude and bedtime habits), relaxation techniques, or a placebo. After 6 weeks the cognitive-behavioral group reduced awake time once asleep by 54%, the relaxation group by 16%, and the placebo group by 12% (Edinger, Wohlgemuth, Radtke, Marsh, & Quillian, 2001). These improvements persisted 6 months later.

Another sleep aid alternative is music. Sixty people aged 60 to 83 who had difficulty sleeping listened to music tapes before bedtime. Sleep improved over a 3-week period in terms of duration, efficiency, and perceived quality (Lai & Good, 2006).

Sleep hygiene is a major component of most sleep interventions. Attention to the environment is important in terms of such factors as noise level and room temperature, and use of the bed for television viewing or working. Attaining a calm mental state is also important; relaxation techniques can be used to deal with mood issues or to avoid perseveration on anxiety-producing topics. Maintaining steady bed and wake times is helpful, as is avoiding certain foods and drink after 4:00 p.m. Finally, it is useful to identify any medical issues that may be in play, such as a medical problem or use of certain medications, and intervening as appropriate.

Although data on the United States are not available, the median amount of time spent on sleep-related issues during medical training in the United Kingdom was 5 minutes (Stores & Crawford, 1998). Not surprisingly, the typical treatment for chronic insomnia by physicians is to prescribe benzodiazepines, which have known side effects, rather than referral to cognitive-behavioral interventions (Montgomery, 2002).

Thus, a widespread approach to sleep problems, and one that is gaining even more popularity due to television advertising, is the use of sleeping pills. Sleeping pill prescriptions increased more than 60% over the past decade. A new generation of sleep aids that reduce neural activity in brain neurotransmitters—products such as Ambien and Lunesta—have been advertised heavily in the United States and have led to substantially increased consumption of sleeping pills. In older patients, however, sedative medications are more than twice as likely to produce an adverse effect as they are to help improve quality of sleep, according to a meta-analysis of 24 randomized, controlled trials (Glass, Lanctôt, Herrmann, Sproule, & Busto, 2005).

Many herbs are reputed to act as sedatives, such as chamomile, exotic passionflower, and valerian extract, but their effectiveness is not supported by randomized, controlled research studies. The same holds true for the popular hormone melatonin, which is found in most health food stores and drugstores. There is little controlled research that supports its use as a sleeping aid, and prolonged use may be unsafe.

RESOURCES

The *American Sleep Association* links people interested in sleep health and sleep disorders, and is a complete source of sleep information communication: www.americansleep association.org.

The *National Sleep Foundation* posts research and lists sleep treatment centers at www.sleepfoundation.org.

To access the June 13–15, 2005, recommendations of the National Institutes of Health State-of-the-Science Conference on the *Manifestations and Management of Chronic Insomnia in Adults*, contact http://consensus.nih.gov.

To find a sleep center near you, visit www.sleepcenters.org. Many centers focus on drugs rather than *cognitive-behavioral therapy*. For online help with cognitive-behavioral therapy approaches, see the website created by Gregg Jacobs of Harvard Medical School, at www.cbtforinsomnia.com.

8

●●●●○○

MENTAL HEALTH

●●● Learning Objectives

- Compare the mental health of older adults with that of younger adults
- Define mental health and mental illness
- Review the causes and consequences of depression in late life, and explain why depression is not a normal part of the aging process

- Examine the difficulties with diagnosing depression in older adults and the consequences of untreated or undertreated depression
- Contrast the pharmacological and nonpharmacological treatments for depression
- Describe the life review process and its impact on mental health
- Apply the life review technique to an older adult
- Explain the purpose of an ethical will
- Identify the stages of Alzheimer's disease, and contrast the pharmacological and nonpharmacological treatments for the disease
- Define preclinical Alzheimer's
- Cite the percentage of older adults between age 60 and age 85+ with Alzheimer's disease
- Explain cognitive fitness and its benefits and limitations
- Analyze the utility of brain games
- Summarize mental disorders that affect older adults
- Review the history of mental health parity in insurance coverage
- Define chronic stress and explain how it is measured and treated
- Explain psychoneuroimmunology
- Critically evaluate the impact of a positive attitude
- Define bright-sided and explain the downside of relentless positivity
- Define the placebo effect and state your opinion on its ethical justification in medicine
- Explain whether trying to look younger in old age is an ageist reaction to a natural process, or an effective way to cope in a youth-oriented society
- Identify mental health and creativity resources useful for older adults

This life is only a test. If this were an actual life, you would have been given better instructions.
—Myrna Neims

Of course, if it does turn out that this is our actual life, it is not surprising that, given the lack of instructions, maintaining mental health can be such a challenge.

MENTAL HEALTH AND MENTAL ILLNESS

Mental health is a multifaceted concept and difficult to define. It may include such ideas and terms as life satisfaction, the statistically normal, the ability to cope, positive functioning, finding meaning and purpose in life, self-actualization, and so forth.

If *mental health* is defined as life satisfaction, researchers consistently report that the vast majority (about 85%) of older adults are satisfied with their lives, and that older adults are at least as satisfied with their lives as middle-aged and younger adults.

Several studies, in fact, have supported the contention that older adults may be better at maintaining good mental health than younger adults, including support for the idea that older adults attend preferentially to positive emotions (Birditt, Fingerman, & Almeida, 2005; Cappeliez & O'Rourke, 2006; Carstensen, Pasupathi, Mayr, & Nesselroade,

2000; Kennedy, Mather, & Carstensen, 2004; Mather et al., 2004; Mroczek & Spiro, 2005; Ruffman, Ng, & Jenkin, 2009; Scheibe & Blanchard-Fields, 2009; Thomas, 2004). The line of reasoning behind these studies varies a great deal, and ranges from physiological changes in the brain with age that have benefit, to greater appreciation of the present in old age given knowledge of a limited amount of time left to live.

Neither the average 50% reduction in income at retirement nor the increases in emotional losses, physical losses, and caregiving responsibilities in later life result in the persistent reduction in life satisfaction among most older adults. Over a quarter century ago, the sociologist Linda George (1986) eloquently stated, "Older adults are apparently masters of the art of lowering aspirations to meet realities" (p. 7).

Although we need to acknowledge the mental health resiliency of older adults, we should also attach importance to the 15% to 20% of older adults who contend with mental disorders of one type or another. A review of the mental health literature in the clinical and research arenas, though, leads one to believe that we pay a disproportionate amount of attention to mental disorders.

Perhaps one reason we pay greater attention to *mental illness* than to mental health is that there is more of a scientific framework associated with it. Operational definitions of mental illness usually follow the specific criteria of the *Diagnostic and Statistical Manual of Mental Disorders (DSM-IV-TR;* American Psychiatric Association, 2000)—a fifth edition of which is scheduled for publication in May 2013. Clinicians and researchers refer to *DSM* guidelines or state how a condition deviates from them. Critics of the guidelines argue, however, that the number of clinical characteristics that identify a mental illness, and the time parameters that are employed, are arbitrary. Flawed that they may be, there are no guidelines for the components of mental health.

This chapter reflects a combination of the two perspectives: mental health and mental illness. As is true of most of the literature, I have organized chapter subheadings largely around mental illness terms. I have also attempted to focus at least as much overall attention on mental health content as on mental illness. Thus, in addition to examining a topic like depression, I explore life reviews; and in addition to examining Alzheimer's disease, I explore cognitive fitness. Additional mental health content is provided in other chapters.

One source of material for the mental disorders component of this chapter was obtained from Chapter 5 on older adults in the 1999 Surgeon General's Report on Mental Health. Though dated, this still remains one of the most comprehensive and evidence-based publications on mental health. The Public Health Reports of the Surgeon General can be accessed through the website www.surgeongeneral.gov.

DEPRESSION

The most likely causes of *depression* in later life are the loss of a spouse or other family support; chronic medical conditions, pain, and loss of functional independence; and difficulty adapting to changing circumstances within the home, family, or living situation. These emotional and physical losses not only can lead to depression, but depression in turn can lead to disease, physical decline, and disability (Brenes et al., 2008). Though the mechanism is not understood, depression increases the likelihood of not only obesity, but also illnesses such as heart disease and diabetes (Vogelzangs et al., 2008). Also, the mortality rate for depressed patients with cardiovascular disease is twice that of those without depression (Lantz, 2002). Even mild depression can weaken the immune system in older persons if it goes on long enough (McGuire, Kiecolt-Glaser, & Glaser, 2002).

Not only does depression lead to disease, but disease can lead to depression. Even among well-functioning older adults, diabetes is associated with a 30% increased risk of incident depressed mood (Maraldi et al., 2007). The reciprocal relationship between depression and disease is not lost on older adults. Interviews with 33 primary care patients age 65 and over revealed clear descriptions of how their heart disease led to depression or how depression led to heart disease (Bogner, Dahlberg, de Vries, Cahill, & Barg, 2008).

Depression also plays a significant role in suicidal behaviors, and older persons have the highest suicide rate of any age group. Older adults account for 25% of all suicide deaths, though they make up only about 13% of the general population. This elevated suicide rate, however, is largely accounted for by White men age 85 and older. The suicide rate of this age/sex category is six times higher than the overall national rate.

Depression Diagnosis

Depression in older adults has often gone undetected until it is too late. It has been estimated that between 63% and 90% of depressed older patients went untreated or received inadequate treatment. One landmark study of older adults who had committed suicide revealed that 51 of the 97 patients had seen their primary care physician within 1 month of their suicide date. Of these 51, only 19 were even offered treatment, and only 2 of the 51 patients studied were provided adequate treatment (Caine et al., 1996).

Videotapes of 385 physician appointments with older patients revealed that more than half of the patients whose responses to survey questions suggested they were depressed never talked with their doctors about their emotional state (Tai-Seale, McGuire, Colenda, Rosen, & Cook, 2007). Even when the older patients let their physicians know about their mental health problems, the physician responses averaged 2 minutes long and were often ineffective.

A substantial proportion of depressed older patients, therefore, receive inadequate treatment from physicians in primary care settings (Alexopoulos et al., 2009). Yet, according to the Surgeon General's report, up to 37% of older adults in the primary care setting (and between 8% and 20% in the community) suffer from depressive symptoms. These figures are higher than those reported elsewhere (see Chapter 2, "Clinical Preventive Services"), and some of this discrepancy may have to do with the definition of major depressive disorder versus depressive symptoms of lesser scope or intensity.

Older adults are less likely than younger adults to report feelings of dysphoria—sadness, unhappiness, or irritability, which is part of the standard criteria for depression in the *DSM-IV-TR*. Older adults are *more* likely to report depressive symptoms—such as the loss of interest or pleasure in activities, weight change, sleep disturbance, agitation or fatigue, feelings of worthlessness, and loss of concentration—but not the scope or intensity of symptoms that qualifies them for a full-fledged major depression. Although these reported symptoms, also referred to as mild depression, are not recognized by *DSM-IV-TR*, they nonetheless are a major clinical concern for older adults and interfere with their performance of social roles and quality of life.

An estimate of the prevalence of depression can vary by the measurement tool being used, and whether clinical depression or depressive symptoms are being measured. *Older Americans 2012: Key Indicators of Well-Being* (Federal Interagency Forum on Aging-Related Statistics, 2012) reports that 18% of older adults have depressive symptoms, compared to 15% of younger adults. Barry Lebowitz, former Chief of the National Institute of Mental Health's aging branch, estimated that 15% of Americans age 65 and over suffered from serious and persistent symptoms of depression, but only 3% were suffering from the clinical diagnosis of major depression as defined by the *DSM-IV-TR*. In other words, though depressive disorders that fulfill rigorous diagnostic criteria are relatively rare, subthreshold disorders, or depression symptoms, are considerably more common; are inadequately diagnosed or properly treated with prescribed antidepressants; and, because they usually go untreated, are likely to become chronic conditions (Beekman et al., 2002).

> **Question:** Given the emotional and physical losses that accumulate in late life, why is depression not considered a normal part of the aging process?

Detection of depression is hampered not only by the underreporting of symptoms by older patients, but also by biases on the part of physicians and family members. In one study, admittedly dated but interesting nonetheless, 75% of physicians thought that depression was understandable in older persons, that is, a normal facet of old age (Gallo, Ryan, & Ford, 1999). Family members may also view the signs and symptoms of depression as "normal aging," when in fact the persistence of depressive symptoms is not normal.

The diagnosis of depression is even more problematic because of cultural factors. African Americans were significantly less likely to receive a depression diagnosis from a health care provider than Caucasians because of greater stigma, shame, and denial, which prevent seeking professional help (Akincigil et al., 2012). African Americans were significantly less likely than Caucasians to have mental health-related office visits to a physician (Wu, Erickson, Piette, & Balkrishnan, 2012).

Diagnosis of depression in older adults has improved in the last few years due in part to better education of primary care physicians. Physicians have been alerted to the need to screen older adults for depression when staff are available for treatment and follow-up, through the recommendation of the United States Preventive Services Task Force. Under the Affordable Care Act, depression screening became part of the free Welcome to Medicare visit for new beneficiaries and also part of free annual wellness visits thereafter.

It is estimated that now up to half of older adults with depression have the condition diagnosed and treated, compared to only 12% to 25% in the late 1990s (Park & Unutzer, 2011). Unfortunately according to the researchers, although depression in elders is diagnosed more and treated more, only 19% of elders showed substantial improvement. The issue is that many elders are not responding to medications because physicians are not adequately trained in trying a series or combination of medications at varying doses to find a drug regimen that works. It can take four or five tries to calibrate the most effective medication, and many primary care physicians are not doing this.

Moreover, some older patients need mental health services in addition to medications, but less than 15% receive it (Unutzer & Park, 2012). It is difficult to steer older patients toward counseling because of the stigma involved, and because insurance coverage is focused more on medications.

Treatments for Depression

There are many modalities for the treatment of depression among older adults, including medication, cognitive-behavioral therapy (CBT), other forms of counseling, exercise, life review, social support, and pet therapy.

The treatment of depression by medication is effective, if properly applied, for up to 80% of older adults, a rate that is comparable to younger adults. Older adults had more frequent and serious adverse reactions than younger adults did to the earlier generation of tricyclic antidepressants, but the subsequent generation of antidepressants, *selective serotonin reuptake inhibitors* (SSRIs), produced fewer side effects among older adults. One side effect that has been documented several times in the literature, however, is the association of SSRIs with bone loss and fracture in older women (Diem et al., 2007) and older men (Haney et al., 2007).

The effectiveness of SSRIs and CBT combined is better than either modality alone (Keller et al., 2000). CBT is designed to alter dysfunctional thoughts, emotions, and behaviors by substituting more effective thoughts, emotions, and behaviors. It can be delivered one-on-one or in groups. The technique has been effective when applied to clinically depressed older adults (Peng, Huang, Chen, & Lu, 2009; Pinquart, Duberstein, & Lyness, 2007), even when administered over the telephone (Simon, Ludman, Tutty, Operskalski, & Von Korff, 2004).

Other psychotherapy techniques have been effective with depressed older adults as well, including problem-solving social skills, interpersonal psychotherapy, psycho-dynamic therapy, reminiscence therapy, and so forth. Some argue that the skill of the provider and the quality of the relationship between the provider and the patient are more important factors than which psychotherapeutic treatment modality is selected.

As noted in Chapter 4 on exercise, physical activity, aerobics, and weight lifting can be effective treatments for depression, or reduce the risk of becoming depressed, among older adults (Blake, Mo, Malik, & Thomas, 2009; Singh et al., 2001; Strawbridge Deleger, Roberts, & Kaplan, 2002). The most common form of physical activity in these studies—walking—reveals that neither high-intensity exercise nor elaborate equipment are necessary for significant results.

Between 1957 and 1995, Americans relied more on nonmedical mental health interventions for mental health problems. Individuals utilized informal social supports, exercise, and counseling rather than medications from their primary care physicians. Between 1996 and 2005, however, the use of antidepressant medications for the treatment of depression increased dramatically, whereas the use of counseling declined (Olfson & Marcus, 2009). It was estimated that antidepressant medication use increased from 6% of the American population to 10%. Analysts speculated that the stigma of depression declined during this time period, but Americans' penchant for treating problems with pills strengthened. Thanks in part to medication advertisements, which quadrupled over the decade 1996–2005 (Szabo, 2009), antidepressant prescriptions doubled, increasing to 164 million in 2008 and resulting in almost $10 billion in US sales (www.usatoday.com/news/health/2010-01-06-antidepressants06_ST_N.htm).

Collaborative care refers to comprehensive care for late-life depression provided in existing physician offices or primary care clinics. It consists of a trained nurse or psychologist serving as a "depression care manager," working with older patients to develop treatments and monitor progress and to refer them to psychiatrists when necessary. The effectiveness of collaborative care is more than 50% over usual care (Unutzer & Park, 2012). The extra cost involved in this treatment is likely to be more than offset by reduced visits to doctors and emergency rooms, fewer hospitalizations, and decreased complications assocciated with diabetes, heart disease, and stroke.

The Life Review Process

A *life review* refers to an autobiographical effort that can be preserved in print, audio, or video. The review is guided by a series of questions in specific life domains, such as work and family. Memories may be further stimulated through a review of the family photo album or other memorabilia, a genealogy, musical selections from an earlier time, or a trek back to an important place in one's past. Life review can be conducted by oneself, in a dyad, or as part of a group process. It is more likely to be conducted by or with an older adult who is relatively content with his or her life and not seeking therapy, than it is to be used therapeutically with an older adult. Nonetheless, life reviews are believed to have therapeutic powers, and they are incorporated into a wide variety of counseling modalities (Haber, 2006).

The psychiatrist Robert Butler first extolled the benefits of the life review process to his colleagues and the public as early as 1961, as a way of incorporating reminiscence in the aged as part of a normal aging process. Dr. Butler described the life review as more comprehensive and systematic than spontaneous reminiscing, and perhaps more important in old age when there may be a need to put one's life in order and to come to an acceptance of present circumstances (Butler, 1995).

The review of positive and negative past life experiences by older adults has enabled them to overcome feelings of depression and despair (Watt & Cappeliez, 2000). Another study of the life review process reported positive outcomes in terms of stronger life satisfaction, psychological well-being, and self-esteem, as well as reduced depression among older adults (Haight, Michel, & Hendrix, 1998). Similar results have been obtained with depressed elders in long-term care institutions (Hsu & Wang, 2009).

Although life reviews are usually helpful for improving the mental health of older adults who are seeking meaning, resolution, reconciliation, direction, and atonement, physicians and other clinic personnel find it is too time-consuming to listen to the reminiscences of older clients in this era of medical care. Health professionals can, however, provide a key role in referring older clients to appropriate forums or helping them obtain relevant life review materials.

One book, *Aging and Biography*, by the internationally acclaimed psychologist James Birren, (Birren, Kenyon, Ruth, Shroots, & Svendson, 1996), helps guide and structure the life review process by suggesting a focus on several themes, such as love, money, work, and family. Birren and his colleagues also suggest in another book, *Telling the Stories of Life Through Guided Autobiography Groups*, that incorporating life reviews into a small-group format can help stimulate the retrieval of memories as well as facilitate the acceptance of memories (Birren & Cochran, 2001). Although life stories are often conducted independently by older adults, they are increasingly being guided by younger persons, perhaps an adult child or grandchild, or by college students (Haber, 2008a; McFarland, Rhoades, Roberts, & Eleazer, 2006).

With careful monitoring, Birren noted that in his many years of experience, he has never had a group member report becoming depressed as a result of a life review. He warns, however, that persons who are already depressed or otherwise needing therapy should be under the supervision of a qualified professional.

> **Question:** Find additional reading material on conducting a life review and then conduct a life review segment (for instance, the development of a hobby, early work career, courting memories, childhood holiday celebrations, the impact of a historical event) with an older adult. What did you learn about aging that was most important to you?

An *ethical will* can be a component of a life review, or done as a separate project. Unlike traditional wills that transfer worldly possessions, ethical wills bequeath values through heartfelt words. Though ethical wills were first described 3000 years ago in the Hebrew Bible, they have become increasingly popular in contemporary America among Jews and non-Jews alike. Ethical wills document the essential lessons that one has learned in a lifetime, or one's hopes and dreams, for future generations. They can be as brief or as long as you like. Here is my ethical will, stated with unique brevity: *I hope you cultivate, and enjoy, the wisdom that aging can bring.*

ALZHEIMER'S DISEASE

For prior editions of this book, I had consistently stated that there were no biological markers for *Alzheimer's disease*, except to examine by biopsy or autopsy the *neurofibrillary*

BOX 8.1   Are You Saved?

The first paragraph below contains an anecdote taken verbatim from the monthly electronic newsletter *Human Values in Aging* (May 2009, p. 1), written by Harry Moody:

I once was sitting in a restaurant with Rabbi Zalman Schachter talking about the search for meaning in old age. Suddenly, Reb Zalman turned to me and said, "You know, this search for meaning all comes down to a simple question: Are you saved?" Hearing this, I was puzzled and I thought to myself, well, he is a clergyman, (and asked) "Is this a theological question?" "No," said Reb Zalman, "I don't mean it in a theological sense but in a computer sense. Are you saved? Have you downloaded your life experience for coming generations? Have you started doing your legacy work?"

This idea contrasts sharply with the attitude of some older adults when I approach them about participating in my Life Review class with students at the local university: "My life is not interesting enough to take up that much of your student's time." Despite this initial attitude, most of these older adults can be persuaded to participate. The students, inevitably, are quite appreciative. Here is one example of what a student reported:

"After two interviews, I thought my older adult was lonely, somewhat depressed and negative. She told me her family does not have time to visit often, and she has serious health problems. I felt sorry for her. By the end of the life review experience I had quite a different impression. She shared great memories, smiled often, and seemed happier than when we started. We shared some great laughs together. She may be a bit lonely, but she is certainly not negative. In fact, she has had an amazing life. I'm glad I was given the opportunity to get to know her. I am thinking about the idea of writing older people's life stories for a living, but I can't believe you can get paid to do something that is this enjoyable!" (Haber, 2008a).

tangles inside cells and the *neuritic plaques* deposited outside cells. That era, though, is coming to a close. Tests to detect Alzheimer's disease are in development.

Preclinical Alzheimer's

A study tracking the progress of a group of patients over an average of a decade found that those who had mild cognitive difficulties with lowered levels of a beta-amyloid protein in their cerebrospinal flud were overwhelmingly diagnosed with Alzheimer's disease by the end of the study period. Specifically, about 90% of patients who exihibited both mild cognitive impairment and the noted changes in spinal fluid composition developed Alzheimer's within 9.2 years (Buchhave et al., 2012). These biomarkers can identify individuals at high risk for future AD at least 20 years before visible symptoms of cognitive impairment (Fleisher et al., 2012).

The original U.S. guideline for detecting Alzheimer's was established in 1984 and consisted of catatastrophic cognitive impairments, such as severe memory loss and personality changes. It took a quarter century, in 2011, for these guidelines to be updated by the National Institute on Aging and the Alzheimer's Association. In addition to the phase when dementia had developed with notable cognitive impairment, now referred to as phase 3 by researchers at the 2012 Alzheimer's Association International Conference that took place in Vancouver, British Columbia, there are two earlier phases identified: (1) phase 1 in which no symptoms are evident but changes are noted in the brain, and (2) phase 2 when mild problems emerge but daily function can still be performed.

The two biomarkers for phases 1 and 2, which are still in development, are abnormal levels of proteins amyloid and tau, and shrinkage of certain brain areas. These biomarkers are not ready for widespread usage because between 10% and a third of the people with these biomarkers do not develop Alzheimer's symptoms by the time they die. These new phases are being referred to in research arenas as *preclinical Alzheimer's*.

Given that clinicians cannot yet identify Alzheimer's with sufficient reliability, and cannot treat it in a meaningful way, the value of these biomarkers is strictly within the research arena. Even if reliability was better, the advantage of family members being better informed about the planning and care of a person with Alzheimer's more than two decades prior to symptoms appearing may be more than offset by the extended period of worry and stigma.

Characteristics of Alzheimer's Disease

The most common symptom in early Alzheimer's disease and other types of dementia is diminished short-term memory. Word finding becomes difficult and may be accompanied by personality changes, emotional lability, and poor judgment. As persons progress to intermediate dementia, their ability to dress, bathe, toilet, and perform other activities of daily living becomes impaired. Persons with severe dementia are totally dependent on others, and the ability to recognize even close family members may be lost.

Alzheimer's disease is the most common form of dementia affecting older adults, accounting for two thirds of cases. Other types of dementia include vascular dementia, alcohol-associated dementia, infection-related dementia, and so forth. There are also reversible conditions that mimic Alzheimer's and other forms of dementia, such as hypothyroidism, depression, and vitamin B_{12} deficiency.

About 8% to 15% of adults over the age of 65 have Alzheimer's disease (Ritchie & Kildea, 1995), but the prevalence is not evenly distributed, it appears to double every 5 years: 1% of persons age 60 to 64; 2% of those age 65 to 69; 4% of those age 70 to 74; 8% of those age 75 to 79; 16% of those age 80 to 84; and 30% to 45% of those persons age 85 and older. Looking at the broader category of cognitive impairment, the rate is 4.65% of 65-to 69-year-olds; 54% of 85-to 89-year-olds; and 84% of those age 90+ (Kukell et al., 2002).

One of the unfortunate correlations with Alzheimer's disease or other forms of severe dementia is that 20% of patients will experience a *burdensome transition*. Examples of a burdensome transition are an unnecessary hospitalization in the last 3 days of life or multiple hospitalizations during the last 90 days of life. Some of the consequences of these types of transitions are double the number of stage IV decubitus ulcers (bedsore with bone exposed), double the likelihood of a stay in an intensive care unit, and a threefold greater likelihood of having a feeding tube inserted (Gozalo et al., 2011).

Exacerbating this problem is that the number of hospitalizations of Americans age 85 and older with dementia rose from 700,000 in 2000 to 1.2 million in 2008 (Zilberberg & Tjia, 2011). Very old demented persons with pneumonia or infections are better treated in a nursing home or hospice than an expensive hospital bed where they are more likely to be confined to their beds and may have to be restrained.

Treatment

Researchers are working on vaccines for the prevention of Alzheimer's disease or the halting of deterioration, with the latest being an immune therapy called IVIG/Gammagard; but these vaccines are likely to be, at best, many years away from fruition. In the meantime, there has been a tremendous surge in the use of medications, particularly two Food and Drug Administration (FDA)-approved drugs for dementia, donepezil and memantine—better known as *Aricept* and *Namenda*. After huge advertisement campaigns (money perhaps better spent on research?), close to $3 billion was spent annually worldwide for Aricept and more than $500 million for Namenda.

Independent research results, however, have been disappointing, with one clinical trial reporting that Aricept is not cost-effective, with benefits below minimally relevant thresholds for delaying entry into institutional care or for slowing the progression of disability (Courtney et al., 2004). Another study reported that Aricept is no more effective than a placebo in treating agitation in patients with Alzheimer's disease, and side effects are problematic (Howard et al., 2007). As Lichtenberg (2009) notes, "many older adults with Alzheimer's disease are prescribed (and continue to be prescribed) drugs that do not benefit them" (p. 8).

In 2010, the situation got worse. The drug, Aricept 23 was approved by the FDA, against the advice of its own reviewers. With questionable benefit to begin with, this new 23-mg version does substantially more harm (Schwartz & Woloshin, 2012). The sole purpose, seemingly, of this odd number, a 23-mg dosage, was that you could not reach it by the combining of the 5- and 10-milligram dosages that were soon to become available in generic form.

Both a clinical and a statistical reviewer for the FDA recommended against approval of the higher dosage. Nevertheless, the drug was approved by Dr. Russell Katz of the FDA who acknowledged that side effects from the higher dose, primarily nausea and vomiting, could lead to significant morbidities and even increased mortality, but concluded that the drug most likely improved overall function even though the study did not show that according to the FDA reviewers.

It is also not uncommon for antipsychotic drugs to be used for controlling agitation and combative behavior in residents with dementia in nursing homes. It is estimated that 185,000 nursing home residents in the United States received an antipsychotic in 2010, which can leave people in a stupor or increase falls or seizures.

Pharmacological therapies (including drugs for depression and anxiety) are not particularly effective for the management of psychiatric symptoms of dementia or for the reduction of disability. Nonetheless, they are prescribed because it is easier to medicate than to engage. A 2002 study by the Kaiser Foundation found that the staffs in a typical nursing home spent a total of only 2 hours and 20 minutes per day with each resident, and relied substantially on medications to manage residents. Perhaps the money spent on dementia medications could be redirected to better social support and more creative interventions, such as music therapy, aromatherapy, and pet therapy (Sink, Holden, & Yaffe, 2005).

Arlene Astell, a researcher at the University of St. Andrews in Scotland, has had good success with improving the mental health of dementia patients in institutional, community, and home settings by showing them familiar movies and photographs, or playing familiar musical selections. Based on the principles used in Montessori schools for children, a training program for older persons with early-stage dementia helps them to better perform simple, but meaningful, tasks (Camp & Skrajner, 2004).

A remarkable video went viral in 2012, showing Henry, a 94-year-old African American man who resides in a Brooklyn, New York, nursing home. Henry, who rarely speaks, became revitalized when listening to an IPod loaded with his favorite music. The video is titled *Alive Inside* and is narrated by neurologist Oliver Sacks and social worker Dan Cohen, founder of a nonprofit organization called *Music and Memory* that has been implemented in 50 nursing homes in 15 states.

From being hunched over in his chair and incapable of answering questions beyond a "yes" or "no," Henry immediately lights up with the music, his eyes wide open, his face full of expression, and he even engages in dialogue when asked what the music means to him: "It gives me the feeling of love, of romance. I figure right now the world needs to come into music, singing. You've got beautiful music here." He then mimics the song of his favorite artist Cab Calloway, scat singing a credible "I'll Be Home for Christmas."

A program called *Meet Me at MoMA* (Museum of Modern Art) in New York City is designed for early- and moderate-stage Alzheimer's patients and their caregivers. This free program is held once a month after the museum is closed, with trained educators escorting groups of patients and caregivers to selected artworks for observation and discussion (www.moma.org/learn/programs/access). Dr. Mary Mittelman, a researcher at New York University, has determined that the program improves overall mood for a majority of participants and is anticipating publication of her findings in the near future.

A program called *TimeSlips*, shows photos to people with memory loss and then asks them to imagine what is going on—not to try to remember anything, but to make up a story. Many of the participants in a Seattle senior center who are participating in this program talk very little to others, including relatives, but become enthusiastic about making up a story of, for example, a photo of a fit elderly man wearing a banana-yellow wet-suit vest who is water skiing. The founder of this program, Anne Basting, directs the Center on Age and Community at the University of Wisconsin, Milwaukee. She reports that it gives people with dementia a low-stress way to communicate with others, including relatives who otherwise have had little communication with a demented loved one.

Persons with dementia in the mild to moderate stages may benefit from cognitive stimulation, such as social day programs that can provide cognitive-stimulating activities that take into account patient and family preferences. A review of 15 randomized controlled trials, mainly with persons with Alzheimer's disease or vascular dementia, reported a consistent benefit on cognitive function (Woods, Aguirre, Spector, & Orrell, 2012).

Regarding diet, high blood levels of trans fats were significantly associated with the impaired mental ability of 104 older adults, average age 87, whereas omega-3, or a combination of vitamins B, C, D, and E, was associated with better mental functioning of the older adults (Bowman et al., 2012). However, this study did not determine whether taking supplements of these nutrients, or decreasing trans fats, would lower the risk for dementia.

Cognitive Fitness

Warner Schaie, a leading researcher in the field of cognitive development, suggested that the "use it or lose it" principle applied not only to muscles, but to brains as well. He reported that by 80 years of age, virtually everybody has some decline in mental function, but how much you slip in your 60s and 70s depends in part on mental stimulation. A higher level of education or greater engagement with cognitively stimulating activities over the life cycle may delay the onset of mental decline (Fritsch et al., 2001; Wilson et al., 2002).

Studies of the brain suggest that educational and social activities, challenging occupations, and brain-stimulating hobbies are stimulants for *cognitive reserve*, the brain's ability to develop and maintain extra neurons and the connections between them through axons and dendrites (Garibotto et al., 2008). The theory is that these connections help compensate for the rise in dementia-related brain pathology that accompanies normal aging. This may explain the studies that reveal that as many as two thirds of people with autopsy findings of Alzheimer's disease were nonetheless cognitively intact in late life.

The research study most widely publicized in the popular media on the factors that may delay the effects of Alzheimer's disease were conducted by Snowdon, Greiner, and

Markesbery (2000), and referred to as the Nun Study. This longitudinal study began with the analysis of handwritten autobiographies of 678 Catholic sisters from seven Notre Dame convents across the country. From a research perspective, these types of religious groups provide the advantage of relatively uniform backgrounds to study, and fewer variations in lifestyle to confound the data.

The participating sisters agreed not only to allow researchers access to their autobiographies, which had been written before they took their religious vows, but to annual mental and physical examinations, as well as to brain donation and autopsy after death. The researchers found that lower linguistic ability in terms of ideas and sentence structure (Snowdon et al., 2000) and greater negative emotional content (Danner, Snowdon, & Friesen, 2001) in early-life writings had a strong association with dementia in later life and premature death.

Another study of 801 older Catholic nuns and priests without dementia at baseline rated their frequency of participation in cognitively stimulating activities. The study results reported that the higher the participation in cognitively stimulating activities, the lower the rate of Alzheimer's disease (Wilson et al., 2002).

In addition to this correlation (not causality) between mental fitness and the expression of Alzheimer's disease, there is evidence to support a relationship between physical fitness and dementia. Dr. Marilyn Albert of Harvard Medical School and her colleagues (1995) conducted interviews with 1,192 people aged 70 to 79 and concluded that not only might mental stimulation—crossword puzzles, reading, and discussion (as opposed to passive television entertainment, idle chit-chat, and doing things from rote)—help stave off dementia and memory loss, but physical stimulation may also. They reported that physical activities may affect the blood flow to the brain and help sustain mental faculties.

People who have been physically active between the ages of 20 and 60 demonstrated a lower risk for Alzheimer's disease in later life (Friedland et al., 2001). A study of 2,200 people over age 65 reported an association between physical fitness and delayed onset of dementia or cognitive decline (Wang, Larson, Bowen, & van Belle, 2006).

However, as noted in Chapter 2, "Clinical Preventive Services," cause and effect are impossible to identify from population studies that are correlational and unable to employ random assignment to treatment and control groups. It is possible, for instance, that some of the persons studied were already in the earliest stage of Alzheimer's disease—before symptoms were detectable—and that this accounted for the association with reduced linguistic ability, the negative emotional content, the lack of participation in cognitively stimulating activities, and the reduced level of physical fitness, rather than the reverse.

In addition, these types of observational studies are still seeking a biological explanation as to how increased mental or physical activity impacts the brain. One study reported that the individual's dementia status at death, that is, the degree of plaques and tangles in the brain, did not correlate with a high versus low cognitive lifestyle score. However, an active cognitive lifestyle was associated with greater neuronal density and cortical thickness in the frontal lobe (Valenzuela et al., 2012).

The U.S. National Institutes of Health convened a 2011 consensus conference and concluded that, at the present time, research is inadequate to determine whether pharmaceuticals, dietary interventions, physical activity, or cognitive engagement prevents or delays Alzheimer's disease or cognitive decline.

Brain Games

Older adults who were trained to perceive greater control over their cognitive functioning improved memory performance (Lachman & Andreoletti, 2006). A 2-week program of memory exercises and lifestyle changes led to improved cognitive function (Small et al., 2006). Older persons in Japan need no additional convincing that they can do something to improve their brain function. Nintendo came out with a video game in Japan called *Brain Training for Adults* in May 2005, then produced a sequel in December 2005; and by March 2006, 3.3 million copies had been sold to eager consumers. Video game players were given performance grades that they could improve upon, ranging from a troublesome score of 80 to an optimal score of 20.

In January 2007 a brain gym opened in Sarasota, Florida. Seniors attempting to prevent or delay the decline of cognitive function are joining these types of brain fitness centers, and engaging in *neurobics*, or exercises for the brain. These centers are like traditional fitness centers in that the member pays a monthly fee, has access to the club's mental exercise equipment, and can pay an additional fee for consultation with a personal cognition trainer.

Although there is evidence that *brain games* and other types of training can help the participant's immediate performance on tasks related to the training, there was no evidence that the effects could be generalized to other areas of cognitive functioning in daily life. Nonetheless, the market for these types of products increased from $2 million in 2005 to about $225 million in 2009 (Papp, Walsh, & Snyder, 2009). Reading, crossword puzzles, and other free activities, however, are likely to be just as effective as a formal and costly brain exercise program.

OTHER MENTAL DISORDERS

Anxiety disorder is associated with at least three of the following symptoms: restlessness or edginess, fatigue, difficulty concentrating, irritability, muscle tension, and sleep disturbance. It is a difficult mental disorder to assess in those who are elderly, and psychological testing is rarely of benefit. The most common anxiety disorders, in order of prevalence, are generalized anxiety disorder, phobia, panic disorder, obsessive-compulsive disorder, and posttraumatic stress disorder (PTSD). PTSD is expected to increase in prevalence among older adults as Vietnam veterans are reaching old age.

Between 3% and 14% of adults age 55 and older meet the criteria for an anxiety disorder, with prevalence rates varying greatly as anxiety definitions overlap with other diagnoses.

Treatment with medications for anxiety disorders tends to be similar between older and younger patients. Benzodiazepines and other anxiety medications, however, are marginally effective in treating chronic anxiety in older patients. For anxiety associated with depression, an antidepressant may be effective. For anxiety associated with mild dementia, a more structured environment may alleviate symptoms. For anxiety associated with bereavement, CBT or an exercise program may be of benefit. However, although CBT may be moderately effective with heping older people's anxiety, it is *less* effective than when it is applied to working-age clients (Gould, Coulson, & Howard, 2012).

Schizophrenia, characterized by delusions, hallucinations, paranoia, disorganized speech, catatonic behavior, and affective flattening, can extend into or first appear in later life. Prevalence of schizophrenia among older adults, however, is only 0.6%, about half the rate for the population aged 18 to 54. Pharmacological treatment of schizophrenia in late life is challenging, as the previous generation of antipsychotic medications have had a high risk of persistent and disabling side effects. The next generation of antipsychotics, such as clozapine and risperidone, may be somewhat more effective with older adults than the earlier neuroleptics.

Alcohol abuse and misuse of medications are also considered to be in the category of mental disorders, but these two topics are examined in Chapter 7, "Selected Health Education Topics." A related mental disorder, *illicit drug abuse*, rarely occurs among today's cohort of older adults, affecting less than 0.1%. This is changing, however, as noted by the Substance Abuse and Mental Health Services Administration which documents the baby boomers' continued use of illicit drugs as they grow older, particularly marijuana and nonmedical use of prescription drugs.

Finally, there are *compulsive behaviors* that are being labeled as mental disorders and treated with antidepressants, SSRIs. These behaviors include such activities as gambling addiction, kleptomania, shopping addiction, and social phobia. Some argue that these are legitimate mental disorders that should be treated medically. Others contend that these behaviors are everyday maladies that are escalated into medical problems by drug company marketing.

With the advent of Prozac, the most popular SSRI, the threshold has been lowered for what constitutes an emotional disorder that needs medication. Prescriptions for the new generation of antidepressants tripled during the 1990s, and sales for these types of drugs doubled between 2000 and 2005. An increasing percentage of Prozac and other SSRI drugs are directed toward compulsive behaviors.

INSURANCE COVERAGE

For many years, advocates have publicly and strongly objected to the unequal Medicare coverage of mental illness and physical illness. Medicare patients paid 50% of Medicare-approved amounts for most outpatient mental health care, but only 20% for medical services for physical conditions. Medicare also imposed a 190-day lifetime limit on inpatient psychiatric hospital care, but there was no cap on care in a general hospital. In addition, Medicare carriers automatically flagged any claims for Alzheimer's disease as subject to the 50% out-of-pocket policy, even when the care warranted 80% coverage. A government memorandum to correct this bias against Alzheimer's disease did not work (Aston, 2002).

Moreover, this disparity in Medicare reimbursement between physical and mental treatments served to further the stigma surrounding mental illness in older adults (Unutzer et al., 2003). This stigma, along with the financial barriers that were erected, led to older Americans accounting for only 7% of all inpatient mental health services, 6% of community-based mental health services, and 9% of private psychiatric care (Persky, 1998). The disparity also fueled the misperception that mental illness could not be treated as effectively as physical conditions in older adults. As noted by the Surgeon General's report on mental health, though, when properly diagnosed and treated, 65% to 80% of depressed older adults improve with medication, psychotherapy, or a combination of both—a success rate higher than many current common medical treatments for nonpsychiatric illnesses.

Well, there is finally good news to report! Full *mental health parity* is now law. The *Medicare Improvements for Patients and Providers Act of 2008* requires equal coverage for mental and physical illness. The reduction in the higher copayment is being phased in over 6 years, to the 20% level in 2014. As has been the case with many Medicare changes, mental health parity in the private sector also became law shortly after Congress eliminated discriminatory mental health insurance practices in Medicare.

Although the 2008 Act only covered employers with 50 or more employees, this has been expanded to everyone, not just larger employers, thanks to the Affordable Care Act. In addition to equal deductibles and copayments, there will no longer be limits on inpatient days and outpatient visits for mental health treatments. Also attributable to the

Affordable Care Act is that Medicare covers annual depression screenings in primary care settings with no cost sharing for beneficiaries, and the gap in Part D coverage for mental health medications will be filled in by 2020.

This is good news for the 7 million older adults in America suffering from depression or depressive symptoms, not to mention the 57 million Americans that the National Institute of Mental Health estimates to be suffering from one or more mental health disorders.

CHRONIC STRESS

Harvard physiologist Walter Cannon coined two terms, homeostasis and fight or flight. *Homeostasis* refers to the body's attempt to preserve the constancy of its internal environment. When cold, for instance, the body shivers to generate heat; and when hot, it sweats to reduce heat. When a challenge produces fear, homeostasis is disrupted and the organism prepares for *flight or fight*. Adrenaline is released, and there is an increase in heart rate, respiratory rate, blood pressure, and blood flow to the brain and large muscles of the extremities.

Fight or flight, in response to a physical challenge, prepares the organism to move more quickly, see better, think better, and reduce blood loss. In modern times, however, stress is more likely to be emotional than the reaction to a physical threat. Fighting or running away is often inappropriate. If you are pressed for time and trapped in big-city traffic, for instance, there is nothing to fight and no way to flee. The fight-or-flight response can be harmful, both physically and emotionally.

Stress research began with Hans Selye. His *General Adaptation Syndrome* consisted of three stages: (1) an alarm reaction, which mobilizes the body's resources; (2) a stage of resistance, in which the body tries to adapt to the stressor; and (3) a state of exhaustion. The trapped commuter, who can neither fight nor flee, is vulnerable to being in a prolonged state of resistance. This prolonged stress response, which is harmful to health, may produce pathologic changes, including hypertension, heart disease, arthritis, asthma, and peptic ulcers.

Chronic stress contributes to depression and anxiety disorders, and with aging it will interfere with normal memory processing (Small, 2002). Several days of exposure to high levels of the stress hormone cortisol leads to memory and learning impairment (Newcomer et al., 1999). One study reported that stressful activity makes older adults more cautious in decision making, but had little effect on younger adults (Mather et al., 2009). The researchers suggest that the stress hormones that accumulate over the life cycle are likely to shrink the brain regions involved in decision making, particularly with decisions involving risk.

Measurement

Perhaps the best-known stress measurement tool of the past half-century is the *Social Readjustment Rating Scale* (SRRS; 1967) developed by researchers Thomas Holmes and Richard Rahe at the University of Washington School of Medicine. The SRRS ranked 43 life-change events according to a score derived from more than 5,000 interviews over two decades. Men and women of different socioeconomic status, age, and marital status were asked to assign numeric values higher or lower than an arbitrary score of 50 for marriage. Ten of the top 15 scores related to the family, with death of a spouse receiving the top score of 100. Surprisingly, the ratings of events were consistent across ethnicities (African Americans and Mexican Americans) and countries (Europe and Japan).

Holmes and Rahe's classic study (1967) correlated the ratings of life-change events over a 12-month period with health risk. Thirty-seven percent of the individuals who scored under 200 underwent an appreciable change of health, compared to 79% of those who scored over 300. An interesting facet of the SRRS scale is its validity, despite its mechanistic approach to life events. The instrument does not, for instance, determine whether the individual's perception of a life event is stressful or not. Thus, the death of a cantankerous and burdensome spouse may be met with relief, whereas a codependent spouse may experience hysteria.

Over the past several decades, researchers have been looking for ways to make stress-measuring instruments more precise and powerful by weighing individual perceptions of stressful events. Lazarus and Folkman (1984) focused on daily hassles (e.g., weight gain, rising prices, losing things) and found stronger statistical associations with health outcomes than those obtained by merely counting life events. It is also clear during this time that the Holmes and Rahe scale was not as responsive to the later years as it could have been, because many of the life events included in the scale are unlikely to have occurred in late life. Age-specific scales are under development.

Perspectives

Stress can be viewed from three perspectives. The first is external, focusing on threatening stimuli from the environment. Measuring stress from this perspective may consist of counting stressful events like widowhood; or calculating hassles, such as being stuck in traffic, that have taken place within a designated time period.

A second perspective on stress focuses on internal forces, such as our psychological response to stressors. Being stuck in traffic, for instance, can produce anger, anxiety, and frustration, or we can perceive the traffic delay as an opportunity to converse with our companions or listen to a few additional audiotapes.

The fact that we do not all perceive events in the same way is illustrated by the well-known picture in Figure 8.1. Do you see a young woman or an old woman? Is it difficult to shift your perception between the two?

From the third perspective, stress is viewed as a transactional process, an interaction between forces in the environment and our perception. For example, because we are in a hurry, traffic triggers a stress response. Our anger and frustration then escalate our stress. In this transactional process, however, we can deliberately take a pause from our escalating stress level and choose to do a deep-breathing exercise. Thus, we can attempt neither to fight nor flee, but rather to flow.

Psychoneuroimmunology

Over the past three decades, researchers have found a number of physiological linkages between the nerve cells of the brain and the immune system, referred to as *psychoneuroimmunology*. These nerve cells connect the brain with the spleen and other organs that produce immune system cells. When the brain perceives a stressful event, for example, immunological changes result, such as a decline in the cells that fight tumors and viral infections. Unfortunately for stress researchers, many other factors can also suppress immunity, such as lifestyle habits (alcohol consumption, smoking, nutritional habits, etc.) and the overall status of the immune system. This latter variable is particularly relevant for older adults, because the robustness of the immune system declines with age.

One landmark study, which examined the relationship between lifestyle stress and the immune system of older adults, compared 69 older caregivers of spouses with Alzheimer's disease to a matched sample of older adults living in the community.

| FIGURE 8.1 | What do you see? |

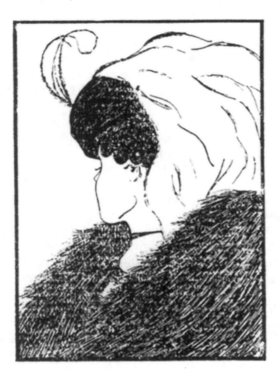

During this 13-month study, the chronic stress of caring for a family member with dementia led to the reduced function of the immune system of the older caregivers, which in turn led to more frequent respiratory tract infections compared to the matched sample in the community (Kiecolt-Glaser, Dura, Speicher, Trask, & Glaser, 1991).

Another study reported that the brain's perception of mental stress may be a better predictor of future heart problems than physical stress recorded through conventional treadmill testing with heart function measured on an electrocardiogram. Persons who responded adversely to mental stress testing (which included reactions to engaging in public speaking or solving math problems on a deadline) were two to three times more likely to suffer a heart attack or progressive chest pain in the future (Jiang et al., 1996).

STRESS MANAGEMENT

Although many Americans report that stress has had some effect on their health, it is less likely to be reported by older adults (about a third) than younger adults (about half). Similarly, in response to the broader question of how much stress they feel in their daily lives, the American Board of Family Practice reported that older adults were less likely to report considerable stress (about half) than younger adults (almost two thirds).

It is possible that older adults manage their stress better than younger adults, either through managing their perceptions of stress better, more frequent prayer, or the practice of other informal stress management techniques. One study reported that stress changes with age, and that older adults get better at managing stress over time (Almeida, Wethington, & Kessler, 2002). The stress focus of young adults is more likely on tension in relationships, middle-aged adults are overloaded by multiple demands on them, and older adults primarily face health problems. Almeida et al. (2002) reported, though, that older adults in their sample reported more stress-free days than middle-aged and younger adults.

It is also possible that older adults are less willing to report stress. They may find it more of a stigma than do younger adults and are reluctant to admit to it; or they may be less able to recognize it, either due to lack of knowledge about what stress is or because the stress is masked by depression, which older adults are more likely to exhibit symptoms of.

Regardless of age, many adults report a great deal of stress from time to time, and the great majority of them consciously take informal steps to control or reduce it. Only a few, however, try formal stress management techniques. The most popular stress management measures are the informal strategies of physical exercise, psychological denial, and avoidance.

Regarding exercise, a group of older adults with arthritis of the knee significantly lowered their depressive symptoms as a consequence of aerobic exercise. The subjects also reduced their disability and pain, and increased their walking speed (Penninx et al., 2002). Another study used a variety of more formal stress management techniques (anger coping, muscle relaxation, deep breathing, etc.) and individualized them according to the needs and preferences of subjects with high blood pressure. The researchers reported that blood pressure level was reduced through stress management, in comparison to a control group in which blood pressure was unchanged (Linden, Lenz, & Con, 2001). Another study implemented a group stress management program and reported clinically significant benefits for patients with type II diabetes (Surwit et al., 2002).

One study examined the effects of *journal writing* on stressful experiences, and subsequent symptom reduction in patients with asthma or rheumatoid arthritis (Smyth, Stone, Hurewitz, & Kaell, 1999). This randomized trial reported significantly greater symptomatic improvement (lung function and disease activity) in the intervention groups, compared with the control groups that wrote about emotionally neutral topics. It is possible that the participants' immune function improved after they unburdened themselves, or that they learned ways to cope better with the current stresses in their life by engaging in journaling exercises. Other controlled studies have demonstrated the short-term benefits of journal writing on patients with high blood pressure (McGuire, Greenberg, & Gevirtz, 2005) or fibromyalgia (Broderick, Junghaenel, & Schwartz, 2005).

Journal writing is a popular method for stress management and personal growth. For information on techniques and workshops, contact the Center for Journal Therapy at www.journaltherapy.com or toll-free 888-421-2298; or the Progoff Intensive Journal Program for Self-Development at www.intensivejournal.org or toll-free 800-221-5844.

A Positive Attitude and an Opposing View

The Harvard Study of Adult Development is a 60-year longitudinal study of 824 persons from adolescence to late life, conducted for the purpose of learning about successful aging (Vaillant, 2002). In addition to looking at privileged men and women from Harvard University and from California, the study examined healthy aging among inner-city men (Vaillant & Western, 2001). The psychiatrist George Vaillant, director of the study, concluded that good mental health with aging, regardless of background, involves a capacity for gratitude, forgiveness, and love; a desire to connect with people and replenish social networks; an interest in play and creativity; and a commitment to lifelong learning.

A longitudinal study of 23 years' duration reported that older individuals with more positive self-perceptions of aging lived 7.5 years longer than those with less positive self-perceptions of aging (Levy, Slade, Kunkel, & Kasl, 2002). This advantage remained after controlling for a number of potentially confounding variables. In other words, a positive perception of aging demonstrated a better survival outcome, regardless of whether participants were young-old or old-old, men or women, higher income or lower income, lonely or not, or better or worse off in functional health. This finding appeared to be a more powerful predictor of longevity than blood pressure level, cholesterol level, smoking, and exercise.

From 1998 to 2007, the psychologist Leonard Poon of the University of Georgia received grant funding to study centenarians through his *Georgia Centenarian Study*. He concluded that mental health is more important to survival than the longevity of your parents or what you have eaten over a lifetime. Poon reported that survivors over the age of 100 appear to be optimistic, to be passionately engaged in some activity, and to have the ability to adapt to repeated losses over time.

The epidemiologist Glen Ostir and his colleagues reported that positive affect predicted subsequent functional independence and survival after a major health event among older Mexican Americans (Ostir, Markides, Black, & Goodwin, 2000) and among older Blacks and Whites (Ostir et al., 2002). Scheier et al. (1999) reported that optimism predicted a lower rate of rehospitalization after coronary artery bypass graft surgery.

Conversely, negative attitudes like anger, pessimism, and gloomy self-perceptions of aging can lead to a host of unpleasant consequences. A high level of anger is associated with subsequent heart disease (Chang, Ford, Meoni, Wang, & Klag, 2002; Williams, Nieto, Sanford, & Tyroler, 2001) and stroke (Ostir, Markides, Peek, & Goodwin, 2001; Williams, Nieto, Sanford, Couper, & Tyroler, 2002b). A 30-year follow-up study of 723 patients revealed that those with pessimistic personalities had a 19% increased risk of mortality (Maruta, Colligan, Malinchoc, & Offord, 2000). A 23-year longitudinal study of older adults reported that negative self-perceptions of aging will diminish life expectancy (Levy, Slade, Kunkel, & Kasl, 2002). Persons aged 60 to 70 took a series of cognitive tests after being given hints that their age might affect their memory results, and it negatively affected their performance (Hess, Hinson, & Hodges, 2009). Persons aged 71 to 82, with more experience at being older, were not as affected by the negative stereotype.

The protective effect of a *positive attitude* on physical health and mental performance may work in a variety of ways. Positive emotions can increase confidence in performance capacity, strengthen social support, stimulate motivation for self-care, and encourage more physical activities that lead to higher-level mental and physical functioning (Penninx, 2000).

It should be noted, though, that many studies of patients with cancer have consistently reported that a positive attitude and social support did *not* affect survival rates (Coyne et al., 2007; Ehrenreich, 2009; Stefanek, Palmer, Thombs, & Coyne, 2009). Perhaps a positive attitude is more important in the prevention process than after disease has come into play. Some argue, though, that even in the realm of prevention we cannot assume that a positive attitude is best.

Researchers surveyed 200 adults age 60 and older and asked them to rate their physical and social expectations. Individuals who had *less* optimistic views of their future well-being had more positive scores on psychological well-being measures. The researchers concluded that the individuals who were able to make more realistic, and even overly negative, estimates of their future health and wellness were more satisfied with themselves than those who were more positive (Cheng, Fung, & Chan, 2009). Perhaps unrealistic expectations of the future, given the well-known physical changes with aging, will lead to disappointment and have a negative impact on psychological well-being. In short, having negative expectations of the future can have a positive impact on health.

Adding to the skepticism toward positive expectations, the well-known investigative journalist Barbara Ehrenreich (2009) wrote the book *Bright-Sided*, with the provocative subtitle: *How the Relentless Promotion of Positive Thinking Has Undermined America*. Her challenging thesis is that being positive is a strong American value, and a virtue that you flaunt at the risk of being stigmatized. In her chapter on breast cancer, Ehrenreich related her personal experience with breast cancer to how she was bombarded with positive thinking after her diagnosis. She received pink ribbons, teddy bears, new terms such as *survivor* rather than *patient*, slogans such as "cancer is a gift and an opportunity," visualization techniques to defeat her cancer, and self-help books. The overriding theme was this message: "A positive attitude is essential for recovery."

Ehrenreich (2009) argued that the relentless positivity "requires the denial of understandable feelings of anger and fear, all of which must be buried under a cosmetic layer of cheer" (p. 41). She concluded the chapter with the following: "What (breast cancer) gave me, if you want to call this a 'gift,' was a very personal, agonizing encounter with an ideological force in American culture that I had not been aware of before— one that encourages us to deny reality,

> **Question:** Do you believe a positive attitude can extend longevity? Explain your answer. Then, argue the opposite.

submit cheerfully to misfortune, and blame ourselves for our fate" (p. 44).

If this doesn't provoke you into thinking more about the benefits and pitfalls of positive thinking, then read *The Antidote: Happiness for People Who Can't Stand Positive Thinking* (Burkeman, 2012).

The Placebo Effect

The *placebo effect* is often referred to as the power of positive thinking. *Placebo* is Latin for "I shall please" and refers to a dummy substance or treatment that is designed to look like the real thing. People may respond favorably to a sham substance or treatment if they do not know it is phony and if they think it is a credible attempt at helping them. For example, patients who believe they are taking painkillers—with doses that contain no medication—release chemicals in their brain that relieve pain (Zubieta et al., 2005).

A survey of 1,200 practicing internists and rheumatologists in the United States reported that half of these physicians say they regularly prescribe placebos to patients. Placebos in this study, however, were not restricted to just inert substances (about 5% used saline or sugar pills), but also analgesics, vitamins, subtherapeutic medication doses, herbal supplements, antibiotics, and sedatives—drugs used for their effect on patients' psyches, but not their bodies (Tilburt, Emanuel, Kaptchuk, Curlin, & Miller, 2008). One interesting study reported that a higher price for a placebo creates the impression of higher value: a $2.50 placebo worked better than one that costs 10 cents (Waber, Shiv, Carmon, & Ariely, 2008).

Placebos provide a standard of comparison for evaluating a new drug or intervention, which must then significantly outperform the placebo. Given that placebos have been known to help about 25% of subjects achieve a normal blood pressure, and improve mental health among 45% of those who were depressed less than a year and 23% of those who were chronically depressed, then a new drug or intervention must exceed this type of a baseline. The power of the placebo is frequently extolled in health newsletters (e.g., "Power of the Placebo Effect," 2000; "Surprising Power of Placebos," 2000).

Then along came two contrarian Danish researchers to dispute the conventional wisdom (see the section on mammograms in Chapter 2, "Clinical Preventive Services," for another attempt by the same Danish researcher, Peter Gotzsche, who relishes a dispute with conventional wisdom). The two researchers examined 114 studies and concluded that with the exception of subjective outcomes, particularly pain outcomes, there was no such thing as a placebo effect (Hrobjartsson & Gotzsche, 2001). They argued that instead of positive attitudes producing positive physical results, spontaneous remission—which occurs naturally in many diseases—accounts for the placebo effect.

> **Question:** Aside from research projects, is it ethical to give someone a placebo? Why do you believe that?

This single study is not the definitive word on the power of the placebo. If it is substantiated, though, there is an upside to debunking the placebo effect, as well as the purported medical advantages in general that are associated with a positive attitude: Those who do not achieve successful medical outcomes do not need to feel guilty about their inability to stimulate the placebo effect.

Proaging: The Botox Alternative

The Botox (botulinum toxin type A) craze came along in 2002 when the FDA approved use of this drug to smooth out aging faces. Small doses of the toxin are injected into the forehead every few months to temporarily paralyze the injected muscle. The drug is expensive, requires repeated application, may have adverse side effects, and can make one look more zombie-like than youthful, but that has not discouraged the generation that has already accepted hair transplants, breast augmentation, collagen injections, chemical peels, and liposuction.

Botox and the cosmetic revolution to keep us looking young were on my mind when I read an essay by Gwenda Blair (2001) called "The Many Faces I See." She wrote about the *matryoshka* doll that comes from Russia: a wooden doll that is hollowed out, with a smaller version of the doll inside, which is also hollowed out with a smaller version inside, and so forth. Ms. Blair wrote about feeling like a matryoshka, with all her earlier *me's* inside and fitted into one another. The rest of the world may only see the wrinkled older woman on the outside, but she knew all the earlier selves still inside her.

Instead of making her external face look younger, Ms. Blair accepted herself as a little girl, a young mother, a middle-aged woman, and an older woman—all rolled into one. Instead of ignoring the old lady with wrinkles and gray hair, she and society can admire the woman who not only knows what it is like to be an old person, but also knows what it is like to be a child, a teenager, a parent, a worker, a mortgage holder, a grandparent, and a retiree.

An interesting video that I show in some of my classes is titled *Let's Face It: Women Explore Their Aging Faces* (Bare Face Productions, 2003, distributed by Terra Nova Films). About a dozen women from age 40 to their early 60s literally explore their faces in the mirror and then discuss their reaction to the effects of aging, comparing their looks to earlier times. These close friends are coming to terms with growing older, with several expressing their disappointment at their diminished beauty (evaluated in terms of societal values), but all of them attempting to be positive and affirming toward the aging process.

I have heard strong arguments that mental health can improve with age if those who so choose change their looks to be more youthful in their appearance. For instance, a more youthful appearance may help a person in his or her 50s land a job or attract a mate. I understand this and support an individual's right to make his or her own decision.

But in general, I make the opposite argument: Mental health can improve more with age if we accept the appearance of old age and all that goes with it, and feel positive about it. This argument would be greatly strengthened, I admit, if there was more societal support of a new genre of elder images, where positive visions of older adults are portrayed frequently in movies, television, theater, books, and popular lyrics. Instead, the title of one scholarly article says it all: "The Aging Woman in Popular Films: Underrepresented, Unattractive, Unfriendly, and Unintelligent" (Bazzini, McIntosh, Smith, Cook, & Harris, 1997).

The same negative stereotype holds true for television. Older Americans are almost 14% of the population, yet constitute only about 3% of the television population. This is true of primetime television characters, individuals portrayed in television advertising, game show contestants, and cartoon figures (Harwood, 2007). Not only are older adults underrepresented, but approximately 70% of older men and 80% of older women seen on television are portrayed disrespectfully, treated with little if any courtesy, and often perceived as "bad" (*Aging Today*, 2009).

Instead of William Shakespeare's description of old age as "second childishness and mere oblivion /sans teeth, sans eyes, sans taste, sans everything," the arts could discover and reinforce the image of old age as one that embodies not just physical diminishment, but also wisdom, joyfulness, spirituality, resiliency, and integrity.

Integrity versus despair is the challenge of the last stage of Erik Erikson's stages of psychosocial development (Erikson, Erikson, & Kivnick, 1987). The task of the elder at this stage of existence is to reflect on his or her life, to review experiences and accomplishments, and to integrate these memories into the belief that he or she has led a meaningful life. Those who accept the aging process and find integrity rather than despair in late life may not only find it personally satisfying, but they may also become positive role models for succeeding generations. Or, there is always botox.

> **Question:** Is trying to look younger in old age an ageist reaction to a natural process, or an effective way to cope in a youth-oriented society? Explain your answer.

MENTAL HEALTH AND AGING RESOURCES

The Geriatric Mental Health Foundation was established by the American Association for Geriatric Psychiatry to eliminate the stigma of mental illness and treatment, and to promote healthy aging strategies for older adults and their families. Contact the Geriatric Mental Health Foundation, 7910 Woodmont Ave., #10050, Bethesda, MD 20814; 301-654-7850; www.gmhfonline.org.

The National Alliance on Mental Illness provides information on mental illness and its treatment, including the publication *Mood Disorders, Depression and Manic Depression*. Referrals are also made to local support groups. Contact the National Alliance on Mental Illness, Colonial Place Three, 2107 Wilson Blvd., Suite 300, Arlington, VA 22201; 800-950-6264; www.nami.org.

For additional information on mental illness and mental health, visit the following two websites: the National Institute of Mental Health at www.nimh.nih.gov, which provides literature and other resources designed for older adults; and National Mental Health America at www.nmha.org, which provides information on advocacy, education, support groups, research, and service.

AARP has, unfortunately, discontinued two national programs with mental health benefits: the Reminiscence Program, for facilitating life reviews; and the Widowed Persons Service, a peer support program of trained volunteers who assisted the newly widowed recover from their losses. Although these programs are no longer offered on a national basis, they may be available through a few state AARP offices. To find out how to access your state office, contact AARP, Social Outreach and Support, 601 E St. NW, Washington, DC 20049; www.aarp.org.

For those who disagree with me and like the idea of spending money on brain-healthy workshops and related resources, contact the Alzheimer's Association's *Maintain Your Brain* program, at www.alz.org/maintainyourbrain/overview.asp; the American Society on Aging's Strategies for Cognitive Vitality, at www.asaging.org/cdc; or AARP, in conjunction with the Dana Alliance for Brain Initiatives, Brain-Health booklets, at www.aarp.org/health/brain/program/staying_sharp_booklets.html.

Civic Ventures promotes the engagement of older adults in civic life in a way that not only benefits society, but also the mental health of older adults. Contact Civic Ventures, 139 Townsend St., #505, San Francisco, CA 94107; www.civicventures.org.

Creativity and Aging Resources

Fostering creativity in older adults can also improve their mental health. "There is some degree of creativity in every person, and the health practitioner's function is to assist the aged person to recognize and believe in his or her full potential. Products of creativity are less important than fostering a creative attitude. Curiosity, inquisitiveness, wonderment, puzzlement, and craving for understanding are creative attitudes. It is possible to help older persons to break free" (Ebersole & Hess, 1990).

To obtain information about the following creative-arts therapies or to identify certified therapists near your location, contact the following nonprofit organizations: the *American Music Therapy Association* at 301-589-3300 or www.musictherapy.org; the *American Dance Therapy Association* at 410-997-4040, or www.adta.org; the *American Art Therapy Association* toll-free at 888-290-0878, or www.arttherapy.org; and the *National Association for Poetry Therapy* toll-free at 888-498-1843, or www.poetry therapy.org. Bonnie Vorenberg is president of Art Age Publications, the purpose of which is to foster Senior Theatre productions around the country; call toll-free at 800-858-4998, or www.seniortheatre.com.

A monograph by McMurray (1990) provides a good source of information for sparking creativity in older persons. Ebersole and Hess (1990) refer to several other guides that encourage creative expression in older adults, including art, music, poetry, humor, and self-actualization. Koch's (1977) account describing how he taught poetry to nursing home residents is a particularly enjoyable and useful resource guide. For an assortment of mental health treatment protocols used by nurses in a variety of practice settings, see Kurlowicz (1997).

The *National Center for Creative Aging*, founded by Susan Perlstein in 2001, is a clearinghouse throughout the United States for information,

> **Question:** Theodore Roszak wrote, "Aging changes consciousness more surely than any narcotic; it does so gradually and organically. It digests the experience of a lifetime and makes us different people—sometimes so different that we are amazed, embarrassed, or even ashamed at the person we once were." Do you think most older adults view their younger selves as someone completely different than who they are now? Why?

research, and training on arts and aging. The mission of the center is to promote creative expression and healthy aging. For additional information, contact the National Center for Creative Aging, 138 S. Oxford St., Brooklyn, NY 11217; 718-398-3870; www.creativeaging.org.

The *Center on Aging, Health & Humanities*, founded by the late Dr. Gene Cohen, has a focus on studying and promoting creativity and aging; it is located at George Washington University, 10225 Montgomery Ave., Kensington, MD 20895; www.gwumc .edu/cahh.

The *Center for Elders and Youth in the Arts* focuses on intergenerational educational programming and community presentations in the visual and performing arts; contact the Institute on Aging, 3330 Geary Blvd., San Francisco, CA 94118; 415-750-4111; www .ioaging.org.

The *Osher Lifelong Learning Institute* (formerly the North Carolina Center for Creative Retirement) promotes lifelong learning and community service opportunities for retirement-aged individuals; contact the University of North Carolina at Asheville, Reuter Center, CPO #5000, One University Heights, Asheville, NC 28804; www.unca .edu/nccr.

9

● ● ● ● ● ●

COMMUNITY HEALTH

● ● ● Key Terms

Area Agency on Aging

senior centers

parish nurses

Shepherd's Centers of America

worksite wellness

Road Scholar

Emeritus Centers

shopping mall-based programs

SeniorNet

National Council on Aging's Center
for Healthy Aging

Healthwise

Chronic Disease Self-Management
Program

Project Enhance

Ornish Program for Reversing Heart
Disease

Benson's Mind Body Institute

Strong for Life

community-oriented primary care

professional associations

community volunteering

Encore Careers

National Senior Services Corps

Retired Senior Volunteer Program

Foster Grandparent Program

Senior Companion Program

Experience Corps

Service Corps of Retired Executives

AARP

Gray Panthers

environmental advocacy

long-term care ombudsman program

BenefitsCheckUp

Red Hat Society

● ● ○   **Learning Objectives**

- Identify your local Area Agency on Aging
- Examine the need for senior centers to be responsive to baby boomers
- Recognize the role that religious institutions and shopping malls can play in providing health-promoting and educational services
- Review the history of worksite wellness
- Examine the evolution of the Road Scholar program
- Describe a shopping mall-based health program
- Identify a computer education program for older adults
- Describe several model health promotion programs for older adults
- Identify more than a dozen professional associations that provide health-promoting services for older adults
- Explain the importance of volunteering for the mental health of older adults and the improvement of society
- Identify model volunteer programs that involve older adults
- Describe the work of community health advocacy programs
- Evaluate the value of the BenefitsCheckUp website

COMMUNITY ORGANIZATIONS

Unless they live in rural settings, older persons are likely to have a wide array of community-based health-promoting programs, resources, and services available to them. Moreover, neither frailty nor disability automatically prevent older adults from gaining access to them. Programs and services for older adults are housed at religious institutions, senior centers, institutes of higher education, public service agencies, AARP (formerly American Association of Retired Persons) chapters, hospitals, clinics, and other community sites, and they are often responsive to the health needs and limitations of older adults.

A logical place for older persons to begin to locate relevant community health resources is the local *Area Agency on Aging* (AAA). These agencies are responsible for providing aging information, as well as coordinating the more than 20,000 organizations around the country that provide services for the aging. Unfortunately, the 629 AAAs do not have uniform names and can be difficult to locate in a telephone directory. The National Association of Area Agencies on Aging (1730 Rhode Island Ave. NW, #1200, Washington, DC 20036; 202-872-0888; www.n4a.org) can provide current information on local AAAs. The Eldercare Locator (800-677-1116; www.eldercare.gov) can provide current information on local caregiver services and resources.

Senior Centers

Older adults seek health information more actively than do younger adults. A major source of information for about 20% of older adults is the neighborhood *senior center*. Almost all of the approximately 13,000 senior centers around the country (half of which receive Older Americans Act funding from the federal government) provide some type of health education or screening program. At one end of the continuum, though, are senior centers that provide a hot meal and bingo only, and at the other end are senior centers that provide not only education and screening, but a variety of exercise and nutrition classes, self-help groups, social services, medical services, and referrals. Senior centers exist in almost every community.

However, when community practitioners were asked where they would locate information on health education and health promotion programs, they identified a wide array of sites, giving no specific emphasis to senior centers. Identified sites included state and local health departments, institutes of higher education, hospitals, public service agencies, and volunteer organizations.

Many senior centers are now vestiges of the 1960s and 1970s, when they focused on hot meals, some health education, and recreational programs, particularly bingo. The sites were, and many still are, dreary looking. In New York City, with a network of 329 senior centers, about half of them are underused, with the mean age of participants rising each year. Mayor Michael Bloomberg wanted to modernize the centers, adding cafes and programs more responsive to today's seniors and the boomers entering the ranks of older adults. These programs would include the latest in exercise fads and health education, and a focus on getting those age 55 to 65 to change their negative views of senior centers.

Conversely, some of the senior centers around the country are excellent places to go to access innovative, health-promoting activities, and I provide summaries of three of these senior centers that I visited when I lived in Texas. The *Geriatric Wellness Center of Collin County* (formerly the Maurice Barnett Geriatric Wellness Center) offers a wide array of health programs, including health assessments, medical screenings and immunizations, health education, caregiving programs, and support groups. In addition, this senior center is unique in three ways: (1) it identifies itself as a comprehensive wellness center to the community, (2) it provides a leadership role for older adults on its board of directors, (3) it matches trained volunteers to older adults discharged from a medical center to provide short-term practical support. Contact Wellness Center for Older Adults of Collin County, 401 W. l6th St. #600, Plano, TX 75075; 972-941-7335; www.gwccc.org.

Retirees not only crafted the native stone wall outside of the *Comal County Senior Citizens Center* but, after a flood, they disassembled, hand-sanded, and reassembled into squares thousands of inch-long pieces of wood for the parquet tile floor. Retirees continue to make contributions to this senior center, including the operation of a thrift shop that provides considerable revenue for center activities. It also has an excellent fitness center. Contact the Comal County Senior Citizens Center, 655 Landa St., New Braunfels, TX 78130; 830-629-4547; www.nbsenior.org.

The *Galveston County Multipurpose Senior Center* offers a variety of health programs, including exercise and country-western dance classes. One innovative aspect of this senior center was an effort 20 years ago to develop leadership among the attending older adults through a senior leadership training program (Grasso & Haber, 1995). However, this effort was phased out after a few years. For more information, contact the Galveston County Multipurpose Senior Center, 2201 Ave. L, Galveston, TX 77550; 409-770-6268.

The *Mather Cafés* are located in the northwest section of Chicago and are based on the premise that there will be nothing in the name, décor, or menu that cries "senior center." The cafe component is stylish, with an open kitchen and inventive foods and drinks that caters to (and is open to) all age groups. It is a neighborhood place, not a senior site. The programs, however, are designed for older adults, ranging from gentle yoga for those with arthritis to computers for shopping online and keeping up with grandchildren. The Mather Cafés are not for retirement, but rather, in their words, for repriorment. Contact the Mather Cafés at www.matherlifeways.com; or the Mather LifeWays Institute on Aging at 888-722-6468. This is an institute that has created ways for older adults to age well, and it has launched a national initiative for educating professionals who serve them.

Religious Institutions

The church, synagogue, or mosque has the potential to be one of the most important sources of health-promoting programs in the community. Congregational members share values, beliefs, traditions, cultural bonds, and the trust and respect that these engender. Among minority groups, religious institutions may be the only community organizations deemed trustworthy of providing health information and social support (Williams, 1996). In addition, religious institutions are able to connect with hard-to-reach older adults, who may be isolated from other sources of health care.

Religious institutions are often called upon to provide a wide array of educational, counseling, and social support services for those persons who are least served by health care institutions: minorities and the poor. It would entail only a small additional step—collaboration with health professionals—for many of these institutions to be able to implement medical screenings and health education programs. Yet the immense potential contribution of religious institutions toward the health promotion of congregation members remains substantially untapped.

More than 80% of Americans past age 65 claim their religious faith is the most important influence in their lives. Of the 5 million persons age 65 and over who do unpaid volunteer work, more than 40% perform most of their volunteer work at religious organizations. According to the U.S. Department of Labor, these older volunteers tend to put in more hours per week and more weeks per year than do younger volunteer workers. Many of these older volunteers could be trained to provide health-promoting services to their peers.

Health programs implemented at religious institutions have contributed to the health of congregation members in a variety of ways. These programs, for example, have improved mammography adherence (Sauaia et al., 2007), prostate cancer screening (Husaini et al., 2008), diabetes and hypertension screening (Boltri et al., 2008), short-term metabolic control (Samuel-Hodge et al., 2009), fruit and vegetable intake (Thorogood, Simera, Dowler, Summerbell, & Brunner, 2007), and weight reduction (Quinn & McNabb, 2001). Many religious institutions have broadened their mission to include mental health–promoting services. Surveys of self-help groups, for instance, reveal that churches and synagogues far exceed any other type of host community site.

Finally, there is the growing role of *parish nurses* (or faith community nurses). Typically, parish nurses are members of a congregation who are either volunteers or salaried part time, and who engage in health screening, health counseling, grief support groups, and community referrals. Though most parish nurses report prior work experience in health settings, only about half of them hold at least a baccalaureate degree in nursing. Many parish nurses focus on the relation between faith and health, and they and their congregational clients are disproportionately over the age of 55. Parish nurses also can provide services that are not accessible in much of the traditional health care system—community case management, community advocacy, and community health education (McGinnis & Zoske, 2008).

The Shepherd's Centers of America

The *Shepherd's Centers of America* is a national association of interfaith organizations, typically housed in local neighborhood congregations that offer older persons an array of educational courses, services, and resources with a wellness approach. Formed in Kansas City, Missouri, in 1972 by Dr. Elbert Cole, this organization originally consisted of six men who delivered hot meals to seven homebound women. In 2011 the organization had 52 centers, 9,000 volunteers, 26,000 persons receiving educational services, and 35,000 older adults receiving caregiving services. The centers provide health education, life enrichment and life review classes, caregiver seminars, bereavement support, exercise and nutrition classes, medical screenings, medication seminars, peer support groups, transportation services, respite care programs, advocacy, and other activities.

The empowerment philosophy of the Shepherd's Centers is embodied in the saying "No one should do for older persons what they can do for themselves." For information on how to join or start a program, contact the Shepherd's Centers of America, One W. Armour Blvd., #305, Kansas City, MO 64111; or contact Sarah Cheney at 816-960-2022; or go to the website, www.shepherdcenters.org.

Other National Resources With a Focus on Religion and Aging

Starting in 1983 as the Interfaith Volunteer Caregivers Program (Haber, 1988b), and continuing in 1993 as the *Faith in Action (FIA) Program*, this Robert Wood Johnson Foundation (RWJF) initiative supported community projects that were designed to expand and support the caregivers of the nation's elders. FIA shared a step-by-step approach to link members of a congregation, or of multiple congregations, in a specific geographic area into a single program to meet specific caregiving needs of older congregation members and others in need. The goal of the project was to enhance the quality of life of older persons in the community who want to avoid premature institutionalization.

With the aid of start-up grants from RWJF, along with continued support and advice, 670 interfaith volunteer caregiver programs were implemented nationwide. In 2005 grants to help launch new congregation-based caregiver programs were discontinued, and in 2008 the 25-year sponsorship of this project by RWJF was concluded. To find out more about the existing network of volunteer caregiver programs, contact FIA at www.fianationalnetwork.org, or contact Rhonda Anderson at 304-907-0428.

The Forum on Religion, Spirituality and Aging is a constituent group of the American Society on Aging. The Forum no longer distributes its newsletter, *Aging & Spirituality*, but it does assist members who want to address their concerns about spirituality and aging. To obtain more information, contact the American Society on Aging, 71 Stevenson St. #1450, San Francisco, CA 94105; 800-537-9728; www.asaging.org. After accessing the website, go to membership, then constituent groups, then the Forum on Religion, Spirituality and Aging.

There is also a journal called the *Journal of Religion, Spirituality & Aging*, which is an interdisciplinary, interfaith professional journal focused on the field of religious gerontology. To obtain information on this journal, contact the editor, James Ellor, Director of the Institute of Gerontological Studies, Baylor University School of Social Work, One Bear Place, Waco, TX 76798-7320.

Worksite Wellness

In 1987, in Omaha, Nebraska, the *Wellness Councils of America* (WELCOA) was founded for the purpose of developing community-based wellness councils to encourage health promotion activities at the worksite. The growth of these councils in cities across America peaked in 1993 with 40 such councils, but the focus has shifted now to membership services rather than councils. There are 5,000 companies that have WELCOA membership, 3,100 employees with national wellness certificates, and a magazine they distribute called *Absolute Advantage,* as well as a variety of how-to books for starting or strengthening worksite health-promoting activities. WELCOA's membership fee is $365 a year.

During the first two decades of WELCOA, there was little emphasis on the health of the *older* worker, despite efforts to encourage such a focus (Haber & Wicht, 1987). Briefly, in 2003–2004, WELCOA included a column in its newsletter that focused on the wellness of aging workers. For additional information on WELCOA, contact David Hunnicutt, President, Wellness Councils of America, 9802 Nicholas St. #315, Omaha, NE 68114; 402-827-3590; www.welcoa.org.

In general, corporate leaders believe wellness programs have both health benefits for their employees and financial benefits for their organization. They have become more knowledgeable about the studies that have correlated participation in *worksite wellness* programs with lower absenteeism and tardiness, fewer medical insurance and disability compensation claims, increased productivity due to higher morale, and lower turnover rates. Almost 20 years ago two meta-analyses (evaluating 51 worksite health programs in total) each reported only one worksite wellness program failing to report a positive return on investment (Pelletier, 1996; Stokols, Pelletier, & Fielding, 1995). In general, though, clinical- and cost-effectiveness studies have rarely employed the gold standard of research methodology—randomized clinical trials (Pelletier, 2009). Thus, some may remain unconvinced.

One of the pioneers in worksite wellness was Johnson & Johnson, the nation's largest producer of health care products. It began its *Live for Life* program more than 30 years ago to improve the health of employees. Johnson & Johnson reported that participating employees became more active, lost more weight, smoked less, showed greater improvement in applying stress management techniques, and lost less time due to sickness. A similar program, Control Data Corporation's *Staywell Program,* began around the same time to provide nutritious foods in the cafeteria and in vending machines, implement no-smoking policies, and provide on-site exercise facilities—and reported similar results.

When the cost of corporate medical plans rose 25% in 1991, some companies took a punitive approach. Turner Broadcasting Systems, for instance, attempted to lower insurance costs by firing or refusing to hire smokers and overweight people. A less extreme response was instituted by companies that raised health care costs for employees who engaged in risky lifestyle behaviors and provided programs to help them reduce risk factors. Hershey Foods employees, for instance, were required to pay $1,400 more in insurance costs per year if they became obese (I wonder if they got a discount if the excess weight was a result of eating Hershey chocolate bars), smoked, remained sedentary, or had high blood pressure or high cholesterol levels.

A positive approach began a short time later when Southern California Edison (SCE) offered insurance premium reductions or reimbursements to employees who underwent screenings or joined risk-reduction programs. SCE was motivated by an internal study that found that employees with three risk factors averaged insurance claims that were twice as high as those with no risk factors.

Both the punitive and positive approaches are still being used. If an employee in the state insurance plan in North Carolina smokes, or is morbidly obese and is not in a weight loss program, an additional 10% in out-of-pocket expenses is assessed. Conversely, Alabama state employees are eligible for a $25 discount off their monthly insurance premiums if their blood pressure, blood glucose, cholesterol, and weight are in the normal range, or if they are actively addressing risk factors in these areas.

One of the major shortcomings of on-site worksite wellness programs has been the tendency for those who need these programs the least—the younger and healthier workers—to utilize them the most. This is due, in part, to the youth of staff members. At General Electric, Campbell Soup, and Johnson & Johnson, the average age of wellness staff members was less than 30. Unless trained or self-educated, youth-oriented fitness center staff will not understand the special needs, interests, and motivations of older employees.

An estimated three fourths of major employers offered preretirement programs that included a wellness component. Even more encouraging, many of these companies do not wait until employees reach their 60s but reach out to employees in their 40s and 50s as well. At the other end of the spectrum, about 15% of companies with wellness programs permit retirees to participate. Retirees may be excluded from worksite wellness programs, however, for such reasons as space limitations, added staff costs, and possible legal liability.

Educational Programs

Less than 9 months after *Elderhostel* renamed itself *Exploritas* it was renamed *Road Scholar*. The first name change was an attempt to rid itself of "elder" in the name and appeal more to younger persons, particularly the huge cohort of baby boomers in their late 40s, 50s, and early 60s. As the average age of an Elderhostel client jumped to 72 in 2008, the number of participants had dropped from 260,000 in 1999 to 155,000 in 2008.

The second name change was due to copyright infringement on the name Exploritas.

Road Scholar (and I'm keeping my fingers crossed that this name sticks by the time you read this), was formerly just a part of Elderhostel, and an attempt to appeal to younger persons with itineraries that offer less structure, more free time, and smaller group sizes (20 people instead of 40) than had been traditional in the past.

Instead of trips limited to those age 55 and over (though younger companions and spouses have always been allowed), the Road Scholar is for anyone age 21 and older. Examples of the new educational travel programs include meeting with Buddhist monks in a monastery in Cambodia and taking a West Virginia rafting trip that includes education about Appalachia. This international program arranges low-cost travel, room and board, and an array of 10,000 educational programs located at more than 1,600 universities, museums, state and national parks, and other community sites throughout the United States, as well as 90 other countries.

There are no homework assignments, no examinations, and no grades. The emphasis is on thought-provoking and challenging programs. Typically, noncredit college courses are 1 to 3 weeks long. Expenses tend to average about $100 a day and are all-inclusive. The older students may live in dormitories and eat in college dining halls, though increasingly they reside in more comfortable lodging in the community. Classes frequently are taught by college faculty and cover many different types of subjects such as music, art, religion, history, health, and astronomy.

Many of the Road Scholar programs are quite innovative. An interesting example that took place at Texas A&M University at Galveston was a sea camp that focused on the coastal environment and endangered species. During the 5-day residential learning program, the students attended classes, took sailing trips, and did netting aboard the *Roamin' Empire*, a 48-foot research vessel. Another program was intergenerational, in which grandparents who wanted to share an experience with their grandchildren (ages 9 through 12) participated in on-the-water activities during 5 days in the summer, and resided in dormitories on campus at night.

The Boston-based company has dominated the business of educational trips for seniors since its founding in 1975. In order to thrive in the future, though, the emphasis is to appeal to people across the age spectrum. For information, contact Road Scholar, 11 Avenue de Lafayette, Boston, MA 02111-1746; or call toll-free at 800-454-5768, or 800-466-7762; or go to www.roadscholar.org. Free catalogs of national and international programs are available.

There are more than 400 *Lifelong Learning Institutes* affiliated with colleges and universities in the United States and Canada. Typically, older adults provide free labor and leadership to these continuing-education programs (Manheimer, 2009). A related initiative is the Osher Lifelong Learning Institutes funded by the Bernard Osher Foundation. These 117 funded institutes are coordinated through a national office housed at the University of Southern Maine, and can be accessed at: http://usm .maine.edu/olli.

Community colleges around the country offer low-cost educational and health promotion programs for senior adults. One long-standing and comprehensive program is the College of the Mainland Senior Adult Program, which provides a variety of educational programs for adults 55+, including arts, crafts, aerobics classes, weight training classes, computer education, area trips, and long-distance travel. For information, contact Alesha Vardeman Aulds at the College of the Mainland Senior Adult Program, 1130 Delmar, La Marque, TX 77568; 888-258-8859, x8432.

Emeritus Centers are bringing retired professors back to campus. These educational programs offer retired faculty members a chance to socialize, discuss topics with fellow academics, teach a course or give a lecture, advise a junior professor or student, or even pursue scholarly endeavors. At Emory University, there is a discussion group for emeriti that focuses on late-life transitions such as relating to adult children, long-term care, and managing a sick spouse. In 2004, representatives of 40 universities attended the first annual meeting of the Association of Retirement Organizations in Higher Education (AROHE). The AROHE conference has been held biannually since then, generating increasing attendance with each new conference. Contact AROHE, University of Southern California, 3715 McClintock Ave. #220, Los Angeles, CA 90089-0191; 213-740-8921; www.arohe.org.

The second established emeritus center, launched in 1974 at the University of Southern California (UCLA started the first one in 1969), is considered to be particularly innovative and comprehensive. In 1993 it began offering retired scholars research stipends up to $2,000, and it also endowed an annual lecture that recognizes continuing achievements in scholarly publications. There is also an off-campus lecture program that allows emeriti to give lectures throughout Southern California. USC's center also serves retired staff members as well as faculty. For a description of USC's program—as well as one at the University of California, Berkeley—see Glazer, Redmon, and Robinson (2005).

There are also college-affiliated retirement communities that have sprung up in approximately 50 college towns across the country, next to such institutes of higher education as Notre Dame, the University of Florida, and the University of Michigan. In addition to socializing with former college classmates—though some choose to retire in communities affiliated with colleges that they did not attend—these retirees can attend classes at reduced rates or for free, and gain priority access to sporting or cultural events.

Finally, many universities offer free online courses to students of all ages, including UC—Berkeley, Massachusetts Institute of Technology, Carnegie Mellon, Utah University, Johns Hopkins, Notre Dame, and the University of Washington. To access these courses, as well as e-books, documentaries, and other materials, visit www. elearningsites.net.

Shopping Mall-Based Programs

OASIS (Older Adult Service and Information System) provides shopping mall-based educational programs at May Company department stores in 40 cities in 24 states, serving about 56,000 adults age 50 and over. OASIS began in 1982 through its founder and president, Marylen Mann, in collaboration with Margie Wolcott May of the May department stores. The founding site and national headquarters is at the May department store in St. Louis, Missouri.

There is only one paid administrator at each OASIS site, with considerable administrative responsibility assumed by older adult volunteers. The courses offered focus on mental and physical health, intellectual stimulation on a wide scope of subjects, and fun. Contact OASIS, 7710 Carondelet Ave., Suite 125, St. Louis, MO 63105; call Marcia Kerz, president, 314-862-2933; or visit www.oasisnet.org.

Given that there is a Jim Smith Society (for men named Jim Smith) and a National Association for the Advancement of Perry Mason (a fictional defense attorney on television who did not lose a case from 1957 to 1966), it is possible that America has a national organization for just about everyone—including shopping mall walkers. The National Organization of Mall Walkers once claimed 3 million members who were racking up miles in malls across America. Some of the shopping mall owners were enticing walkers to their malls with gifts, provided they accumulated sufficient mall mileage.

Not all has been bliss in mall-walking America, however. The National Organization of Mall Walkers, alas, appears to have bitten the dust, and there was a *New York Times* article ("Sneaker-Clad Army," 2001) that reported on a mall owner in suburban Chicago who was attempting to get rid of its older mall walkers. He complained that they rarely did any shopping and, to boot (so to speak), he believed that the walkers got in the way of the real shoppers. This story had a happy ending, though, as the mall walkers successfully advocated for their right to walk in this mall. They were able to accomplish this victory without the support of a national mall-walking organization.

Computer Education

Ball State University's Fisher Institute for Wellness and Gerontology runs a community center for older adults in downtown Muncie, Indiana. This center is a learning laboratory for its graduate students, who organize and implement a variety of wellness and learning programs at the Community Center for Vital Aging (CCVA) (contact www.bsu.edu/wellness). The first program implemented at the Center was *SeniorNet Computer Training*, a class for older adults to learn how to use a computer. Each of the computer classes at the CCVA had met its maximum enrollment over the first 5 years of the center's existence, and the older students who had completed their classes reported that they felt more connected with family members by learning to use e-mail, and more connected in general through access to the Internet.

SeniorNet is an award-winning national program, and the largest trainer of adults age 50 and older on computers. The organization began in 1986 with 22 members, and now has educated 1 million older adults at 130 learning centers in communities around the country. SeniorNet provides training for

Question: Can you locate a model health program in your community, oriented toward older adults, and describe it in sufficient detail to satisfy the curiosity of an interested older adult? Choose a program that is located at one of the following sites: hospital, senior center, AARP chapter, religious institution, retirement community, university, community college, Area Agency on Aging, or shopping mall.

teaching staff; offers hardware, software, and course curricula; and shares strategies with community organizations for effective marketing to seniors. SeniorNet also provides online computer courses, discussion rooms for computer users, discounts on computer hardware and software, and newsletters. For more information, contact SeniorNet, 12801 Worldgate Dr. #500, Herndon, VA 20170; 571-203-7100; www.seniornet.org.

MODEL HEALTH PROMOTION PROGRAMS

Although there is no certain method for determining whether a health promotion program is a model program deserving of replication, there has been no shortage of attempts to promote such programs through directories that include summaries of model programs and contact information. Many of the model health promotion programs identified in these catalogues have been developed over the years with the aid of federal grants and other funding sources, have gone through multiple program evaluations, and can be helpful to health professionals who are interested in launching or improving their own programs.

National directories of model health programs for older adults began in the 1980s, when a directory of 40 programs was compiled by the Administration on Aging and distributed by the National Council on Aging. Another directory was published in 1992 and included 24 model health promotion programs, which were selected by a panel of experts through a cooperative project between AARP and the U.S. Public Health Service's Office of Disease Prevention and Health Promotion.

A third effort began in 1999 by the Health Promotion Institute (HPI) of the National Council on Aging. The author of this book had two programs listed in their best practices manual: the Healthy Aging Exercise and Health Education program, which has been conducted in churches, senior centers, and other community sites, and is described in Chapter 4, "Exercise"; and the Health Assessment and Intervention program, which used health contracts/calendars and has been offered in conjunction with geriatric primary care clinics, and is described in Chapter 3, "Health Educators: Collaboration, Communication, and Health Behavior Change."

The National Council on Aging (NCOA) Center for Healthy Aging

The latest effort to list model health promotion programs is focused on *evidence-based programs*, with 16 model programs summarized by the *National Council on Aging's (NCOA) Center for Healthy Aging*. To obtain more information, contact the National Council on Aging, Center for Healthy Aging, 1901 L St. NW, 4th floor, Washington, DC 20036; 202-479-1200; www.ncoa.org. This resource center provides other healthy-aging materials as well, such as manuals, toolkits, and links to other healthy-aging websites, contact www.healthyagingprograms.org.

The center also serves as a support entity for the Administration on Aging's (AOA) Evidence-Based Disease Prevention Grants Program. AOA competitive awards were given to community organizations to develop and promote evidence-based model programs around the nation, some of which are described in this chapter.

Healthwise

The best-known older adult medical self-care program is a model program called *Healthwise*, located in Boise, Idaho. The Healthwise program relies mostly on the *Healthwise Handbook,* which in 2012 was in its 18th edition, and provides information and prevention tips on 190 common health problems.

The handbook includes physician-approved guidelines on when to call a health professional for each of the health problems that it covers. Some Healthwise community programs have supplemented the distribution of the handbook with group health education programs or nurse call-in programs. There is a Spanish language edition of the *Healthwise Handbook*, called *La Salud en Casa*, and a special self-care guide for older adults called *Healthwise for Life*.

With the assistance of a $2.1 million grant from RWJF, Healthwise distributed its medical self-care guide to 125,000 Idaho households, along with toll-free nurse consultation phone service and self-care workshops. Thirty-nine percent of handbook recipients reported that the handbook helped them avoid a visit to the doctor (Mettler, 1997). Blue Cross of Idaho reported 18% fewer visits to the emergency room by owners of the guide.

Elements of the Healthwise program have been replicated in the United Kingdom, South Africa, New Zealand, Australia, and Canada. In British Columbia, the *Healthwise Handbook* was distributed to every household, and all 4.3 million residents had potential access to the Healthwise content through a website and a nurse call center.

Additional information can be obtained from Donald Kemper or Molly Mettler, Healthwise, Inc., 2601 N. Bogus Basin Rd., Boise, ID 83702; 800-706-9646; or go to www.healthwise.org.

Chronic Disease Self-Management Program

Kate Lorig and colleagues at the Stanford University School of Medicine have been evaluating community-based, peer-led, *chronic disease self-management programs* (CDSMPs) for many years, beginning with the Arthritis Self-Management Program. This program has since evolved into a curriculum that is applicable to a wide array of chronic diseases and conditions.

Typically, each program involves about a dozen participants, led by peer leaders who have received 20 hours of training. The peer leaders, like the participants, are typically older and have chronic diseases that they contend with. The program consists of 6 weekly sessions, each about 2.5 hours long, with a content focus on exercise, symptom management, nutrition, fatigue and sleep management, use of medications, managing emotions, community resources, communicating with health professionals, problem solving, and decision making. These topics are contained in the textbook *Living a Healthy Life with Chronic Conditions* (Lorig et al., 2006). The program is delivered in community settings such as senior centers, churches, and hospitals.

The theoretical basis of the program has been to promote a sense of personal efficacy among participants (Bandura, 1997) by using such techniques as guided mastery of skills, peer modeling, reinterpretation of symptoms, social persuasion through group support, and individual self-management guidance. In addition to improving self-efficacy, Lorig et al. (2001) reported reduced emergency room and outpatient visits, and decreased health distress, fatigue, and limitations in role function.

The CDSMP is housed at Stanford University's Patient Education Research Center, 1000 Welch Rd. #204, Palo Alto, CA 94304; 650-723-7935; http://patienteducation.stanford.edu/programs/cdsmp.html.

With the help of the AOA Evidence-Based Disease Prevention Grants Program, the National Council on Aging's Center for Healthy Aging, and the nationwide network of Area Agencies on Aging, the CDSMP has gone nationwide. In the past 2 years 75,000 older adults have participated in the CDSMP. Under the Affordable Care Act, there is $10 million additional funding to implement the CDSMP. Finally, there is an online version of the CDSMP, with funding from The Atlantic Philanthropies, to help people with arthritis, asthma, diabetes, lung and heart disease, stroke, and other chronic conditions.

Project Enhance (Formerly Senior Wellness Project)

Senior Services of Seattle/King County began the Senior Wellness Project in 1997 at the North Shore Senior Center in Bothell, Washington. It was a research-based health promotion program that included a component of chronic care self-management that was modeled after Kate Lorig's program. The program also included health and functional assessments; individual and group counseling; exercise programs; a personal health action plan with the support of a nurse, social worker, and volunteer health mentor; and support groups. A randomized controlled study of chronically ill seniors affiliated with the Senior Wellness Project reported a reduction in number of hospital stays and average length of stay, a reduction in psychotropic medications, and better functioning in activities of daily living (Leveille et al., 1998).

The Senior Wellness Project represented a demonstration of a partnership among a university, an Area Agency on Aging, local and national foundations, health departments, senior centers, primary care providers, older volunteers, and older participants. Versions of this model program are being replicated at senior wellness sites around the country (80+ sites in the United States) and two sites in Sweden to test its effectiveness in a variety of communities, in an assortment of sites, serving a diversie of clientele. One study of this program demonstrated higher levels of physical activity and lower levels of depression among its participants (Dobkin, 2002).

The Senior Wellness Project converted to *Project Enhance,* which was divided into two components: Enhance Fitness and Enhance Wellness. *Enhance Fitness* is an exercise program that focuses on stretching, flexibility, balance, low-impact aerobics, and strength training. Certified instructors have undergone special training in fitness for older adults. Classes last an hour, involve 10 to 25 people, and participants can track their progress through a series of functional evaluations. Participants who completed 6 months of Enhance Fitness improved significantly in a variety of physical and social functioning measures, and also reported reduced levels of pain and depression. There was also a reduction in health care costs (Ackerman et al., 2003).

Enhance Wellness focuses on mental health, with an emphasis on lessening symptoms of depression and other mood problems, developing a sense of greater self-reliance, and lowering the need for drugs that affect thinking or emotions. Enhance Wellness typically consists of a nurse and social worker working with an individual. An analysis of the effectiveness of the program found that it reduced depression when measured 1 year after the program was completed, and improved exercise readiness, physical activity levels, and self-reported health (Phelan et al., 2002).

Project Enhance programs have been replicated in 28 states, with over 20,000 participants. To learn more about Project Enhance, contact Susan Snyder, Program Director at Senior Services of Seattle/King County, 2208 Second Ave. #100, Seattle, WA 98121; 206-448-5725; www.projectenhance.org.

Ornish Program for Reversing Heart Disease

Dr. Dean Ornish, a physician at the University of California at San Francisco and founder of the Preventive Medicine Research Institute, has developed a program for reversing heart disease that has been replicated at several sites around the country. Dr. Ornish has recommended a vegetarian diet with fat intake of 10% or less of total calories, moderate aerobic exercise at least three times a week, yoga and meditation an hour a day, group support sessions, and smoking cessation.

Dr. Ornish and his colleagues have reported that as a result of their program, blockages in arteries have decreased in size, and blood flow has improved in as many as 82% of their heart patients (Gould et al., 1995). A 5-year follow-up of this program reported an 8% reduction in atherosclerotic plaques, whereas the control group had a 28% increase. Also during this time, cardiac events were more than doubled in the control group (Ornish et al., 1998).

The applicability of Ornish's program to nonheart patients is still of uncertain utility. It may take highly motivated individuals (e.g., patients with severe heart disease) and significant medical and health support (requiring significant resources) for the program to be generalizable. It is exceptionally difficult, for instance, to maintain a diet on one's own with a fat intake of 10% or less of total calories. For additional information, contact Dean Ornish, Preventive Medicine Research Institute, 900 Bridgeway, Suite 1, Sausalito, CA 94965; www.pmri.org. As noted in Chapter 6, "Complementary and Alternative Medicine," the Ornish program and Benson's Mind/Body program are covered by Medicare for qualified patients seeking intensive cardiac rehabilitation.

Benson's Mind/Body Medical Institute

Herbert Benson is a physician affiliated with Harvard Medical School and is known for his best-selling books on the *relaxation response* and for popularizing the term *mind/body medicine*. For individuals feeling the negative effects of stress, Benson's program teaches them to elicit the relaxation response, a Western version of meditation. The *Benson–Henry Institute* for MInd Body Medicine's clinical programs treat patients with a combination of relaxation response techniques, proper nutrition and exercise, and the reframing of negative thinking patterns.

Benson's nonprofit scientific and educational institute conducts research, provides outpatient medical services, and trains health professionals, postdoctoral fellows, and medical students. The Benson–Henry Institute for Mind Body Medicine is located at 151 Merrimac St., 4th floor, Boston, MA 02114; 617-643-6090; www.massgeneral.org/bhi.

Strong for Life

The *Strong for Life* program is a home-based exercise program for disabled and nondisabled older adults. It focuses on strength and balance, and provides an exercise video, a trainer's manual, and a user's guide. The program was designed by physical therapists for home use by older adults, and relies on elastic resistive bands for strengthening muscles. The exercise program led to a high rate of exercise adherence among older participants, as well as increased lower-extremity strength, improvements in tandem gait, and a reduction in physical disability (Jette et al., 1999).

The program was developed at Boston University and is listed as an evidence-based best practice by NCOA's Center for Healthy Aging. To order a DVD, contact www.strongforlifeworkout.com.

The American Geriatrics Society/Foundation for Health in Aging (FHA)

The American Geriatrics Society is the leading professional organization for geriatricians. It developed the Foundation for Healthy Aging (FHA) to help older adults and their caregivers become active participants in their own health care. The website, www.healthinaging.org, provides a wealth of high-quality educational material that can be downloaded without cost. One such resource is *Eldercare at Home*, a document that helps informal caregivers meet the needs of medically or functionally compromised older adults at home. Another resource provides up-to-date guidelines on diabetes, incontinence, pain management, fall prevention, and other important topics. This information is separated into professional practice guidelines for physicians and other health care providers, as well as easy-to-read versions for patients and caregivers.

The American Geriatrics Society/Foundation for Health in Aging is located at 40 Fulton St., 18th Fl., New York, NY 10038; 212-308-1414; www.healthinaging.org.

Community-Oriented Primary Care

Over a 4-year period (1992–1996), I participated in two *Community-Oriented Primary Care* (COPC) interdisciplinary teams, one housed in a Public Health Service Section 330 community health clinic for patients who are indigent, and the other in a university-affiliated outpatient clinic (Thompson, Haber, Fanuiel, Krohn, & Chambers, 1996; Thompson et al., 1998). COPC refers to the activities of primary care health professionals who go out into the community on their own initiative to gain more understanding of individual clients, as well as the community from which they come. This contrasts with a traditional primary care practice, where individual patients seek medical care at a clinic site.

Thus, in addition to the traditional focus on the individual patient, COPC also makes the family and the community the focus of diagnosis, treatment, and ongoing surveillance (Nutting, 1987). The practitioner of COPC moves from the narrow, biomedical, physician-led, clinic-based, one-to-one form of medical care, to a new vision of providing health care that includes the social environment that shapes an individual's health and behavior choices.

The two most popular definitions of a community are (a) individuals who share a geographical area, and (b) a group of persons who share values and/or lifestyles. The concept of community from a COPC perspective, however, typically focuses on the community of clients of a health professional or health facility that has a specific type or set of health problems (e.g., diabetes, noncompliance, cancer, alcohol abuse). A COPC project also tends to take a broad view of community and to systematically examine the status or perceptions of the wide variety of community members who interact with patients (e.g., spouses, ministers, curanderos, pharmacists, peers).

In addition to identifying relevant persons in the community who can shed light on a specific health problem, the COPC practitioner reviews extant data or collects new data. The county health department or other city and county agencies may provide relevant demographic, social, economic, mortality, and morbidity data. Other sources of data include chart reviews of clients or surveys of residents in the community. Health problems in a local community that are documented through data and are of unusual magnitude tend to stimulate COPC projects.

Often, health or disease data at the local community level are compared with data from similar populations in other parts of the country, or with Healthy People 2020 data or projections. Another good source of comparative risk factor data is the Behavior Risk Factor Surveillance System (BRFSS) (www.cdc.gov/brfss). The BRFSS is a continuous telephone survey that examines patterns in eating habits, physical activity, and other individual behaviors that affect health. There is risk-factor data compiled in all 50 states and for selected local areas.

The goals of a COPC project are to (a) identify measurable objectives for reducing a health problem or the risk factors that contribute to it; (b) focus on health education, disease prevention, or health promotion; (c) inform providers and consumers that they have the opportunity and the responsibility to be advocates of change and to make the health care system more responsive to their needs; and (d) recognize that health professionals can be more effective in teams, including primary care physicians, clinical nurses, community health nurses, physician's assistants, epidemiologists, public health specialists, social workers, medical sociologists, and health educators.

Without a mechanism for reimbursement of its activities, the COPC model may have only a modest impact on the average clinical practice in the community. At least two abbreviated elements of the COPC model, however, can supplement any traditional clinical practice in a cost-effective way: (a) define a health problem that affects a significant number of clients, and (b) develop a small project in the community that systematically addresses this problem. The leader of the COPC movement to integrate community health and medicine has been Dr. Paul Nutting, Center for Research Strategies, 225 E. 16th St. #1150, Denver, CO 80203-1694; 303-860-1705.

> **Question:** Which one of the model health promotion programs summarized in this chapter is of most interest to you? Find out more information about this program (or a similar health and aging program), and describe it in sufficient detail to adequately inform a health professional.

A Model Health Program in a Chinese Community

I observed what may have been the best example of a model health promotion program—a self-led Tai Chi class—while on an early morning jog in China in 1978. Tai Chi is a nonstrenuous sequence of physical movements derived from the ancient Chinese martial arts. Tai Chi attempts to increase energy, improve balance, and enhance mental and spiritual health. The participants I observed in the community, over half of whom were older adults, had maximum accessibility to this program—they had only to exit their front doors. There were no fees to be paid and no professionals to depend on. Figure 9.1 shows people practicing Tai Chi.

FIGURE 9.1   Chinese Tai Chi.

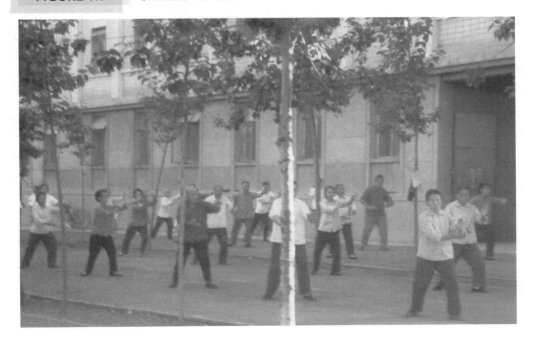

I later observed similar groups of older persons in China participating in Tai Chi in community parks (Haber, 1979). Since that time, several studies have reported that Tai Chi is beneficial for older adults with balance problems (Wolf et al., 1996; Wolfson et al., 1996), and it is now being taught at many senior centers and other community sites throughout the United States.

PROFESSIONAL ASSOCIATIONS

Health promotion and health education programs are sponsored by many disease-specific *professional associations*. The *Arthritis Foundation*, for example, offers several health education programs, among them self-help and peer support programs, including the Arthritis Self-Help Course, PACE Exercise, arthritis clubs, and aquatic programs. All programs are taught by trained volunteer instructors, many of whom cope with arthritis.

It is estimated that everyone over the age of 60 has some degree of osteoarthritis, and about 40% of older Americans recognize some of its symptoms. Osteoarthritis, the most common form of arthritis, is the gradual wearing away of tissue around the joints of the hands, feet, knees, hips, neck, or back. Arthritic pain may vary from mild to severe, and it may come and go. Arthritis cannot be prevented nor cured, but the function of arthritic joints can be improved and the pain often can be alleviated.

More than 100 local chapters of the Arthritis Foundation offer a 6-week course that provides information on medications, exercise, nutrition, relaxation techniques, coping skills, and the practical concerns of daily living. Practical information can range from the identification of places to purchase Velcro-modified clothing, to the location of aquatic exercise programs.

Many of the Arthritis Foundation programs were developed and evaluated at the Stanford Arthritis Center over many years and are offered around the country. Participants are typically asked to pay a small fee for courses and instructional materials. Besides health education programs, local arthritis chapters distribute free booklets on arthritis as well as information about most arthritis medications. For additional information, contact the Arthritis Foundation, P.O. Box 96280, Washington, DC 20077-7491; 800-283-7800; www.arthritis.org.

Many other professional associations also offer health education programs and materials. If you cannot locate a state or local chapter of a specific professional association, contact one of the following national headquarters for information on local educational opportunities and support groups, as well as for resource materials:

Alzheimer's Association (24-hour toll-free telephone link to access information about local chapters and community resources, free catalog of educational publications, and research program): 225 North Michigan Ave., Floor 17, Chicago, IL 60601; 800-272-3900; www.alz.org

American Cancer Society (education and support programs, workshops, transportation programs, publications, and financial aid): 250 Williams St. NW, Atlanta, GA 30303; 800-227-2345; www.cancer.org

American Diabetes Association (local chapters for support and referrals, outreach programs for minority communities): 1701 North Beauregard St., Alexandria, VA 22311; 800-342-2383; www.diabetes.org

American Heart Association (cookbooks, guides on treatment and prevention, and research funding program): 7272 Greenville Ave., Dallas, TX 75231; (800) 242-8721; www.americanheart.org

American Lung Association (education; advocacy; and research on asthma, emphysema, tuberculosis, and lung cancer): 1301 Pennsylvania Ave. NW, # 800, Washington, DC 20004; 202-785-3355; www.lung.org

National Stroke Association (survivors, caregivers and family, and medical professionals): 9707 E. Easter Lane, Centennial, CO 80112; 800-787-6537; www.stroke.org

American Parkinson's Disease Association (local chapters, educational materials, referrals, and research): 135 Parkinson Ave., Staten Island, NY 10305; 800-223-2732; www.apdaparkinson.org

Better Hearing Institute (information on medical, surgical, and rehabilitation options): 1444 I St. NW #700, Washington, DC 20005; 202-449-1100; www.betterhearing.org

National Association for Continence (advocacy, education, and support): 62 Columbus St., Charleston, SC 29403; 843-377-0900; www.nafc.org

National Association on Mental Illness (support groups, education, advocacy, and research): 3803 North Fairfax Dr., #11, Arlington, VA 22203; 703-524-7600; helpline: 800-950-6264; www.nami.org

National Council on Alcoholism and Drug Dependence (advocacy, information, and referrals): 217 Broadway, #712, New York, NY 10007; 212-269-7797.; www.ncadd.org

National Council on Problem Gambling (guides to counselors, support groups, and treatment facilities): 730 11th St. NW, # 601, Washington, DC 20001; 202-547-9204; www.ncpgambling.org

National Digestive Diseases Information Clearinghouse (support groups; referrals; and fact sheets on gastroesophageal reflux disease, hemorrhoids, constipation, ulcers, and irritable bowel syndrome): NIH, 2 Information Way, Bethesda, MD 20892; 800-891-5389; www.digestive.niddk.nih.gov

> **Question** Visit the website of one of the professional associations listed in this section. What is the most innovative or interesting component of this program that involves older adults that you can find? Please describe it and why you chose it.

National Osteoporosis Foundation (research, education, and advocacy): 1150 17th St. NW, # 850, Washington, DC 20036; 800-231-4222; www.nof.org

COMMUNITY VOLUNTEERING

The United States finds itself with two parallel phenomena that invite convergence. On the one hand, the country has vast unmet community service needs; on the other hand, the United States draws only partially on the large and growing productive potential of older people.
—Caro and Morris (2001)

Although many analysts see the rapidly growing older adult population in the United States in terms of being a financial burden on future generations, others see a vast, untapped social resource for improving the health and well-being of older adults and society itself. An AARP survey reported that over half of Americans age 50 to 75 are planning to incorporate community service into later life (Freedman, 2002).

The Bureau of Labor Statistics of the U.S. Department of Labor, however, reported that in that same year the volunteer rate for people age 65 and older was less than half of that (22.7%).

If the potential tidal wave of *community volunteering* could be unleashed, there would likely be greater fulfillment in, and purpose to, the latter part of the life cycle. A meta-analysis of 37 independent studies reported that the sense of well-being among older volunteers was consistently enhanced as a consequence of their volunteer efforts (Wheeler, Gorey, & Greenblatt, 1998). The authors also noted that while this mental health phenomenon was taking place, significant experience and energy were being directed toward the service needs of society's more vulnerable groups.

About a century ago, many services in America—education, law enforcement, fire fighting, hospital care, social service—relied upon volunteers. Over time, however, community services began to be dominated by paid personnel, with the more affluent obtaining services privately and the less affluent relying on publicly funded services. In addition, volunteering in the public sector became less attractive and peripheral to the main work of paid staff. Volunteer responsibilities were not only becoming marginal to the mission of public organizations, but when volunteers were utilized, they were often lacking in training, supervision, and recognition.

Marc Freedman, president of Civic Ventures, described the volunteer opportunities available to most older adults as "incapable of capturing the imagination of a new generation of older Americans." In his book *Prime Time: How Baby Boomers Will Revolutionize Retirement and Transform America*, Freedman (1999) argues that we need to "learn how to tap the time, talent, and civic potential of the group that is our country's only increasing natural resource." To accomplish this goal, volunteers need to be adequately trained and offered ongoing support, including stipends (Morrow-Howell, Hong, & Tang, 2009). Persons of low socioeconomic status report the most benefit from their volunteer experience.

Encore Careers, at www.encore.org, is a follow-up initiative by Marc Freedman to help individuals transition out of their work careers and into jobs in the non-profit and public sectors. Encore careers are those that are extended into personally fulfilling public service opportunities, providing modest but continuing income. Freedman (2007) provides many examples in his book *Encore: Finding Work That Matters in the Second Half of Life*. Encore careers have a positive impact on society's greatest problems.

Encore, along with AARP, has encouraged older adults to join the *Peace Corps*. Established in 1961 under the initiative of a baby boomer role model, President John F. Kennedy, the Peace Corps over time has been reaching out more to older adults. Beginning with Lillian Carter, former President Carter's mother, who volunteered in India at the age of 68, those age 50 and older now constitute 7% of Peace Corps volunteers. Older Americans can serve a traditional 2-year period or take part in shorter assignments.

Regardless of one's impact on the community, the volunteer experience seems to be consistently beneficial to one's mental health (Morrow-Howell et al., 2002). The beneficial effect of volunteering may be particularly timely during widowhood. People who have experienced spousal loss report a greater likelihood of volunteering a few years after the death of their spouse. The volunteer experience then appears to be protective against depressive symptoms while enhancing one's confidence in oneself (Li, 2007).

Another study reported that volunteer opportunities produce mental health benefits in nursing homes. These were not volunteer opportunities to help nursing home residents, but volunteer opportunities performed *by* nursing home residents. Residents from five long-term care facilities were given the opportunity to tutor students in

English-as-a-second-language. The treatment participants improved their psychological well-being in comparison to nursing home control groups (Yuen, Huang, Burik, & Smith, 2008).

Federal Volunteerism

The following community volunteer programs represent model programs that provide training, supervision, and recognition. Program evaluations, though limited, support the contention that these programs not only enhance the lives of the persons they serve, but also the mental health of the older volunteers themselves (Morrow-Howell, Hinterlong, Rozario, & Tang, 2003).

The *National Senior Services Corps* (also known as Senior Corps) was established in 1973 and is the principal vehicle for federal volunteerism for Americans age 55 and older. About 500,000 older Americans, most of whom are low income, participate in the corps and accept a small stipend for their effort. Volunteers serve primarily through one of the following three programs:

1. The *Retired Senior Volunteer Program* (RSVP), which matches the personal interests and skills of older Americans age 55 and over with opportunities to solve problems in their local communities.
2. The *Foster Grandparent Program*, which trains low-income adults age 60 and over to serve 20 hours a week helping children with special needs (for example, a seriously ill child with cancer).
3. The *Senior Companion Program*, which trains low-income adults age 60 and over to support their peers who are frail and disabled (for example, a stroke victim who is confined to a wheelchair and suffering from depression), in order to help them remain as independent as possible. In 2011, 13,600 older volunteers in 220 programs served 61,000 clients.

For additional information on these programs and other federal volunteer opportunities, visit www.seniorcorps.org.

There are two intergenerational programs that receive substantial federal support: Experience Corps and the National Mentoring Partnership (NMP) program. The goal of *Experience Corps* is to place adult volunteers age 55 and older in elementary schools and youth-focused organizations, particularly in the inner city. Experience Corps has 2,000 older volunteers in 19 cities serving 20,000 students, with the goal of going nationwide. Older adults who serve at least 15 hours a week receive a stipend ranging from $100 to $200 a month. For additional information, contact Experience Corps, 401 9th St., NW, Washington, DC 20004; 888-687-2277; www.experiencecorps.org.

Unlike the Experience Corps, the NMP program is not focused exclusively on the training and placing of older volunteers. However, many older adults participate in this program. The NMP program provides the information and tools that volunteers need to mentor young people in their communities. This organization has seeded and nurtured programs in 23 states. For additional information, contact MENTOR, 1680 Duke St., 2nd floor, Alexandria, VA 22314; 703-224-2235; www.mentoring.org.

The *Service Corps of Retired Executives* (SCORE), in conjunction with the Small Business Administration, helps retired executives and business owners who have the time to counsel younger entrepreneurs who are launching America's small businesses. There are 347 SCORE chapters with 13,300 older volunteer mentors who provide free counseling and low-cost workshops in local communities. SCORE consultants are in the 55+ age range and average 40 years of business experience. If you are interested in obtaining additional information, contact SCORE at 800-634-0245; www.score.org.

AARP

More than 70 years ago, the founder of AARP, Ethel Percy Andrus, said that the way to lead a life with purpose and meaning was "to serve, and not to be served." This tradition can be found among the large minority of AARP's 37 million members who volunteer annually. In addition, AARP has more than 3,200 local chapters dispersed among the 50 states, through which community service programs are implemented. These programs reach about 3.5 million people annually. To locate one of these local chapters, contact AARP at their toll-free number, 888-687-2277.

Three of the most popular AARP community volunteer programs are the following:

1. AARP's *55 Alive Driver Safety Program* is implemented by volunteers who are trained to provide driver education. This program helps older adults drive safely, and can significantly lower their automobile insurance rates. It has been offered to older adults for over 30 years, producing several million graduates. To contact, call toll-free 888-227-7669.
2. AARP's *Tax-Aide* provides free tax counseling and preparation service for middle- and low-income taxpayers age 60 and older. Volunteer tax counselors are trained and certified by the Internal Revenue Service. The Tax-Aide program assists more than 2 million people each year and is staffed by more than 30,000 AARP volunteers. Contact them at the toll-free number 888-227-7669.
3. AARP's *Senior Community Service Employment Program* (SCSEP) is implemented in conjunction with the Department of Labor. This program trains and transitions low-income older people into paid employment. There were about 100 sites in the United States and Puerto Rico in 2004, serving almost 22,000 people. To contact SCSEP at AARP, go to www.aarp.org, then enter Search: Senior Community Service Employment Program.

Question: Describe a volunteering experience you have had. Were you trained, supervised, and recognized? Was it a satisfying experience? How could your experience have been improved? If you have never done volunteer work, become a volunteer and report on your experience.

Founded in 1958 as the American Association of *Retired* Persons, it eventually became an organization with less than half of its members *retired*. Given universal recognition of its name, though, a compromise was struck and rather than giving up entirely on its name, it shifted to AARP. Anyway you call it, its influence is great. The bimonthly *AARP The Magazine* is mailed free to 22.4 million households with AARP members, the largest circulation of any magazine in the United States. Regarding its future, in 2014 every one of the 76 million baby boomers is eligible for AARP membership.

COMMUNITY HEALTH ADVOCACY

Gray Panthers

The best-known role model for community health advocacy in aging was Maggie Kuhn (1905–1995), founder of the *Gray Panthers*, an intergenerational advocacy group. I took a photograph of Maggie in 1978 (see Figure 9.2) on, literally, a slow boat to China, when Chinese relations with the Soviet Union were very strained. Ever the feisty one, Maggie

FIGURE 9.2	Maggie Kuhn, founder of the Gray Panthers advocacy group.

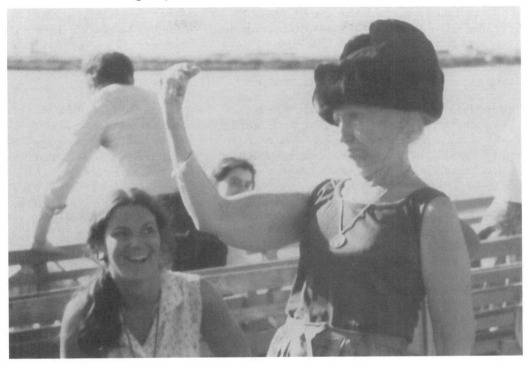

thought posing in a Russian hat might amuse our Chinese guides. The expressions on the faces of our guides, however, were inscrutable.

To find out about the advocacy issues that the Gray Panthers are currently interested in, contact Gray Panthers, 1319 F. St. NW, #302, Washington, DC 20004; 800-280-5362; 202-737-6637; www.graypanthers.org.

To purchase or rent an excellent and creative video on Maggie Kuhn's life, called *Maggie Growls*, e-mail orders@wmm.com; or visit the website at www.wmm.com. For an interesting review of this video, see *The Gerontologist*, 2005, vol. 45, no. 4, pp. 565–566.

Environmental Advocacy

Environmental advocacy is a strong interest among many older adults, perhaps as part of their quest to leave Planet Earth in as good of a condition as when they were born into it. Unfortunately, several environmental advocacy organizations listed in a prior edition of this book no longer are active. Perhaps that is the nature of advocacy groups involving older adults. They come and go.

One that still seems to have survived, though it has moved and changed leadership, is Great Old Broads for Wilderness, founded in 1989 by Susan Tixier of Escalante, Utah. She was concerned about motorized vehicles in designated wilderness areas, and rampant grazing and mining that were scarring the Utah landscape. She organized an annual hike (the Broadwalk), published a newspaper (the *Broadside*), declared that women members younger than 45 would have to be called "Great Old Broads-in-Training," and organized a variety of environmental advocacy efforts.

In 2003 the organization moved to Durango, Colorado, under the leadership of Ronni Egan and Rose Chilcoat. They now work with 22 chapters—called Broadbands—in nine states; they have become more inclusive, with the statement "There are broads of all ages and both genders in every state of the Union." For more information, contact: Great Old Broads for Wilderness, 605 E. 7th Ave., Durango, CO 81301; 970-385-9577; www.greatoldbroads.org.

Granny Peace Brigade/Occupy Wall Street

In a *New York Times* article (April 28, 2006, p. A21) there was a summary of a trial of 18 women between the ages of 59 and 91. Some of the women used canes, one was legally blind, and one used a walker. They called themselves the Granny Peace Brigade, and they had been arrested for blocking the entrance to a military recruitment center in New York City's Times Square when they *tried to enlist*. They claimed they wanted to join the armed forces and spare the lives of younger soldiers in Iraq.

The judge, sensing a public relations disaster, found grounds to claim that the frail older women had been wrongly arrested, and that they had left room for people to enter the recruitment center. When the trial was over, the Granny Peace Brigade sang the song "God Help America," composed by a member of a sister group in Tucson, Arizona, called the Raging Grannies. The song goes like this: "God help America, we need you bad, 'cause our leaders are cheaters, and they're making the world really mad."

On a related note, when Occupy Wall Street was active in the fall of 2011, Frances Goldin decided to join in, holding a sign that stated: *"I'm 87 and mad as hell."* She also decided to get arrested because she was fed up with the growing gap between rich and poor, and wanted to call attention to the issue. The police refused to cooperate. NBC reported that she asked one officer: "What if I socked you in the eye?" He responded, "I'd give you a free shot." Goldin followed up: "Well, what if I kneed you in the groin?" He replied: "You are *not* going to get arrested!"

Seems to me older adults can play a unique role on the front lines of protest movements.

The Long-Term Care Ombudsman Program

Long-term care ombudsmen are advocates for residents of nursing homes, board and care homes, assisted living facilities, and similar adult care facilities. Roughly two thirds of ombudsmen are older adults (based on conversations with state ombudsmen directors and my own experience), and about 90% of the persons served by ombudsmen are older adults.

Question: If you were to start up an advocacy group in retirement, what would you focus on and how would you go about it? What would be the advantages and disadvantages of recruiting older adults into this advocacy group?

Begun in 1972 as a demonstration program and continued under the federal Older Americans Act, every state is required to have an ombudsman program that addresses resident complaints and advocates for improvements in the long-term care system. In 2004 there were 8,400 certified volunteer ombudsmen and more than 1,000 paid staff who investigated 264,000 complaints made by 135,000 individuals. The most frequent complaint they investigated was lack of care due to inadequate staffing.

There are 53 state long-term care ombudsman programs that are linked to 600 regional/local ombudsman programs. About 75% of the states have included trained volunteers. For additional information contact the National Long-Term Care Ombudsman Resource Center, 1001 Connecticut Ave., NW, #425, Washington, DC 20036; 202-332-2275; www.ltcombudsman.org.

BenefitsCheckUp

BenefitsCheckUp was launched nationally in June 2001 by the National Council on Aging. It is the first national website for older adults and service providers to look for federal and state program benefits that older adults are entitled to, but are not currently receiving. The site includes information on more than 1,350 public benefit programs and has 40,000 local entry contacts. Seniors may be eligible for Supplemental Security Income, food stamps, utility bills assistance, home weatherization, vocational rehabilitation, in-home services, caregiving support services, legal services, nutrition programs, training and education opportunities, and so forth. In 2003, BenefitsCheckUpRx was launched, a national website to allow older adults to find out which of 250+ programs can help them save money on their prescriptions.

Users receive a printed report that tells them which programs they may likely qualify for and where to enroll. What may have taken the older consumer or a helper days or weeks to ascertain, BenefitsCheckUp can do in minutes. They claim to have helped more than 3 million people find $12 billion worth of benefits. To access this service, go to the website www.benefitscheckup.org.

BOX 9.1	Red Hat Society

The Red Hat Society is an advocacy group, but it is like no other. This group advocates for fun and a sense of humor. In 1997 Sue Ellen Cooper gave a friend a crimson fedora and a copy of Jenny Joseph's poem "Warning," which encourages old women to wear purple with a red hat that doesn't match. In some mysterious way, this led to a loose-knit social movement of 41,000 Red Hat chapters in more than 30 countries, with 1.5 million members. The chapters are for women age 50 and over who are willing to organize social functions and attend them in a red hat and a purple outfit. Many local chapters have adopted memorable names, like "Red Hot Mamas" and "RedNReady." The primary rule for each chapter is that the women who organize social events must attend them dressed in "full regalia."

To find out more, contact the Red Hat Society, 431 S. Acacia Ave., Fullerton, CA 92831; 866-386-2850; www.redhatsociety.org.

10

● ● ● ● ● ●

SOCIAL/EMOTIONAL SUPPORT, LONG-TERM CARE, AND END-OF-LIFE CARE

● ● ● **Key Terms**

social support and social network	informal versus formal caregiving
social/emotional support	nursing home and culture change
lay support	nursing home alternatives
online support	Eden Alternative
social networking	Green House
pet support and therapy	home care alternatives
religious or spiritual support	long-term care insurance
sage-ing	advance directives
peer support	POLST
empowerment theory	hospice
intergenerational support	palliative care
physician and allied health support	Buchwald phenomenon
long-term care	Death with Dignity Act

● ● ● **Learning Objectives**

- Differentiate social support, social network, and social/emotional support
- Examine the impact of social/emotional support on health and longevity

- Discuss whether there is more social isolation in America today than in generations past
- Recognize the involvement of boomers and older adults in electronic social networking
- Review the influence of pet support on the mental health of older adults
- Critically evaluate whether religious activity promotes physical health and extends longevity
- Identify aging and religious and spiritual resources
- Discuss whether health professionals should concern themselves with the religious beliefs and practices of clients
- Review the peer support movement and its implications for older adults
- Explain empowerment theory
- Analyze the role of health professionals in the peer support movement
- Discuss the strengths and weaknesses of peer support groups
- Cite examples of model intergenerational support programs
- Summarize ways to compensate for inadequate physician support with health objectives
- Define long-term care
- Distinguish between informal and formal caregiving
- Compare traditional nursing home care with culture change in long-term care
- Examine the variety of long-term care alternatives
- Review home modifications and home care alternatives
- Analyze long-term care insurance
- Examine advance directives and Physician Orders for Life-Sustaining Treatment (POLST) in particular
- Describe the growth of the hospice movement and discuss the barriers and opportunities for growth in the future
- Define palliative care
- Discuss your opinion of the Buchwald phenomenon and its impact on hospice use
- Describe and analyze the Death with Dignity Act

Most older Americans express a clear preference for spending their last years at home, surrounded by the people they love.

—*William Thomas*

This quote links the three sections of this chapter, as social/emotional support is the bedrock of good long-term care and end-of-life care. It's not just older Americans but all Americans who prefer home to institution, family and friends to staff, and comfort to unnecessary aggressive intervention.

DEFINITION OF SOCIAL/EMOTIONAL SUPPORT

Social/emotional support can be defined as the perceived caring, esteem, and assistance that people receive from others. Support can come from spouses, family members, friends, neighbors, colleagues, health professionals, or pets. The literature is rife with elaborate taxonomies of support, yet it can be reduced to three basic types:

1. *Emotional support* provides people with a sense of love, reassurance, and belonging. When individuals feel they are being listened to and valued, they develop a healthy sense of self-worth. Emotional support has a strong and consistent relationship with health status. Clearly, emotional support is the foundation of *social support* in general.
2. *Instrumental support* refers to the provision of tangible aid and services that directly assist people who are in need. Examples are financial help and household maintenance. Good instrumental support has been correlated with a decrease in psychosomatic and emotional distress, and with greater life satisfaction.
3. *Informational support* is the provision of advice, feedback, and suggestions to help a person address problems.

Social networks are defined in terms of structural characteristics: the number of social linkages, the frequency of contacts, and so on. Although the characteristics of people's social networks do not reflect on the quality of their social support, they do correlate with positive health outcomes.

There is a tendency, however, for social networks to shrink with age—older adults have about half as many friends and associates as younger people—because older persons cease relating to people who are not as close or important to them. With older adults, the quantity of relationships may decrease over time, but the quality of social relationships may be better and lives may be more satisfying (Lang, 2001). I refer to this as *social/emotional support* because, unlike social networks, it includes the emotional quality of the social support.

One study refuted the popular stereotype that older adults become more socially isolated with age. Although the size of one's social network declines with age, older age is positively associated with frequency of socializing with neighbors, religious participation, and volunteering (Cornwell, Laumann, & Schumm, 2008). The authors speculate that major later-life transitions, such as retirement and widowhood, may prompt greater social/emotional connectedness through other venues.

Social/emotional support appears to lower the risk of mortality in older adults (Eng, Rimm, Fitzmaurice, & Kawachi, 2002; Obisesan & Gillum, 2009). A population study of social and productive activities that involved little or no physical activity among older Americans reported that social/emotional support is as important as fitness when it comes to affecting mortality (Glass, de Leon, Marottoli, & Berkman, 1999). In the United States, older persons who were satisfied with the social/emotional support available to them were twice as likely to report better health as those who were not satisfied (White, Philogene, Fine, & Sinha, 2009).

Social/emotional support can be helpful in trying times. It can lower the risk of late-life depressive symptoms (Isaac, Stewart, Artero, Ancelin, & Ritchie, 2009), reduce anxiety and depression in older cancer patients (Lien, Lin, Kuo, & Chen, 2009), improve self-rated health after a disaster such as a hurricane (Ruggiero et al., 2009), and encourage older women to exercise while recovering from a hip fracture (Casado et al., 2009). Social strain, on the other hand, can discourage older adults with osteoarthritis from exercising (Cotter & Sherman, 2008).

Social influence may even affect obesity. One study reported that people with obese friends are significantly more likely to develop obesity themselves (Christakis & Fowler, 2007). Friendship, perhaps, provides permission to overindulge in an unhealthy consumption of food. This 32-year longitudinal study (part of the rigorous Framingham Heart Study), however, could not explain why obesity transmission is stronger in male–male friendships than in female–female friendships. Also, this finding may encourage additional blame on obese people and their choice of companionship, rather than on the overall environment in the United States that promotes obesity.

FAMILY, FRIENDS, CHURCH, AND OTHERS

Large-scale epidemiological studies have shown that membership in a social network of family, friends, church, and other support structures is correlated with lower mortality risk. The classic research endeavor in this area, led by the epidemiologist Lisa Berkman, was a study of 7,000 residents of Alameda County, California. The research team found that residents who were married, had ample contact with extended family and friends, belonged to a church, and had other group affiliations were half as likely to die over the course of the 9-year study as those with less adequate social supports (Berkman, 1983).

Over the next decade, research findings on the relationship between social/ emotional support, social networks, and mortality were replicated by other large studies (Goodwin, Hunt, Key, & Samet, 1987; House, Landis, & Umberson, 1988; Williams et al., 1992) that controlled for other factors possibly affecting mortality, such as lifestyle, socioeconomic status, age, race, and access to health care. These studies have shown that social/emotional isolation has as strong an effect on mortality as does smoking or high cholesterol.

More contemporary studies have reported on the influence of social/emotional support, or the lack of it, on morbidity and mortality. For example, loneliness in people over age 50 greatly increased their risk of high blood pressure, comparable to the risk of being overweight or inactive (Hawkley, Masi, Berry, & Cacioppo, 2006). Inadequate social support among older adults is comparable to smoking and surpasses inadequate diet and exercise as a known risk factor for mortality (Holt-Lunstad, Smith, & Layton, 2010).

A spouse or supportive family member is very important in helping people adopt or sustain good health habits. Using 8-year longitudinal data from the Health and Retirement Study, researchers found that when one spouse improved his or her health behavior, the other spouse was likely to do so as well (Falba & Sindelar, 2008). These behaviors ranged from smoking, drinking, exercising, cholesterol screening, and obtaining a flu shot.

Another study reported that lifestyle interventions targeted at men and women as couples, rather than as individuals, resulted in a greater reduction in cardiovascular risk factors like cigarette smoking, systolic blood pressure, and cholesterol level (Pyke, Wood, Kinmonth, & Thompson, 1997). The authors reported that targeting the couple may strengthen outcomes through the mutual reinforcement of lifestyle changes.

Elderly, community-dwelling men and women were more likely to have obtained preventive care when they lived with their spouse than when they lived alone or with adult offspring. Specifically, those living with a spouse were more likely to obtain an influenza vaccination, cholesterol screening, colorectal cancer screening, routine physical checkup, and routine dental care (Lau & Kirby, 2009). Data from a focus group revealed how spousal support influences dietary changes following a diagnosis of type II diabetes in middle-aged and older adults (Beverly, Miller, & Wray, 2008).

An interesting study reported that the greater the marital strain over time, the steeper the decline in health for both men and women. When the researchers separated study participants into three age groups—those ages 30, 50, and 70—only the oldest group showed negative health effects (Umberson, Williams, Powers, Liu, & Needham, 2006). The researchers speculated that there may be a cumulative effect over time among couples unhappy with their marriage, combined with age-related declines in immune function and a higher rate of health problems such as heart disease.

The loss of a spouse or loved one can be quite severe and in one study the risk of a heart attack in the week after death is six times greater than normal (Mostofsky et al., 2012). The death provokes bereavement, which is accompanied by depression, anger, and anxiety, all of which can elevate heart rate and blood pressure and increase the risk of blood clotting.

> **Question:** Do *you* think there is more social isolation in America today than in generations past, and on what do you base your assertion?

Spouses as a source of support, though, are increasingly unavailable with age, particularly among older women. Although 84% of males and 67% of females live with their spouses during late middle age, the percentages drop to 65% of males and 21% (!) of females at age 75 and over. Fortunately, older women living independently manage pretty well psychologically and may fare even better than women living with a spouse, provided they have supportive relationships from other relatives and from friends (Michael, Berkman, Colditz, & Kawachi, 2001).

Adult children can be a primary source of social support for older adults, though their support for parents often has to compete for time and energy with their own needs and those of their children. Because of the limitations of spousal and child support, friendships take on increasing importance in late life. In one study, support from friends was found to be more important for preventing depression than support from children (Dean, Kolody, & Wood, 1990). In another study of 1,500 Australians age 70 and older, friends rather than children or other relatives were most important in lengthening survival (Giles, Glonek, Luszcz, & Andrews, 2005). Qualitative interviews with 40 unmarried women ages 40 to 75 led to the recommendation that nurse practitioners who routinely prescribed exercise to improve the health of older adults may be more effective if they enlist the support of older friends and other older adult peers (Dorgo, Robinson, & Bader, 2009).

| BOX 10.1 | Bowling Alone? |

In 1995, Robert Putnam published an article titled "Bowling Alone: America's Declining Social Capital," and then followed up subsequent criticism of his article with a book, *Bowling Alone: The Collapse and Revival of American Community* (Putnam, 2000). Putnam argued that both television and a generation that is less civically engaged than their parents has created more social isolation—to the detriment of themselves and society. His conclusion generated much discussion, including from those who argued that there has only been a change in type of social support (e.g., cyberspace, nontraditional small groups like book clubs and support groups, and prayer fellowship) in contemporary America, rather than the quantity or quality of social involvement.

The question of whether there is a trend toward less social support or to different types of social support in American society remains unanswered. However, Putnam's writing has emphasized the importance of monitoring social activity in America, and it has stimulated discussion on what we should do to sustain or improve it.

The variety of relationships to consider will be greater among boomers than is the case with the present cohort of older adults. Because of the boomers, the number of older people who *live together romantically*, for instance, more than doubled in the decade from 2000 to 2010 (Lin & Brown, 2012). Are these cohabitants friends, or something more comparable to spouses? They may not marry in order to protect their individual nest eggs to pass on to their children, or they may not want to jeopardize a pension or Social Security payment earned through a former relationship, or they may not want to be financially responsible for taking on the other person's medical debts, or something else may motivate them.

Another category likely to need more analysis is *divorce*. Only 10% of people who got a divorce in 1990 were over 50, versus 25% in 2010. Divorce and choosing to remain single have contributed to about a third of boomers being unmarried today versus just 20% at a comparable age in 1980.

LAY SUPPORT

Health professionals rarely take the time to assess the ways that ordinary people help one another, or learn how to strengthen the helping process that is referred to as *lay support*. Different terms and definitions are used to describe lay support, but the commonalties tend to crosscut these differences.

One such definition is that of *lay health advisors*, referring to "people to whom others naturally turn for advice, emotional support, and tangible aid. They provide informal, spontaneous assistance, which is so much a part of everyday life that its value is often not recognized" (Israel, 1985). A concept similar to lay health advisors is *natural neighbor*, coined even further back in history by Collins and Pancoast (1976), referring to people who are prompted by empathy or a desire to help others in the neighborhood, often through volunteer work at churches or community organizations.

Some lay health advisors or natural neighbors may not be as "natural" or as skillful as others, but are willing to participate in paraprofessional training programs to increase their skills and to better identify persons who are in need of support. Two such programs, sponsored by the federal government, are the *Senior Companion Program*, in which low-income persons age 60 and over receive a small stipend (below minimum wage) to provide companionship to peers in need; and the *Foster Grandparent Program*, in which low-income persons 60 and older receive a small stipend to provide companionship and guidance to children with exceptional needs, especially in hospitals, centers for those with mental retardation, correctional facilities, and other institutions that serve children. Government assessments of these programs and independent researchers report that in addition to providing benefits to the young and old in need, older volunteers improve their *own* mental and physical health as well.

ONLINE SUPPORT

There are thousands of different social support, self-help and health information groups available online. With appropriate cautions, clinicians may find these services to be a useful adjunct to their care. The American Self-Help Clearinghouse's *Self-Help Group Sourcebook* (www.selfhelpgroups.org) provides online information about 1,100 national and international self-help support groups for addictions, bereavement, physical health, mental health, disabilities, caregiving, and other stressful life situations. Information on starting and sustaining a group is also provided.

Patients are forming *online support* groups on a daily basis. Type in a disease-specific support group in your search engine of choice. Once you locate one group, you can ask participants for names of other relevant online support groups. To share symptoms, medications, treatments, results, and other medical data with people with similar medical conditions, consider PatientsLikeMe Inc., or CureTogether (www.patientslikeme .com or www.curetogether.com).

One helpful online resource is the *Association of Cancer Online Resources* (ACOR) at www.acor.org. This is the largest online cancer information and support repository (plus a few noncancer groups), with more than 160 groups representing more than 55,000 members. Interestingly, although patients can find *peer support* and health providers through ACOR, researchers are finding subjects through ACOR. Clinical research trials on cancer can often expedite their recruitment process through contacting ACOR (Dolan, 2007b).

When facing a serious illness, there are often issues relating to sex, incontinence, death, and other sensitive topics that may be hard to share with family members. Online support gives one the freedom to be more anonymous and, therefore, more candid. On the downside, chat rooms and bulletin boards are not monitored or professionally facilitated; on the Internet, there is rarely a professional expert available to intervene when bad advice, faulty information, or inappropriate support is being given.

Also, online support does not permit a warm embrace when you need it. It is not uncommon to spend an excessive amount of time on the Internet to the exclusion of being with people who are important to you, or meeting other significant responsibilities. Ironic as it might seem, there are Internet addiction support groups on the Internet to help people with such afflictions.

There are Internet sites that are national in scope, but locally oriented, and help people connect to each other on more than just medical or health concerns. One Internet company that makes a business out of connecting people to each other is *Meetup.com* (www.meetup.com). This organization helps people set up face-to-face meetings anywhere in the country to discuss politics, environment, caregiving, hobbies, and so forth. In its first 2 years—2002 to 2004—Meetup. com signed up 2 million users. *I-Neighbors. org* (www.i-Neighbors.org) helps Internet users set up neighborhood websites. This nonprofit initiative has helped 5,900 neighborhoods share information about local services, events, and personal interests.

The two largest *social networking* sites are *Facebook* and *Twitter*. (MySpace was the number one site a few editions ago, but has been far surpassed by these two sites.) Facebook began in 2004. It allows users to exchange information, growing to more than 900 million users worldwide in 2012. Twitter began in 2006. It allows you to send and read messages of up to 140 characters, and in 2012 there were 340 million tweets daily. Facebook is used more for relationship building, whereas Twitter lets you briefly know what someone is doing.

According to a survey conducted by Princeton Survey Research Associates, social networking use grew by 13% between April 2009 and May 2010 among persons age 18 to 29; but 100% among those age 65 and older. In 2010, 26% of older adults were connected to social networking sites.

An increasing number of boomers have joined Facebook, partly for the purpose of checking up on children, but increasingly for connecting with long-lost friends or to establish new ones. In 1 month alone, July 4, 2009, to August 4, 2009, the number of Facebook members who were age 55 and older increased by 25%, according to Facebook's Social Ads Platform (i.e., user profiles).

Another trend for boomers was to join their own electronic networking sites. However, most of the sites listed in the 2010 edition of this book, like eons.com, boomj .com, secondprime.com, and others, terminated rather quickly. A few like boomspeak .com and eldr.com have continued. The twin purposes of these electronic sites are for boomers to meet others with similar interests and as an information portal to topics of relevance for this age group.

MyWay Village (www.mywayvillage.com) offers a similar service, except that it is directed (a) toward older adults (not boomers), and (b) to a specific senior living community. This older-adult technology company helps seniors get online and not only communicate more effectively with other residents, as well as family and friends, but also keeps them posted on events at that particular senior living community site. This service is being offered to retirement communities around the country.

PET SUPPORT AND THERAPY

It is estimated that between one third and one half of all households in the English-speaking world contain pets, yet there has been limited empirical research on the effects of animal companionship. Though meager (and not rigorous), the research results that get published suggest that the positive effects of pet ownership on human health should be taken seriously (McNicholas et al., 2005). Many of the studies have focused on older persons, who are believed by some researchers to have the greatest need for companionship. For example, pet attachment among older women living in the community served as a mediating effect on the relationship between loneliness and general health (Krause-Parello, 2008).

Pet therapy in long-term care facilities reduced loneliness in comparison to older residents in a control group (Banks & Banks, 2002). A more unique pet therapy program teamed up mildly to moderately depressed patients with dolphins at a marine science institute in Honduras (Antonioli & Reveley, 2005). Compared to a control group who got the same relaxation regimen, minus the dolphins, the intervention group enjoyed longer relief from their depression symptoms, with improvement still evident 3 months later. The researchers reported that no side effects are likely with this intervention, though accidental injuries may occur. Conservationists argue that these programs may not be so benign for the dolphins.

The majority of the evaluations of pet intervention programs have not been rigorous, even to the extent of including control groups. Also, the positive effects of pet companionship have not been separated out from the fact that many community interventions incorporate pets as only part of a novel or intriguing activity. Many such pet support programs also involve children or young adults. One study, though, did control for other factors by comparing volunteer visitors who brought a dog to a long-term care facility to volunteers who visited without a dog. The former elicited significantly more positive mood changes in participating residents (Lutwack-Bloom, Wijewickrama, & Smith, 2005).

Although not particularly rigorous overall, the research evidence to date has been consistently positive and suggests that it would be desirable if more community and volunteer organizations would play a constructive role in increasing pet visitation and pet ownership. One such organization that does just that is the *Pets for the Elderly Foundation*, which pays the fees to 58 animal shelters in 30 states for adults age 60 and older to adopt a companion dog or cat from a participating shelter. See www.petsfortheelderly.org, or call 866-849-3598.

Other Pet Support and Therapy Options

In contrast to live animals is the unique (and not as heart-warming) idea of robotic dogs that was hatched by two researchers from the veterinary school at Purdue University. They pilot-tested robotic dogs with older adults in retirement homes, and reported there were positive psychological effects on the older residents. The researchers noted that the older adults not only responded well to the robot dogs, but also they did not have to worry about remembering to feed them or about being fit enough to walk them (Eisenberg, 2002). The downside of this experiment might be the novelty of the situation producing immediate results that do not survive more than a few encounters, and the less-than-ideal tactile sensation that the robot dog provides.

Although much less common than nursing home and retirement home programs, pet therapy programs based in *hospital units* under the leadership of nurses have been implemented as well. A pet therapy intervention with 50 hospitalized patients reported that patients had significant decreases in pain, respiratory rate, and negative mood state, and a significant increase in perceived energy level (Coakley & Mahoney, 2009). As is typical of many pet therapy programs, the research initiative did not include a control group.

There are organizations that promote pet ownership and visitation on a national basis, many of which—like Jeff's Companion Animal Shelter, which provided isolated older adults with companion dogs—survive only a few years. The *Delta Society*, however, has been in existence for 35 years. It is an international not-for-profit organization that provides training for volunteers and animals in visiting and therapy programs. Its program, Pet Partners, brings volunteers and their pets to nursing homes, hospitals, and schools. The society sponsors an annual conference and publishes a bimonthly magazine. For more information, contact the Delta Society, 875 124th Ave., NE, Ste. 101, Bellevue, WA 98005, www.deltasociety.org. To observe the effects of one visiting dog, see Figure 10.1.

FIGURE 10.1   **Dog from a pet companion program visiting an older adult in the author's community health education class.**

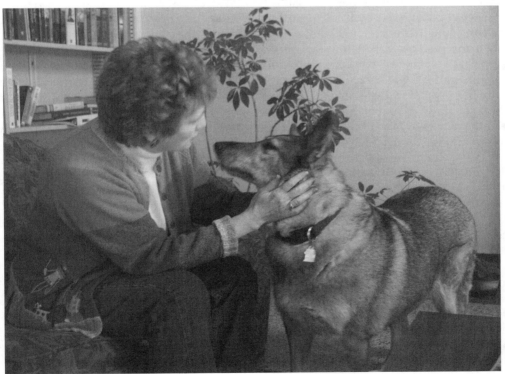

Another national program, called *Home for Life*, provides a sanctuary for pets if an older pet owner has to move into a nursing home or another residence that does not allow pets, or if the pet owner dies. The animal is guaranteed a home for life in this pet sanctuary. This program not only provides a safe and affordable residence for pets, but can arrange for travel to the sanctuary. For contact information, visit www.homeforlife.org.

RELIGIOUS OR SPIRITUAL SUPPORT

Religious and spiritual activities are often not differentiated in research, though when quantitative methods are employed the variables tend to be measured by way of religious beliefs or practices (Atchley, 2009). When a distinction is made, *spiritual activity* is more varied in its manifestations and focused on the internal process, whereas *religious activity* is considered to be more organizationally based and more traditional in its manifestation.

In the 1990s there was widespread belief that religious or spiritual people not only live longer, but they also have stronger immune systems, are physically healthier, and are less depressed than those who are not (Koenig et al., 1997, 1999; Larson, 1995; Strawbridge, Cohen, Shema, & Kaplan, 1997). The relationship between religious activities and good health remained even when researchers controlled for potentially confounding variables, such as chronic illnesses, functional abilities, age, race, and other health and social factors. Explanations for the positive relationship between religion and health included the impact of religion on healthy lifestyles (e.g., less addiction to smoking and drinking); positive and supportive social relationships; positive ideologies and prayer, which lower harmful stress hormones; and more stable marriages.

One interesting study during that decade on the effect of religious involvement on longevity reported that Christians and Jews tended to die less frequently in the month before their own group's major religious holidays (Idler & Kasl, 1992). Another remarkable—and considerably more controversial—study reported that intercessory prayer (praying long distance for others) was an effective adjunct to standard medical care, when analyzed as part of a randomized, controlled, double-blind, prospective, parallel-group trial—in other words, as part of an allegedly rigorous study (Harris et al., 1999). Patients in the coronary care unit treatment group, who were the ones receiving intercessory prayer, had lower overall adverse outcomes than control group patients. Even more startling, the patients in this study were unaware that they were being prayed for, and those who did the praying did not know and never met the patients for whom they were praying. (I'll get back to this later, hold off with making a conclusion here.)

A less controversial study on prayer reported that people who engaged in private prayer before surgery were more optimistic on the day before surgery than those who did not; and people who were optimistic before surgery for coronary heart disease recovered from surgery more effectively than those who were not (Ai, Peterson, Bolling, & Koenig, 2002). Conversely, sick patients who were pessimistic about their religious faith had a higher risk of mortality within 2 years (Pargament, Koenig, Tarakeshwar, & Hahn, 2001).

Harold Koenig, a physician and leading researcher on religion, spirituality, and medicine, reviewed 350 studies on the impact of religious involvement on physical health and reported that the majority of the studies support the finding that religious people are physically healthier and require fewer health services. Moreover, an additional 850 studies examined the relationship among religion, spirituality, and mental health, and about 70% of these studies reported that people experience better mental health and adapt more successfully to stress if they are religious (Koenig, 2000).

And Now for the Rest of the Story

Led by two psychologists from Columbia University, researchers now state that there is *no* compelling evidence of a relationship between religious or spiritual activity and health and longevity. The psychologists reviewed all 266 articles published during the year 2000 on religion and medicine, and reported that only a few demonstrated the beneficial effects of religious involvement on health (Sloan & Bagiella, 2002).

One of the common mistakes made by the researchers in the studies they reviewed—including the one on intercessory prayer—is the failure to control for multiple comparisons, commonly referred to in research as a fishing expedition. In other words, if you examine enough variables you will find some of them significant on the basis of chance alone. When studies with multiple dependent variables are statistically corrected for—a standard practice in statistical analysis when examining multiple comparisons—the significance levels of these variables commonly disappear.

The psychologists also noted that many studies were correlational rather than causal, and that religious behavior can be the product of good health, rather than its cause; and the lack of religious behavior can be the product of poor health, rather than its cause. In other studies that were examined, the analysts reported that improved physical and mental health functioning was based solely on self-report with no independent assessment; that researchers were not blinded to the data collection process, which can compromise objectivity; and that analyses of covariates that might explain the relationship between religion and health were omitted from many studies (Sloan & Bagiella, 2002).

One particularly rigorous study that supported these contentions was a 14-year longitudinal analysis that carefully controlled for potentially confounding covariates. Over this length of time, religious activity no longer had predictive value in terms of physical health or psychological well-being (Atchley, 1998).

Also, there was a follow-up study on the research that I reported on earlier, on intercessory prayer and cardiac bypass patients. This follow-up research took almost a decade to complete, involved 1,800 patients at six hospitals, cost $2.4 million in funding, and was rigorously conducted. The result: Prayers offered by strangers had no effect on the recovery of people who were undergoing heart surgery (Benson et al., 2006). In fact, patients who knew they were being prayed for had a *higher* rate of postoperative complications. This result may have been a chance finding, suggested the researchers, or perhaps it was due to the heightened awareness and anxiety over the realization that their condition needed to be prayed for.

The research battles wage on, and there are still some who believe religious and spiritual activities improve physical health or extend longevity. In the meantime, perhaps it is reasonable to endorse the idea that health professionals who work with older clients should be sensitive to their religious and spiritual needs and provide the time to listen to, and empathize with, their concerns. In addition, health professionals can strengthen the mental health of their clients by finding out whether they have an interest in, and access to, a pastor, rabbi, or religious study group. If the client is primarily home-bound, the health professional can encourage the client to inquire about receiving visits from volunteers at the client's previously attended religious institution.

Finally, it should be noted that religious activity may not affect all older adults equally. It may, for instance, be especially important as a source of social support for Black elders (Krause, 2008). Holding strong religious or spiritual beliefs appeared to protect elderly African Americans from contemplating or committing suicide (Cook, Pearson, Thompson, Black, & Rabins, 2002). Involvement in religious activity correlated with greater self-esteem and personal control in a sample of older African Americans (Krause, 2008). African American caregivers were found to be more likely than White caregivers to use religion as a means of coping and to receive greater consolation in the face of adversity (Ferraro & Koch, 1994). Finally, a national sample of 1,500 older adults, equally divided between Blacks and Whites, concluded that "older Black people are more likely than older White people to reap the health-related benefits of religion" (Krause, 2002).

Aging and Spirituality Resources

An important academic journal in this field is the *Journal of Religion, Spirituality, & Aging* (formerly titled the *Journal of Religious Gerontology*, and before that the *Journal of Religion & Aging*), which is published four issues per year by Routledge, the academic branch of Taylor & Francis, Inc., 325 Chestnut St., Suite 800, Philadelphia, PA 19106; 800-354-1420.

In an earlier edition of this book I described two model programs on spirituality and aging, neither of which survived for very long. A brief description of each program reveals how innovative they were.

1. Naropa University in Boulder, Colorado, housed a master's degree program in gerontology. This unique gerontology program focused on infusing future administrators of elder programs and long-term care facilities with the capacity for compassionate care. This program not only paid attention to the knowledge and skills required to be an effective gerontology professional, but also to the student's inner development and his or her attitude of service toward older adults. Alongside coursework, gerontology students engaged in contemplative practices like meditation and yoga.
2. The Spiritual Eldering Institute, which was also located in Boulder, Colorado, was a multifaith organization that focused on the spiritual dimensions of aging and provided a variety of workshops and other educational opportunities on this topic. The Institute sponsored a training program to help produce leadership in spiritual eldering. The impetus for this program had emerged from a book written by its founder and president, Rabbi Zalman Schachter-Shalomi (1995), titled *From Age-ing to Sage-ing: A Profound New Vision on Growing Older.* Although the Institute closed in November 2005, it was replaced by The Sage-ing Guild, a networking organization for approximately 300 professionals trained and certified in the Sage-ing philosophy, summed up by the phrase "Changing the paradigm from Aging to Sage-ing." For more information, send an email to info@ sage-ingguild.org, or access www.sage-ingguild.org.

A book suggestion for those interested in the spiritual aspects of aging is *Still Here: Embracing Aging, Changing and Dying* by Ram Dass (2000). Ram Dass, a well-known spiritual leader and former Harvard professor, suffered a crippling stroke while in the midst of writing this book, and the septuagenarian managed to eloquently integrate this experience into the rest of his writing. As he notes in his book, "These days I'm the advance scout for the experiences of aging, and I've come … to bring good news. The good news is that the spirit is more powerful than the vicissitudes of aging" (Ram Dass, 2000, p. 204).

PEER SUPPORT GROUPS

Growing older presents the challenge, for most people, of coping with chronic conditions—either their own or those of loved ones. A significant number of these people are discovering the benefits of belonging to a peer support group. Such groups unite people with common concerns so that they can share their ideas and feelings, exchange practical information, and benefit from knowing they are not alone. In short, they attempt to help members learn to live as fully as possible, despite the limitations that accrue with age.

A peer support group can be organized around a health-promoting theme (e.g., weight reduction, exercise, alcohol restraint, stress management, or smoking cessation), or it can exist to cope with almost any chronic health condition—Alzheimer's caregiving, cancer, arthritis, heart disease, lung disease, stroke, hearing or visual impairment, and others. It appears that seeking support is a higher priority for persons with stigmatizing illnesses or conditions such as alcoholism, breast cancer, depression, and widowhood, than it is for less stigmatizing problems like heart disease (Davison, Pennebaker, & Dickerson, 2000).

Peer support groups have certain commonalties: most operate informally, meet regularly, and do not charge fees. Most distribute leadership responsibilities among their peer members, and many involve health professionals in educating members. Peer support groups, however, can differ widely in the way they operate. Most Alzheimer's groups, for example, focus primarily on the emotional needs of caregiving members. Other groups may emphasize education, whereas others focus on health advocacy in the legislative arena. Some groups meet in an institutional setting, such as a hospital, with strong professional leadership that differs markedly from groups that meet in a home or church and do not include professional involvement.

Research on support groups, focused on older adults or not, tends to be qualitative. The samples are small, and few utilize a control group. The results are almost always that groups reduced isolation, provided practical information, and participants felt empowered. We know little about ineffective or damaging groups. Almost all the groups that I have visited appeared to be helpful to participants, but one that I attended included a peer leader who made inappropriate comments regarding medical care and medications, and expressed unusual ideas about what constitutes good coping practices.

By any standard, the self-help group movement is a phenomenon to be reckoned with. By as far back as 1979, there were an estimated 15 million participants in almost 500,000 groups, and growth has been steady since then. Three decades ago, based on a probability sample of over 3,000 households, self-help groups had already become the number one source of assistance to persons with mental health problems. More individuals in the United States participated in self-help groups (5.8%) than sought help from mental health professionals (5.6%) or consulted with clergy or pastoral sources (5%) (Mellinger & Balter, 1983).

Fitzhugh Mullan (1992), a physician and former director of the Bureau of Health Professions, suggested that newly diagnosed patients "... instead of simply going to that white-coated doctor and medical establishment (go) to people who have already 'been there' in some way ... people who have already had the condition, or who are coping with it."

Empowerment Theories

There are a wide variety of untested theories on how peer support empowers its participants. One way is through the "helper" principle: helping others brings mental health benefits upon oneself. Another way is through modeling behaviors: giving encouragement and advice to others may help us clarify our ideas and become increasingly conscientious about our own health behaviors. Yet another way that peer support groups may empower is through the exchange of information about community resources, assistance with transportation needs, and encouragement to be assertive with health care professionals and within the health care system.

Support group members may also empower each other by validating their feelings in a sympathetic environment and by developing new behaviors, attitudes, and identities. Support group members with medical disabilities, for example, may view outsiders as "temporarily able-bodied" or as potential victims of future disability, thereby questioning the superiority of others and enhancing their own self-image and ability to accept adversity.

The peer support group may also empower its members by providing them opportunities to participate voluntarily in group advocacy activities, to share leadership functions, and to work for causes that are larger than themselves. For example, one support group in New York City, Friends and Relatives of the Institutionalized Aged, blocked the New York State Health Department's attempt to relax standards for nursing home care, and pressured the New York State Department of Social Services into revising regulations to allow more residents access to nursing home beds following hospitalization.

Another example of advocacy in peer support groups was initiated by a member of the Self-Help Group for the Hard of Hearing in Omaha, Nebraska. One older man expressed frustration with a recalcitrant hearing aid provider who refused to stand behind his promise of "satisfaction guaranteed." The subsequent threat of picketing this provider's establishment by a dozen support group peers quickly led to the successful resolution of the hearing aid consumer's problem.

Age-Related Peer Support Groups

Peer support groups, at least theoretically, may be especially appropriate for aging persons who need chronic care and their caregivers. Age-related peer support groups may provide support when younger family support persons are geographically distant and/ or involved with their children. Declining birth rates after the baby boom generation means that fewer children and grandchildren are available to serve as support persons. Job mobility, retirement relocation, and neighborhood growth and renewal result in the dispersion of family, friends, and neighbors. An increasing percentage of women—who constitute almost two thirds of the caregivers in America—have entered the workforce over the past few decades and have reduced the number of caregiving hours available to assist frail older adults.

Butler et al. (1998) noted before the turn of the century that older persons tended to be reluctant to seek help from mental health professionals, due to a perceived stigma and an unwillingness to access large, impersonal, and highly bureaucratic organizational structures. This is likely to change with the new cohort of educated and more assertive boomers entering the ranks of older adults. Conversely, some mental health professionals perceived mental health problems as irreversible in old age, and were less enthusiastic about treating older adults. This too is likely to change as more health professionals are exposed to geriatric training and education.

In response to shrinking family support systems, I built a peer support group component into many of my earlier research and demonstration grants that focused on older adults and health promotion, health education, or caregiver training (Haber, 1983b, 1984, 1986, 1989, 1992a; Haber & Lacy, 1993). Some participants in these peer support groups continued to provide social support and practical assistance to each other for years after the funded project—and the participation of health professionals—had terminated. One health promotion class, for instance, continued to meet a decade later as a monthly peer support group. A member of the group sent me the letter that appears in Figure 10.2.

FIGURE 10.2	"Dear David" letter.

April 1

Dear David,

    You might already know - but the outgrowth of your classes is a continuation of socialization among nearly 20 persons. The "Prime Timers" are going strong - we meet once a month.
    We are never at a loss for agenda! April 24, we will meet at Kountz Memorial Church for Fred Aliano's famous spaghetti, and a relaxation tape to improve our mental health.
    Everyone sends love and we miss you. From your friends....

Jackie Devaney,
secretary for the day

Health Professionals and Peer Support

In its early years, the peer support movement met with resistance from many health professionals. The groups were labeled nonprofessional or antiprofessional, and were accused of potentially causing harm by "practicing medicine without a license." Fortunately, these attitudes have changed—indeed, many health professionals now initiate or are actively involved in self-help groups.

Peer support groups are best labeled as *non*professional, as are most individuals who comprise them. Although nonprofessional, peer support groups are rarely antiprofessional. The role of the groups is to complement the services of health professionals. A few self-helpers may rail against professionals, but the overwhelming majority do not. Self-help group members are just as likely as those who do not join self-help groups to seek, or to encourage other people to seek, professional assistance.

Peer support group members may help health professionals by meeting existing service gaps, uncovering new knowledge, providing the ongoing social/emotional support that health professionals cannot provide, and helping to identify individuals who need a referral to a health professional.

Health professionals may aid peer support groups by improving their effectiveness through training in facilitation skills, providing current research knowledge or resource materials, providing feedback through evaluation studies, and making referrals to existing support groups or starting new groups or peer pairings.

Many health science students come into contact with mutual-help groups during their educational process. Students who visit a single group, though, need to be concerned about whether they are adequately informed about groups in general. Groups differ in the unique personalities of their members, how they are run, where they are located, and so forth. What can students and health professionals do to educate themselves about peer support groups?

1. Visit different types of groups, especially those that represent problems that are typical of their (future) clientele. Most groups welcome observers who want to educate themselves.

2. Volunteer to make presentations to some of these groups, allowing plenty of time for questions.
3. Refer clients to these groups, and get feedback from them on the groups' effectiveness.
4. Start a specific group if none currently exist, or arrange for peer support between two willing patients. A person who has effectively coped with a health problem for a long time may find it satisfying to advise a newly diagnosed patient; and the newly diagnosed person may appreciate first-hand experience from someone who has successfully incorporated the health problem into a satisfying lifestyle.

> **Question:** Visit a peer support group and then describe your experience in neutral terms—respecting the anonymity of the participants—to an older adult. What is the older adult's opinion of the peer support group you visited, and what does it reveal about his or her attitude toward this type of support?

To find a peer support group in your community, contact your local Area Agency on Aging. If you cannot locate your Area Agency on Aging (because there are 629 of them, and few if any have "Area Agency on Aging" as part of their name) contact the Eldercare Locator, National Association of Area Agencies on Aging, at 800-677-1116, for assistance, or access the website, www.eldercare.gov.

INTERGENERATIONAL SUPPORT

Generations often live far away from one another. Grandparents and grandchildren may be both geographically and emotionally separated from each other. If personal interactions occur infrequently, they can at least be memorable. There were two travel companies that specialized in intergenerational travel (mostly grandparent/grandchild) that I listed in the last edition, both of which went out of business. Too bad. Neat idea.

Travel experts report that the best age for traveling with a grandchild is when he or she is between 11 and 14 years old. A grandchild at that age is old enough not only to appreciate the trip, but to be responsible as well. The child is also not so old as to be set in his or her ways or to be totally into his or her own thing.

Older adults can also be a tremendous source of support to children who are unrelated to them. The *Foster Grandparent Program* is a national program that trains volunteers age 60 and over to serve 20 hours a week with children in hospitals, shelters, and special-care facilities. Low-income volunteers receive a small stipend. For more information, contact the Foster Grandparent Program, Senior Corps, 1201 New York Ave., NW, Washington, DC 20525; 202-606-5000; www.seniorcorps.org.

The *Off Our Rockers* program is a model program that I visited and was very impressed with. It trains volunteers age 50 and over to visit for 1 hour with kindergarten through third-grade students in the Dallas area schools. In 2008, 91 older volunteers served 508 elementary-school students who needed individualized attention. For more information, contact the RSVP director, 3910 Harry Hines Blvd., Dallas, TX 75219; 214-823-5700.

In Bend, Oregon, through the Central Oregon Council on Aging, a *TECH (Teenager Elder Computer Help)* program was born (www.councilonaging.org). High school students sign up to teach local senior citizens about Facebook, Skype, smartphones, taking and sending digital pictures, and other tech challenges.

For information and ideas about intergenerational programs and projects, contact the *Center for Intergenerational Learning* at Temple University. The center has a toolkit for intergenerational program planners titled *Connecting Generations, Strengthening*

| FIGURE 10.3 | Older adult assisting student with her reading comprehension. |

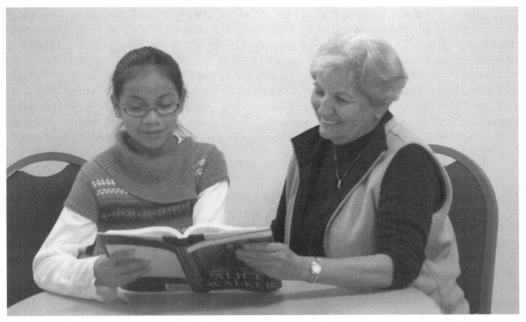

Communities. The toolkit consists of a handbook, video/DVD, and CD-ROM. Contact the Center for Intergenerational Learning, Temple University, 1700 North Broad St., Philadelphia, PA 19122; 215-204-6970; www.Templecil.org (see Figure 10.3).

To order a free copy of the *Intergenerational Projects Idea Book*, contact AARP Fulfillment, 601 E St. NW, Washington, DC 20049, and request stock #D15087.

PHYSICIAN AND ALLIED HEALTH PROFESSIONAL SUPPORT

Nearly 80% of the American population visits their physician at least once a year, with older adults visiting their physician more than any other age group (Federal Interagency Forum on Aging-Related Statistics, 2000). Because of their unusual degree of access to the older adult population, and the fact that 85% of adults say a doctor's recommendation would motivate them to get more involved in positive health practices, physicians are uniquely positioned to promote the health of older patients.

The physicians' potential for providing targeted social support to older patients and helping them change their health behavior is not being realized. National surveys of primary care physicians reveal several barriers to counseling patients on health topics and providing them support, including lack of time, training, teaching materials, knowledge, and reimbursement. With older patients, physicians are even less likely to discuss changing a health behavior habit than they are with younger patients (Callahan et al., 2000).

The Council of Scientific Affairs of the American Medical Association concluded that although physicians are well situated to play a leadership role in health promotion, they either do not act on these opportunities or are ineffectual in their daily practice. The council has suggested, therefore, that physician involvement with patient education should be embedded in a cost-effective framework by using allied health personnel and paraprofessionals to provide advice in small-group settings to reduce costs.

There is research support for the council's recommendations to use allied health personnel and to provide advice in small-group settings. Physician counseling to change the health behaviors of older patients has demonstrated more effectiveness when supplemented by cost-effective allied health personnel (Calfas et al., 1996; Goldstein et al., 1999). Clinic patients with similar chronic diseases who attended a group outpatient visit reported positive health outcomes (Beck et al., 1997; Clancy, Cope, Magruder, Huang, & Wolfman, 2003; Dorsey et al., 2011).

As part of funded demonstration projects earlier in my career, I created *physician prescription forms* to refer older patients to community exercise classes, and personally distributed them to interested physicians (mostly geriatricians). In this way, I have involved physicians with community health promotion projects run by graduate students in allied health, health education, and gerontology (Haber et al., 1997, 2000; Haber & Lacy, 1993).

LONG-TERM CARE

Long-term care is part of the final chapter in most people's life histories. It refers to the personal care and assistance needed on a chronic basis due to disability or illness that limits the ability of the individual to function independently. Perhaps the ideal goal for long-term care was articulated best by William Thomas, the founder of the Eden Alternative and the Green House (to be reviewed later), who stated that we should seek home- or community-based long-term care options developed on a cornerstone of love (Thomas, 1996).

The actuality of long-term care today, however, is still predicated on institutional care, which is based on rigid control over resident routines and safety regulations. As noted by Kane (2001), the "bulk of [long-term care] public dollars go where older people do not want to go." Despite the overwhelming preference of older Americans to remain in their own homes, Kane lamented that we spent 80% of public dollars on the care provided by nursing homes. Fortunately, in the decade-plus since Kane made these comments, there has been steady progress away from nursing home care.

Two thirds of the nation's 17,000 nursing homes are for-profit homes, which tend to be less concerned about quality of care and more concerned about keeping costs down and profits up (Duhigg, 2007b; Harrington, Woolhandler, Mullan, Carrillo, & Himmelstein, 2001). One study (Comondore et al., 2009) reported that not-for-profit nursing homes deliver higher-quality care than for-profit nursing homes, and if all nursing homes in the United States were converted to not-for-profit homes, residents would receive 500,000 more hours of nursing care per day. At the present time, though, about 90% of nursing homes have too few workers per patient (Pear, 2002).

Staff–patient ratios are not all that is wrong with nursing homes. One egregious example of cost cutting in a for-profit nursing home occurred in the Evergreen Gridley Health Care Center in Northern California in 2002. An investigation reported that this institution spent an average of $1.91 per day at that time to feed residents, about $1 a day less than California spent on food for inmates in state medical prisons. This was also about $2 a day less than the U.S. Department of Agriculture cited as the minimum necessary for a nutritious diet for older adults (Schmitt, 2002).

Treatment of dementia in nursing homes is also not ideal. According to Dr. Patrick Conway, chief medical officer for the Centers for Medicare and Medicaid Services, almost 40% of nursing home patients with signs of dementia were receiving antipsychotic drugs at some point in 2010, even though there was no diagnosis of psychosis. The inappropriate use of this medication was for the purpose of calming down agitated behavior, but as a consequence it also increased the risk of significant mental and physical health problems as well as an increased risk of death.

In eight states, nursing homes are encouraged to improve through incentives. In Ohio, for instance, almost 10% of the Medicaid payments to nursing homes depend on factors like residents' satisfaction, rates of medical complications, and the number of nurses on staff. The problem with these incentive programs is that standards are low. Ohio requires meeting only 5 of 20 quality standards and almost all nursing homes qualify for the incentives. The states argue that low standards made these initiatives politically feasible, and eventually they plan on raising the standards.

There are many good nursing homes in the United States, populated by dedicated and competent staff who alleviate the institutional and bureaucratic feel of these facilities. Yet remaining in one's own home is the ideal way to get long-term care as reported by almost all Americans. The problem is that adequate in-home assistance is hard to obtain and even harder to afford. We will, therefore, summarize a variety of long-term care options, some of which are innovative, attractive, and promising, whereas others represent slight improvement over the traditional nursing home.

But first we examine informal versus formal caregiving, and culture change in nursing homes.

INFORMAL CAREGIVING

There are only four kinds of people in the world—those who have been caregivers, those who currently are caregivers, those who will be caregivers, and those who will need caregivers.
    —Rosalynn Carter, former First Lady of the United States

Informal caregivers are family and friends who support their loved ones facing chronic illness or disability. They, not paid caregivers, are the primary source of help to the frail elderly. The Family Caregiver Alliance (www.caregiver.org) reports that if informal caregivers had to be replaced by paid services, it would more than triple the amount we currently spend on home health care and nursing home care combined.

Ascertaining precisely how many informal caregivers there are in America is a daunting proposition. On the one hand, the Bureau of Labor Statistics will include a grandchild as a caregiver if she paid two 20-minute visits to a grandparent over the past 3 months. On the other hand, many caregivers provide substantial help with household chores, like doing laundry, preparing meals, and shopping for groceries, but don't view themselves as caregivers and are undetected.

Given these limitations it is estimated that 40 million Americans over the age of 15 provide unpaid care to someone over age 65 because of a condition related to aging. Fifty-six percent are women, a smaller majority than found by past surveys by the Bureau of Labor Statistics; and female caregivers spend an hour more on elder care on their caregiving days than men do.

The most commonly used measure for the functional health of the care recipient is termed *activities of daily living* (ADL). This measure summarizes an individual's ability to perform basic personal care tasks such as eating, bathing, dressing, using the toilet, getting in or out of a bed or chair, caring for a bowel-control device, and walking (the latter being the most common ADL limitation for older adults).

Instrumental activities of daily living (IADL) summarizes an individual's ability to perform more complex, multidimensional activities in the environment, such as home management, managing money, meal preparation, making a phone call, and grocery shopping (the latter being the most common IADL problem). These limitations typically precede the limitations associated with ADL.

It is estimated that the average nursing home resident needs help with four ADL, but some care recipients who need this amount of help are still cared for at home, and well short of that amount of care, the strain on family caregivers and other informal caregivers can be substantial. Informal caregiving for an older adult often has a negative impact on health, personal freedom, employment, privacy, finances, and social relationships (Hooyman & Kiyak, 2011).

Yet even this onerous task has its intimate and positive qualities. Two separate studies of older caregivers stated that about 70% reported they had positive feelings toward at least one aspect of caregiving for an older adult (Cohen, Colantonio, & Vernich, 2002b; Wolff, Dy, Frick, & Kasper, 2007). Some of the positive aspects included companionship, fulfillment, enjoyment, and the personal satisfaction of meeting an obligation. One group of researchers went so far as to report that under some circumstances, caregiving behaviors are associated with *decreased* mortality risk among those caregivers (Brown et al., 2009). The lead researcher, Stephanie Brown, speculated that helping a person you love may relieve some of the harmful stress effects of seeing that person suffer.

There is a national trend toward increasing the amount of long-term care provided in the home, rather than in the nursing home. At the state level this has been manifested in *Medicaid Managed Long-Term Care* programs to shift the care of frail elders from nursing homes to homes. In addition, Congress allocated $4 billion in extra funds (over half of that amount through the Affordable Care Act) through a program called *Money Follows the Person*, which gives states Medicaid dollars to help this transition.

Also at the federal level, Medicare regulations adopted in October 2010 mandate that every 3 months every nursing home resident is asked *The Question*: Do you want to talk to someone about the possibility of returning to the community?" A later modification of this regulation stipulated that the resident can decline a quarterly question, and hear it only annually. If the resident responds "yes" at any time, a contact with an outside agency is mandated along with a discussion of how this might be put into operation. Obviously, the transition out of a nursing home is not always possible.

Yet, some progress has been made. At the turn of this century 73% of Medicaid dollars went to institutional care versus home or community services. By 2010 that percentage declined to 55%. One has to realize, though, that much of this decline in nursing home occupancy has been due to the expansion of assisted living facilities (ALFs). Although the cost is lower and the regulations less burdensome in these facilities, most people believe the clearest long-term care distinction is between living in a large facility like a nursing home or ALF, versus living in one's home.

To alleviate some of the medical strain on informal caregivers who attempt to keep older relatives at home, rather than transferring them to an institutional setting with greater medical oversight, there are increasing *telehealth* and *telecommunication* support options. Telehealth allows health information to be transmitted electronically from the person's home to his or her physician's office. Medication compliance, blood pressure, weight, blood glucose, and other vital information can be monitored. Technology can also transmit information to adult children, alerting them through motion sensors to unusual patterns of activity that might signal a health problem or emergency. (More on this in Chapter 13, A Glimpse Into the Future and a Look Back.)

For those who want information on informal caregiving, there is a website created by *AARP's Caregiver Resource Center*, and can be accessed through www.aarp.org/home-family/caregiving. There is also a hotline at 877-333-5885. Other resources are www.eldercare.gov (800-677-1116); www.caregiver.org (800-445-8106); and www.alzheimers.org (800-438-4380).

Informal Caregiving for Dementia

Owing to the protracted period of decline with Alzheimer's disease, older adults with Alzheimer's are at risk for abuse by caregivers, and caregivers in turn are at risk for depression, anxiety, and somatic problems. Nonetheless, about 75% of cognitively impaired older adults are cared for in a home setting, with limited outside support.

Cognitive-behavioral therapies, which help caregivers identify, plan, and increase positive activities for the patient, can improve the mood and reduce depressive symptoms of Alzheimer's caregivers and care recipients alike. These therapies are incorporated into a variety of venues, including caregiver education and social support, and can lead to reduced caregiver burden, depression, and dysphoria (Lee, Soeken, & Picot, 2007; Mittelman, Roth, Coon, & Haley, 2004). This support option can be effectively provided over the Internet as well (Marziali & Garcia, 2011). Caregiver support, in turn, can lead to the delay of institutionalization of older persons by almost a year (Andren & Elmstahl, 2008).

There is a reciprocal relationship between the health of the older adult, particularly the older adult with dementia, and the health of the caregiver. The more debilitating the person's dementia, the greater the mortality risk of the caregiver (Christakis & Allison, 2006). Conversely, when the caregiver of a demented person gets increasingly depressed, it increases the psychiatric symptoms of the demented person (Sink, Covinsky, Barnes, Newcomer, & Yaffe, 2006). Moreover, caregiver depression is not alleviated when the patient is institutionalized (Schulz et al., 2004).

An interesting facet to caregiving for dementia was reported in a recent Alzheimer's Association survey. During the past 15 years, the number of men caring for loved ones with Alzheimer's or dementia had doubled, from 19% to 40%. This trend paralleled the higher number of women over the age of 65 in the United States with the disease—3.4 million compared to 1.8 million men. The Alzheimer's Association also reported that these demographics have changed the tone of local support group meetings by adding a male perspective. This perspective is focused both on how to do caregiving chores well, and how to seek out appropriate help when needed. In turn, men are learning how to be better nurturers through these groups.

FORMAL CAREGIVING

Formal caregiving refers to paid caregiving in the home or in the institutional setting. In 1974, Congress decided to exempt paid domestic workers who provided services in the home from wage and overtime protections. The intent of the law was to exempt the babysitter or neighbor who provided the occasional support, but the law also included professional home care aides. This "companionship exemption" was finally rectified by Congress almost 30 years later when nearly 2 million home care workers were finally protected (Butler, 2012).

The irony of home health care workers averaging about $21,000 a year, and leading to 40% of them relying on public benefits like Medicaid and food stamps, was not lost on Congress. Also not lost on Congress was the projection by the Bureau of Labor Statistics that about 13 million older adults will need daily assistance to live outside of a nursing home by 2030 and the projected number of caregivers available to them would be woefully inadequate (Solis, 2011). Increased wage and benefits, and receiving a time-and-a-half premium when working more than 40 hours a week, may make a small dent in this increasing shortage problem.

Another problem with formal caregiving, though, is the lack of background checks at many health care agencies (Lindquist et al., 2012). A survey of 180 agencies in seven states revealed that some of the agencies resorted to recruiting random strangers off of Craigslist. Overall, only 55% of the agencies did a federal background check on their employees, 33% did a drug test (particularly problematic given that many older adults have pain medication, including narcotics, in the home), and only 33% administered a test for caregiver skill competency, including cardiopulmonary resuscitation (CPR) certification, lifting and transfer skills, behavioral management, cognitive support, or help with ADL. Only 30% of agencies sent supervisors to a home to check on caregivers, with some not checking with the care recipient at all, and most relying on asking the caregiver over the telephone about how things are going.

What about converting informal family caregivers into formal paid caregivers? One study reported that when states allow spouses to become paid personal care providers, there were fewer nursing home admissions compared with the use of nonfamily paid caregivers (Newcomer et al., 2012). The fear, of course, is that paying for unpaid family care would increase public costs. If it resulted in fewer nursing home admissions, though, this could be a cost-effective alternative for the state.

The Older Americans Act mandates that every state has a *long-term care ombudsman program* to help families and older adults navigate the bureaucracy of nursing home care, to mediate conflicts, and to advocate for residents and family members fighting for better care. The recommended caseload by the federal government is that each ombudsman is responsible for 2,000 nursing home residents. The national average, however, is responsibility for 2,500 residents. There is also a recommendation that each nursing home be visited four times a year, but this too is generally not met.

Ombudsman positions are funded jointly by the state and federal government and each program develops a system of recruiting volunteers to help make up for the shortfall in funding to meet the recommended standards for oversight. In 2010 there were 1,167 full-time equivalent paid staff nationwide in ombudsman offices, and 8,813 trained volunteers.

Although older people overwhelmingly want to remain in their homes, the availability of family members to provide care for them continues to decline due to smaller family size, greater mobility among adult children, a higher percentage of single-parent families among adult children, and rising employment rates among women. There are demonstration grants, both as part of the Affordable Care Act and through separate funding agencies, that are experimenting with adequate pay and benefits for both formal and informal caregivers to see whether this problem can be alleviated in a cost-effective way.

NURSING HOMES AND CULTURE CHANGE

Nursing homes are institutions licensed by the state to offer room, board, 24-hour nursing care, and therapy in a medical setting. There are also detailed federal regulations covering every aspect of nursing home care. Consequently, nursing homes are expensive, averaging more than $80,000 per resident per year. Despite the growth of the frail older adult population in America, the number of nursing homes is not growing. Instead, less expensive and less regulated options like ALFs are growing.

Despite the industry's attempt to change the term "nursing home" to "skilled nursing facility," the nursing home term still prevails. That's unfortunate. No one thinks a nursing home is a home. The needs of a large number of residents must be met, and this is done as most large institutions must do it, through numerous bureaucratic rules and regulations.

Large-scale food service, for instance, is not organized to meet individual preferences for food or how it is prepared, much less when and where residents might want to eat it. There are also rules for bathing, waking, sleeping, and even the choice, or lack of such, for a roommate. There are long corridors, medication carts, nursing stations, and huge dining rooms in nursing homes. Staff are not family; instead, they are underpaid and underappreciated workers. They take care of bodily and medical needs, and they tend to do it short-staffed in most nursing homes. Activities are scheduled and initiated by staff. Many residents have few or no visitors from outside. Precisely what about this description reminds you of *home*?

Culture change, or *person-centered care*, in long-term care is focused on choice, self-determination, dignity, respect, and purposeful living. As noted by the gerontologist Sonya Barsness, when she walked into a nursing home, there was a prominently displayed sign: "Residents do not live in our facility. We work in their home" (Stone, Bryant, & Barbarotta, 2009). Even with this conscious effort, institutions rarely look homelike, and bureaucratic relationships rarely encourage a feeling of shared humanity.

Nonetheless, the Commonwealth Fund 2007 National Survey of Nursing Homes reported that almost a third of nursing homes engaged in some type of culture change effort to promote choice and self-determination by residents, though only 5% indicated that they are completely engaged in this effort.

The *Pioneer Network* (www.pioneernetwork.net; also access www.residentcentered care.org and www.planetree.org) began in 1997 to advocate for more person-directed care, that is, long-term care models that emphasize flexibility and self-determination. The network sponsors workshops and conferences to promote caring and loving communities, no matter what type of housing it is located in. Perhaps the closest we have come is the Green House, one of the nursing home options to be described in the next section.

There are specific state government initiatives that could foster culture change in nursing homes. These initiatives cost money at a time when funding for long-term care is in short supply. Nonetheless, here are a few such ideas:

- Mandate increased wages and benefits, and better training, for nursing home aides to improve quality of care and reduce exceptionally high turnover rates.
- Provide financial awards to exemplary long-term care settings.
- Give stiff fines to owners of long-term care settings that consistently perform poorly.
- Require choice for nondemented long-term care residents when it comes to eating, bathing, waking, and going to bed.
- Eliminate forced roommates.
- Establish state long-term care clearinghouses for information and support.

NURSING HOME ALTERNATIVES

The basic premise of the *Eden Alternative* is that nursing homes should treat residents as people who need attentive care in a homelike setting. To accomplish this goal, nursing homes need to consider the involvement of pets, plants, and children (see Figure 10.4), and other amenities that make life worth living. Regarding dogs, cats, and other pets, they can live permanently with residents in long-term care facilities through some Eden Alternative programs. This enhances the bonding potential.

The Eden Alternative was initiated by Dr. William Thomas in 1991 when he was medical director at a nursing home in New York. Since then, more than 300 nursing homes have been registered in this movement (in the United States, Canada, Europe, and Australia). Studies that support the benefits of the program—lower mortality rates, urinary tract infections, respiratory infections, staff turnover, resident depression, and medication costs—are reported in Thomas's book *The Eden Alternative* (1994).

An Eden Alternative Train-the-Trainer program was launched in 1996. The 3-day program demonstrates how to create a long-term care environment that supports

FIGURE 10.4   The author's son visiting a resident in a nursing home (1984).

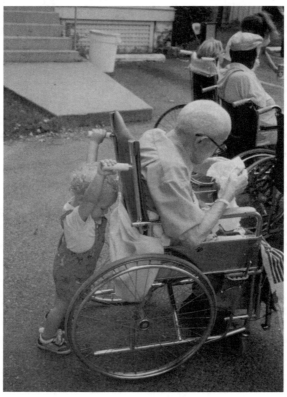

residents emotionally and spiritually as well as physically. To find out about the training, or the location of Eden Alternative sites in your state, go to their website, www.edenalternative.com.

A radical remake of the nursing home industry along the lines of the Eden Alternative, however, has been slow and difficult. Over the past two decades, the 300 nursing homes that have adopted some aspects of the Eden Alternative comprise only about 2% of all nursing home care in the United States. Moreover, most institutions remain pretty much an institution, no matter how much you humanize it.

William Thomas, therefore, moved on from the Eden Alternative to create the *Green House Project*, a home environment for long-term care. Small (10 to 12 persons) "Green Houses" are erected to serve frail older persons with skilled nursing needs who desire an alternative to the larger nursing home institution and the medical model. The Green House Project (www.thegreenhouseproject.com) takes place in a home—not a "home-like" institution.

Dr. Thomas and colleagues have implemented many innovations in these group homes, including architectural ones, policies for staff empowerment that help reduce turnover, and ideas to promote as much resident autonomy as possible. (More detail is provided in Chapter 13, "A Glimpse Into the Future and a Look Back.") If Green Houses can approach the cost of nursing homes, yet provide so much more in the way of autonomy and choice to residents, this could become the long-term care model of the future.

A more traditional alternative to the nursing home, ostensibly for those persons who are not at the level of nursing home care (though many are), are ALFs, which are currently the fastest growing alternative. There is no federal oversight, but about 85% of the states require state oversight and 60% require licensing. ALFs have room and board, 24-hour supervision, housekeeping, meal preparation, and assistance with ADL, but more autonomy and privacy, and fewer regulations, than can be found in nursing homes. The decline in nursing homes, at a time when the older adult population is increasing substantially, has a lot to do with the growth in ALFs.

> **Question:** What are three reasons that a nursing home administrator might offer in resistance to the idea of converting his home into an Eden Alternative? How would you address these barriers and help change the mind of this administrator?

The challenge for ALFs is that although they tend to be smaller institutions with fewer regulations, they are still institutional in appearance and bureaucratic in function. In many states they are primarily private pay and not affordable for most people of modest means. Also, the policies for transferring residents to nursing homes when health care needs become increasingly burdensome are typically unclear and can lead to confrontations among residents, family, and ALF administrators. For more information, contact the National Center for Assisted Living, 1201 L. St. NW, Washington, DC 20005; 202-842-4444; www.ncal.org.

There are about 2,400 *Continuing Care Retirement Communities* (CCRCs) serving about 750,000 older adults. The focus of CCRCs is on the private-paying client who may be independent at first, but may need more care and assistance in the future and wants to be able to stay in the same area where his or her spouse and friends remain. Many CCRCs have a large entrance fee with monthly maintenance expense, though there are à la carte arrangements that are fee-for-service packages as well.

The challenge for these "step-down" facilities is that when transferring from independent living to assisted living or nursing home care, the concept of remaining emotionally close in the same geographical vicinity as spouse and friends can be undermined by the different living circumstances, policies, and schedules among the different levels of care in a CCRC. Also, affordability is not even a possibility for someone making do on limited means.

HOME CARE ALTERNATIVES

Naturally Occurring Retirement Communities (NORCs), or *Virtual Villages*, are living facilities and neighborhoods that were initially designed for young families and healthy adults, but over time have turned into communities that contain mostly an older adult population. NORCs receive financial support from the state's aging network or through federal grants, and Virtual Villages are community-directed through self-imposed fees. These living options have increased to about 100 nationwide in an attempt to sustain accessible and safe housing and neighborhoods, as well as affordable places to grow old. Rather than having older adults transfer prematurely to supportive institutions, the support is brought to where the older adults are living.

In these communities residents pay yearly dues for prescreened home health aides, carpenters, cooks, computer experts, and whatever other help is needed. These self-help initiatives have proven effective in keeping older adults in place, provided the residents can continue to afford the services. If not, some states like New York provide additional financial support to intentional communities through NORC programs. The challenge is how to make these programs work for residents who are afflicted with complicated medical needs. More on this housing option is presented in Chapter 13, "A Glimpse Into the Future and a Look Back."

Granny flats—also known as accessory dwelling units, ECHO housing (Elder Cottage Housing Opportunity), or mother-in-law suites—are modified interior parts of a dwelling, or add-ons to the main dwelling, that allow for an older adult to have a separate but supportive unit to live in and yet be close to family members when support is needed. The challenge centers around zoning that attempts to avoid excessive population density in a community, that is, permitting "duplexes" where single-family homes now exist.

Adult foster homes (AFHs) are located in residential neighborhoods and serve between one and five residents. Costs are usually far lower than nursing home care, and resident autonomy is far greater as well as being in a home environment. AFHs are licensed and regulated. The challenge is that it is not always clear when, or if, the resident needs to be transferred to a more institutional environment because of the increased physical or mental decline of a resident.

The goal of *Guided Care* is to keep frail older adults in the home and reduce costs by delaying or avoiding hospital and nursing home care. It is based on a specially trained registered nurse in a primary care practice working in partnership with two to five physicians in order to provide high-quality care for 50 to 60 chronically ill patients with particularly heavy health care use based on prior insurance claims. The model includes assessing the patient and primary caregiver at home, providing them with a patient-friendly action plan, promoting patient self-management, monitoring conditions monthly, coordinating the effort of all health care providers, smoothing transitions between sites of care (particularly in and out of hospitals), educating and supporting family caregivers, and facilitating access to community resources (Leff & Novak, 2011).

At 20 months, Guided Care patients experienced 21% fewer hospital readmissions, 16% fewer skilled nursing home days, 30% fewer home health care episodes, with only 4% more emergency department visits (Boult et al., 2011). In addition, all participants ranging from older adults, to caregivers, to physicians, to nurses, reported improved quality of care. Guided Care will be expanded and evaluated under the Affordable Care Act.

Foreign-based home care has been an option for some newly retired boomers. Americans head down to Mexico or another location in Central or South America, where they rent an apartment, receive three meals a day, laundry and cleaning service, and 24-hour home health care from an attentive staff person at a fraction of what it would cost in the United States. An estimated 60,000 American retirees live in Mexico under these conditions. The downside to this home care solution is that you live in a foreign country far from family, and there is little government regulation to protect the consumer.

LONG-TERM CARE INSURANCE OPTIONS

Long-term care insurance plays a minor role in financing home care and other long-term care alternatives. Although estimates vary, the American Association for Long-Term Care Insurance estimates that 3% of Americans have long-term care insurance. This type of insurance is expensive, and premiums increase as the beneficiary ages.

There are numerous limitations in coverage, along with many other pitfalls. In California in 2005, nearly one in every four long-term care insurance claims were denied, many for technical and questionable reasons. Moreover, many policy-holders found the policy details to be confusing and not what they expected. This prompted an investigation in Congress by the House Committee on Energy and Commerce, which called for federal oversight of the industry rather than relying on lax state regulations (Duhigg, 2007a).

In 2012, long-term care insurance rates rose between 6% and 17%, according to the American Association for Long-Term Care Insurance. Plus, new policies were being written with even more restrictions to limit insurers' risks. The greater cost and limitations were based on greater unpredictability of claims with growing life expectancies and uncertainty over the prevalence and duration of Alzheimer's and other forms of dementia.

Exacerbating this problem were extraordinary declines in interest rates that limited the insurers' ability to generate financial returns on their income, sufficient to pay claims. Despite double-digit rate hikes and additional restrictions, many of the major insurance companies decided to drop out of providing long-term care insurance altogether, including Prudential, MetLife, and Unum.

From this author's perspective it makes more sense to build up a retirement savings account than to spend money on expensive long-term care premiums that are constantly going up with greater restrictions on what is covered.

An alternative to private long-term care insurance is a *public insurance program*. Shortly before he died, Senator Ted Kennedy and his congressional colleagues proposed the *Community Living Assistance Services and Supports (CLASS) Act*, part of the Affordable Care Act, which would create a premium-funded insurance program. Working-age adults could become eligible for a cash benefit after paying into the program for 5 years. Coverage could then be maintained long term by continuing to pay premiums. Despite the 5-year waiting period and the initial buildup of revenues, the projected premium costs would escalate rapidly at around the 10-year mark, leading to insolvency of the program.

Because it was belatedly decided that premiums costs would have to be raised significantly and perhaps benefits capped, the program would likely be less appealing to healthier and younger clients, making the program even less financially viable. As CLASS was a stand-alone provision of the Affordable Care Act, it was terminated before it was scheduled to be launched.

For those of us who support public long-term care insurance, it has become clear that the only option is for it to be mandatory and include more healthy and younger persons. It is not clear if this will ever become politically feasible in the United States.

Programs of All-Inclusive Care for the Elderly (PACE) is an integrated model of both insurance and care that targets individuals who are eligible for nursing home care, but are able to live in the community with the help of PACE supportive services. By combining Medicare dollars, state Medicaid funds, and individual resources, a more comprehensive range of services is provided, including prevention. Services and resources are targeted toward the home (e.g., grab bars and ramps) or provided at adult day health centers. There are 75 PACE organizations serving 23,000 people age 55 or over in 29 states. The average age of participants is 80 (Bloom et al., 2011).

The adult day health center is the heart of the PACE program. It includes a health care clinic, occupational and physical therapy services beyond what traditional Medicare or Medicaid would provide, and various other resources. The average PACE participant attends an adult day health center 2.5 days a week, with some spending 5 days a week if they live with a family member who works, and others attending only a few times a month (Greenwood, 2002a).

The upside to the PACE program is that more individualized care may be provided at lower cost (Wieland et al., 2000). Evaluations have shown that PACE can achieve a substantial reduction in the use of institutional care (Kane, Homyak, Bershadsky, & Flood, 2006). Outcome studies have reported that PACE improves functional status and overall health, and reduces patient death rate (Hansen, 2008).

The downside to this innovative program is that state governments must be active partners, and the financial risks of starting and maintaining a program are still not

> **Question:** Why is long-term care more of a health promotion issue than a medical care issue? Or, if you believe otherwise, support your position.

well understood (Greenwood, 2002b). Another concern is that some individuals who are *not* eligible for nursing home care *are* deemed eligible for the PACE program and included in the evaluations that have suggested, perhaps unrealistically, cost savings to the state.

For more information about PACE, contact the National PACE Association, 801 N. Fairfax St., # 309, Alexandria, VA 22314; 703-5351565; or visit www.npaonline.org.

END-OF-LIFE CARE

Advance Directives

Effective communication is important up to the end of life. Some health care professionals and family members believe that discussing end-of-life care issues upsets older adults, but most older adults are not upset by such a discussion once they are aware of their benefits. It is important that clients' views be clearly communicated and recorded before an unexpected crisis develops. Clear thinking is more likely when a patient is relatively healthy and not suffering from anxiety.

Unfortunately, this type of communication is still the exception rather than the rule. Among older respondents, 87% thought cardiopulmonary resuscitation (CPR) should be discussed routinely with health professionals, but only 3% had engaged in such discussions. Interestingly, videos may be more persuasive than words. When it comes to making advance care decisions, older persons who view a video rather than hearing a verbal description are much more likely to not only communicate their wishes, but to choose comfort over unnecessarily aggressive treatment (Volandes et al., 2008).

Another example of communication failure is the fact that although most older adults understand the idea of an *advance directive*, the vast majority have neither signed one nor discussed the issue with a health professional. Even when an advance directive has been signed it may not be specific and clear enough to help physicians and family members decide what to do. Geriatrician Joanne Lynne, director of George Washington University's Center to Improve Care of the Dying, laments the inadequacy of advance directives and end-of-life communication between health professionals and clients.

One advancement in this regard is the POLST form, which stands for *physician orders for life-sustaining treatment*. This document is voluntarily signed by the individual and a physician, physician's assistant, or nurse practitioner, and has two advantages over the better-known *living will*. First, a POLST addresses potentially unwanted emergency medical care by directing medical personnel on which actions to take, or not to take, in the event of an emergency. The directive is electronically accessed quickly by emergency personnel or physicians in an emergency situation through an online statewide database. The digital version is available around the clock with one call.

Second, it is more detailed about desired medical intervention. For instance, a person can choose to have CPR, or full treatment, or can choose to not attempt resuscitation (DNR), and allow natural death. There is also a third choice, limited additional intervention, that includes comfort care, and may or may not include intravenous fluids, antibiotics, and/or transfer to a hospital. Other issues are also addressed, such as the circumstances under which artificially administered nutrition is acceptable.

Oregon was the first state to use the POLST form in the mid-1990s, followed by 14 states that have adopted it and 20 more that are considering it.

The need for POLST was revealed in one study in which 1,200 seriously ill Medicare beneficiaries were interviewed at five U.S. teaching hospitals. Only 40% of the study patients requested a preference for treatment focused on extending life, whereas 60% expressed a preference for comfort care. However, although 86% of the patients who wanted aggressive treatment reported that their care was consistent with their preferences, only 41% of those who preferred comfort care reported consistency with their preferences (Teno, Fisher, Hamel, Coppola, & Dawson, 2002).

A video seen by older adult patients admitted to a skilled nursing facility was created to better inform them about medical options at the end of life. Among those who viewed the video, over 90% preferred to forgo aggressive interventions to die at home; of those who did not see the video, 75% chose to die in hospitals (Volandes et al., 2012). The video did not attempt to scare patients with alarming images, as more than 95% who saw it would recommend it to other patients. The video is available through a nonprofit foundation (www.ACPdecisions.org).

TERMINALLY ILL

Initial research efforts reported that not only did peer social support improve quality of life among terminally ill persons in comparison with persons in control groups, but also that survival rates improved as well. Subsequent research has not supported these findings. Peer support groups, for instance, did not prolong survival in women with metastatic breast cancer, but it did improve mood and the perception of pain (Goodwin et al., 2001). Researchers affiliated with the Behavioral Research Center of the American Cancer Society concluded that there is no evidence that social support or psychological intervention improves survival (Stefanek et al., 2009).

Dr. David Spiegel, one of the researchers who initially reported that peer support may prolong survival (Spiegel, Bloom, Kraemer, & Gottheil, 1989), has since retracted his optimism. In response to the subsequent wave of research studies that did not support extended survival, he reminded us that although there may have been an overreach, there is consistent evidence of a mental health benefit. As he aptly stated, "Curing cancer may not be a question of mind over matter, but mind does matter" (Spiegel, 2001, p. 1768).

While support group research has not substantiated extended survival rates, there are studies reported on in the next two sections that suggest that hospice and palliative care patients *do* live longer than patients not receiving such care.

HOSPICE SUPPORT

The philosopher (and humorist) Woody Allen once said, "I don't mind dying. I just don't want to be there when it happens." This sentiment may be shared by many Americans. For those who *are* willing to be there and who want an open acknowledgment of the experience surrounded by family, friends, and compassionate caregivers, there is *hospice.*

St. Christopher's Hospice, near London, was established in 1967 by the physician Cicely Saunders, who wrote about her experiences launching a hospice (Saunders, 1977). The St. Christopher's Hospice prototype was an independent institution that provided inpatient care for dying patients. The first American hospice, Connecticut Hospice in New Haven, was founded a few years later in 1974 and modeled after the London exemplar.

Hospice programs have since expanded their service sites, providing not only care in a hospice inpatient unit (now serving only a small percentage of hospice patients) but also to care in private homes, nursing homes, and other settings. Hospice has evolved into a type of care, rather than the site of care. Its distinguishing characteristic is the emphasis on psychosocial and spiritual support over medical procedures. By focusing on psychosocial and spiritual support, hospice attempts to improve the mental health and quality of life of clients, even as their physical bodies deteriorate.

The growth of the hospice movement in the United States has been tremendous. Between 1990 and 2010, the number of hospice programs in America increased from 1,800 to 5,000; the number of terminally ill persons served, from 210,000 to 1.6 million. During the first decade of this century, Medicare dollars spent on hospice increased from $2 billion to more than $12 billion (84% of persons receiving hospice care in America were covered by Medicare). The percentage of all deaths in the United States under the care of hospice has increased from no one in 1973 to 41% of the American population in 2011. The growth of hospice care has been consistent and unrelenting.

The Centers for Disease Control and Prevention looked at the deaths of people over age 65 and noted encouraging trends. The proportion of older adults who died in a hospital dropped from 49% in 1989 to 32% in 2009; and the proportion who died at home increased from 15% to 24% during that same time period. The increase in home deaths is more significant than the decline in hospital deaths, because accompanying the latter was a substantial increase in nursing home deaths. Although death in a nursing home is likely to be more humane than in a hospital (where an unnecessary end-of-life aggressive procedure may occur), some may not consider it to be a marked improvement.

One of the more startling statistics is that although 10% of older people on hospice visited an emergency room in their final month, among those who were not enrolled in hospice 56% visited the emergency room (Smith et al., 2012). Why is this important? (1) Emergency personnel are unfamiliar with patient histories, goals, and preferences; (2) emergency rooms are places to fix problems, some of which are not able to be fixed, rather than provide comfort; (3) emergency rooms are frightening places, often followed by intensive care or care in the hospital, rather than care at home where most people prefer to be; and (4) emergency care is expensive, and one of the biggest contributors to why 25% of Medicare expenditures happen in the final 6 months of life.

One component of hospice that can stand improvement is length of service. The majority of hospice patients die within 2 or 3 weeks of enrollment and, in 2009, 34% were in hospice fewer than 7 days. This means that hospice, despite its growing usage, is lagging behind in acceptance in a timely manner. Hospice is being thought of by too many as a very last resort. Ira Byock, director of palliative care medicine at the Darmouth–Hitchcock Medical Center, quips: "This is brink-of-death care rather than end-of-life care."

There are several barriers to why more persons do not receive more time in hospice care, or hospice care at all. First, many physicians are still reluctant to refer patients to hospice, seeing it as an admission of defeat. Many family members also see it in the same negative way. Second, most insurance companies, including Medicare, require that the physician certify that the patient has fewer than 6 months to live. The problem is that only late-stage cancer tends to be that predictable. Emphysema, congestive heart failure, Parkinson's disease, dementia, and other conditions are not as predictable. (Consequently, the Affordable Care Act will fund several pilot "prehospice" programs that eliminate the need to predict 6 months to live or less.)

Third, older minority adults are less likely to use hospice services due to fewer minority staff and volunteers, less trust of the health care system, and cultural beliefs that discourage the use of hospice care (Haber, 1999). In 2009, 44% of White decedents received hospice services in the last 30 days of life, versus 34% of Blacks, and 31% of other minorities. Conversely, 26% of White decedents used intensive or critical care units in the last 30 days of life, versus 32% of Blacks, and 33% of other minorities.

Finally, a major difficulty facing hospice clients and their families in the future may be the lack of a sufficient number of caregivers, especially for clients who choose to stay at home. Eighty percent of hospice clients are age 65 or over, and 83% are living in a private residence. Their spouses and increasingly their adult children are elderly themselves and physically unable to bear the exhausting burden of supporting the terminally ill in conjunction with hospice support (which plays a supplementary, not a primary, role). It is problematic whether we will be able to find sufficient numbers of volunteers and paid staff to help meet the additional social support needs of the family of the terminally ill elderly who desire to remain at home with hospice support

> **Question:** Do you think it is likely that in 15 years the majority of Americans will die with hospice support? What would it take for this to happen?

Inadequate social support not only prevents some older adults from participating in hospice, but it may also characterize the situation of those who die in a hospital setting. Dying in a hospital largely means dying by oneself. According to one hospital study that used video cameras taped to patient doorways, seriously ill hospital patients were spending 75% of their day alone (Sulmasy & Rahn, 2001).

Related to hospice care are *palliative care programs*, which are designed for the purpose of alleviating pain from serious illness. Unlike hospice, palliative care is targeted toward all patients, not just those in terminal care situations. These programs are increasing in number, but by 2006 only 30% of the 4,100 hospitals had such a program. In 2008, though, medical boards began to recognize palliative care as an official subspecialty for the first time, and it is anticipated that these types of programs will increase.

Why are palliative care programs important? One study of patients with metastasized lung cancer reported that those getting palliative care from the start of their diagnosis reported less depression, pain, nausea, mobility, worry, and other problems (Temel et al., 2010). Moreover, even though substantially fewer opted for aggressive chemotherapy, they lived almost 3 months longer than the group getting standard care.

The Art Buchwald Phenomenon

Many people are scared off by hospice because they feel it is a death sentence. To be eligible, patients must be certified by two doctors as having 6 months or less to live, assuming their illness runs a normal course. Yet there are two mitigating factors that make hospice less of a death sentence. First, hospice patients, in one study, lived an average of 29 days longer than comparable nonhospice patients (Connor, Pyenson, Fitch, Spence, & Iwasaki, 2007). This may be due less to the social/emotional support provided by hospice and more to the lethal nature of aggressive treatment on the terminally ill.

Second, there are many terminally ill diagnoses that are not very predictable, certainly much less so than the gold standard of predictability—late-stage cancer. In fact, 17% of the 1.3 million hospice patients in 2006 were *discharged*. One of those hospice patients was Art Buchwald, the Pulitzer Prize–winning newspaper humor columnist who in his prime was published in more than 550 newspapers. After 5 months in hospice, Buchwald left hospice care in 2006 and eventually died the following year, at the age of 81.

After kidney and vascular problems forced physicians to amputate one of his legs, Buchwald decided to refuse dialysis and enter hospice. Expecting to die in a few weeks, Buchwald, to the amazement of himself, his physicians, family, and friends, experienced his kidneys starting to work again. After leaving hospice he wrote about his 5-month experience in a book titled *Too Soon to Say Goodbye* (2006). Once back in the community he began to make the rounds of appearances necessary to support the sales of his book.

Although this is an unusual case, to say the least, publicizing it may reduce the stigma of hospice as a death sentence (but, on the negative side, strengthen our culture's denial of death). As Buchwald noted in his book, hospice provides as much comfort and support as possible and, if one should die, allows the person to die with dignity. An entire team consisting of volunteers, a physician, nurse, social worker, bereavement coordinator (for the survivors), and others are dedicated to the goals of comfort, support, and dignity. Until Americans change their attitudes toward dying and death, perhaps publicizing the *Buchwald phenomenon* can make the hospice option more palatable.

Resources

Since 1983, Medicare has covered hospice care provided by Medicare-approved agencies or facilities for terminally ill older persons who elect it in lieu of standard hospital treatment. Most private health insurance plans and some state Medicaid programs also pay for hospice care. For more information on hospice, including where to locate the one closest to you, contact the *National Hospice and Palliative Care Organization*, 800-658-8898; www.hospiceinfo.org. Or contact the *Hospice Foundation of America*, 800-854-3402; www.hospicefoundation.org.

DEATH WITH DIGNITY ACT

In October 1997, after 3 years of legal challenges, the state of Oregon legalized physician-assisted death through the *Death with Dignity Act*. In 2006, the United States Supreme Court *rejected* an effort by the Bush Administration to prevent Oregon and other states from creating Death with Dignity Laws. In November 2008, voters in the state of Washington passed the second statewide Death with Dignity Act.

In 2009, Montana approved the act by judicial decision through a state district judge. Legalization efforts failed, however, in California, Hawaii, and Maine. In 2012, voters narrowly rejected (51%/49%) the Death with Dignity Act in Massachusetts after opposers outspent supporters by 4 to 1.

Those in favor of the law are not just progressive Democrats, but conservative Republicans as well. Libertarians in particular are supportive because they do not want government meddling in their final days. Those against the law are the Roman Catholic Church, other religious groups, and the American Medical Association. The latter's opposition is a bit ironic given their tardiness in opposing cigarette smoking, a practice that hastens death and without much dignity.

The Oregon Department of Human Services espouses that the term *physician-assisted suicide* is incompatible with the Death with Dignity Act, and will use only the terms *physician-aid-in-dying* or *physician-assisted death*. Physician-assisted death legislation is a rigorous process for determining which individuals are eligible to take advantage of it.

The Oregon statute mandates that an adult resident makes two separate requests more than 15 days apart, orally and in writing, with the written request signed by two witnesses—at least one of whom is not related to the patient, and that two physicians affirm that the patient has no more than 6 months to live and does not suffer from any mental disorder, including depression, that might impair judgment. The prescription, usually a lethal dose of barbiturates, cannot be administered by a physician and must be self-administered. (There are a few more requirements, but you get the point, it can't be done on a whim.)

During the first 15 years of Oregon's law, 596 Oregonians availed themselves of it, about 40 persons per year, or 0.2% of dying Oregon patients, nearly all of whom were on hospice care. Among terminally ill persons who requested a prescription for lethal medication, less than half actually ended up taking their lives (Hedberg, Hopkins, & Southwick, 2002). Oregon residents who requested assistance spent more time communicating about the issue through discussions with nurses, social workers, and physicians.

According to participating nurses and social workers, the primary reason patients make such a request is to be able to control the circumstances of death if they so choose, not to end their lives because they are depressed, lack social support, or fear being a financial drain on family members (Ganzini et al., 2002). In a later study of 56 Oregonians who requested physician-assisted death, few rated pain as a primary motivation. The primary reasons were a desire to be in control, to remain autonomous, and to die at home (Ganzini, Goy, & Dobscha, 2009).

Although a good death is subject to interpretation, few would define it as an individual who is hooked up to machines in a hospital under the control of medical personnel, and subjected to futile, painful, and extremely costly attempts to extend life. The Death with Dignity Act allows patients to place limits on their emotional and physical pain and to be in control of the decision-making process.

About 80% of those who have died through the Death with Dignity Act were cancer patients, and the diagnosis with the next highest percentage was amyotrophic lateral sclerosis (ALS, also known as Lou Gehrig's disease). This latter disease makes it difficult to comply with one component of the law, to self-administer the lethal dose of barbiturates. Dr. Richard Wesley, a retired pulmonologist and critical care physician with ALS, said he would find a way to meet this requirement even though he had lost the use of his limbs. He added: "I don't know if I'll use the medication to end my life, but I do know that it is my life, it is my death, and it should be my choice" (Hafner, 2012).

11

●●●●●●○

DIVERSITY

old old

young old

sex and gender

minority, race, ethnicity, or
  disadvantaged

African American elders

Hispanic American or Latino elders

Asian and Pacific Islander elders

ethnically oriented assisted living
  facilities

Native American elders

culture

cultural competence

ethnogeriatrics

acculturation

socioeconomic status

gay aging

spirituality and religion

Jewish aging

rural aging

global aging

international cinema

●●○ Learning Objectives

- Compare the young old and the old old
- Describe the different circumstances of aging men and women in the United
  States
- Examine the role that race/ethnicity plays in aging in the United States
- Describe characteristics of being an African American elder in the United States

- Describe characteristics of being a Hispanic American elder in the United States
- Describe characteristics of being an Asian/Pacific Islander elder in the United States
- Describe characteristics of being a Native American elder in the United States
- Define culture and the field of ethnogeriatrics
- Examine the influence of socioeconomic status on the aging of Americans
- Compare the influence of race/ethnicity and socioeconomic status on aging
- Examine how gay baby boomers may change the institutions that serve them in old age
- Describe SAGE and the LGBT Aging Issues Network
- Describe spiritual and religious resources for older adults
- Recognize the unique support that Jewish Americans provide their older adults
- Describe the challenges facing rural elders
- Examine global aging and contrast old age in developed and developing countries
- Discuss the role that the international cinema can play in improving the understanding of aging and old age

Over a lifetime, people of similar ages can be expected to become increasingly diverse. As they grow older, some people will become ever more learned and wise, while others will make little progress in knowledge and wisdom. Some will discover fitness to be a rewarding hobby and persist in it as they grow older, while others will become increasingly sedentary and frail. Some will appreciate each day more and more as the number of remaining days become fewer and fewer, whereas others will view aging as a depressing decline into decrepitude.

Despite the increasing diversity with age, much of the content of this book reports on what we can expect will happen to most of us as we age. If the author qualified every statement with "depending on a person's age, race, socioeconomic status, religion, gender, geographical location, sexual orientation, and so on . . ." this would be a ponderous book indeed. (Pardon the author's assumption that it is not.) This chapter, therefore, is intended to draw the diversity that accompanies aging to the attention of the reader, and to allow the reader to contemplate how difficult it is to make general statements about how we age.

AGE

The very definition of being old is not obvious. The onset of old age can be anywhere from age 40 to age 85. At age 40 workers are old enough to be deemed in need of protection from age discrimination as defined by the 1967 Age Discrimination in Employment Act. At age 50 people become eligible for membership in AARP (formerly the American Association of Retired Persons). At age 60 individuals are eligible to participate in activities at most senior centers. At age 62 residents can live in public housing for elders and receive early Social Security retirement benefits. At age 67—for those born in 1960 or later—you can qualify for full Social Security benefits. At age 75 a patient is eligible for treatment at some geriatric primary care clinics. Many demographers use age 80 or 85 as a cutoff point for gerontological analysis.

Nonetheless, the more or less official chronological designation for old age in America is 65. This tradition began in Germany in 1884, when Chancellor Otto von Bismarck established age 70 as the standard retirement age, hoping, perhaps, that few if any would qualify for benefits. And few did. The qualifying age was eventually reduced to 65 in 1916. When Social Security was enacted in the United States, in 1935, the practice of establishing 65 as the eligibility age was continued. Thus, age 65 was instituted as a de facto national definition of old age.

Gerontologists began to realize, however, that few meaningful statements can be made about the population in general over age 65. They began to argue over the tendency to write about adults age 65 and over as if they were all the same when, in fact, the population has become increasingly diverse past this age marker.

Many gerontologists began to divide the older adult population into two groups for analysis, the *young old* and the *old old,* with age 75 as the dividing point at first—then age 80; and now it is not unusual to use age 85. Perhaps as the number of centenarians increase to a million or more when the baby boomers become of age, another dividing line will be added at age 100, in order to differentiate among the young old, middle old, and old old.

Dividing the older population into two or more categories is helpful for making more specific statements about being older. The old old are consistently different physically and cognitively from the young old, even if these differences are affected by changes in society from one decade to the next.

Take, for example, the decline in nursing home use among the old old over the past 15 years. Using age 85 as the dividing line for the old old, 25% of the 85+ population resided in nursing homes in 1985; by 1999 this percentage had been reduced to 18%. Though the percentage may have been reduced, this age group was still 18 times more likely to be institutionalized than those age 65 to 74 in 1999, the same ratio as in 1985.

Thus, although less likely to be institutionalized over the past 15 years, the old old, in comparison to the young old, are subject to institutionalization at a constant ratio. Economic, political, and lifestyle realities may change over time, but differentiating between the young old and the old old is likely to remain useful for researchers and clinicians.

Among those 85 and older, about 96% have at least one chronic condition, disability, or functional limitation, versus 76% of those age 65 to 69. Among those age 85 and older, about 30% to 45% have Alzheimer's disease, versus 2% among those age 65 to 69. Among the noninstitutionalized, the average health care expenditures for those 85 and over are almost twice as high as it is for those age 65 to 74. The old old are considerably more physically, mentally, and financially vulnerable than the young old.

Before the reader gets too carried away with the differences between the old old and the young-old, we end with the reminder that even when we divide older adults into more specific age groups, we still fail to account for the considerable variability that remains. As noted in Chapter 1, "Introduction," in the section on extraordinary accomplishments and aging, some nonagenarians are recording new works of music and producing hit singles, whereas others are completing marathons and climbing mountains. Some sexagenarians, on the other hand, are looking forward to becoming decreasingly active as they enter retirement.

SEX AND GENDER

It seems to me the most challenging part in writing this section was selecting the title. I shifted from *gender* to *sex* before finally deciding that both apply. *Gender* refers to the psychological and cultural aspects of being male or female, whereas *sex* refers to the biological attributes. *Intersex* refers to having an atypical combination of male and female physical features. This section will focus on the first two categories.

As the population ages, it becomes decidedly more female. Life expectancy of a male born in the United States is 76.2 years, and that of a female is 81.3 years. Women represent 56% of the population age 65 to 74, and 72% of those over age 85. To make these percentages more comprehensible, I offer the example of Edgewater Pointe retirement community in Boca Raton, Florida, where slightly over 70% of the 9,000 seniors in the 23-home chain are female. In order to ensure that women in this retirement community have a chance for a spin on the dance floor, management must hire male dancers, or occasionally attract male volunteers from a local college fraternity.

The Institute for Health Metrics and Evaluation, though, has reported the gender gap is closing. Between 1989 and 2009, U.S. male life expectancy increased 4.6 years, whereas female life expectancy increased 2.7 years. The institute staff speculated that males have been smoking less, are less inclined toward obesity, and their hypertension and high cholesterol levels are more likely to be detected and treated than is the case with women.

Though women are more likely to reach older ages, the prevalence of disability is consistently higher among women than men. More than half of women 70 and older report difficulty with mobility, such as walking across a room or climbing stairs, compared to 36% of men. Women age 70 and older are more than twice as likely as men (57% vs. 28%) to have difficulty with routine strength activities.

In addition, older women have higher rates of illness, physician visits, prescription drug use, acute illnesses, and chronic conditions. Among the chronic conditions that both women and men can acquire, osteoporosis is the most unfair to women, with 80% of those who have this condition being women. Men, however, are more likely to encounter life-threatening acute conditions and to require hospitalization (Hooyman & Kiyak, 2011). Thus, Medicare, with its emphasis on hospital coverage and its weaknesses in providing nursing home care, community care, and home care, favors the profile of older men's medical status over older women's. (Just a coincidence that men designed it?)

Older women are more likely to be unpaid caregivers. Older wives are more likely to care for their spouses than are older husbands. Among adult children who care for their elderly parents, about 75% are daughters. And about two thirds of the 2.4 million grandparents who are raising grandchildren are women (Health Resources and Services Administration [HRSA] 2002).

The greater responsibility for caregiving is due primarily to cultural expectations. Society expects women to leave the workforce when family obligations beckon. Not only have women been viewed as less essential than men in the workforce, but they have been expected to accept substantially less money in the workforce as well. For most of the life cycle, the current cohort of older women have been considered the primary caregivers for family members, whereas men have been considered the primary breadwinners.

Unpaid caregiving responsibilities and lower wages for women are complicated by widowhood. Because women generally marry men older than themselves, live longer than men, and infrequently remarry in their 50s and older, it follows that 52% of women 65 and over are widowed, in contrast to 14% of men. Consequently, it is not surprising that women are more likely to experience economic insecurity in old age than are men.

According to the 2011 Profile of older Americans, the median income of female older adults was $15,072, versus $25,704 for older men. The poverty rate of older women was 10.7% versus 6.7% for men. The average monthly Social Security benefit was 25% smaller for women than for men. As noted by the late Tish Sommers, founder of the Older Women's League, "Motherhood and apple pie may be sacred, but neither guarantees economic security in old age." This economic disparity, however, will diminish in the future if the higher percentage of women graduating from an institute of higher education results in the lessening of the wage disparity between the sexes.

There is an ever-increasing ratio of women versus men enrolled in college. The proportion of men age 18 to 24 enrolled in college declined slightly, from 33.1% to 32.6%, between 1967 and 2000, whereas the proportion of women *doubled*, from 19.2% to 38.4%! Women currently make up 57% of all college students.

Despite some of the disadvantages that accrue to women, older women are more health conscious and more resilient. They are twice as likely as men between the ages of 45 and 64 to have a regular physician, almost three times more likely to have seen a physician in the past year, and more likely to seek immediate medical care if they are sick or in pain (Shelton, 2000). They are also more likely to eat a healthful diet and to take a supplementary vitamin pill. In addition, older women have more frequent social contacts and more intimate relationships compared with older men.

Perhaps some combination of these factors contributes to greater resiliency and a lower likelihood of committing suicide. Between the ages of 65 and 69, male suicides outnumber female suicides by 4 to 1; by age 85, this ratio increases to 12 to 1.

It seems ironic that for many years clinical research trials sponsored by the National Institutes of Health focused almost exclusively on male subjects, though men in general demonstrated little interest in their own health. This practice of excluding women from clinical trials was ended in 1991 by Dr. Bernadine Healy, the first woman to head the National Institutes of Health. Also in 1991, Dr. Healy created the Office on Women's Health in the Department of Health and Human Services. There has been no interest on the part of male leadership to create a counterpart office. While women's health centers are commonplace in the community, men's health centers are a rarity.

Question: Women live longer, are better connected socially, and commit suicide less often in late life. On the other hand, they appear to have more health and financial burdens. Who is better off in America, older women or older men? Why?

A final note on the sex and age issue: Not only do differences between men and women increase with age, but aging women themselves are becoming more diverse. An article in the *Journal of the American Medical Association* reported that there is now no medical reason for excluding women in the sixth decade of life from attempting pregnancy on the basis of age alone (Paulson et al., 2002). No group is more diverse than women in their 60s, some of whom are new mothers, some of whom are grandmothers, and some of whom have never mothered.

RACE AND ETHNICITY

Definition

The following are several terms that overlap in meaning and are often used without definitions: minority groups, racial groups, ethnic groups, and the disadvantaged. The term *minority groups* tends to refer to subgroups within a population that are subject to discrimination, usually on the basis of race, ethnicity, or national origin. *Racial groups* are categories based on parentage and physical appearance, and are increasingly problematic because of widespread genetic diversity. *Ethnic groups* include individuals who share a sense of race, religion, national origin, or other cultural feature. The term *disadvantaged* refers to subgroups with fewer resources than the mainstream, and is often associated with minority groups, racial groups, or ethnic groups.

Other terms have increased in usage as well, particularly in academic settings, including *people of color, multicultural,* and *diversity.*

Perhaps in deference to the difficulty of defining racial or ethnic categories, the census form was revised to allow Americans to select more than one racial or ethnic category. Nearly 7 million Americans took this opportunity to identify themselves as a blend of two or more races. The category of multiracial, available for the first time in 2000, was selected by 2.4% of the country's population. In the 2010 census, this increased to 3% (though President Barack Obama stated he was not one of the census participants who chose this category).

Although Americans were finally allowed to select more than one racial category in the 2000 or 2010 census, it did not solve all problems. People of Middle Eastern descent were considered White by federal census officials, whereas people from India, once classified as White, were placed into the Asian category. One education professor at the University of Phoenix wondered why a Pakistani in America is not considered Black, but a biracial adult with blond hair and blue eyes is permitted to choose Black on the census form (Briggs, 2002). The situation was even more confusing in the 1960s, when the Census Bureau did not even count Hispanic people separately, Asian Indians were classified as White, and many in the general population did not consider the Irish, Italians, and Eastern European Jews to be White.

Though most biologists and anthropologists now deny the legitimacy of creating distinct racial categories, the reality for older adults in America is quite different. Most minority elders have grown up without equal rights and protection under the law. Job discrimination over the years has left minorities with fewer resources to cope with their old age, and a legacy of poverty, poor nutrition, and substandard housing that contributes to poor health in old age. This history of discrimination has also affected the minority older adult's ability or willingness to access the health care system over the life cycle, though the advent of Medicare corrected this problem in old age.

During their work years, many minority elders had labor-intensive jobs, inadequate access to health care, poor diets, and substantial stress. Not surprisingly, therefore, elderly minorities experience greater health problems than do elderly Anglos. One consequence is that minority elders are more likely to consider "old age" as beginning in the early 50s.

Racial Disparities In Health Care

The Institute of Medicine, an independent research institution that advises Congress, reported in March 2002 on the first comprehensive examination of racial disparities in health care among people who have health insurance. Previous studies reported on the lack of access to health care by minorities, as well as on how the lifestyles of minorities contribute to poor health. This study tackled the delicate issue of racial prejudice in health care.

The report reviewed more than 100 studies conducted over a decade and concluded that racial disparities contributed to higher death rates among minorities. It cited that minorities were less likely to be given appropriate medications for heart disease; less likely to be offered bypass surgery, angioplasty, kidney dialysis, or transplants; less likely to receive the most sophisticated treatment for HIV; and more likely to have lower limbs amputated as a result of diabetes (Stolberg, 2002).

The authors believed that a racial bias, perhaps subconscious, contributed to a reduced opportunity for minority patients to receive the latest and most sophisticated treatments. The explanation of why this takes place is complex and may include that there are disproportionately fewer minority physicians, minority patients are less likely to have a long-lasting relationship with a primary care physician, and physicians may assume that minority patients are less likely to comply with follow-up care.

Racial And Ethnic Distribution

As noted in Figure 1.9 in Chapter 1, "Introduction," the U.S. older adult population is becoming more ethnically diverse. The majority White, non-Hispanic population will have declined from 80% of the older adult population in 2010 to 58% in 2050. Sixty percent of the projected growth in the older adult population will be among older minorities. The Hispanic older adult population alone will increase from 7% of the total older adult population in 2010 to 20% in 2050.

This growth in minority older adults, particularly Hispanic older adults, reflects the overall population trends in America. By 2042, the White, non-Hispanic population will become a minority of the overall population. Although the absolute number of the White population remains fairly stable at just over 200 million people, the Hispanic population is projected to almost triple, from 50 million in 2010 to 133 million by 2050.

African American Elders

African Americans have a higher incidence of cancer and a significantly lower cancer survival rate than any other population group in the United States. African Americans are about 40% more likely to die from *colon* cancer than are Whites, because they are diagnosed at a later stage and respond worse to standard chemotherapy regimens (Dimou, Syrigos, & Saif, 2009). African American women are twice as likely to experience invasive *cervical* cancer due to diagnosis at a later stage of cancer (Patel et al., 2009). African American men have up to a fivefold increased risk of *prostate* cancer deaths in comparison to White men (Cheng et al., 2009). Blacks are about 40% less likely to receive surgery or chemotherapy for *lung* cancer (Hardy et al., 2009), or chemotherapy for *breast* cancer (Bhargava & Du, 2009).

Moreover, Blacks are at higher risk of developing *diabetes* than Whites (Maskarinec et al., 2009b); Black male deaths from *stroke* are nearly twice as high as those among White males; Black women have twice the rate of *coronary heart disease* as White women; and Blacks have a greater risk of *hypertension* than any other ethnic group in the United States, with medication nonadherence playing a large role (Bosworth et al., 2008). Nonadherence is common among African Americans even when they are insured, and it results in greater use of emergency rooms by Blacks than by any other racial/ethnic group in comparable insurance plans (Roby, Nicholson, & Kominski, 2009).

Older African Americans are much more likely to rate their health as fair or poor (48%) than are older Whites (28%), and are almost 50% more likely to be burdened by illness or injury that restricts daily activities. For reasons not clearly understood, however, there is evidence of a *crossover phenomenon* once Blacks reach age 85—that is, the remaining life expectancy for Blacks is higher than that of Whites. At age 65, White people can expect to live an average 1.3 years longer than Black people, but at age 85, life expectancy is 3 months higher for Black people.

African American patients are more likely to die after major surgery than White patients, controlling for patient characteristics such as severity of illness (Lucas et al., 2006). Hospital factors account for much of the difference, as Black patients are more likely to undergo surgery in very low-volume hospitals, and low volume is a risk factor for mortality. Another study reported that African American hospital patients have had a higher mortality rate than non-Blacks after abdominal aneurysm repair due to their receiving care in lower quality hospitals that have fewer resources (Osborne, Upchurch, Mathur, & Dimick, 2009).

Another study concluded that Black and White patients are, to a large extent, treated by different physicians. The physicians who treat Black patients may have less clinical training and less access to important clinical resources (Bach, Pham, Schrag,

Tate, & Hargraves, 2004). In yet another study, Black patients were found to be more likely than Whites to have a less experienced surgeon, and more likely to have complications from surgery to remove blockages from the carotid arteries (Halm et al., 2009). When African Americans with chest pain arrived at the emergency department, they were significantly less likely to receive electrocardiography or a chest radiology than Whites (Pezzin, Keyl, & Green, 2007). The researchers did not speculate on the causes of these disparities.

Nursing homes remain relatively segregated, roughly mirroring the residential segregation within metropolitan areas. As a result, Blacks are much more likely than Whites to be located in nursing homes that have serious deficiencies, lower staffing ratios, and greater financial vulnerability (Smith, Feng, Fennell, Zinn, & Mor, 2007).

When it comes to breast cancer, though, environmental factors may take a back seat to genetic differences. African American women may have significantly lower survival rates compared with White or Hispanic women because of genetic differences in likelihood of tumor types. A study of 2,140 breast cancer patients with no evidence of metastasis was part of a closely regulated trial of chemotherapy drugs (Woodward et al., 2006). The participating women had similar access to medical attention and similar treatment, and almost 10 years of follow-up care. African American women had a higher mortality rate from breast cancer due in part to a higher likelihood of a particular type of breast cancer called estrogen receptor–negative disease, which is more difficult to treat.

Discrimination over the years leads to mistrust, and this, in turn, may play a role in the differences in health care utilization between African American elders and White elders. African Americans represent about 12% of the population, but only 7% of those who receive hospice care. The California HealthCare Foundation issued a report in 2007 that stated Blacks may view hospice care as a way for doctors to deny them the medical care they have been fighting to get. This lack of trust is exacerbated by the scarcity of minority employees in hospices. Similar distrust of health providers extends outside the area of hospice (and it is shared by Hispanics and Asians). African Americans perceive an environment of health provider discrimination in general, which partly explains why their health care needs go unmet (C. Lee et al., 2009).

Regarding diet, it is important to acknowledge and support ethnic food preferences. Yet Black elders are susceptible to eating foods high in fat and sodium, including pork products such as bacon, sausage, and pig's feet; foods fried in animal fat; smoked foods; and pickled foods. Because Blacks are more likely than others to be salt-sensitive and to have high blood pressure, it is important that sodium intake be limited. African Americans need to change their seasoning to use more products such as herbs, spices, lemon juice, garlic, pepper, and ginger.

African Americans are also disadvantaged by neighborhood grocery stores that are more likely to be well stocked with processed foods and to be short on fruits and vegetables. A high number of neighborhood fast-food restaurants do not offer low-income older Blacks many healthy alternatives to a high-fat and high-salt diet.

Question: Black elders appear to have the greatest amount of homogeneity among the four minority categories recognized by the U.S. Census Bureau. Is that an advantage or disadvantage when it comes to community advocacy? Why?

On the bright side, caregiving appears to be less of a mental health burden on Black grandmothers who are raising grandchildren in their households compared with White grandmothers. A study of 867 grandmothers reported that Black grandmothers are more likely to embrace the prospect of raising grandchildren and consider this an important role in holding kin networks together (Pruchno & McKenney, 2002). Grandparent caregivers are increasing rapidly in number in the United States, reaching 6.7 million in 2009.

In addition, older African Americans may be better able than Whites to cope with the death of a spouse (Elwert & Christakis, 2006). This may be due in part to family connections, as older Black adults are much more likely to live with relatives, or it may be related to having deeper ties to religious life and more emotional support from fellow church members.

Hispanic American Elders

Hispanic Americans (*Latinos* is the preferred term in some areas) recently became the largest minority group in the United States. They are not homogeneous in that they include Mexican Americans (49%), Cuban Americans (15%), Puerto Ricans (12%), and people from Central America, South America, and Spain (25%). Although the Hispanic populations share the Spanish language, there is much diversity in their dialects, their ability to speak English, and length of time spent in the United States.

Hispanics in general have high rates of heart disease, diabetes, and cancer; and certain subgroups disproportionately fall prey to higher disease rates and lower functionality levels, as well as to poor eating habits, smoking, lack of exercise, and alcohol excess. This vulnerability is enhanced by a language barrier that is experienced by many Hispanics (Johnson-Kozlow, Roussos, Rovniak, & Hovell, 2009), especially those with a lower acculturation level (Janz et al., 2009).

Hispanics would benefit from eating a higher proportion of traditional foods that are rich in fiber and complex carbohydrates, such as chickpeas, fava beans, pinto beans, plantains, cassavas, sweet potatoes, taniers, mangos, guavas, papayas, and corn tortillas. Even in Mexico, however, the traditional diet of fresh foods is vanishing and is being replaced by imported fast foods, home-grown junk foods, and soft drinks.

In 2007, 42% of the Hispanic population age 65 and older had finished high school, compared to 76% of the total older adult population; and 9% of older Hispanic Americans had a bachelor's degree or higher, compared to 19% of all older persons.

AARP's National Eldercare Institute on Health Promotion (now defunct) conducted a study that examined the barriers to community health promotion programs among primarily Spanish-speaking Hispanic elders. A list of significant barriers follows:

1. Many Hispanic elders are unfamiliar with senior centers, whereas others who visit the centers find the programs to be culturally insensitive to them.
2. Hispanic physicians, followed by Spanish-speaking or bilingual health professionals, are preferred but are in short supply. The belief in folk medicine and the healing power of God can often result in the postponement of timely doctors' visits.
3. Lack of knowledge of (and experience in) the American health care system, compounded by financial limitations and lack of transportation, constitute a major barrier to timely health care services.
4. The most credible source of health information for Hispanic elders is Spanish-language television and radio—40% of Hispanic elderly speak Spanish only—followed by the extended family, churches, community groups, and Hispanic social clubs and organizations.

Health education programs need to involve the extended family, in both program development and implementation. Program presenters need to be sensitized to the spiritual beliefs and folk medicine of Hispanic elders and, when possible, to focus on ideas from both folk and Western medicine. The role of the *curandero*, a traditional healer who provides physical, psychological, social, and spiritual support for the Hispanic family (not just the individual), also needs to be understood and incorporated into health education programs. Curanderos believe that morbidity and mortality are associated with strong emotional states, such as *biles* (rage) and *susto* (fright).

Hispanic women who care for older relatives with dementia delay longer in placing them in nursing homes than do White caregivers (Mausbach et al., 2004). The findings probably reflect cultural values that emphasize the importance of family and the expectation that family members will care for each other. Participants in the study also report greater benefits from, or more positive aspects of, caregiving. Hispanic women who were more acculturated to U.S. society, however, were more likely to institutionalize their relatives.

Asian and Pacific Islander Elders

Asian and Pacific Island Americans encompass at least 16 ethnic and cultural groups, many of which have little in common in terms of language, culture, religion, and immigration history. The largest group of older Asian Americans are Chinese (30%), followed by Japanese (24%), Filipino (24%), Koreans (8%), Asian Indians (5%), and other backgrounds (Vietnamese, Cambodian, Laotian, Hmong, Thai, Pakistani, and Indonesian). The largest group of Pacific Island Americans are the Hawaiians and Samoans, followed by Polynesians, Micronesians, and Melanesians. There are many other smaller islands that could be included as well.

It is difficult to generalize within this diverse group. The poverty rates for older Japanese, Filipino, and Asian Indian Americans are low, whereas the poverty rates for older Southeast Asians are very high, reaching 47% among the Hmong elders. Within this diverse group is the highest proportion of people with less than a ninth-grade education, but also the highest proportion of those with a bachelor's degree or more.

Interestingly, the prevalence of diabetes in this diverse ethnic group is more than double that of Whites, and this prevalence holds up regardless of body weight. The higher prevalence applies to native Hawaiians, who suffer from high rates of obesity, as well as to the Japanese, who have a relatively low body weight (Maskarinec et al., 2009b).

Among Southeast Asian Americans, only 2% of the population is elderly because the refugee experience limited the number of elders who could immigrate, and some still have not reached age 65 since their arrival. At the other end of the spectrum are the Japanese elders, who currently constitute 7% of their American population. The percentage of Japanese elders is expected to grow due to current limits on the immigration of younger persons from Japan.

After the Japanese attack on Pearl Harbor in 1942, 110,000 Japanese Americans living in the Western states were incarcerated. It is believed that many of these now-elderly Japanese Americans tried to suppress their Japanese ancestry, often teaching their children to do the same. This is one example of the dramatic differences in the life experiences of older adults among the various Asian American and Pacific Islander ethnic groups.

Asian and Pacific Islander cultures traditionally emphasize the importance of family bonds and the unquestioned authority of elder family members. The extent to which younger family members abide by these traditional values and beliefs, however, is varied. In fact, among Southeast Asian American elders the traditional family roles are often reversed. More than 85% of the elders live with younger family members, who provide almost all of their economic and social support. This transfer of authority to the younger generation is one example of the difficulties that these elders have had in adapting to American culture.

TABLE 11.1 Percentage of Persons Age 45–55 Caring for Parents, by Ethnicity

ETHNICITY	% PROVIDING CARE
White	19
African American	28
Hispanic American	34
Asian American	42

Source: AARP. (July 2001). *In the middle: A report on multicultural boomers coping with family and aging issues.* Washington, DC.

In general, though, it appears that Asian American baby boomers provide more caregiving support for their parents than do other ethnicities (see Table 11.1).

Yet the erosion of family caregiving support over the past decade has been revealed in other ways. Vietnamese elders, for example, are now being placed in nursing homes in America, something that was not condoned 20 years ago.

An interesting alternative that has begun to emerge in the Asian American community are *ethnically oriented assisted living facilities*—sprouting up across America from Seattle to the Lower East Side of Manhattan—that cater to older Asian immigrants (Kershaw, 2003). These facilities provide ethnic foods, like miso soup, soba noodles, and dark-roasted teas, which are staples of the older Japanese American diet; and traditional games such as *rummi kub*. Even among Asians who were brought up to believe that they have a duty to take care of their aging parents in their homes, assisted-living facilities that provide ethnic support for older residents are becoming an increasingly attractive option.

> **Question:** Vietnamese elders are now being placed in nursing homes in America, something that was not condoned 20 years ago. From the perspective of *Vietnamese adult children caregivers*, do you think this trend is a positive or negative contribution to their lives? Why do you believe that?

Native American Elders

Native Americans are defined by the Bureau of the Census as American Indians, Eskimos, and Aleuts. As members of 562 federally recognized tribes (and about 100 nonrecognized tribes), Native Americans are exceptionally diverse both culturally and linguistically.

Native Americans have the smallest percentage of adults living to age 65—only 5.4%—among all ethnic groups. A study by the National Indian Council on Aging found that at age 45, reservation-dwelling Native Americans had the health characteristics of the average American at age 65. Urban-dwelling Native Americans demonstrated these elderly characteristics at age 55.

Because many do not live long enough to develop them, Native Americans have less heart disease and cancer than the general population, but have more pneumonia, influenza, diabetes, accidents, chronic liver diseases, septicemia, gallbladder disease, and hypertension (Butler et al., 1998). Since 1955 the Indian Health Service has focused its resources on treating infectious and acute diseases that occur in infancy through young adulthood, with few resources available for managing the chronic diseases of aging.

There is widespread poverty among Native Americans, and as recently as 1984, 25% of them lived in households without plumbing. Elderly Native Americans have a work history of high levels of unemployment and low-wage jobs, with 65% having worked as semiskilled workers, unskilled workers, or farm workers. Only about 22% graduated from high school, and 12% have no formal education at all.

National Organizations with an Emphasis on Minority Aging

American Society on Aging, Network of Multicultural Aging, 71 Stevenson St., #1450, San Francisco, CA 94105; 415-974-9630; www.asaging.org

Asian & Pacific Islander Health Forum, 450 Sutter St., #600, San Francisco, CA 94108; 415-954-9988; www.apiahf.org

Asociación Nacional Pro Personas Mayores, 234 E. Colorado Blvd., #300, Pasadena, CA 91101; 626-564-1988; www.anppm.org

Association of Asian Pacific Community Health Organizations, 300 Frank H. Ogawa Plaza, #620, Oakland, CA 94612; 510-272-9536; www.aapcho.org

National Caucus and Center on Black Aged, Inc., 1220 L. St. NW, #800, Washington, DC 20005; 202-637-8400; www.ncba-aged.org

National Hispanic Council on Aging, 734 15th St. NW, #1050, Washington, DC 20005; 202-347-9733; www.nhcoa.org

National Indian Council on Aging, 10501 Montgomery Blvd. NE, #210, Albuquerque, NM 87111; 505-292-2001; www.nicoa.org

Office of Minority Health Resource Center, The Tower Building, 1101 Wootton Pkwy., #600, Rockville, MD 20852; 800-444-6472; www.omhrc.gov

CULTURE

Culture has been defined as our entire nonbiological inheritance. Among those who believe that cultural differences among older adults are at least as important as socio-economic differences are the academicians who refer to themselves as *ethnogeriatricians*. The field of *ethnogeriatrics* focuses on the ability to provide health care in ways that are acceptable to older adults because they are congruent with their cultural backgrounds and expectations. One study concluded that when the *cultural competence* of the health care organization is compatible with the clients' perception of cultural need, there are cultural congruence and better treatment outcomes (Constantino, Malgady, & Primavera, 2009). Specifically, when older Hispanic clients received mental health services from culturally competent clinicians, depression, anxiety, and suicidal thoughts declined.

One topic of particular interest to ethnogeriatricians is the degree to which the *acculturation* of the older person—the incorporation of mainstream cultural values, beliefs, language, and skills—affects health care and health behavior. In other words, to what extent does identification with one's ethnic category, versus identification with mainstream culture, affect one's belief in allopathic medicine and the efficacy of scientific treatments, one's ability to work with a health care provider of a different cultural background, one's need for dependence on family for decision making in health care, one's belief in control over health outcomes, and one's willingness to negotiate with a complex medical bureaucracy?

Communication between persons with different cultural identifications can be problematic. Some people prefer a slower pace of conversation in a health care setting, whereas others prefer a fast-paced conversation and expect to be interrupted. Some patients prefer close physical proximity when communicating, whereas others prefer to be an arm's length away. Some cultures prefer eye contact, whereas others may consider this disrespectful. Some cultures value stoicism or mask their emotions with laughter or a smile, whereas others encourage open expression of pain, sorrow, and joy.

The etiquette of touch, hand gestures, and finger pointing is highly variable across cultures. There is also a diversity of attitudes toward the subjects of death and dying, ranging from a preference for direct communication to the belief that these topics are inappropriate for discussion.

Communication is also hampered by the lack of appropriate foreign-language access in medical clinics and health care settings around the country, as cited in the Institute of Medicine's Report on Unequal Treatment. This situation is particularly burdensome for Hispanic elderly, because 40% do not speak English.

When offering health care, health education, disease prevention, or health-promotion programs to ethnic older adults, the following precautions are recommended by AARP:

1. Ethnic communities need to establish their own health priorities and be involved in program development and implementation.
2. Factors affecting health care accessibility within a community must be identified and addressed.
3. Language should be familiar, nontechnical, concise, factual, and specific.
4. Nonprint formats, such as videotapes, audiotapes, slide shows, songs, games, and plays, should be encouraged.
5. Printed materials should use large type, be attractive, and make generous use of photographs and drawings of older peers.
6. Communication should acknowledge and incorporate cultural beliefs, and visual images should include familiar people, settings, and symbols.
7. Efforts toward cultural sensitivity must be sustained and reinforced over time.

Just as there is diversity among cultural groups, there is diversity within cultural groups. A Spanish-speaking grandmother with limited formal education may have little in common with an English-speaking, college-educated, gay older male, though both came from Cuba and are presently living in Miami. Cultural insensitivity can just as easily come from stereotyping the older person's cultural affiliation as from ignoring the person's cultural affiliation completely. One's degree of ethnic identification may be affected by educational level, one's primary language, religion, gender, year of immigration, and so forth.

When communicating with diverse older persons in a medical or community health setting, cultural sensitivity may be enhanced by asking a series of questions:

1. In times of illness or need, to whom do you turn for health information or care?
2. What help or assistance do you expect from your family members?
3. Are there ideas that you grew up with that help you to explain your specific illness or health problem?
4. What types of traditional medicine, or alternative medicine, do you use?
5. Do your health beliefs or practices differ from what you find in medical care or community health settings?
6. What are your attitudes toward medicine in this country, and how soon in the course of an illness do you seek to access it?
7. What roles do traditional foods play in your health? Are these foods geographically accessible and affordable?
8. What advice would you give to health care providers about your health care?

For additional health education questions that may be asked of culturally diverse older adults in the areas of nutrition, exercise, social support, folk medicine and religious healing, and trust and communication, see the article by Haber (2005a).

Physicians in New Jersey must take cultural competency training before they can get medical licenses from the State Board of Medical Examiners. State legislators in Arizona and New York have proposals to require medical schools to teach a course in cultural competency as a graduation requirement. California legislators have proposed a continuing-education requirement for doctors in cultural and linguistic competency. In short, states are taking steps, or thinking about taking steps, to reduce health care disparities and to make sure that physicians are more responsive to cultural and language differences among their patients. For additional information on how culture and language affect the delivery of health care, go to the website www.diversityrx.org.

The Commonwealth Fund issued a report titled *Cultural Competence in Health Care* (Betancourt & Carrillo, 2002), highlighting exemplary practices. For example, the Family Practice Residency Program at White Memorial Medical Center in Los Angeles provides 30 hours of cross-cultural training for all family practice residents that includes topics like the role of traditional healers. The state of Washington provides reimbursement for certified interpreters and translators for Medicaid beneficiaries, with eight languages readily available. The Kaiser Permanente Medical Center in San Francisco encourages workplace diversity, on-site interpreters, and an emphasis on culturally competent care delivery. The Sunset Park Family Health Center Network at the Lutheran Medical Center in Brooklyn, New York, trains China-educated nurses to upgrade their clinical skills in order to pass state licensing examinations, provides language and interpretation services, and celebrates a variety of religious and cultural holidays.

SOCIOECONOMIC STATUS

At retirement, the Black median household income is only 48% of the White median household income, and the Hispanic median household income is only 40%. Social Security benefits account for more than half of Black and about two thirds of Hispanic median household retirement income, in comparison to a little more than a third of White median household retirement income. Viewed another way, 8% of White older adults live in poverty, versus approximately 25% of Hispanic and Black older adults.

This leads to a major question in sociology in terms of health care and health behavior: Which has more explanatory power, ethnic differences or socioeconomic status? Though the evidence leans strongly toward socioeconomic status, ethnicity plays a role as well.

The effects of ethnicity on severity of disease and mortality rate typically disappear or are greatly reduced when socioeconomic status (i.e., income level and education) is taken into consideration. People with low income and educational levels do not engage in screenings in a timely manner or seek treatment later in the course of their disease; are less likely to follow the treatment plan; are more likely to cut back or discontinue medication because of cost; and are more likely to have higher disease rates and disease severity, higher disability rates, and higher mortality rates (Chu et al., 2009; Dimou et al., 2009; Fuller-Thompson, Nuru-Jeter, Minkler, & Guralnik, 2009; Link & McKinlay, 2009). One demographer estimates that socioeconomic differences account for 80% of the life expectancy divide between Black and White men and 70% of the imbalance between Black and White women (Geruso, 2012).

Type II diabetes patients who are disadvantaged by education and income, for instance, are more likely to have problems reading prescription bottles, educational brochures, and nutrition labels. Consequently, they have more difficulty with blood sugar control and experience more diabetes-related complications than persons with higher income and literacy levels (Schillinger et al., 2002).

Environment also plays a factor in fostering a healthy lifestyle. Low-income adults are much more worried about the safety of walking in their neighborhood than are higher-income adults, and they report less access to safe parks and recreational facilities. Low-income residents also report that fresh fruits and vegetables are not readily available where they shop in their neighborhood, and when they are available they cost too much. Low-income families eat more processed foods because they are more accessible and cheaper than healthier foods.

Yet a few studies report that ethnic factors are more important than socioeconomic factors when it comes to health care behaviors or health status. After controlling for potential confounding variables, including socioeconomic status, Blacks were less likely than Whites to seek eye examinations when coping with diabetes, to receive beta-blocker medications after heart attacks, and to follow up after being hospitalized for mental illness (Schneider, Zaslavsky, & Epstein, 2002). A study of Medicare patients reported that when patient income, education, and attitudes were controlled, race was still a factor when only 46% of Black Medicare patients sought free flu shots, versus 68% of White Medicare patients (Schneider, Cleary, Zaslavsky, & Epstein, 2001).

In one study culture was more important than genetic make-up. The researchers concluded that the racial disparity in hypertension had more to do with discrimation than any evidence of a destructive "hypertension gene" in African American groups (Gravlee & Mulligan, 2012). It appears that culture, independent of socioeconomic status and DNA, may be influential in specific health care realms.

GAY AGING

Gay refers to people who are sexually attracted to members of the same sex, and usually refers to both lesbians and gay men, though sometimes just to the latter group. LGBT is the commonly used acronym for lesbian, gay, bisexual, and transgender, but there is very little research on the latter two groups and they will not be focused on here.

Gay aging as a topic does not appear in many gerontology textbooks (including, unfortunately, the first four editions of this book) or research articles in gerontology journals. In part this is due to the invisibility of the gay lifestyle among today's cohort of older adults. This is beginning to change because the baby boomers started to become the gerontology boomers in 2011 and will become more visible in the gerontology field (Haber, 2009). A brief description of two historical events may explain why the boomers will be different than the current cohort of older adults.

The Stonewall Inn in Greenwich Village in New York City was the site of riots that began in the early morning of June 28, 1969, and lasted for several days. These riots were spontaneous and violent demonstrations incited by a police raid of a bar that catered to the gay community. These types of raids were routine for police, where they would shut down the bar and customers would be arrested and exposed in newspapers. The riots in 1969, however, led to the beginning of the gay liberation movement in the United States.

The Stonewall riots were the first time in American history that gays fought back against government-sponsored persecution. Immediately following the riots two gay activist organizations emerged in New York City (Gay Liberation Front and Gay Activists Alliance), and three newspapers were launched to focus on the promotion of the rights of gays and lesbians (*Gay Power, Come Out!*, and *Gay*; for more information see Carter, 2004). Within the following year, gay rights groups were launched in most major American cities. On the 1-year anniversary of the riots, the first Gay Pride marches took place in New York City and Los Angeles.

In commemoration of a quarter century of gay rights activities implemented after the riots occurred, the Gay Pride march in New York City in 1994 drew more than 1 million people. In 1999 the U.S. Department of the Interior designated the Greenwich Village area where the riots occurred as a National Historic Landmark, the first of significance to the LGBT community.

The second historical event took place in 1973. Prior to that, the American Psychiatric Association listed homosexuality in the *Diagnostic and Statistical Manual of Mental Disorders (DSM)* as a sociopathic personality disturbance (American Psychiatric Association, 1952). This diagnosis was based on alleged research studies that supported the idea that homosexuality was a pathological fear of the opposite sex caused by traumatic parent–child relationships. The stigma of being gay, therefore, was reinforced by the prominent scientific societies of the era.

A more rigorous study by Evelyn Hooker (1957), however, found no differences between the happiness and adjustment of the homosexual men in her sample versus the heterosexual men. Despite subsequent research studies with similar benign results, it was not until 1973 that homosexuality as a pathological disorder was removed by the American Psychiatric Association from the *DSM*. This was followed by a similar reversal by the American Psychological Association in 1974. In the scientific community, being gay was finally declared normal.

Implications of Two Historical Events for Gay Aging

In the early 1970s, Gay Pride became a national movement in the aftermath of the Stonewall riots, and additional support for gay adults was derived from the two major health professional associations removing the pathological label associated with being gay. One can further argue, though, that this emerging Gay Pride movement in the early 1970s came too late for many adults who are age 65 and over today. This cohort was already in their mid-30s and older during that critical era. Subsequent lifestyle and attitude change, as well as advocacy efforts, would prove to be difficult for them to embrace.

The youngest baby boomer, however, was only age 5 at the time of the Stonewall riots, whereas the oldest was 23. They were young enough to assimilate a change in attitude and behavior. This was reflected in a 2006 national survey conducted by Zogby International and released by MetLife, which reported that 44% of LGBT boomers were "completely out" and 32% were "mostly out" (MetLife Mature Market Institute, 2006).

Now, as a cohort on the verge of becoming gerontology boomers—the leading edge of the boomers reached age 62 in 2008, with an estimated 1.7 million of them collecting early Social Security benefits that year—they are likely to be very different than the current cohort of older adults in their willingness to advocate for more supportive age-related programs, organizations, agencies, and services. If the boomers are more likely to assert their rights as older gay Americans, it will be essential that health care professionals in the gerontology field become aware of practices and policies in community organizations and service agencies that affect the quality of life of gay Americans. It is also imperative that greater acceptance of this lifestyle be encouraged in the field.

Lesbians and Gay Men

Although there are no accurate statistics on the percentage of LGBT people in the United States population, researchers estimate that approximately 3% to 7% of the population is self-identified as such, most of them lesbians and gay men. This translates to between 1 million and 3.5 million older lesbians and gay men and, thanks to the aging of the large cohort of baby boomers, this number will double by 2029 (Jackson et al., 2008).

Today's older gays grew up in an environment where they were vilified as sinful and considered undeserving of constitutional protection. They were "viewed as perverted by society, evil by the church, sick by the medical and psychiatric professions, and criminal by the police" (Reid, 1995, p. 217). Many of today's older lesbians and gay men have internalized these negative cultural attitudes and beliefs (Orel, 2004). The oppression and disempowerment that older lesbians and gay men have endured has unquestionably affected their mental health and, for many, their physical health as well.

A survey of 2,560 LGBT adults aged 50 to 95 across the United States revealed greater rates of disability, depression, and loneliness, and increased likeliness to smoke and binge-drink compared with heterosexuals of similar ages (Fredriksen-Goldsen, Kim, & Barkan, 2012). A survey of California gay and bisexual men between the ages of 50 and 70 reported higher rates of hypertension, diabetes, physical disability, and psychological distress than similarly aged heterosexual men (Wallace, Cochran, Durazo, & Ford, 2011).

Another major concern for gay and lesbian elders is lack of support from significant others who live with them. Singlehood in late life is correlated with a variety of negative physical and mental health outcomes (Blank, Asencio, Descartes, & Griggs, 2009). A study by Anderson (2008) of gay older adults reported that they were twice as likely as nongay elders to live alone in the latter part of the life cycle, four times less likely to have children to help them, and half as likely to have a significant other or close relative to call on for help. A self-administered survey of 416 older gay men and lesbians in America reported that physical and mental health was less likely to suffer if the individual lived with a partner (Grossman, D'Augelli, & O'Connell, 2001). Unfortunately, most did not; only 29% in this sample lived with a partner.

Research studies consistently point out differences between lesbians and gay men. Lesbian sexuality tends to be more relationship focused, with an emphasis on the sharing of emotions. Gay men are more sexually focused, with hypermasculinity not uncommon when young—a characteristic that does not age well. There is speculation that lesbians are less vulnerable than gay men to the changes that aging brings to the body over time. Body image allegedly becomes less important for aging lesbians than gay men. Others argue that aging gay men become more adaptable with age as well (Wierzalis, Barret, Pope, & Rankins, 2006).

Another difference between gay men and lesbians is the differential impact of the AIDS epidemic on male boomers coming of age in the 1980s and 1990s. By 2002 there had been approximately 460,000 U.S. adult deaths from AIDS or AIDS-related causes, with the number of adult male deaths being about 400,000 (Knauer, 2009). The promise of the Stonewall rebellion and its aftermath was interrupted by the AIDS devastation, particularly in the larger cities such as San Francisco, New York, and Washington, DC.

One can argue, however, that the decimation from AIDS—the brunt of which was borne by male boomers—inspired several positive trends, such as a growing number of long-term monogamous relationships, the mass community outreach that took place during the mid-1980s, a wide spectrum of community services that humanized the face of a deadly epidemic, and acceptance and integration into one's neighborhood (Knauer, 2009). Gay men were significantly more likely than lesbians to bring gay concerns to the attention of the general public (Oswald & Masciadrelli, 2008).

Minority gay aging is more challenging to understand and deal with than gender issues, because it is complicated by additional societal discrimination, lower income levels, more chronic impairment, greater concerns about financial and functional independence, and even less research targeted to gay minority aging. Lesbians and gay men of color have demonstrated higher rates of victimization than White lesbians and gay men (Balsalm & D'Augelli, 2006). Despite this inequity, a literature search through MEDLINE reported that 85% of the studies on gay persons omitted the participants' race/ethnicity (Boehmer, 2002).

Discrimination and Legal Concerns

More than a third of gay youth have been victimized by an immediate family member or by their peers at school. By the time a gay person reaches old age, the likelihood of victimization at home, in school, at work, or in the community by acquaintances or strangers is very high. The fear and stress of expecting discrimination or experiencing actual discrimination can lead to low self-esteem, depression, involvement with risky sexual partners, alcohol abuse, drug abuse, or other types of victimization (Balsalm & D'Augelli, 2006).

Access to programs and services is hampered by sexual orientation, including entrée into senior centers, meal programs, food stamps, domestic-violence shelters, counseling programs, and medical care. A study conducted by the U.S. Department of Health and Human Services reported that gay seniors are only 20% as likely as heterosexual elders to access needed services. A survey of federally funded Area Agencies on Aging revealed that half of the senior centers would not welcome gay men and lesbians if their sexual orientation were known; and 72% of gay elders reported they were tentative about using such services, with only 19% participating in a senior center (Knauer, 2009).

Gelo (2008) reported that only 25% of gay older adults are completely open about their sexual orientation to health care workers. The average medical school allocates less than half a day within the 4-year curriculum on GLBT issues (Bonvicini & Perlin, 2003). Even gay boomers are highly skeptical and fearful of the medical profession caring for them in an unbiased manner (MetLife Mature Market Institute, 2006).

Compounding these inequities is the lack of eligibility for Social Security spousal benefits, as well as 401(k) and other pension plans, health insurance, and inheritances associated with one's partner. Also, there is great likelihood that gay elders will experience unwelcoming housing options such as retirement communities and nursing homes, and community sites such as senior centers (Knauer, 2009). Given the concern that facilities will be insensitive to the needs of gay elders, the lack of gay-only facilities has been troubling to this community.

In addition to gay individuals receiving no federal benefits in the United States, there is little help for older adults with HIV/AIDS. In 2005, 15% of new HIV/AIDS diagnoses were among people over the age of 50, according to the Centers for Disease Control and Prevention, yet federal government recommendations for routine HIV/AIDS screening goes up only to age 64. Another issue of nationwide relevance is the lack of Medicaid protection for the assets and homes of same-sex partners that are otherwise provided to married spouses. Also, the Family and Medical Leave Act guarantees leave to employees to care for parents, children, or spouses, but not for domestic partners.

On the state front, there are an increasing number of laws that recognize same-sex partners as having rights when it comes to hospital visitation, inheritance, funeral arrangements, and so forth. It should be noted, though, that even legally married same-sex couples are not eligible for Social Security spousal and survivor benefits, because the federal government does not recognize these marriages under the 1996 Defense of Marriage Act.

Nonetheless, nine states have legalized gay marriages through legislation enacted in 9 years: Massachusetts (since November 2003), Connecticut (October 2008), Iowa (April 2009), Vermont (April 2009), New Hampshire (July 2010), New York (July 2012), and Maryland, Maine, and Washington (November 2012). On May 9th, 2012, President Barack Obama became the first sitting president to endorse the legalization of same-sex marriage. Also, three states recognize civil unions (New Jersey, New Hampshire, and Washington), which provide comparable rights and responsibilities as legal marriage. Civil unions can allow insurance coverage, health care decision-making powers, and survivor benefits.

The future of gay marriage in the United States looks bright. A 2012 ABC/*Washington Post* survey reported that while only 31% of those age 65 or older support gay marriage, about half of those between ages 30 and 64, and 66% of adults under age 30, support it.

There have been promising state legal victories for gay individuals. In November 2008 Florida's strict law banning adoption of children by gay people was found to be unconstitutional by a state judge, who stated there was no legal or scientific reason for sexual orientation alone to prohibit one from adoption. In a November 2008 settlement with New Jersey's Civil Rights Division, eHarmony agreed to launch a new website catering to same-sex singles. In 2012, Minnesota rejected a proposed constitutional amendment to define marriage as between a man and a woman.

There have been state legal defeats as well for gay individuals. In November 2008, Arkansas prohibited people who are cohabitating outside a valid marriage from serving as foster parents or adopting children. By 2010, 31 states had passed bans on same-sex marriages, and 19 banned same-sex civil unions as well. California (in November 2008) and Maine (in November 2009) repealed same-sex marriage legalization at the ballot box, after its passage by state legislators and endorsement by governors in the respective states.

It is not clear how effective legal documents will be, given the controversial nature of gay marriages or civil unions. A living will or a power of attorney for health care may still be contested when it comes to granting rights to gay partners or spouses. These legal documents can always be contested by biological family members. Moreover, municipal laws differ from area to area, and statewide protections are diverse when it comes to nondiscrimination ordinances and litigation remedies (Dubois, 1999).

In addition, as these state laws are increasingly proposed and contested, there has been an accompanying increase in hate crimes based on sexual orientation. The number of these types of crimes rose from 1,017 in 2005 to 1,265 in 2007 ("Many Suffer From," 2008). Aging LGBT people face many barriers and challenges that require thoughtful planning to ward off some of the unexpected and undesirable events that often occur in the United States. Discrimination is even more severe in nonmetropolitan areas that have no gay neighborhoods or gay-identified businesses and services (Oswald & Masciadrelli, 2008).

Community Programs

SAGE (Services and Advocacy for Gay Elders) is a model community program in New York City that has existed for 30 years (Kling & Kimmel, 2006). SAGE offers gay seniors in the five New York boroughs access to innovative clinical and social services, including access to professional social workers for crisis intervention and ongoing assistance.

Services provided by SAGE include support groups, programs targeted to HIV/AIDS individuals, volunteers who provide a wide range of assistance to older LGBT adults, friendly visitor programs, and ongoing training and workshops that are problem oriented. A recently implemented SAGE educational initiative has encouraged self-reflection and an examination of culture and society for the purpose of creating a more meaningful aging experience. The curriculum covers fears of aging, changing self-definitions, sexuality and aging, losses and gains with aging, religion and spirituality, physical and mental health, and community building. Another innovative program is an interactive online resource that lists LGBT-friendly housing options.

Many of SAGE's social, cultural, intellectual, legal, financial, political, spiritual, and recreational programs are being replicated by community programs throughout the United States. SAGE encourages local advocacy through professional conferences and workshops conducted nationwide. One of the goals of SAGE is to increase practitioner sensitivity and to provide information on how agencies and organizations can replicate or create policies and practices that support LGBT elders. In 2012, SAGE released a guide called: *Inclusive Services for LGBT Older Adults: A Practical Guide to Creating Welcoming Agencies.*

In 2008 SAGE organized the fourth National Conference on LGBT Aging, which drew more than 600 participants to New York City. The conference was also notable for being sponsored for the first time by AARP. Additional information on SAGE is available through their website, www.sageusa.org.

The American Society on Aging (ASA) sponsors the LGBT Aging Issues Network (LAIN). This network's goal is to raise awareness about the concerns of LGBT elders and about the unique barriers they encounter in gaining access to housing, health care, long-term care, and other needed services. It should be noted that the name of this network was the Lesbian and Gay Aging Issues Network until 2008, when it was pointed out that its title overlooked the needs of aging bisexual and transgender individuals.

LAIN provides a bimonthly online update entitled OutWord Online, which publishes brief news items and timely announcements about relevant events nationwide, at www.asaging.org/lain. LAIN also publishes a quarterly newsletter entitled *OutWord*, which bills itself as the most comprehensive ongoing source of information about LGBT aging. It provides information on books, periodicals, videos, websites, reports, factsheets, and listservs. For information on more than 400 service providers, community organizations, websites, and articles on LGBT aging, visit ASA's LGBT Aging Resources Clearinghouse at www.asaging.org/larc.

The ASA Joint Conference on Aging (with NCOA, the National Council on Aging) was held in the spring of 2010 in Chicago. There was a full track of 15 LGBT-related research and practice sessions; a meeting for an ongoing LGBT peer interest group; a site visit to the Center on Halsted, a highly visible symbol for the LGBT community of Chicago; and several informal opportunities for networking and socializing (see www.asaging.org). This professional conference is held annually in March.

How will the aging network respond to the challenges of meeting the diverse needs of gay boomers? Will the Area Agencies on Aging begin to provide training and education to meet the needs and desires of gay boomers? Will they advocate for more responsive policies in senior centers, nursing homes, assisted living facilities, and retirement communities? Will the medical profession provide a curriculum for medical residents and fellows, as well as continuing education opportunities for existing health providers, to address the health care needs of gay boomers? Will the federal government modify Social Security survivor benefits so they are available to same-sex couples?

Since the time of the Stonewall riots and the elimination of the pathological definition of homosexuality, the group identity of gay boomers has been significantly enhanced. Gerontologists of all stripes—educators, researchers, and practitioners—need to be sensitive to the needs and aspirations of the coming cohort of gay boomers.

SPIRITUALITY AND RELIGION

Historical evidence of people's involvement in spiritual or religious activities dates as far back as 300,000 to 400,000 B.C. Moreover, some form of spirituality or religion may be found in virtually every culture in the world today (Krause, 2008). Spiritual and religious beliefs and practices, therefore, must serve some basic human function(s), due to their unrelenting prominence in history and continued prevalence around the world today.

In America an estimated 85% of the population report that they are spiritual or religious. The evidence that a person becomes spiritual or religious upon reaching a certain advanced age is not supported by research, but such beliefs and practices appear to become more important as older adults rely on their faith to cope with the challenges and losses of late life (Idler, McLaughlin, & Kasl, 2009).

Two caveats are in order. To tackle the issue of diversity within the topic of religiosity and spirituality, one should also include information on nonbelievers (atheists, agnostics, and the apathetic) in association with aging or old age. This author, unfortunately, could not find research on this topic. Also, diversity might suggest that the different religious denominations or spiritual domains might reveal important differences in the way people age, but this topic also did not lead to fruitful research investigation. There is evidence, limited though it is, to suggest that religion may provide more support for aging Blacks than aging Whites, and more support for aging women than aging men (Krause, 2008), something to consider when contemplating the diversity of race and gender.

This section combines spiritual and religious activities together, even though there are important distinctions to be made. Many people associate *spirituality* with inner experiences and *religion* with external experiences linked to organized institutions. Spirituality often takes the form of "intense awareness of the present, transcendence of the personal self, or a feeling of connection with all of life, the universe, a supreme being, or a great web of being" (Atchley, 2009, p. 2). Religion, in contrast, is primarily connected to institutions, and the teachings in these institutions "place boundaries on the beliefs and behaviors of the people who worship there" (Krause, 2008, p. 9).

Given this distinction, it is harder for researchers to measure the great variety of spiritual beliefs and practices that emanate from innumerable settings, and easier to measure such ubiquitous religious activities as attendance at a religious institution or self-reported frequency of prayer. Not surprisingly, therefore, the vast majority of research is conducted in the realm of religion rather than spirituality. Nonetheless, the two topics are related in their quest for meaning and purpose, and it does not feel right to leave out the realm of spirituality in this section despite the scarcity of research in this domain.

One important consideration within the topic of religious and spiritual diversity and aging in America is, in my opinion, whether or not older adults with strong spiritual or religious beliefs and practices, whatever they may be, draw life-affecting support from them. As noted previously, the evidence on whether spiritual or religious beliefs or practices affect whether we live substantially longer or healthier is weak at best. On a more limited time basis, sick patients who are pessimistic about their spiritual or religious faith have a higher risk of mortality within 2 years (Pargament et al., 2001), whereas those who are strong in their faith and are seriously ill can extend their mortality beyond the date of an important religious holiday (Idler & Kasl, 1992). The overall impact on longevity and health, though, has not been substantiated convincingly by researchers (Sloan & Bagiella, 2002).

What is likely, however, is that spiritual and religious resources have the potential to improve one's quality of life, particularly after age 65, when issues such as the meaning of life and death come to the forefront. Aging patients (Ehman, Ott, Short, Ciampa, & Hansen-Flaschen, 1999) and physicians (Duenwald, 2002) agree that religious and spiritual concerns are of great importance in late life because of proximity to death, and the need for living wills, durable powers of attorney for health, end-of-life counseling, and emotional support.

In this section I will summarize the spiritual and religious resources cited throughout the chapters of this book, and then discuss the potential to maximize the quality of life of older adults through religion and spirituality using the example of Jewish aging.

Spiritual and Religious Resources

There are a number of spiritual and religious resources that can be of help not only to older adults, but also to their health educators, community practitioners, chaplains, and health care providers. As cited earlier, there is an academic journal, *Journal of Religion, Spirituality & Aging*, published by the Haworth Press, and two (among many) important books on this topic are *From Ageing to Sage-ing: A Profound New Vision on Growing Older* (Schachter-Shalomi, 1995) and *Still Here: Embracing Aging, Changing and Dying* (Ram Dass, 2000).

Also noted earlier are many religious institutions providing a wide array of education, counseling, social support, disease prevention, and health promotion services. These services include support groups, pastoral counseling, parish nurses, and medical screenings. There are national networks of religious-based wellness activities, such as the Shepherd's Centers of America and the Interfaith Volunteer Caregiver Program. The latter program continues to provide congregation-based caregiving support services around the country even though the Faith in Action program that implemented it was discontinued by the Robert Wood Johnson Foundation, which is not funding new programs.

Also reported earlier are religious-based nutrition and weight-loss programs, such as the Weigh Down Diet and First Place programs; and there are religious-oriented health, wellness, and sports programs that are associated with the Jewish Community Centers and with Beliefnet.

Religious institutions provide fellowship, trust, and support that are foundations for health-promoting programs and services, and they offer ideological content that promote healthy lifestyles through strengthening marriages, lowering stress during crises, and avoiding risk factors such as smoking, drinking, and infidelity. It is not surprising that spiritual and religious resources for aging Americans are plentiful.

Jewish Aging

I selected Jewish aging as a model for aging Americans and their caregivers (Haber, 2011) for a few reasons. I am a nonobservant Jew who wanted to learn more about his heritage. Also, with limited space, I wanted to focus on one sector of aging Americans and summarize the breadth of resources and services available to them. In addition, according to the National Jewish Population Study, there is a uniquely high percentage of American Jews age 65 years and older (19%), compared to American elders overall (13%), making this a particularly important topic for this denomination (Address, 2005).

The challenge for American Jews extends beyond this group's disproportionate number of aging adults. Jewish boomer adult children have above-average educational levels, which are associated with lower fertility rates and greater geographical mobility in their careers. These combined factors—fewer adult children caregivers, spread over a wider geographical area—create additional caregiver challenges for Jews. At the same time, though, old age is greatly valued in Jewish tradition for its wisdom, and a long life is considered to be a reward for righteous living. This particular religious group should, therefore, be highly motivated to effectively engage the community in the support of its aging population.

This is, in fact, the case. The Jewish community has a strong legacy of supporting elders through excellent nursing homes and supportive housing for the aging, family service agencies, and Jewish community centers. New challenges, however, bring forth the need for new and innovative community initiatives. Some examples follow.

The Mitzvah Model. Rabbi Dayle Friedman defines mitzvah as an act of kindness, and the Mitzvah Model expects all Jews, regardless of age, to perform them. Even impaired older adults can ask: What can I contribute? As Rabbi Friedman writes, "We are called to invite and facilitate elders' contributions so that they may not only experience meaning but also actually help to repair our broken world" (2008, p. 20).

An example of this is the *Hands and Hearts* program, which allows nursing home residents to reach out to newcomers with hand-made gifts and a personal visit. With these acts of kindness the residents convert a collection of strangers into a caring community. This program was created by the chaplain Sheila Segal, and her colleagues at the Abramson Center for Jewish Life (formerly the Philadelphia Geriatric Center).

This center was founded in 1959 and was the first research center in the United States sponsored by a geriatric facility. For more information about the Abramson Center for Jewish Life, contact the Polisher Research Institute, 1425 Horsham Rd., North Wales, PA 19454; 215-371-1890; www.abramsoncenter.org.

Lilmod: Elders as Students of Torah. *Lilmod* is the Hebrew word for learning and studying. Rabbi Friedman believes that aging is enriched by the study of the Torah, the Talmud, and other Jewish texts. The Torah is the five books of Moses, referred to by non-Jews as the Old Testament. The Talmud refers to the vast body of Jewish law and traditions. Elders are not only students who study the Torah and the Talmud, but they are teachers and mentors to the young as well.

The enthusiasm for Jewish study among elders is widespread. One example of older adult participation in Jewish education is the Florence Melton Adult Mini-Schools, located at 49 sites in 26 cities in the United States. The content of this 2-year program is divided among Rhythms of Jewish Living, Purposes of Jewish Living, Ethics of Jewish Living, and Dramas of Jewish Living. Thirty percent of the students in this community-based adult education program are 50 to 59 years old, and 28% are over age 60. These percentages are mirrored in many synagogues' adult education programs. For more information, contact Judy Mars Kupchan, Florence Melton Adult Mini-Schools, 601 Skokie Blvd., Suite 1A, Northbrook, IL 60062; 847-714-9843.

Rabbi Friedman notes that the *andragogical* approach to education (see Chapter 3, "Health Educators: Collaboration, Communication, and Health Behavior Change") is practiced at these adult learning sites. Adult learners are encouraged to talk about their life experience in order to build from the known to the unknown, to encourage personal reflection and sharing with others, and to set their own learning objectives and evaluation criteria.

There is also an ancient Jewish technique for learning that is quite compatible with the andragogical approach to education, called the *Hervuta Method*. The Hervuta Method is based on the idea that each person has access to a piece of the truth, and we need to talk with a partner or small group to get closer to the truth. Partners or individuals in a small group rotate reading text, then discussing it, and sometimes following that up by sharing in a larger group. For more information, contact a synagogue that uses this technique: Rabbi Steven Sager, Beth El Synagogue, 1004 Watts St., Durham, NC 27701; 919-682-1238.

L'Dor Vador. This Jewish term means "from generation to generation." The actualization of L'Dor Vador is through intergenerational activities, encounters, or messages between older adults and the young. One such example is the *ethical will*, first described in the Hebrew Bible 3,000 years ago in Genesis. Initially, these wills were transmitted orally, but over time they evolved into written, video, or audio recordings. Whatever form it takes, the ethical will fulfills a Jewish mandate: "You shall teach them diligently to your children" (Deuteronomy 6:7).

The purpose of an ethical will is to share values, lessons, hopes, dreams, loves, and the benefits of forgiveness with succeeding generations. The richest sharing of life occurs in the last stage, when an older adult is able to assimilate all of life's lessons over the life cycle, and the younger generation can contemplate on a full life and its lessons. One resource to contact for learning about the ethical will is www.ethicalwill.com, a site that also provides a monthly e-mail newsletter.

A related intergenerational activity frequently practiced in the Jewish community, is the *life review* (see Chapter 8, "Mental Health," and Chapter 13, "A Glimpse Into the Future and a Look Back"). By listening attentively and perhaps helping older adults to record their life stories, younger people can help these adults come to terms with their lives and teach succeeding generations about their roots.

DOROT. This organization was established to enhance the lives of Jewish and other elderly in the greater New York Metropolitan area. It fosters interactions between the generations, including volunteer opportunities for youth to serve and enhance the lives of elders. DOROT provides training and consultation, and has published a manual, *Friendly Visiting Plus: A Proven Method for Enhancing Connections between Older Adults and the Community*. DOROT is located at 171 W. 85th St., New York, NY 10024; 212-769-2850; www.dorotusa.og.

Generation2Generation. This intergenerational program won the 2009 Programming Award from the Association of Jewish Aging Services. It is housed at the Hebrew Home at Riverdale and provides a group of 30 young Jewish students an opportunity to work with older residents. The students learn about Jewish attitudes on aging and how to improve understanding between generations.

The Hebrew Home at Riverdale is a not-for-profit geriatric care center that provides a continuum of care for more than 3,000 older people. The nursing home houses the 5,000-square-foot Derfner Judaica Museum, a collection of 1,400 objects of Judaica that dates back centuries, and is a part of the lives of about 900 nursing home residents, average age 87. There are also about 5,000 paintings (by Warhol, Picasso, Matisse, etc.), sculptures, drawings, prints, and photographs distributed throughout the many buildings that constitute the continuum of care at the Hebrew Home. For more information contact the Hebrew Home at Riverdale, 5901 Palisade Ave., Riverdale, NY 10471; 718-581-1000.

The Art of Jewish Caregiving. This is a unique program designed to educate caregivers and health care professionals about the diversity of the Jewish culture and traditions in order to enhance well-being at a critical time in a person's life. Jewish Home and Aging Services in Detroit provides caregiving videos, resource guides, and retreats; contact Jewish Home and Aging Services, 6710 West Maple Rd., West Bloomfield, MI 48322; 248-661-2999. The Jewish Eldercare of Rhode Island Outreach Program offers in-service caregiving training for nursing home staff on Jewish observances, traditions, and dietary customs; and similar training to visitors to private residences. The 8-week curriculum for volunteers is referred to as CHAVER (the Hebrew word for friend, and an acronym for *Caring Helpers and Visitors Empower Residents*). Contact the Jewish Seniors Agency of Rhode Island, 100 Niantic Ave., Providence, RI 02907; 401-351-4750.

Spiritual Eldering refers to the movement to recognize the potential for aging with wisdom, or *sage-ing*. This movement was founded by Rabbi Zalman Schachter-Shalomi (1995) and sprung from his book *Age-ing to Sage-ing: A Profound New Vision on Growing Older*. Although the Spiritual Eldering Institute he founded had a short life and terminated in 2005, the training programs he created and that produced about 300 leaders in sage-ing continue. For more information, send an e-mail to info@sage-ingguild.org, or visit www.sage-ingguild.org.

Reb Zalman, as he is commonly referred to, was born in 1924 in Poland. He was ordained as an Orthodox rabbi in 1947, but received a doctorate from the Reform-run Hebrew Union College. Although Reb Zalman's lack of convention became controversial among some sectors of Judaism, he was able to promote interfaith dialogue; the integration of the physical, emotional, intellectual, and spiritual realms; a commitment to feminism; and the full inclusion of LGBT people within Judaism—along with his innovative work in spiritual eldering and encouraging older adults to become mentors for younger adults.

Perhaps the best definition of spiritual eldering was provided by another rabbi, Abraham Joshua Heschel: "There is a realm of time where the goal is not to have but to be, not to own but to share, not to subdue but to be in accord" (1951, p. 4).

Sacred Aging has been promoted by Rabbi Richard Address, director of the Department of Jewish Family Concerns at the Union for Reform Judaism. Rabbi Address's goal for sacred aging is to re-vision how to help older adults become a meaningful part of the congregation, community, and family. He has written on how to incorporate Jewish values into end-of-life decision making, caregiving for aging parents, and developing programs and resources for older adults.

As a leader in the Reform Jewish tradition, Rabbi Address has created new rituals for older adults who are experiencing loss, transition, or personal growth. Some of these rituals focus on becoming a grandparent, reaching an unusually advanced age or wedding anniversary, entering retirement, moving into a retirement home, and completing a year of mourning. For more information on Rabbi Richard Address's perspective on Jewish Aging, contact the Department of Jewish Family Concerns, Union for Reform Judaism, 633 3rd Ave., New York, NY 10017; 212-650-4294.

The Hebrew Rehabilitation Center (HRC) provides 625 long-term care hospital beds, 50 short-term skilled nursing beds, and 46 post acute beds, along with adult day health care, home health care, outpatient specialty clinics, and community-based health and wellness programs. Nearly one third of the 1,200 employees have been with the organization for more than 10 years, highly unusual for the health care field today. The volunteer corps includes nearly 300 individuals, age 13 to 90+, who receive on-the-job training and supervision.

HRC is part of Hebrew SeniorLife, which has a tradition of caring for seniors that spans more than a century. HRC is currently launching a 162-acre, multigenerational campus that will provide housing options for seniors amidst a K–8 school and an early childhood education program. HRC is also affiliated with Harvard Medical School, training about 500 students in 13 geriatric care professions per year. Additionally, HRC houses the Institute for Aging Research (IFAR), the largest gerontological research facility located in an applied setting. IFAR is in the top 11% of overall institutions receiving National Institutes of Health funding, and is number one among long-term care facilities. Among its many research accomplishments, it sponsored the ground-breaking weight training program with very-old older adults (Fiatarone et al., 1990; see Chapter 4, "Exercise"). HRC is located at 1200 Centre St., Boston, MA 02131; 617-363-8392.

Menorah Park Center for Senior Living (MPC) is dedicated to the health of older adults through its nursing home, housing options from independent to assisted living, adult day care center, rehabilitation center, home health agency, and community services. In 2009 MPC helped 10 women between the ages of 89 and 96 achieve their Bat Mitzvah at these advanced ages (see Chapter 1, "Introduction"). Also in 2009 MPC sponsored the *Chutzpah Mission*, which sent 10 residents, age 77 to 94, with their wheelchairs, oxygen tanks, and nebulizers, to Israel for educational and tourism purposes. For more information about these and related health services and programs, research endeavors, and educational pursuits, contact Menorah Park for Senior Living, 27100 Cedar Rd., Cleveland, OH 44122; 216-831-6500.

The Association of Jewish Aging Services (AJAS) of North America was founded in 1960 to support not-for-profit elder services delivered in the context of Jewish values. There are 115 member organizations representing 95% of Jewish-sponsored nursing homes, housing communities, and outreach programs throughout the United States and Canada. AJAS sponsors the *Journal on Jewish Aging*, which reports on practical and operational information unique to Jewish aging services, and hosts an annual conference. For more information, contact AJAS, 316 Pennsylvania Ave. SE, #402, Washington, DC 20003; 202-543-7500.

RURAL AGING

Rural Americans are spread out over four fifths of the land area but in 2010 made up only 16% of the U.S. population. Among older adults the percentage was higher, with 23% residing in rural areas. Living in a rural area increases the probability of living in poverty; income levels for older rural families are about one third lower than those for older urban families. In 2007 food stamps were obtained by 10.3% of rural Americans versus 7.3% of urban Americans; 31% of rural grade-schoolers got a free or reduced lunch versus 25% of urban grade-schoolers.

Rural living is associated with a higher ratio of convenience stores stocked with less variety and fewer healthy foods than supermarkets; substandard and dilapidated housing; a larger number of health problems; greater likelihood of living in a community without a doctor, nurse, or medical facility; inadequate caregiving support complicated by the migration of children to cities in search of work; challenging transportation issues due to longer distances to drive to needed services, lack of public transportation, and poor roads; and greater likelihood of having an attitude of distrust toward the health care system, or to have been instilled with an attitude of independence and self-reliance and a reluctance to demand needed health services (HRSA, 2002).

Nurses, social workers, physicians, and other health professionals are in short supply in rural settings. This is due in part to health policies, such as lower reimbursement for health providers in rural settings (based on operating costs that are assumed to be less), but also to the lack of community and health care resources in many rural locations. Health professionals are concerned about locating in rural areas that may lack quality public schools, cultural opportunities, job opportunities for a spouse, and sophisticated hospital equipment. Consequently, there are 10 internists per 100,000 population in rural areas, compared to 52 per 100,000 in urban areas (Elliott, 2001b).

Elderly persons who live in rural areas receive fewer services per home health care visit, and they have poorer health outcomes than their city-dwelling older adult counterparts (Schlenker, Powell, & Goodrich, 2002). These findings may represent accommodation of rural home health providers to rural realities, such as the lower availability of certain health care personnel like physical therapists or longer travel distances.

On a variety of measures, rural populations are in poorer health and at higher risk for poor health due to harmful health behaviors. Adults living in rural areas are more likely to smoke and have limited activity levels due to chronic conditions (HRSA, 2002), to be overweight (Wisconsin Study, 1996), and to have a higher rate of self-reported depression and a more negative self-appraisal of health (Thorson, 2000) than their counterparts in urban areas.

Rural elderly exhibit a larger number of medical problems than urban elderly, problems that also tend to be more severe. They are more likely than their urban elder counterparts to rate their health as poor or fair, to be heavy drinkers, and to *not* be "uniquely advantaged by embeddedness in strong, supportive kin networks" (Lee & Cassidy, 1986, p. 165), even though the rural stereotype of strong kin support suggests the contrary.

Inadequate accessibility of health care services makes it especially important that rural residents engage in prevention and health-promoting behavior. The adoption of health-promoting practices by older adults in rural areas may be enhanced through the encouragement of health care professionals. A survey of family and general practice physicians in rural Mississippi revealed that such encouragement is more likely if a staff person is assigned by the physician to preventive medicine education, and if flow charts are used to direct physician attention to needed prevention activities (Bross, Hartwig, & Herring, 1993).

Rural Resources

The *Rural Assistance Center* (RAC) makes referrals to federal and state agencies, provides publications, and serves as a clearinghouse for rural information. The RAC is the repository of rural information on more than 225 different federal health programs and additional private programs. The website includes searchable databases, congressional bill tracking, and quarterly newsletters. Contact the Rural Assistance Center, School of Medicine and Health Sciences, #4520, 501 North Columbia Road, Stop 9037, Grand Forks, ND 58202; 800-270-1898; www.raconline.org.

Inquiries can also be directed to the Office of Rural Health Policy, Health Resources and Service Administration, 5600 Fishers Lane, 9A-55, Rockville, MD 20857; 301-443-0835; www.ruralhealth.hrsa.gov.

> **Question:** If you were launching a health promotion program for older adults, what are some of the details you would need to consider that are unique to a rural setting?

The *National Rural Health Resource Center* is a nonprofit organization that provides technical assistance, information, tools, and resources for the improvement of rural health care. Contact the National Rural Health Resource Center, 600 E. Superior St., #404, Duluth, MN 55802; 218-727-9390; www.ruralcenter.org.

GLOBAL AGING

The average age of the world's population is increasing at an unprecedented rate. Between 2009 and 2040, the percentage of older adults will double from 7% to 14% of the total world population, according to the U.S. Census Bureau. Although *developed countries*, those with the most economic development, have the largest proportions of older people—of the 25 countries with the oldest populations, 23 are found in Europe—*developing nations* have the most rapidly growing senior cohorts.

Figure 11.1 highlights this differential growth. In 1950, there were 205 million people worldwide aged 60 and over, increasing to 606 million people in 2000, and projected to increase to 2 billion people worldwide in 2050. In other words, tripling between

| **FIGURE 11.1** | Population aged 60 or over: World and developing regions, 1950–2050. |

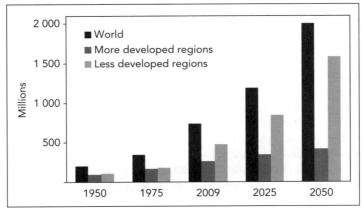

Source: United Nations, World Population Aging, 1950–2050.

1950 and 2000, and more than tripling between 2000 and 2050. However, in developing countries, the growth rate is quite a bit faster during this century, reaching 15 times the population it was in 1950 compared to 2050, versus only a fourfold increase during that century for developed countries.

The major source of diversity in global aging is whether a country is economically developed or not. In addition to the greater growth in older adults among developing countries, there is a much lower standard of living. This translates into almost a 20-year difference in life expectancy between India, a developing country, and Sweden, a developed country.

Let us look at one rapidly developing country, at least in its urban areas, and that is China. Due to a significant decline both in fertility and in adult mortality, persons age 65 and over now constitute about 7% of the Chinese population, but are projected to rise to 13% by 2025 and to 25% by 2050.

As Chinese elders increase in number, the number of caregiving children is declining dramatically due to the one-child policy—a policy that limits married couples to one child in urban areas—which was implemented in 1979. For most Chinese elderly, social security means relying on extended family, but the rapidly escalating older adult population in China is being paralleled by an equally rapid decline in children caregivers as a result of an estimated 350 million fewer births since 1979, because of the one-child policy.

The increase in the percentage of older adults in developing countries presents additional challenges for the future. The economist Young-Ping Chen noted that "the developed countries got rich before they got old; the less developed countries are getting old before they have a chance to get rich" (AARP, 2001). Thus, the rise in the number of countries with old-age disability or survivors programs—from 33% in 1940 to 74% in 1999—may not keep pace with the growing number of older adults in developing countries. Conversely, these developing countries may have to rely even more heavily on a less prosperous informal network of family and community to support their burgeoning older adult population.

In China, for instance, 70% of older adults are supported by their families, and only 16% rely on the government's troubled pension system. Yet China's traditional extended family is dispersing more rapidly than ever before, and grown children are now leaving their elderly parents to fend for themselves. China's urban population has increased from 20% in 1980 to 47% in 2009. Rural elderly, however, are the most resistant to this urbanization trend. As the young move toward urban jobs, socialized medicine in rural areas has collapsed. In less than a generation the rural population, which consists of many older Chinese, went from universal health coverage to 79% uninsured.

Japan, a developed country, has other challenges. In 2010, Japanese women had been at the top of global life expectancy for 26 consecutive years, reaching 86.3 years. Men were near the top of their gender in global life expectancy, achieving 79.6 years. Both sexes, however, slipped in life expectancy in 2011, due in part to the tsunami that claimed 20,000 people dead or missing, two thirds of whom were age 65+.

There were other challenges to life expectancy in Japan as well. With 22.7% of the population over the age of 65 in 2010, and the time-honored tradition of adult children living with and caring for Japanese elders weakening, two trends occurred: (1) the number of Japanese seniors living alone or with just their spouse doubled over the prior decade, and (2) the cost of government assistance to the elderly increased more than 70% over the prior decade, amounting to 12% of Japan's annual gross domestic product.

As the Japanese elderly continue to increase and the birth rate drops, seniors are expected to account for 29% of the population by 2025. Smaller families, combined with adult children seeking jobs in cities, lead to lack of space, desire, and financial ability to care for parents in urban settings. Although many retirees are drawing pensions, fewer and fewer working-age people are paying into them. Consequently, premiums are expected to rise in Japan at the same time that older adult benefits are to be curbed.

Many other developed countries are being challenged as well. As the number of working-age individuals for each older adult shrinks, we are learning about the magnitude of the economic strains that this increasing dependency ratio produces. There is a potential, for instance, for conflict over funding for pensions and health care for older adults versus a country's need to support public schools and unemployment benefits for younger adults.

In the United States, women can expect to live to 81.3 years, and men to 76.2 years. Though the country has been getting older, the United States is still absorbing many young immigrants. As a consequence, the *dependency ratio* of workers to older adults in the United States is declining more slowly than in countries that are aging without much immigration. This has slowed down the decline in workers contributing to Social Security and Medicare.

> **Question:** What are the lessons that developed and developing countries can offer each other when it comes to both the role of older adults in society, and the care of these older adults?

BOX 11.1   Aging and the International Cinema

An interesting analysis of 14 international feature-length films between 1988 and 2003 provides those interested in the field of cross-cultural aging with models of successful aging by elders valued within their communities (Yahnke, 2005). Elders serve as role models and mentors for the young and middle-aged, and they apply experience and wisdom to the crises that they discover—and sometimes create. In general, old age in international cinema is viewed as a time of strength, and the old as an integral part of family and community.

I have seen 11 of the following 14 films, and I can personally recommend them to you as an excellent way to sensitize yourself to cross-cultural aging. These wonderful films highlight the hope, joy, and inspiration that can be found in old age. Too bad we have fewer examples to draw on from American cinema, but old age role models in the American cinema have been increasing lately, perhaps an appeal to the growing number of gerontology boomers.

- *Antonia's Line* (Holland, 1995)
- *Babette's Feast* (Denmark, 1989)
- *Central Station* (Brazil, 1998)
- *Cinema Paradiso* (Italy, 1990)
- *Eat Drink Man Woman* (Taiwan, 1994)
- *The King of Masks* (China, 1996)
- *Last Orders* (United Kingdom, 2001)
- *Minor Mishaps* (Denmark, 2002)
- *Shower* (China, 2000)
- *Since Otar Left . . .* (France and Belgium, 2003)
- *Spring, Summer, Fall, Winter . . . and Spring* (South Korea, 2003)
- *Tea with Mussolini* (UK and Italy, 1999)
- *Waking Ned Devine* (Ireland, 1998)
- *Yi Yi: A One and a Two* (Taiwan and Japan, 2000)

This trend delays the inevitable crisis in the dependency ratio but does not prevent it, especially with pressure to limit immigration from Mexico. As the dependency ratio increases along with the huge baby boomer cohort becoming eligible for Social Security and Medicare, there will be greater challenges to maintain benefits.

To find out more about international policy and research on aging, a free biannual e-mail newsletter, *AARP International*, can be obtained by contacting AARP's Office of International Affairs at www.aarpinternational.org.

Aging and the International Cinema

In addition to the films listed on the previous page, two films received positive reviews in the June 2006 issue of *The Gerontologist*. *Ladies in Lavender* (2004) is an English film that was reviewed by Bradley Fisher and is about an older woman who converts a potentially foolish love experience into one of self-knowledge and inner peace. *Autumn Spring* (2003) is a Czech film, reviewed by Howard Schwartz, about an older husband full of mischief and an older wife ready to disengage from life, and how they reconcile, thankfully, toward the husband's perspective on life. I enjoyed both of these films, and another international film reviewed in the October 2012 issue of *The Gerontologist*, the Iranian film *A Separation*. This excellent film tackles several themes, including the challenge of middle-aged caregiving for an increasingly frail parent.

A film I have not yet seen, *Amour,* won the Palme d'Or in 2012, the highest prize awarded at the Cannes Film Festival. *Amour* is about an octogenarian couple facing their mortality. It has become quite commonplace recently for gerontological films to gain international recognition. I encourage you to take advantage of these opportunities to learn about cross-cultural aging in such an enjoyable way.

12

●●●●●●

PUBLIC HEALTH POLICY

●●● Learning Objectives

- Describe the role of public health in the United States, and how healthy aging can be strengthened through it
- Discuss the idea of a Wellness General of the United States
- Define *wellness*
- Critically evaluate the policy of implementing junk food and drink taxes

- Outline the components of strengthening wellness research
- Outline the components of monitoring wellness utilization
- Cite the most influential Surgeon General's Reports
- Explain the importance of linking medical clinics and community health
- State and support your opinion on the role of government in health promotion
- Evaluate the future of Social Security
- Assess the future of Medicare
- Summarize the Affordable Care Act, and its impact on Medicare and Medicaid
- Assess the necessity of rationing
- Critically evaluate the need for a government-coordinated, single-payer managed health care system
- Critically evaluate Medicare Part D
- Differentiate between patented and generic drugs
- Identify and summarize several important public health policy issues
- Assess the future of geriatric medicine and research
- Examine the importance of comparative effectiveness
- Assess the likelihood of winning an age-discrimination-at-work suit
- Document support for your opinion on public health policy issues of interest to you
- Argue the case that Oregon does, or does not, deserve to be held up as a model state for health promotion
- Describe a green burial

Americans live more than 30 years longer than they did a century ago; this is mostly due to triumphs in public health, such as improvements in sanitation, water and air quality, hygiene, immunization, and health education. *Public health* differs from medicine in that it focuses on preventing disease and promoting health in whole populations rather than treating disease and injury in a single patient.

Most Americans today, however, have much less awareness of public health care in this country than they do of medical care. The best-known aspects of public health relate to the goals of maintaining clean water and a clean environment, food safety, and control of communicable diseases. These public health roles come to the attention of the public only when there is a threat to water or food safety or an outbreak of a drug-resistant infection.

Even less well known is the role that public health plays in gathering health information, conducting screenings and immunizations, providing health education, and conducting health interventions. These types of activities reflect public health's concern with a broad range of health factors that influence the quality of life of individuals, families, groups, and communities.

The public's lack of awareness of these endeavors is probably due to the fact that relatively little funding (minuscule in comparison to what we spend on medical care) is targeted to support these types of public health activities. Ironically, in 2002, when there was a modest infusion of federal funds into public health departments for bioterrorism preparedness, cash-strapped state and local governments were forced to slash their public health budgets for health education and health interventions by a substantial amount. Another factor that contributes to the anonymity of public health efforts in the areas of community health education and intervention in the gerontology field is that its diminutive budget is focused on low-income young mothers, adolescents, and children. Public health has largely ignored aging adults, despite the steady increase in the average age of the American population. One report concluded the following:

> The new challenge for public health is to develop a focus on healthy aging. . . . Inadequate resources and attention are focused on health promotion and prevention of disease or secondary disability for older adults, the very population that experiences the highest rates of chronic disease and disability. (Palombo et al., 2002)

The study authors also noted the lack of collaboration between public health departments, which attempt to improve overall health in the community, and the small network of practitioners in aging agencies, who strive to improve the quality of life for aging persons. This raises the question: What if this collaboration between public health and aging was strengthened as well as backed by substantial resources?

Additional questions are then raised: How would public health policy foster healthy aging in American society? What practices would it attempt to implement? How would additional funding be generated, and how would escalating medical expenditures be reduced? I will examine these questions next, beginning with the section that proposes the establishment of a *Wellness General* of the United States.

At the end of an earlier edition of this book, in the final chapter, the concluding subsection was entitled "President Haber." In the last two paragraphs of that edition I proposed my health promotion platform for the country. It consisted of four sentences on three moderately controversial priorities: universal health care coverage, reimbursement for health promotion that has demonstrated effectiveness, and federal resources to help promote more physical activity among Americans.

For this edition of my book, I continue to expand my platform to dozens of proposals and escalate the controversial nature of some of them. I attribute this change to the aging process. I may or may not be growing wiser with age, but it does appear that I am growing bolder.

My boldness does not extend to predicting the future success of the Affordable Care Act. However, I will express my preferences and hopes regarding this landmark legislation that is reviled by many, but I disagree with them heartily. I believe it is an adequate first step and like other landmark legislation, such as *Social Security* and *Medicare*, it has the potential to get better over time.

WELLNESS GENERAL OF THE UNITED STATES

My first task as president will be to convert the position of the Surgeon General of the United States to Wellness General of the United States. The designation *surgeon general* refers to the chief medical officer of a military, state, or federal public health service. At the federal public health service level, the position of Surgeon General of the United States is filled by a physician selected by the president for a 4-year term, for the purpose of leading the nation toward better health. The physician primarily uses this office as a bully pulpit, exhorting policymakers, community leaders, and citizens toward healthier lifestyles.

The proposed Wellness General of the United States will have new resources and responsibilities (Haber, 2002b). The resources will be generated by a junk food tax. The responsibilities will be to (1) strengthen wellness research, and (2) increase wellness utilization at the state, community, family, and individual level. Before examining these two responsibilities, the term *wellness* and the generation of resources through a controversial junk food tax will be reviewed.

WELLNESS

Surgeon general is a military term that can be disconcerting to advocates of wellness. The *general* part of the term may be accepted within the narrow definition of a leadership position. The word *surgeon*, however, is not as easily salvageable. It is derived from the domain of medicine and narrowly linked to an operation or a manual procedure relating to physical disease or injury. *Wellness*, on the other hand, is a broader term that includes not only disease and injury, but also health promotion and disease prevention—not only the physical realm, but the emotional, social, intellectual, and spiritual domains.

Although the term *wellness* has had many supporters in the health professions over the past 25 years (Jonas, 2000), it tends to be less recognized than the terms *health promotion* and *disease prevention*. Health promotion, also referred to in the medical domain as *primary prevention*, refers to mainstream interventions like exercise, nutrition, and stress management that have relevance to a variety of diseases or disabilities, and to immunizations that are targeted to prevent specific diseases.

Wellness, however, conveys one additional important message—that good health is more than physical well-being, and that it is more than a response to actual or potential disease or disability. Ardell's (2000) definition is the most cogent: optimal health and life satisfaction that includes physical elements (exercise and nutrition), psychological aspects (stress management and emotional intelligence), social and intellectual elements (connectedness to significant others and passionate ideas), and spiritual components (seeking meaning and purpose in life).

Although exercise, nutrition, and stress management are the most familiar and practiced components of wellness (and its cousin, health promotion), it tends to be the more alternative activities—herbal medicine, chiropractic, acupuncture, massage therapy, spiritual healing, aroma therapy, relaxation techniques, self-help groups—that are associated with wellness. Perhaps this is due to the tremendous growth in these approaches over the past three decades and the significant amount of media attention devoted to them.

Since a Wellness General will have to cover more territory than a Surgeon General and will have more responsibilities (to be examined later), it will be necessary to increase the stature and resources of the position. Stature can be increased by elevating the position to cabinet-level status, complementary to the Secretary of Health and Human Services. Resources can be increased by legislating a wellness budget, and funding it through junk food taxes.

JUNK FOOD TAX

One way to create a budget for the Wellness General is to craft federal legislation that mandates a small tax on junk food—candy bars, cookies, cakes, pastries, ice cream, soda, corn chips, tortilla chips, potato chips, and the remaining high-fat, high-sugar, or high-salt junk foods, which constitute over 20% of Americans' calories. Jacobson and Brownell (2000) estimate that a national tax of 1 cent per 12-ounce soft drink would generate about $1.5 billion annually, and 1 cent per pound of candy, chips, and other snack foods would raise more than $100 million annually. A more recent analysis reported that a 1-cent-per-ounce tax on sugar-sweetened beverages would generate $14.9 billion in the first year alone (Chaufan, Hong, & Fox, 2009).

This is not a strategy without controversy. The main argument against junk food taxes is that the government should not pry into people's personal business. More than a decade ago, a *Washington Post* editorial belittled then–Agriculture Secretary Dan Glickman, who had announced that "it is the government's role to guide Americans into adopting a healthier lifestyle." The editor of the *Post* argued that we should tackle obesity and inactivity with common sense and self-discipline rather than expecting government to do it for us. The editor also asserted that a tax on unhealthy foods "sounds like something the government-always-knows-best social engineers in Washington, D.C. could feast upon." Other newspaper editorials argued, in similar fashion, that a tax on junk food is a bad idea.

Civil liberty concerns are raised as well. Wellness advocate Donald Ardell asks, "Don't we have a right to choose what we eat? Should we also tax those who do not exercise enough? What about those with no sense of humor? Now there's a group to sock with a big tax hit!" (personal communication). Those opposed to junk food taxes ask: If government gets more involved with promoting individual health, will it interfere with individual freedom and personal responsibility (Callahan, 2000)?

Those in favor of junk food taxes respond that there are long-time precedents for this. Of the main risk factors that enter our mouths, two are regulated and taxed—tobacco and alcohol (first implemented by President George Washington and continued over two centuries); and three, for the most part, are not—sugar, salt, and fat. If government gets more involved with improving nutrition (and reducing obesity), the health outcomes will enhance individual freedom and responsibility as well as the financial and humanitarian interests of society. These differing opinions and values are difficult to reconcile.

Philosophical concerns aside, there are "sin" taxes that work. As noted in Chapter 7, "Selected Health Education Topics," cigarette taxes reduce smoking and are followed by a reduction in lung cancer rates. It may be unreasonable to assume, however, that taxes will also reduce the consumption of junk foods. There is little doubt that these foods are unhealthy and costly to our health care system—with an estimate of $147 billion in annual medical expenditures for diet-related diseases (Finkelstein et al., 2009). But food consumption habits are probably shaped more by advertising dollars than by food taxes. Unlike tobacco products, there are no regulations to curb food product advertising.

Quite the opposite situation exists, in fact. McDonald's and Coca-Cola's marketing budgets are each more than $1 billion annually. Many additional billions of advertising dollars encourage the consumption of high-fat, high-sugar, and high-salt products. In contrast to this spending spree, the National Cancer Institute spent $1 million to promote its 5-a-Day (fruits and vegetables) campaign.

Even if a junk food tax could counter the effect of advertising and lower the consumption of junk food, wholesalers and retailers could regain sales levels by absorbing the tax burden through price reductions. If the taxing authority countered these price reductions with additional tax increases, low-income persons would bear the highest tax burden.

The implementation of small, not very burdensome taxes on junk food, however, could be instituted for the purpose of raising revenue rather than curbing consumption. Nineteen cities in the United States levy taxes on some nutritionally deficient foods such as soft drinks, candy, chewing gum, potato chips, and so forth. Much of these tax revenues, though, are spent on nonhealth activities. Another problem is that raising taxes on junk food at the state, county, or city level—no matter how modest—can provoke junk food industries to fight back. In response to industry threats or incentives (e.g., not to build, or to build, manufacturing or distribution centers), 12 cities, counties, or states reduced or repealed their junk food taxes (Jacobson & Brownell, 2000). When the state of Washington imposed a 2-cent tax on soft drinks, the food and beverage industry spent $16 million on the referendum that repealed it.

Question: Examine the pros and cons of the idea to tax junk foods. What is *your* opinion of this idea, and why?

It makes more sense, therefore, to implement junk food taxes at the federal level, rather than at a lower level of government. This won't be a picnic to accomplish either. When a sugar tax was proposed as part of the Affordable Care Act, the food and drink industry spent $58 million and blocked it.

Also, it makes more sense to implement junk food taxes for the purpose of supporting community health programs that have undergone research scrutiny, than for the goal of reducing the consumption of junk food or raising revenue for nonhealth purposes.

STRENGTHEN WELLNESS RESEARCH

One of the two primary responsibilities of the Wellness General will be to *strengthen wellness research* (left side of Figure 12.1). Wellness, health promotion, and disease prevention have not been high research priorities in the American research community (Woolf & Johnson, 2000). Moreover, the research that has taken place has been scattered among the various institutes of the National Institutes of Health (NIH) as well as other funding sources. The wellness movement will benefit, therefore, if funding for research is not only increased in amount through a budget generated by a junk food tax, but also consolidated into, and coordinated through, one of the institutes of health.

A good candidate to house wellness research would be the NIH's National Center for Complementary and Alternative Medicine (see Chapter 6, "Complementary and Alternative Medicine"), which can be renamed the *National Center on Wellness*.

NIH'S NATIONAL CENTER ON WELLNESS

The Wellness General of the United States could authorize the conversion of the NIH's National Center for Complementary and Alternative Medicine into the National Center on Wellness (NCW). The NCW will continue to fund research on complementary and alternative medicine therapies, as well as proven mainstream therapies like exercise, nutrition, immunizations, and smoking cessation. More research is needed on how to implement these strategies more broadly and effectively.

United States Preventive Services Task Force

The National Wellness Center will not only fund mainstream and alternative research topics, but it will also be coordinated with the *United States Preventive Services Task Force* (USPSTF). The USPSTF will publish a summary of the state of wellness research every 4 years, and ways to convert research findings into practice recommendations. Also, instead of the USPSTF serving as an advisory council, with health policy decisions made by Congress and the lobbyists who influence them, it will be given the authority, with the Wellness General's oversight, to link recommendations to practical reimbursement decisions.

Monitor Wellness Utilization

The second goal of the Wellness General of the United States will be to *monitor wellness utilization* (right side of Figure 12.1), and encourage its utilization at all levels of society, from state government, to private insurance, to work, to community, to clinics, to family, and to individuals.

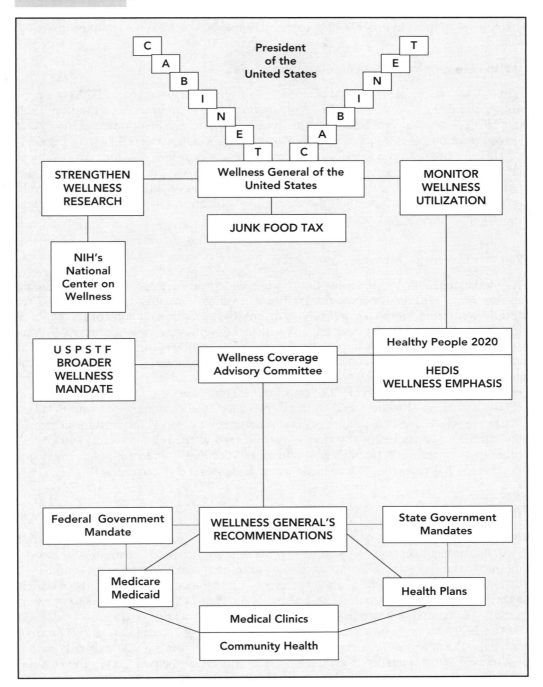

FIGURE 12.1   Wellness General of the United States.

Healthy People 2020

Healthy People 2020 is a public–private effort to promote health over the decade 2010 to 2020 (see Chapter 1, "Introduction"). Although health goals have been established, the data compiled, and progress monitored, the financial support to achieve Healthy People

2020 goals is largely missing. The percentage rates of physical inactivity and obesity among Americans, for instance, has been monitored, but it nonetheless has increased over the past decades. The Wellness General will need to set priorities that are backed by financial support in order to help Healthy People 2020 achieve its wellness goals.

Health Plan Employer Data and Information Set

In the private sector the National Committee for Quality Assurance (NCQA) is a non-profit watchdog of managed-care organizations that also provides accreditation. Each year NCQA issues a report card on the quality of managed health care plans that is derived from the Health Plan Employer Data and Information Set (HEDIS).

HEDIS is based on 50 performance measures, only a few of which are wellness activities. The Wellness General will encourage more wellness services to be evaluated under HEDIS and to measure whether managed-care organizations are effectively reaching out to beneficiaries and increasing the utilization rate of these wellness services (Asch, Sloss, Hogan, Brook, & Kravitz, 2000).

Wellness Coverage Advisory Committee

The Medicare Coverage Advisory Committee, which was created in 1998 to evaluate new therapies, will now become the Wellness Coverage Advisory Committee (WCAS) (middle column of Figure 12.1). WCAS will link the recommendations of the USPSTF to practical reimbursement decisions. It will make reimbursement recommendations to the Wellness General based on (a) the research findings funded by the National Wellness Center, (b) the recommendations made by the USPSTF, and (c) the percentage of persons needing to be engaged in such activities as determined by the Healthy People 2020 initiative and the HEDIS performance measures.

The WCAC will recommend to the Centers for Medicare and Medicaid Services whether to reimburse new treatments under Medicare as well as forward these recommendations for consideration by state governments and the private sector. The WCAC will employ consumer advocates who will make sure that the research on a new wellness therapy has relevance to low-income and under served populations.

Wellness General's Reports on Health

The Wellness General will continue in the tradition of the Surgeon General and attempt to publish a major report each year or two to heighten America's awareness of important public health issues. The impact of some of these reports have been profound.

The 1964 *Surgeon General's Report on Tobacco*, for instance, summarized the research on the health hazards of tobacco use, and many analysts believe it was a major factor in the 50% reduction in tobacco use that took place over the next three decades.

The 1979 *Surgeon General's Report on Health Promotion and Disease Prevention* became one of the most, if not *the* most, widely cited documents on the role that risk factors play in morbidity, mortality, and medical costs. This report helped launch the Healthy People 1980 initiative, and the subsequent decade-long initiatives: Healthy People 1990, 2000, 2010, and 2020.

The 1996 *Surgeon General's Report on Physical Activity and Health* did an excellent job of summarizing the research on the importance of moderate-intensity physical activity or exercise, the value of accumulating physical activity or exercise over the course of a day, the importance of resistance training along with aerobic exercise, and the utility of establishing an exercise habit of 30 minutes a day, most days of the week. These recommendations helped to change practices.

The 1999 *Surgeon General's Report on Mental Health* reported on the surprising prevalence of depressive symptoms among older adults and the inability of health professionals to identify and treat this problem. It also highlighted the reimbursement discrepancy between mental health and physical health problems, which was finally corrected a decade later.

The 2004 *Surgeon General's Report on Bone Health and Osteoporosis* warned that by 2020, half of all American citizens older than 50 will be at risk for fracture if no immediate action is taken. There has been much scientific progress in the prevention and treatment of osteoporosis that can be systematically applied to alleviate this serious health problem.

The 2006 *Surgeon General's Report on the Health Consequences of Involuntary Exposure to Tobacco Smoke* reported that there is no risk-free level of exposure to secondhand smoke. Nearly half of all nonsmoking Americans are still regularly exposed to secondhand smoke, which increases their risk of developing heart disease by 25% to 30% and lung cancer by 20% to 30%. This report further spurred state restrictions on tobacco usage in public places.

Question: Access one of the Surgeon General's reports. What do you find to be the most interesting or important age-related idea in this report, and why do you believe that?

For additional information on these and other surgeon general's reports, access the Web site www.surgeongeneral.gov.

The Wellness General will not only continue this important educational mission, but will also disseminate these reports to academic faculty who are training health care professionals, to health insurance administrators who are establishing health insurance policies, and to health practitioners who are implementing programs in medical clinics and community health organizations.

Federal and State Mandates

In addition to Medicare prevention at the federal level, the Wellness General will encourage state and local governments to follow the federal government's lead on prevention, on the basis of cost savings as well as promoting health. One study, a national survey of community-dwelling Medicare beneficiaries, reported that improved health behaviors lowered Medicare costs (Stearns et al., 2000). Another study reported that positive changes in physical activity, weight management, and smoking cessation significantly lowered health plan expenditures within 18 months (Pronk, Goodman, O'Connor, & Martinson, 2000).

The first state-mandated comprehensive wellness program, the *New Jersey Health Wellness Promotion Act* (NJHWP), was implemented on November 6, 2000. The NJHWP required most managed-care and fee-for-service insurers in New Jersey with 50+ employees to provide health and wellness treatments. Health plans in New Jersey initially opposed the legislation, attempting to extract extra fees to adopt wellness activities. Their opposition stalled the program for 7 years, until they were successful in establishing a financial cap on expenses.

A follow-up study of the NJHWP investigated whether the 18 specific preventive tests (medical screenings and immunizations) and physician interventions (counsel on smoking, exercise, weight) were implemented. It turned out that many of the mandates were unnecessary, as they were already being covered by existing insurance policies.

Moreover, only sigmoidoscopy, mammography, and Pap smear testing were consistently used by recipients, and the adoption of the other tests and interventions fell short of desired usage goals (Sheffet, Ridlen, & Louria, 2006).

Other state health insurance mandates have primarily taken the form of mandatory coverage for specific cancer screening tests. In 2008, 49 states and the District of Columbia mandated coverage for breast cancer screenings, 28 for cervical cancer, 27 for prostate cancer, and 26 for colorectal cancer. The pervasive mandates for prostate cancer (see Chapter 2, "Clinical Preventive Services") raise the concern that evidence-based medicine can be trumped by medical lobbyists. Also, states should consider coverage for counseling or behavioral interventions to address unhealthy behaviors like tobacco use, alcohol use, sedentary behaviors, and poor nutritional habits.

Linking Medical Clinics and Community Health

Health insurance primarily covers treatments in hospitals and medical clinics. Unfortunately, the link between these medical institutions and community health programs barely exists. The Wellness General of the United States will strengthen this relationship.

American adults visit or consult with their physicians on a regular basis, and the older they get the more frequent the contact. On the basis of access alone, therefore, it is a good idea to involve medical clinics not just in medical care, but also in the wellness of Americans. Medical personnel can be helpful when it comes to recommending lifestyle changes. The unassisted quit rate for smoking is about 1% to 3%, but brief physician advice can increase the quit rate by an additional 1% to 3% (Stead, Bergson, & Lancaster, 2008). If every primary care provider in the United States offered a smoking cessation intervention to smokers, therefore, an additional 1 million persons would quit each year.

Unfortunately, clinic staff rarely find the time for even brief wellness counseling, much less to provide adequate follow-up. In this era of rising health care costs, additional time spent on patient health education at the medical clinic seems to be an unaffordable commodity. It is more feasible for clinicians to refer clients to less expensive health education specialists or trained peer leaders who conduct community-based health programs.

These community-based programs are likely to be more accessible, affordable, and effective when embedded in trusted institutions like the church, the school, the community center, or the senior center; and more likely to be affordable and sustained when led by trained peers who provide ongoing social support.

The previously described model program, the *Chronic Disease Self-Management Program*, (in Chapter 9, "Community Health") is one example in which referrals from medical clinics can have both health and financial payoffs. A 6-month randomized controlled trial with almost 1,000 adults at churches, community centers, and other sites reported that the program cost $70 per participant and saved $750 per participant, primarily through fewer days in the hospital (Lorig et al., 1999). Another previously described model program, the *Senior Wellness Project* (since renamed Project Enhance), involved 201 adults in a randomized controlled design, and the $300 cost per participant saved $1,200 per person (Leveille et al., 1998).

> **Question:** What do you like and not like about the proposal to appoint a Wellness General and change the health care system to accommodate wellness?

Given the government's emphasis on revenue-neutral legislation when proposing new programs, "evidence of effectiveness should be supplemented when possible by information on cost-effectiveness," according to the USPSTF.

The Wellness General will establish guidelines for collaboration between medical clinics and community health programs. The guidelines will establish which interventions are reimbursable, what the criteria should be for client eligibility, and what type of provider expertise is necessary (Haber, 2005b, 2001a). Coverage policies will be updated to reflect the latest scientific evidence, and to emphasize the need to reach low-income and other underserved components of the patient population.

The link from community health programs back to medical settings is also essential. Even seemingly benign wellness interventions, such as a walking program, can affect medications and alter physiological parameters that determine medical treatment.

An Opposing Point of View (Sort of)

Fire the Wellness General! Get government off our backs! If the government is going to be involved in health promotion at all, let it focus on the social, environmental, and particularly the economic contexts in which health behaviors are shaped. Improve living conditions, and health behaviors will follow suit. Give individuals freedom and self-responsibility, instead of creating a backlash against health-promoting initiatives through government meddling.

Hire a Wellness General, and where will Big Brother intrude next? Should government encourage a downhill skier to take a 30-minute walk instead? Should government add to the stigmatization of overweight Americans by singling them out for ineffective interventions? Should government encourage insurance plans to be punitive toward smokers? If so, should it add overweight people, sedentary people, and, oh yes, those pesky downhill skiers to the list of scofflaws?

If this argument and these questions appeal to you, read Daniel Callahan's (2000) *Promoting Healthy Behavior: How Much Freedom? Whose Responsibility?*

Shortly after reading Callahan's book, though, I read *Food Politics* (Nestle, 2002) and *Fast Food Nation* (Schlosser, 2001). Another set of questions arose in my mind: Is it fair that the food and drink industries spend billions of dollars a year advertising high-fat, high-sugar, and high-salt products that influence our eating behaviors, while the federal government spends only a few million dollars on nutrition education? Or, as stated by Kelly Brownell, director of Yale University's Center for Eating and Weight Disorders: "The entire federal budget for nutrition education is equal to one-fifth of the advertising costs for Altoids mints."

Is it fair that diet-related diseases resulted in $147 billion in annual medical expenditures in 2008 (Finkelstein et al., 2009)? This comes to just over 9% of all medical expenditures in that year. For Medicare beneficiaries, normal-weight

> **Question:** Clearly the author supports a strong government role in promoting the health of an aging society. State the advantages and disadvantages of such a strong-government approach. Do you agree or disagree with this governmental emphasis, and why?

persons averaged $4,700 a year in medical costs, whereas obese persons averaged $6,400. Sedentary behaviors may cost society a similar amount. Is it fair that research on increased physical activity and exercise reports a significant effect on disease protection, improved functionality, and lower medical costs, yet we do so little to dislodge Americans from sitting in front of their television sets and computer screens?

And was it *un*fair that the federal government played such an important role (or meddled, depending on your point of view) in reducing the number of Americans who smoked cigarettes by 50%, in about three decades? Clearly, this is no longer an opposing view. I believe government must play a big role in promoting the health of Americans, and I offer three landmark pieces of legislation to make my case.

SOCIAL SECURITY

As noted in the first chapter, few can argue that inadequate income is irrelevant to health. A pending publication in *Social Science Quarterly* by Rice University and University of Colorado professors reports that in the United States its poorest citizens not only live their later years in worse health, but live approximately 5 years less than affluent persons.

It is important, therefore, in a chapter on public health policy, to examine the future of Social Security. Social Security is indisputably one of the most successful pieces of legislation ever created, with a longevity of almost 80 years. Moreover, without access to Social Security, 58% of women and 48% of men above the age of 75 would be living below the poverty line. The Center on Budget and Policy Priorities estimates that 20 million Americans are kept above the poverty line through Social Security benefits.

The future of Social Security depends on its solvency. The good news is that compared to Medicare, fixing Social Security is a walk in the park. Yes, the percentage of people over age 65 has grown, from 6% of the population in 1935 to 13% today. And, yes, the number of Social Security beneficiaries is expected to rise from 57 million in 2012 to 90 million in 2033. And, yes once again, the number of workers contributing into Social Security has decreased, from approximately 4 workers per beneficiary in the 1960s, to 2.9 workers in 2012, and the number of contributing workers is expected to decline further to 2.1 workers in 2036.

But fixing Social Security is not that hard. Here are five ways, with the last one solving somewhere around 80% of the problem all by itself.

1. Raise the retirement age.
2. Reduce the amount of money Social Security pays out to the highest earners.
3. Change the cost-of-living adjustment formula.
4. Increase the money Social Security collects in payroll taxes or (the simplest, easiest, and most politically palatable solution . . .)
5. Remove the payroll tax cap from Social Security ($110,100 in 2012).

The last option is politically feasible because the vast majority of wage earners are unaffected, and the lowest wage earners with the greatest need continue to be helped as much as before. But every year delayed, the problem becomes more daunting. This last option would have solved 100% of the problem if enacted in 2010.

What about privatizing Social Security? There is nothing social and nothing secure about this. If you became eligible for a privatized Social Security system just before the stock market crashed in 2008, you were (insert your own dismal word here). Moreover, the cost of converting to a privatized plan is in the trillions, and where would we get this funding?

More than two thirds of respondents in their 20s and 30s in a 2011 Wells Fargo survey said they were not confident in the stock market as a place to invest for retirement, which is a likely destination for funds in a privatized Social Security alternative. In addition, pension plans outside of Social Security are rapidly disappearing with only 10% of workers now having a pension plan in the work setting. Most everyone else relies on a 401(k)-type plan that, like privatized Social Security, places the burden on workers to plan for their own retirement rather than the greater predictability of a defined-benefit-type pension similar to Social Security. In other words risk would be added on to risk in a privatized system. Ignore all this and perhaps you can believe privatizing Social Security is a good idea.

If we do nothing? At around 2033 we will only have enough revenue to pay out 77% of promised benefits. (Although bad, this is not as dire a circumstance as most young people have been led to believe today—about 30% of whom do not expect any income at all from Social Security during their retirement years.) If we fix the problem? The last half of the 21st century is clear sailing. The percentage of the population that is older goes down, the percentage of the population contributing to Social Security goes up.

MEDICARE

I can appreciate that perhaps a few readers may believe that I have minimized the magnitude of the Social Security problem in the prior section (I respectfully disagree), but you won't find me doing that with Medicare. First let me state that Medicare is widely and enthusiastically popular, and justifiably so. There are 40 million adults age 65 and over who are covered, along with 8 million under age 65 with disabilities. Without Medicare, many of these individuals would not be able to afford health care.

But after half a century of success Medicare needs change. Back in 1970, astronauts on the Apollo moon flight reported back to base: "Houston, we have a problem!" Well, a few years earlier, in 1965, Medicare was created and "America, we have a problem! A BIG problem!"

Let us start with the rising costs. Between the years 2000 and 2030, Medicare beneficiaries will double, from 40 million to 80 million. Medicare costs, which constituted about 14% of total spending in 2012, is projected to increase to 32% by 2025, and left unchecked would be an astonishing 90% of all federal income taxes by 2075.

The federal government spent about $600 billion on Medicare expenditures in 2012, and it was far from being a self-sustaining program, that is, paid for through taxes from Medicare users. Instead, half the amount spent on Medicare was *not* funded through payroll taxes but by federal income taxes on all Americans or shoved into the future as debt. The average out-of-pocket health care costs for a person with Medicare is a substantial $4,600 a year, but would be a lot higher without the general taxpayer subsidy of more than $5,000 a year per Medicare beneficiary.

During the first decade of this century, medical costs went up close to 10% a year, considerably higher than the overall inflation rate. The reasons were simple: utilization of medical services rose partly due to a steady introduction of *increasingly expensive new technologies and treatments*, and partly due to an *aging population* that has more medical issues than younger adults. The reason was *not* due to administrative mismanagement. Quite the contrary. Medicare's administrative costs are 2% to 3% per year, versus 15% to 20% that is typical of private-insurance plans.

Americans under the age of 65 pay an average of 3% of their total income on health care; Americans over the age of 65 spend 16% of their total income on their health needs. Why is that? Not only do medical costs rise with age due to greater need, there are considerable costs borne by the Medicare beneficiary in terms of premiums, copayments, and deductibles. Medicare also does not cover dental expenses, hearing care, or vision care. In addition, Medicare does not cover long-term nursing home care or routine assistance with daily activities at home.

The most common strategies proposed for reigning in Medicare costs are higher premiums for higher-income older adults (already begun), increase cost-sharing (i.e., copayments and deductibles) by beneficiaries to reduce discretionary use of medical care, and higher eligibility age (to coincide with higher Social Security eligibility ages).

An even more stringent strategy is a *voucher* or *premium support plan*. Some analysts make a distinction between the two, but they both basically give beneficiaries a set amount of money and/or tax credits to buy private insurance policies. This has the advantage of planners knowing how much will be spent on Medicare but the disadvantage of shifting more costs to beneficiaries. A greater concern is that the voucher plan will not increase in amount over the years, commensurate with the rise in medical care inflation.

Another plan for curbing costs places the emphasis on providers. It phases out *fee-for-service* Medicare, which encourages more medical tests and procedures ordered by providers. The more tests and procedures ordered, the more profits for providers, not to mention the motivation to protect oneself more against potential lawsuits for not doing enough for their patients. Instead, this system shifts to *managed care,* in which all providers are paid fixed sums and then let the physician decide—with government oversight—on how to make do within the budgetary limit.

The bottom line is that we spend more than double the amount of what most European countries spend on health care, and do not get longer health expectancy. Part of the problem is that we have more than a 2-to-1 ratio of specialists to primary care physicians (PCP); whereas in other countries the ratio is 1 to 1. Consequently, nearly 40% of primary care services are provided by specialists in the United States, due to the well-documented shortage of PCPs and willingness of specialists to take on this role.

Specalists not only get paid more, but they use more expensive interventions. One such intervention is the MRI scanner. The United States has 4.2 times more MRI scanners than Canada, and our utilization of them has been astonishing (as I will explain under "Rationing").

The Affordable Care Act was developed to cover more people with health insurance, to reduce costs, to increase prevention, and to maintain quality of care—all ambitious goals, to say the least.

AFFORDABLE CARE ACT

On June 28, 2010, the Supreme Court allowed states to opt out of expanding the *Medicaid* component of the *Affordable Care Act* (ACA), but otherwise left the legislation in tact. The primary goal of the ACA is to reign in medical care costs while expanding insurance coverage to the younger-than-age-65 population. The act, as we will examine in the next section, substantially affects older Americans as well.

The full name of the ACA is the Patient Protection and Affordable Care Act, and its pejorative political name is "Obamacare." Any way you want to call it, this could be the start of something good, despite its unpopularity among the majority of Americans, which began before its passage. Massive negative advertising by the health care insurance industry and relentless bashing by Republican opponents and some Democrats in conservative states have taken its toll.

It is not a single-payer, universal health care system, which I prefer and will examine later, but it is the start of a system of health care that can reach many of the 50 million uninsured, improve quality of care, and, miracle of miracles, has the potential to start to make health care more affordable. The last goal is popular only in theory and will be exceptionally difficult to achieve.

The ACA requires most U.S. citizens to have health insurance, and those without insurance coverage will be required to pay a special tax on their returns. A fundamental component of the ACA is that it creates *state-based health insurance exchanges.* Instead of a single individual with no negotiating power approaching a mammoth insurance company, individuals can purchase insurance coverage from competing health plans through these state exchanges. If states fail to set up an exchange, the federal government will do it.

Subsidies to help people attain insurance are available to individuals/families with income levels between 133% and 400% of the federal poverty level. It also expands Medicaid to 133% of the federal poverty level. The ACA also creates separate insurance exchanges through which small businesses can purchase coverage for employees.

The ACA is a huge document with many interesting ideas in it for promoting quality and reigning in costs, a few of which will be analyzed here. It continues a role for private insurance companies, however, which I do not believe adds to the effectiveness of the act, but which made it (barely) politically feasible to be signed into law on March 23rd in 2010.

Affordable Care Act's Impact on Medicare

Those on Medicare stay in Medicare, but ACA impacts it in several ways. By 2020 the donut hole—described later, but it basically refers to a coverage gap—in Part D Medicare, which is the prescription drug benefit, is phased out. ACA offers better prevention coverage under Medicare such as an annual wellness visit with no coinsurance (previously offered only the first year that the beneficiary entered the Medicare program). It waives deductibles and copayments on medical screenings, making mammograms, bone scans, depression screenings, diabetes screening, and colonoscopies free. It increases payments for office visits to primary care physicians, who are in increasingly short supply because of much lower reimbursements compared to specialists.

There are also Medicare savings strategies as part of ACA, with the goal of extending the Medicare Trust Fund's solvency for 8 additional years, to 2023. One step taken is a payment reduction for Medicare Advantage plans, the private insurance option that averaged 14% more than what it costs the government to provide traditional Medicare. This extra payment for private insurers was never justified in the first place when put into effect during the Bush Administration.

To help curb excessive administrative costs or profits, consumers will receive rebates if a private insurer spends less than a required percentage on medical care from collected premiums—85% for large group plans and 80% for small groups and individuals. About $1 billion in refunds was expected in 2012, averaging about $150 per eligible family.

There are also income-related beneficiary premium increases, including for Medicare Part D. The rate of growth in Medicare payments will slow for skilled nursing care, home health care, outpatient and inpatient hospital services, laboratory services, durable medical equipment, inpatient rehabilitation, and hospice care.

Through the ACA, Medicare will now link hospital reimbursements to the quality of patient care during their stays. Hospitals will get financial bonuses for patient satisfaction, how quickly they provide anticlotting medication to heart attack patients after they arrive at the hospital, and provide antibiotics to surgery patients just before an operation, and take steps to avoid blood clots. Patient rankings on nurse/physician communication, how clean their rooms and bathrooms were, and how well their pain was controlled will also be assessed.

However, with more than 20% of Medicare patients returning to the hospital within a month of discharge in 2011, one of the ACA's cost-saving measures is a financial penalty to hospitals whose Medicare patient readmission rate with heart attacks, heart failure, or pneumonia is higher than expected. Hospitals that serve a high percentage of poor patients may be unfairly affected, as low-income patients often cannot afford the medications they are prescribed or the healthful food they are directed to eat, or understand the complex instructions they are expected to follow, to keep them from returning to the hospital.

In the first 2 years—2010 and 2011—that hospitals were warned that these penalties were coming into effect in October 2012, many hospitals took initial steps to see whether they could lower the readmission rates before penalties were administered. Some of these steps consisted of ensuring that released patients get follow-up checkups, medications, and doctors' appointments to keep them from being hospitalized again. Barnes-Jewish Hospital in St. Louis even sent nurses to patients' homes within a week of discharge to check up on them. Overall, initial actions by these hospitals resulted in only a minimal readmission rate drop of 0.1 percentage point.

Nonetheless, about 2,200 hospitals are expected to be penalized $280 million in total for excess readmissions in the first year of implementation, with the penalty amounts becoming increasingly severe in subsequent years. Critics argue that the overall amount of money at play—bonuses minus penalties (or vice versa)—is too small to change the way hospitals behave.

Although the ACA's CLASS act (Community Living Assistance Services and Supports) provision never got off the ground (see Chapter 10, Social/Emotional Support, Long-Term Care, and End-of-Life Care), other long-term care initiatives to keep more people out of nursing homes are included in the ACA. The *Community First Choice Option* assists states with the costs of in-home programs for people who would otherwise be institutionalized, and the *Balancing Incentive Program* increases federal matching Medicaid funds in states with less coverage for home and community services. Also, ACA helps husbands and wives hold on to more of their assets if a spouse must spend down to qualify for Medicaid assistance with long-term care.

One cost-containment strategy impacts on all persons, though perhaps more significantly on older adults with their greater medical expenses. The ACA establishes a *Patient-Centered Outcomes Research Institute* to encourage study on how well alternative treatments or drugs work. Critics argue this is a stealth strategy for the *rationing* of care. Proponents like myself are in favor of not spending money on expensive options that do not do better, and sometimes even worse, than more cost-effective strategies. Wouldn't you want to be sure that the medical procedure or drug you take is the most effective option and, if possible, not excessively costly?

Finally, an *Independent Payment Advisory Board* is a 15-member Medicare commission established under the ACA that operates independently to help keep Medicare spending from growing excessively. Starting in 2019, the board makes recommendations to curb growth in Medicare spending to the gross domestic product (GDP) per capita plus 1% (i.e., limits spending to 1% over the growth of the economy). This can be problematic in times of recession, which affects GDP but not necessarily the need for health care. Also, medical innovations can be costly in the short term, but save money in the long term. Congress retains the right to overrule the board's recommendations.

Affordable Care Act's Impact on the Younger-Than-Age-65 Population

If individuals have medical care coverage and are satisfied with it, they stay on it. However, Americans who have no medical care coverage will now have it, and those with poor coverage will now have a better option. Those with preexisting medical conditions can no longer be denied health insurance coverage. Those with moderate incomes receive insurance subsidies and those with low incomes are eligible for an expanded Medicaid program. There are state-run (or federal-run for those states refusing to do it) exchanges offering private insurance plans for people who are uninsured, self-employed, or between jobs.

Businesses with fewer than 50 employees are exempt from penalties that otherwise are imposed for not covering their workers. Small businesses with fewer than 25 workers and average wages of less than $50,000 get tax credits to help cover their workers. The state health insurance exchanges for individuals to purchase insurance will also allow small businesses to buy coverage.

These changes in the health care system will allow all Americans to participate in a health care plan similar to the excellent ones that have long been available to U.S. congressmen. Insurance plans must meet certain ACA standards, and insurance plan details must be posted online so consumers can compare costs and benefits before enrolling. Enrollees are allowed to switch insurance plans each year if desired.

No one can be sure how the ACA will turn out. One thing *is* for sure. If nothing had been done, U.S. health care insurance would continue to become a growing financial disaster, and about 50 million Americans would be without health insurance.

Affordable Care Act's Impact on Medicaid

Medicaid is the nation's health care program for low-income persons. It is a joint federal–state program, but the states set the eligibility rules. The Affordable Care Act originally called for every state to expand Medicaid to low-income adults under age 65, starting in 2014, but the Supreme Court decision in 2012, which upheld the rest of the Affordable Care Act, did not mandate that states expand their Medicaid coverage, but rather made it voluntary for states.

If a state opts out, this can create a subset of people who earn too much to qualify for Medicaid, but not enough to qualify for the tax credit that would help them pay for health care insurance. Consequently, due to this part of the Supreme Court's decision, the ACA will likely fall short of its initial goal of covering an additional 34 million uninsured Americans.

More specifically, Medicaid expansion was projected to cover an additional 16 million uninsured. If any of the dozen governors weighing their course of action as of this writing decide to opt out of Medicaid expansion, this will reduce the number of uninsured expected to access medical care insurance through an expanded state Medicaid program.

RATIONING

As noted previously, the ACA establishes both a Patient-Centered Outcomes Research Institute and an Independent Payment Advisory Board. Both are considered by political opportunists as a negative step toward rationing. So be it. We need to ration, and we need to do it *explicitly*. In other words, we need to ration and be *rational about*, medical care.

Rationing was already being done prior to the Affordable Care Act, but haphazardly. We excluded the uninsured, for instance, and this is a form of rationing. We prohibited preexisting conditions from being covered; again, a form of rationing. We raised premiums to such a high level that many were underinsured or had such high deductibles that they were reluctant to utilize medical services. Once again, a form of rationing. We also rationed through excessive rejections of individual medical claims by health insurers.

It appears more reasonable, to me at least, to discuss rationing in a more explicit way. For example, when $100,000+ medical procedures are being done on patients who have 6 weeks left to live (Singer, 2009), we need a rationing plan to prohibit this. When there are 62 million CAT scans (computerized axial tomography, or three-dimensional images from X-rays) in 2008 for a nation of only 300 million people, we need to ration these scans. Other countries allow many fewer scans and still have better health expectancy results.

Perhaps we also need to ration the number of specialists we train, and give incentives to encourage more medical students into primary care. There were twice the number of specialists and twice the rate of use of medical technologies in New York City than in Albany, New York, and—you guessed it—Medicare spent twice as much treating each patient in New York City as in Albany. Yet the medical outcomes were the same.

We have allowed unlimited electrocardiograms (EKGs) in this country. For healthy people with no symptoms of heart disease, the EKG is more likely to lead to unnecessary medications or surgeries than it is to identity early disease. Excessive EKGs also drive up the number of unnecessary CAT scans. We do annual blood work for people who feel well. This will more likely lead to unnecessary and expensive follow-ups than to identify previously undiagnosed disease.

Evidence-based medicine suggests we offer medical screenings too frequently (e.g., Pap smears every year or 2), too soon in the life cycle (e.g., mammograms in the decade of the 40s), too late in the life cycle (e.g., colonoscopies in the 80s and 90s), and too routinely (prostate specific antigen tests). Rationing on the basis of scientific evidence makes sense in a country with run-away medical costs.

Rationing does not mean that you cannot acquire the medical care that you want, if you can afford to pay for it on your own. If you want *proton beam treatment*, an expensive therapy for prostate cancer, fine, pay for it. Proton beam therapy requires a particle accelerator in a football-field-sized building, and costs Medicare $50,000 to $100,000. This therapy does not cure more people or reduce side effects; in fact, the side effects may be greater (Leonhardt, 2009).

And it is definitely not the cheapest alternative. A targeted form of radiation is half the cost. Surgery to remove the prostate gland is even less, and watchful waiting costs only a few thousand dollars in follow-up doctor visits and tests. There are no studies to show that the high-technology treatment does better at keeping men healthy or keeping them alive longer. In fact, most of these men will die of something other than prostate cancer. Yet which option is growing most rapidly? You guessed it. Proton radiation therapy usage rose tenfold from 2002 to 2006, resulting in several billion dollars spent in a medically unjustified fashion.

Because these treatments are so profitable for the provider it does not matter that the nine existing proton beam centers are currently underutilized, there are 20 more in the planning or construction stages (Emanuel & Pearson, 2012).

In 2008, Medicare paid for 480,000 injections for Avastin to treat macular degeneration, at a cost of $20 million. It also paid for 337,000 shots of Lucentis at a cost of $537 million. The National Eye Institute sponsored a 2-year clinical trial with first-year results that suggest the cheaper Avastin is just as effective as Lucentis at preventing vision loss. There were no significant differences in mortality or morbidity. If the second year of research substantiates these findings, no one benefits—other than the drug maker—from Medicare's inability to require more expensive drugs to be paid for out-of-pocket.

There are harsher forms of rationing. In the United States, for instance, the Transportation Department values a life at $6 million when deciding on road safety improvements. If the cost of a project is more than the value of the lives expected to be saved by the improvements, the project is deemed too expensive. The Environmental Protection Agency (EPA) also makes decisions on a cost-benefit analysis, valuing a life at $9 million (Porter, 2012). In Britain, the National Health Service recommended against paying for a therapy that costs more than $31,000 to $47,000 for each year of life gained, adjusted for quality. In Australia and New Zealand, the government decided not to pay for a pneumococcal vaccine until its price fell to justify spending $20,000 for each year of life gained, adjusted for quality.

One quarter of all Medicare expenditures are spent on the last year of life, costing more than six times what is spent on other Medicare beneficiaries. Should we place a value on how much we are willing to spend to prolong an older person's life by a month?

We have reached a point where approximately 50% of all the health care spending is now government spending in the United States (Medicare, Medicaid, Veterans Affairs). If we cannot control these tax-payer supported costs, it will crowd out funds for infrastructure maintenance, such as repair of roads and bridges. It will crowd out support for public school education. It will crowd out funds for public safety. It will crowd out funds for medical research. Let individuals who can afford it spend as much money on health care as they want, but public spending on health care needs to be capped and rationed in an explicit way, or it will completely take over federal, state, and local budgets.

> **Question:** There will likely be quite a lot of ongoing change in our health care system in the near future. Where will we be 20 years from now? Will there be a single-payer universal health care system? What else might happen by then? Why do you believe that?

THE POTENTIAL OF A GOVERNMENT-COORDINATED, UNIVERSAL, SINGLE-PAYER, MANAGED HEALTH CARE SYSTEM

I would go one step further than the Affordable Care Act, and get rid of private insurers. Although competition in many commercial markets in the United States drives costs down, in health care it appears to drive costs up. There are additional costs for maximizing profits, for advertising among competing private plans, for executive salaries, and for individual practitioners to hire staff to decipher the rules among multiple plans. None of these expenditures inspires improvements in health care quality.

A private insurance component of Medicare, called Medicare Advantage, has not produced savings. Before the financial subsidy legislated to private insurers through the Bush Administration is finally phased out through the ACA, more than a quarter of Medicare beneficiaries had signed up for it. Costs for Medicare Advantage's private insurers were about 12% more expensive than costs under traditional Medicare.

The lack of cost savings occurred even though private insurers were more effective at attracting the healthier and less costly Medicare enrollees, thereby leaving more of the frail and more costly beneficiaries for traditional Medicare to take care of. As I noted in an earlier book (Haber, 1989), this is called "adverse selection." Despite this advantage, it was more than offset by the higher administrative costs of private insurers, who were also less effective than Medicare at negotiating lower rates from hospitals and doctors.

Although Sweden's health care system is far from perfect (this applies to all countries), it has a government-funded, single-payer system that provides quality care at only 9% of the GDP (about half of the GDP devoted to health care in the United States). This percentage has remained relatively stable since 1977, versus a steadily increasing percentage in the United States over this time period.

Sweden's system is quite a bit different from the U.S. system, but let us focus on just one of these differences. They provide cost savings for physicians who link to its one system for implementing electronic medical records. Thus, 90% of their physicians did so. In the United States, however, only a small minority of physicians had adopted a cost-effective electronic medical record on their own. In addition, we have had hundreds of payment systems, requiring untold costs in training and deployment of personnel to sort through all the unique regulations.

Although the Affordable Care Act is not a single-payer system, it does have managed care elements to it. For instance, electronic medical records are mandated for physicians and medical offices by 2014, or there are financial penalties. According to the national coordinator for health information technology in the Obama administration, Farzad Mostashari, the growth in medical record-keeping had increased dramatically in 2011 and 2012 due to this impending mandate, with primary care doctors doubling in electronic medical use in 2 years time, to 40%, and to more than one third of the nation's 5,000 acute care hospitals converting to its use.

A few years ago the physician Benjamin Brewer lamented that he had 301 different private insurance plans to deal with. He wrote in an online column for the *Wall Street Journal* that he had to employ two full-time staff members for billing, and two secretaries who spent half their time collecting insurance information. "I suspect," Dr. Brewer wrote, "I could go from 4 people in the paper chase to only one with a single payer system."

The Department of Veterans Affairs is an exception in the United States in that it is a single-payer, managed care system with an integrated delivery system, salaried physicians, and medical information that is coordinated and tracked electronically. This system is not only cost-effective, but each physician has access to a detailed electronic record of every patient visit, test, medication, and surgery. It allows patients to access their electronic medical records as well, and encourages their interest and involvement in their own health care. Medicare is another single-payer exception in the United States. It spends only 2% to 3% on administrative expenses, whereas large private insurers spend about 15% to 20%.

Question: The author is clearly against a market-driven, fee-for-service, profit-oriented health care system. And yet markets, profit, competition, and other elements of capitalism have proven their worth over the years in contributing to quality products at affordable costs. Are these elements of capitalism helpful or a hindrance in encouraging quality health care for all in America? Explain your answer.

Not only does competitive, nonintegrated care raise costs in the health care industry, it is impossible for the health consumer to figure out which health care plan among the competing plans is the best one to suit their needs. It may sound good politically to give consumers "choice." But even if consumers were given educational assistance in making this choice, they would have to be clairvoyant to know which health care plan, with its unique set of benefits and costs, will best meet their upcoming medical needs.

MEDICATION ISSUES

Medicare Part D: A Critical Analysis

On January 1, 2006, *Medicare Part D,* a medication reimbursement program, was launched. Unsuccessful with an attempt to privatize Social Security, Part D was a step for the Bush administration toward privatizing Medicare. A major component of this legislation was the inclusion of a mandated middleman, private insurers, to cover the cost of medications. These private insurers offer different premiums and copayments, and cover different drugs. Beneficiaries need to figure out which private plan among many in their geographical area is best for them. One study reported that older adults were "very confident" that they had chosen the right prescription drug plan that minimized total annual cost, when in fact they had not (Hanoch, Rice, Cummings, & Wood, 2009).

Comparing the different plans is a complicated process. In 2006, investigators from the nonpartisan Government Accountability Office (GAO) placed 900 telephone calls to 10 of the largest companies offering drug coverage to Medicare Beneficiaries. Insurers failed to provide complete and accurate cost information more than 70% of the time. Trained operators at the same insurance company gave different answers to the same question. Even when GAO investigators were able to correctly identify the least costly plan, the insurance representatives provided a quote that was less than the actual cost to the beneficiary. The GAO investigators found that some of the private insurers referred callers to a toll-free government telephone number, 800-MEDICARE (633-4227). The Medicare office, according to the GAO investigators, was able to give accurate answers to consumer questions only 61% of the time.

Complexity is only part of the problem; cost is an issue too. Medicare Part D does not allow the federal government to negotiate lower prices directly from drug manufacturers. This has not been the case with another government agency, the U.S. Department of Veterans Affairs, which pays nearly 50% less for drugs overall than does Medicare Part D. As a consequence, immediately after Medicare Part D was passed, drug prices rose sharply by 3.4%, three times the rate of inflation. Prices rose even more during the first quarter after the Medicare prescription drug benefit went into effect, by 3.9%, which was almost four times the rate of inflation. Prices did start to go down a couple of years later, but, according to analysts, not as a consequence of competition in the private sector. Instead, a number of lower-cost generic drugs that had been released into the open market (see pay-for-delay in the next section), were having an effect.

It is not surprising that in comparison to five countries—Australia, Canada, Germany, New Zealand, and the United Kingdom—Americans were more likely to fail to fill a prescription medicine, or to take it regularly, due to its cost (Monaghan, 2006).

An added benefit to the pharmaceutical industry that was negotiated by lobbyists was the transfer of 6.5 million dual-eligible, low-income elderly and younger disabled poor from the lower-paying Medicaid program to the higher-paying Medicare Part D program. It is estimated that pharmaceutical companies received an additional 30% for comparable prescription drugs than they did through Medicaid (where it was possible to negotiate, and achieve, deeply discounted drug prices), and which led to a $2 billion annual windfall from this transfer—paid for by the American taxpayer.

Complexity and cost are not the only problems. Private plans can decide to end coverage of a particular drug during the year, and the consumer may be stuck paying the full amount for the rest of the year. Or they may raise premiums after the beneficiary has signed up, while the beneficiary is locked in and unable to change plans during that year. This turned out to be the case. In 2006 insurers raised premiums 13% *after* retirees signed up and, not surprisingly, the private plans raised costs 15% more than traditional government programs. Consumers Union (www.consumersunion.org) reported that more than 25% of insurers raised enrollees' annual costs after members were locked in for the year. This unseemly policy in the business world is known as "bait and switch."

The beneficiary can also develop an illness during the year that requires a drug that their health plan does not cover. In addition, the beneficiary may reach the "donut hole," an uncovered gap in medication costs in which case a beneficiary is on his or her own. In the first year, 3 million older adults reached this donut hole, and by 2009 there were 4 million in the donut hole. (The Affordable Care Act eliminates this donut hole by 2020.)

Finally, the Medicare Part D premium and deductible did not pay for the additional cost of medications generated by this benefit. So, among this legislation's many problems, therefore, was perhaps the most serious one: increasing debt passed along to future generations of taxpayers.

Much of the formulation for this public policy was created by lobbyists, rather than by the efforts of nonpartisan analysts. A congressional aide who helped write Medicare Part D, John McManus, formed his own lobbying firm the year after its passage and received $620,000 from drug companies and trade associations. Thomas Scully, the chief administrator of Medicare, was a hospital industry lobbyist *before* being appointed, and a lobbyist for the drug companies *after* he left government upon the passage of Part D. He was given a special ethics waiver to make this quick transition.

A leader on Capitol Hill in the creation of Part D, Representative Billy Tauzin, left Congress once Part D was passed to become the well-paid president (with a pay package estimated to be over $2 million a year) of a powerful drug industry lobby, the Pharmaceutical Research and Manufacturers of America.

Drug companies lobbied intensely in the development of this legislation. The health care industry spent $325 million to influence Congress, with drug companies leading the way with $87 million. Families USA, the major voice for health care consumers, spent $40,000. AARP attempted to influence the legislation in favor of the health care consumer, but it had a divided loyalty. After Part D was passed, AARP and its partner, the UnitedHealthcare Insurance Company, quickly became the number one insurance provider of medications through Part D.

The lobbying efforts paid off for insurers and drug companies; we'll have to wait and see how well Medicare beneficiaries make out, along with subsequent generations footing the unpaid bill. A survey of health care opinion leaders, conducted by the Commonwealth Fund in June 2006, reported that only 30% of respondents (mostly from the business and insurance sectors) agreed that making Medicare drug coverage available only through private plans was good for beneficiaries. On the bright side, though, researchers from a RAND Corporation study reported that, particularly among the poor and disabled, out-of-pocket spending for prescription medications dropped among beneficiaries, and there was an increase in the number of prescriptions filled. Also, most agree that Medicare Part D can be good for beneficiaries, though basic changes to the law—particularly giving Medicare the authority to negotiate drug prices—are needed.

> **Question:** I believe that if we become more responsive to the health care needs of older adults, we will probably provide better health care for people of all ages in America. What do you think is the logic behind this belief?

Patented Versus Generic Drugs

One potentially good policy component of Medicare Part D stated that the use of a brand name drug by a beneficiary required approval from the Medicare Part D private insurer, even when a doctor believed that a less expensive generic drug might not work as well for the patient. Unfortunately, insurers were looking to accomplish the exact opposite of this policy.

When the White House negotiated an agreement with the pharmaceutical industry in 2009 to lower the cost of drugs in the donut hole by 50% as part of a health care reform package, it allowed an important element inserted into the proposal by the pharmaceutical industry. The 50% discount on donut hole drugs would apply only to brand name medicines (a much smaller discount, 14%, was later added for generics). Thus, the pharmaceutical companies would not only gain income from many seniors who otherwise could not afford the drugs in the donut hole, but they also encouraged more expensive brand-name drugs into the Part D program.

There is a similar set of conflicting priorities outside of Medicare Part D. A cheaper generic drug can come on the market only after a patent expires on a drug that has the same active ingredients. Generic drugs usually cost 60% to 90% less than brand-name versions, and the prices fall more as each new competitive generic drug enters the market. Unfortunately, drug companies producing brand-name medicines are able to pay generic drug makers to delay the marketing of less expensive generic products. These anticompetitive *pay-for-delay* settlements keep generic drugs off of the market at the expense of American consumers.

In addition, the Food and Drug Administration (FDA) had a backlog of more than 800 applications to bring new, cheaper generic drugs to the market. Despite an FDA statute that generic drugs need to be reviewed within 6 months, it took 20.5 months to review each application in 2004. Only 200 employees were available to review 800 new generic applications. There were 2,500 employees, however, to review 150 applications for the nongeneric drugs that manufacturers attempted to bring to the market. Most of these new drugs were not only very expensive, but they were also not particularly innovative.

According to Marcia Angell (2004) in her book *The Truth About the Drug Companies: How They Deceive Us and What to Do About It,* few of these drugs contained new active ingredients that would make them better than drugs already on the market to treat the same condition. Of the 78 new drugs that the FDA approved in 2002, for instance, only 7 were truly innovative, and not one of those came from the major American pharmaceutical companies.

Rather than the $800 million on average that the drug companies claim it costs to bring out a new drug, these "me-too" drugs are likely to cost a small fraction of that amount. Nexium, for instance, was a me-too, patented drug that took the place of Prilosec, which went generic and was reduced in price. Nexium was heavily advertised as something new and improved, and this expensive drug was promoted through such modalities as television and print advertising, and through "education" for, or marketing to, physicians. Spending on marketing and administration constitutes about 30% of pharmaceutical revenues.

Effective lobbying is what allows drugs like Nexium to continue to be compared to placebos during clinical trials, rather than being compared to existing drugs on the market. If a new medication had to be superior to an existing drug, most of them could not be successfully navigated through the clinical trials to gain FDA approval.

We need to: (1) either allow the federal government to negotiate costs with American pharmaceutical companies, or allow Americans to shop in Canada and other countries where the cost of prescription drugs is much less and safety precautions are comparable to those of the United States; (2) eliminate pay-for-delay, that is, the loopholes for patented medications that delay the cost-effective generics from coming to the market; (3) counter the influence of pharmaceutical detailers, and encourage states to hire their own staff (referred to as counter detailers) to visit physicians and persuade them to prescribe generics whenever possible; and (4) prohibit the advertisement—to the tune of $4.3 billion in 2008—of (expensive, new) prescription drugs, based on the evidence that advertising promotes the purchase of unnecessarily expensive medications (as well as unnecessary medications) over generics.

AND, BRIEFLY, THE REST OF MY PUBLIC HEALTH POLICY CONCERNS

Leaning once again toward the side of a strong federal or state government role in promoting the health of an aging society, I recommend the following public health policies:

1. **Tobacco.** Now that tobacco is finally regulated by the FDA through the Family Smoking Prevention and Tobacco Control Act, it is important that the FDA set new

standards to reduce the nicotine content of cigarettes and to regulate chemicals in cigarette smoke. Smoking in all public places should be banned throughout the United States. Federal and state taxes on tobacco products should continue to increase.

2. **Alcohol**. Establish uniform drinking-and-driving laws for all states, including a legal blood alcohol content limit for drivers of .08%. Increase the federal excise tax on alcoholic beverages, and use the additional revenue to promote responsible drinking practices. Continue the prohibition of advertisements for liquor on television.

3. **Physical Activity and Exercise**. For the benefit of future cohorts of older adults, require daily physical education classes in elementary through high school, and provide exercise options so that children can engage in the physical modality they enjoy. Give recognition—perhaps through certification as a *heart-friendly location*—to shopping malls that promote walking and stairway use, communities that promote the use of bicycle and walking paths, and worksites that promote exercise for sedentary employees. Require commercial building codes to include safe, attractive, and accessible stairways (i.e., build stairwells in the centrally located sites where most elevators are now situated, pipe music into them, and hang attractive artwork on their walls). Recognize and reward transportation planners who shift their focus from cars to bike paths and sidewalks. Provide subsidies (OK, this one is a bit far-fetched) for the manufacturers of electronic games and television sets powered by exercycles.

4. **Nutrition**. For the benefit of future cohorts of older adults, pass an amendment to the National School Lunch Act that requires high nutritional standards for all food and drinks sold on school premises, including cafeterias, vending machines, and at school-related events. Prohibit the marketing of junk foods directed at children. Add a 1-cent tax on high-fat, high-sugar, and high-salt junk foods, and use the resources for health-promoting initiatives. Require all restaurant menu boards and menus to state the caloric content of foods and drinks. Set limits on the amount of salt allowed in processed foods and restaurant meals. Change nutrition labels so that sugar and trans fats are included in the percentage of the daily value that they represent, and, most significant, *apply the percentages to the specific product* (e.g., "this product is 40% sugar"), and not just to the daily intake for the day. Limit the sugar content of certain products such as breakfast cereals, or else relabel them (e.g., "breakfast candy"). Shift federal agriculture subsidies from grain farmers to fruit and vegetable growers. Develop statewide policies to expand and support farmers markets that sell locally grown organic food.

5. **Geriatric Medicine**. There was an initial burst of enthusiasm in the 1970s when geriatric training programs were established, and again in 1988 when the first examination in *geriatric medicine* was administered. After that, many who were grandfathered in for a period of time, and who needed to take the examination to remain qualified, opted not to do so, and the number of physicians specializing in geriatrics began to decrease—from 8,800 board-certified geriatricians in the United States to 7,100 in 2012. One expert predicted that by 2030 we will need 36,000 geriatricians (Olson, 2012). Despite high career satisfaction among geriatricians (Leigh, Tancredi, & Kravitz, 2009), there was only one trained geriatrician for every 5,000 Americans age 65 or older in 2005. With the large number of baby boomers turning 65 each year, that ratio will increase to one for every 8,000 older patients in 2030.

In 2007 only 253 of 400 geriatric fellowship slots were even filled, and only 91 of those physicians had graduated from a medical school in the United States. Not only is quality care compromised by the lack of geriatricians but so is cost-effectiveness. One study reported that geriatricians were more efficient than other physicians in managing hospitalized older patients, with shorter length of stay and lower costs per admission (Sorbero, Saul, Liu, & Resnick, 2012).

The best way to increase the supply of geriatricians is to provide better reimbursement for "high-touch" medicine versus "high-tech" procedures, and to elevate the income of geriatricians, who have been consistently ranked as the lowest-paid medical specialty. In the short term, something similar to the proposed *Geriatricians Loan Forgiveness Act* would also help. This Act, if passed, would forgive $35,000 of educational debt incurred by medical students for each year of advanced training to obtain a certificate of added qualifications in geriatric medicine or psychiatry. More standardized geriatric training across all medical specialties would be helpful as well.

Equally challenging is the nursing shortage in our health care system—a deficiency that directly affects the quality of geriatric care, given the importance of nursing to the field of geriatrics. In 2008 an estimated 116,000 registered nurse positions were unfilled at U.S. hospitals, and nearly 100,000 jobs went untaken in nursing homes. The shortage was not due to the lack of interest in nursing careers, but to the lack of faculty in schools of nursing. A nurse with the graduate degree needed to teach can earn, on average, $14,000 more per year as a practicing nurse than as a teacher. Consequently, almost 50,000 qualified applicants to professional nursing programs were turned away in 2008 due to lack of faculty, according to the American Association of Colleges of Nursing.

6. **Geriatric Research**. The problem of meager funding for geriatric training spills over into the geriatric research arena as well. In 2003 there were only 62 physician-fellows nationwide who were in their second or subsequent year of training in geriatric research. There is also a need for increased funding for geriatric research evaluating the effectiveness of counseling and other behavior-changing strategies focused on increasing physical activity, improving nutrition, reducing problem drinking, and encouraging smoking cessation. An innovative funding initiative would be to evaluate whether older adults can become effective public health advocates—particularly in the areas of environmental protection and strengthening elementary school education. When health behavior change strategies are supported by research, incorporate these health strategies into Medicare; and encourage state legislatures and private health care plans to mandate reimbursement for them as well.

7. **Comparative Effectiveness**. Comparative effectiveness is an important research consideration in the Obama administration's Affordable Care Act. This term refers to research that provides unbiased information to make the best medical choices for a given patient. Congress, through the ACA, set aside a down payment of $1.1 billion to improve medical decisions that affect patients. Many of the studies on the priority list developed by the Institute of Medicine affect older patients. Despite the persuasive logic of such a program, lobbyists of all stripes are seeking to discontinue this program to determine best medical practices, as these decisions may negatively affect the practices and products they represent.

This type of lobbying has been effective in the past. In December 2002 a rigorous research trial, costing $130 million and involving 42,000 patients over 8 years, produced what appeared to be solid evidence that generic diuretic pills for high blood pressure cost only pennies a day and were more effective and safer than newer drugs that were 20 times more expensive. However, pharmaceutical giants making big money on patented hypertension drugs managed to suppress the purchase of the inexpensive diuretics over the following 6 years. Their strategy consisted of heavy marketing of patented drugs, highlighting the limitations of the research results (no studies are flawless), and paying pharmaceutical representatives to convince physicians that the studies were fatally flawed. Only after some of the patents expired on the expensive hypertension drugs did the pharmaceutical companies relent (Pollack, 2008).

A more general example of the need to evaluate effectiveness and cost-effectiveness is provided by the Dartmouth Atlas study of Medicare beneficiaries. There are large regional differences in spending and utilization that do not improve quality of care (Sutherland, Fisher, & Skinner, 2009). In high-spending areas, Medicare patients are seen by physicians more often, are admitted to hospitals more frequently, and are the recipients of more screening tests of unproven benefit than in low-spending areas. Patient outcomes are not improved in the high-spending areas, and older adults do not feel they are being denied necessary care in the low-spending areas.

8. **Age Discrimination at Work**. Discrimination of any type (e.g., on the basis of gender, race, religion, or age) is bad for worker health. There are eight types of discrimination prohibited by law, and age discrimination has the lowest success rate—14%—when it comes to charges filed with the Equal Employment Opportunity Commission.

In a 5-to-4 ruling in 2009 (*Gross v. FBL Financial Services*), the Supreme Court shifted the burden of proof in cases of age discrimination at work. Previously, if a worker could show that age was *one* of the factors in a layoff or other adverse employment decision, the *employer* was required to show it had acted for a legitimate reason and not on the basis of age bias. Now, the *worker* must bear the more difficult burden of proving that age was the *deciding factor*. Congress needs to act once again to pass a bill, the *Protecting Older Workers Against Discrimination Act*, to reverse the 2009 Supreme Court decision that has guided the lower courts to apply this onerous standard of proof to deny thousands of age-discrimination claims.

The same five socially conservative Supreme Court justices blocked the gender pay discrimination claim of Lilly Ledbetter on the basis that it took place more than 180 days prior to her complaint—despite the fact that this was due to her lack of prior knowledge rather than to tardiness on her part. Congress reversed this injustice by passing the *Lilly Ledbetter Fair Pay Act* of 2009.

As the percentage of the workforce age 55 and older rose from 13% in 2000 to about 19% in 2012, strategies such as advocacy and education are not likely to be sufficient for protecting the older worker. Legal action is important to prevent employers from forcing workers to retire simply because of age, rather than because of reduced ability and desire. This is an injustice that is not good for the mental health of older adults and can limit potential contributions of older workers to society. Moreover, the burden of proof for older workers who claim age discrimination should be the same as for workers who claim discrimination on the basis of gender or race.

9. **Income Security**. Low income and poor health are strongly correlated, and both depend on a solvent Social Security system. Eliminate the maximum amount of earnings that can be subjected to the Social Security payroll tax, and include state and local government workers who are now exempted from Social Security payments. This will make Social Security solvent for the foreseeable future, and preserve a safety net for low-income elders. Social Security needs to live up to its name and be secure. Conversely, privatization of Social Security not only entails huge start-up costs, but would also make Social Security payments less predictable in the future.

Require employees to opt out of their retirement program rather than requiring them to opt into it; currently only 40% of eligible workers in organizations that offer

401(k) plans actually enroll in them. Eliminate the option of, or place restrictions on, lump-sum removal of retirement benefits when one is changing jobs or at any time prior to an age that makes one eligible for Social Security benefits.

So-called registered or certified financial advisors for older adults, who now may obtain this title through minimal educational effort, should be required to pass a universal accreditation standard for financial advisors working with older Americans.

OREGON AS THE MODEL STATE FOR HEALTH PROMOTION

Yes, I now live and work in Oregon, but I don't think this should compromise my credibility on selecting Oregon as a model state for health promotion, for two reasons. First, I had a similar section in an earlier edition of this book about Oregon being a model state for health promotion, many years before I even thought about moving here. Second, I decided to reinsert this section because, well, let's face it, this state is impressive, as the following legislative accomplishments attest to.

- 1967—A bill designated Oregon's beaches as public highways, resulting in the creation of many coastal state parks for recreational and meditative purposes, and granting public access to its residents to the entire coastline.
- 1971—The "Bottle Bill" required that deposits collected on beverage containers when sold in Oregon be refunded when returned empty. Many other states followed suit to encourage recycling, reduce litter, extend landfill capacity, and decrease the incidence of glass lacerations.
- 1973—Oregon decriminalized simple possession of marijuana, from a jail sentence to a fine, which was followed by several other states in order to reduce the arrests of young people and to better use the limited resources of law enforcement.
- 1973—An Oregon bill required every city and county to prepare a comprehensive land use planning program to comply with statewide goals. Farmers and wine growers in the Willamette Valley (my home now), barricaded by the Coast Range on one side and the Cascades on the other, prevented suburban sprawl and private developers from infringing on the finite valley's agricultural industry. A number of states later developed similar statutes for growth management.
- 1981—Oregon was the first state to acquire a Medicaid waiver to create foster care homes as an alternative to nursing homes. This long-term care option is situated in a private home in a residential area in order to serve one to five adults. Add assisted living beds to adult foster care home beds, and Oregon ranks first per capita in nursing home alternatives.
- 1990—The Physician Orders for Life-Sustaining Treatment (POLST) was developed in Oregon. It is more comprehensive and accessible than other advance directives, and continues to be adopted by other states.
- 1994—The Oregon Health Plan implemented a novel system of allocating scarce Medicaid funds (some years, obviously, funds are much more scarce than others) to cover as many poor residents as possible each year, as well as prioritize medical services through an independent commission that receives public input.
- 1994—Death with Dignity in Oregon was the first legislation to legalize physician-assisted dying (summarized in Chapter 10, Social/Emotional Support, Long-Term Care, and End-of-Life Care).

1998—Oregon was the first state to institute a medical marijuana registry along with its Medical Marijuana Act, to allow the medical use of marijuana.

1998—Oregon became the first state in the nation to require all elections be conducted by mail. Expanding voting access can be thought of as a community mental health issue. Unfortunately, in 2012, many states made voting less accessible for low-income people without driver's licenses.

2006—Oregon became a national model for significantly reducing methamphetamine abuse by requiring key ingredients to become prescription drugs, expanding drug treatment, and reducing doctor shopping.

2009—Oregon became the first state to make POLST electronically accessible, and able to be accessed quickly in emergency situations.

2011—(OK, this one was a failed piece of legislation, and Oregon was *not* the first state to propose a single-payer system, but) Oregon may be the most persistent advocate for a single-payer system, with 2011 being its latest attempt. ("Single payer" is summarized earlier in this chapter.)

BOX 12.1   Green Burials (and Lifestyles)

Eco-friendly burials have been popular in Britain for years, with about 200 Green cemeteries, but they are just starting to catch on in the United States, specifically in California, Florida, New York, South Carolina, and Texas. The movement consists of biodegradable coffins costing as little as $100 (or the body is wrapped in a shroud alone), with no embalming or vaults, and the designation of Green cemeteries with natural burial sites.

The first Green cemetery in the United States was established in 1998 in Westminster, South Carolina, and is called the Ramsey Creek Preserve. There is no embalming and no use of vaults, just biodegradable materials and bodies that replenish the Earth. For additional information about Green cemeteries and burials, contact www.memorialecosystems.com.

The U.S. funeral industry, which generates an estimated $11 billion in revenue annually, is against the idea. Many individuals also find the idea unacceptable, relying on the comfort provided by funeral services, floral displays, vaults, and traditional burials and grave sites. But as Mark Harris (2007) notes in his book *Grave Matters*, each year in the United States 800,000 gallons of formaldehyde are injected into embalmed bodies. Formaldehyde is a carcinogen that eventually leaches into the environment. Also, there is enough metal buried with coffins and vault linings to rebuild the Golden Gate Bridge each year.

Cremations are considerably less expensive and use far fewer resources than traditional burials. The more orthodox advocates of the Green movement argue, however, that they too involve hazardous emissions such as carbon monoxide.

AARP reported in 2007 that more than half of the boomers in the United States, about 40 million adults, can be classified as *Green boomers*. These ecologically minded boomers are buying organic foods and goods produced locally (to reduce gasoline usage and air pollution), financially supporting Green companies and nonprofit environmental groups, buying compact fluorescent light bulbs that use less energy, purchasing gas–electric hybrid cars, using solar-powered water heaters, recycling, and monitoring their thermostat settings at home. Eventually, some of these boomers will also join the ranks of those who opt for *Green burials*.

CONCLUSION

Let us return to the question that began this book (Chapter 1, "Introduction"): "Did you know that the federal government establishes goals for healthy aging?" My response is "Yes, but it is not enough; we need a three-dimensional vision of healthy aging":

1. Make one of these health goals the appointment of a Wellness General, and provide sufficient funding and a health care structure to make the role effective.
2. Provide government-coordinated, universal, single-payer, managed health care coverage.
3. Truly make it *health* care coverage, with a twin focus on medical care *and* health promotion.

13

●●●●●●

A GLIMPSE INTO THE FUTURE AND A LOOK BACK

● ● ● Learning Objectives

- Ponder questions about the future of being an older adult in America
- Speculate on a gerontological or geriatric job in the future
- Analyze the factors contributing to the reengagement of boomers during the traditional retirement period
- Explain the need for a reengagement counselor
- Identify the institutional changes that make reengagement more likely
- Examine the higher educational aspirations and achievements of boomers and older adults, and their implications
- Review the need for the transformation of senior centers
- Explain the movement toward chronic disease self-management
- Define medical, social, and emotional management
- Examine the ideas about why emotional health may improve with age
- Define socioemotional selectivity and gerotranscendence
- Define generativity and ego integrity
- Discuss the role that life review can play in the mental health of older adults
- Define elder cohousing and provide an example of it
- Identify several creative trends in the supportive housing movement
- Differentiate a Green House from a nursing home
- Define virtual village and differentiate it from a Naturally Occurring Retirement Community
- Define niche retirement communities and give examples
- Examine innovations in smart homes and telehealth
- Identify your own top three health promotion priorities

Enjoy the freedom of being old. There are fewer social pressures, and far more opportunities for growth and engagement.

—Ken Gergen

Gerontology and geriatrics are a tough sell to students, despite the emergence of the gerontology boomers. The following anecdote is typical of this challenge. I gave a talk to 40 undergraduate nurses, mostly seniors, some juniors, and began by asking how many of them planned on working primarily with older adults. Five hands were raised. That's 12.5% of the class.

Just down the block from this classroom, not more than 100 yards away, was a regional hospital where my wife works. I asked the students what percentage of the patients in that hospital are older adults. No takers. I told them that my wife reported almost 50% were Medicare patients. This is a typical percentage for hospitals in America. The same percentage of older patients holds true for the outpatient medical clinics surrounding this hospital. As the leading edge of the baby boomers are moving into their late 60s, these percentages will go up—dramatically. In short, I told them, many more of you will be working primarily with older adults than you now realize.

The 76 million boomers won't just be creating jobs for nurses. If you are interested in marketing, who do you think you will be selling products to? If you are interested in education, who believes most strongly in lifelong education? If you are interested in social work, who will be most in need of your services? If you are interested in science, who will be the subjects of an increasing number of research studies?

BOX 13.1	Questions About the Future

The five content areas selected for this concluding chapter caught my fancy, but if you skim through this book you will see many innovative and creative ways to work in the fields of gerontology and geriatrics. Perhaps those topics will appeal to you more than the examples that I provide. Many career paths are just beginning to emerge, like the ones in this chapter, but others have not even been conceived of yet.

You will find the content in this chapter introduced in prior chapters. Besides providing additional details on these topics, I want you to ponder questions that are broader than the ones I raised in earlier chapters, and some of them are more personal as well. The questions are:

How will old age be different for boomers than for the present cohort of older adults?

How will old age be different for the current cohort of college students?

What aspects of old age are you looking forward to?

What gerontology or geriatric job possibility appeals to you the most?

Does this job already exist, will you have to transform an existing one, or will you have to create a new one?

Can this job opportunity allow you to help transform some aspect of society?

I believe the fields of gerontology and geriatrics are in the beginning of a revolution. The topics in this book are appearing on the front page of the daily newspaper, each evening on network and cable broadcasts, and every day on the Internet (e.g., see Haber, 2008b). I cannot imagine any student selecting a different field to work in. And yet, many of them do.

Students do not make career decisions based exclusively on job opportunity. What also motivates them is the prospect of entering a field that excites them. Many believe this means working with the young. Young persons are energetic, attractive, and have a long future ahead of them. These are qualities that the students themselves share.

Boomers are energetic and attractive too. While they do not have most of their lives ahead of them, they will be dramatically revolutionizing society in their later years. I believe students can be convinced that gerontology and geriatric careers will encompass innovative and creative ways to be a part of this revolution. The variety of emerging careers in these disciplines will stir their emotions and imagination.

I have selected five unique career paths with which to do the stirring: reengagement, wellness center, physical health, mental health, and supportive housing. All five of these career options relate to the reengagement of older adults that will take place among the coming cohort of boomers.

REENGAGEMENT

[An older adult] who no longer has to worry about raising a family, pleasing a boss or earning more money will have the chance to join with others in building a compassionate society where people can think deep thoughts, create beauty, study nature, teach the young, worship what they hold sacred and care for one another. Once we realize that, we should have no difficulty understanding the most important thing about the longevity revolution: It has given the remarkable generation of the boomers the chance to do great good against great odds.

— T. Roszak (1998, p.8)

In 2011 baby boomers began to turn age 65 and started becoming the gerontology boomers. Most of them will not retire, if by retirement is meant a type of disengagement. Instead, they will be much more likely to reengage. Why will these gerontology boomers be different from the current crop of retirees?

1. The boomers will be the *longest-lived cohort* of older adults. They may have 25 or 30 years of life to negotiate after giving up their main line of work. How many of them will be comfortable with the idea of a quarter century without additional earnings? How many will be comfortable letting go of education, exploration, and engagement, in order to retire?

2. The boomers will be the *best-educated cohort* of older adults. Between 1950 and 2000 the percentage of Americans age 65 and over with a high school diploma leaped from 18% to 66%; and college graduates from 4% to 15%. When all the baby boomers reach age 65 and older (replacing the current cohort of older adults), these percentages increase to 89% who have completed high school and 36+% who graduated college. The number of college students age 40 to 64 increased 20% in the last decade, to almost 2 million students. During the 1990s alone, the percentage of Americans age 60 to 64 involved in adult education almost doubled, jumping from 17% to 32%. They say a mind is a terrible thing to waste: not only from the individual's standpoint, but from society's as well—76 million minds, to be precise.

3. The boomers will be the *healthiest cohort* of older adults. Although there is some evidence that boomers report more functional impairment than earlier cohorts at the same age, much of this data may be due to higher health expectations from the boomers as well as better medical diagnoses and improved medical literacy (Martin, Freedman, Schoeni, & Andreski, 2009). The reality is that boomers have been the recipients of substantial advances in medicine and public health, higher standards of living, and significant increases in educational attainment, all of which correlate with good health. Almost 90% of Americans age 65 to 74 report that they have no disability, and the disability rate for older Americans continues to decline. An increasing number of older adults are exercising in late life, with brisk walking for exercise becoming commonplace among the old. Strength training increased substantially between 1998 and 2004 in the United States, particularly among women age 45 and over (Swan, 2005). Not only is a mind a terrible thing to waste, so is a healthy body.

4. The boomers will be the *largest cohort* of retirees ever. The number of Americans age 65 and older will increase from 35 million in 2000 to more than 70 million in 2030. When these boomers came into the world they revolutionized hospitals and health care just through their sheer numbers; they then created similar upheaval in the public schools, followed by the housing market. A sizable number of them protested against the Vietnam War and civil rights injustices. Not only is this cohort large in size, but it also has a history of making change, and it is unlikely that retirement as we know it will remain unscathed.

5. Last but not least, the boomers are likely to become the *most engaged cohort* of older adults. A national survey by Hart Research Associates reported that about 60% of boomers believe that retirement is a "time to be active and involved, to start new activities and to set new goals." A survey by Civic Ventures and the MetLife Foundation reported that 58% of leading-edge baby boomers—those age 51 to 59— said they want to take jobs that serve their communities. This desire of many midlife and older adults to be engaged in the community appears to produce health benefits. Older volunteers, for instance, report higher levels of physical, cognitive, and social activity (Fried et al., 2004), as well as improved psychological well-being (Morrow-Howell et al., 2003; Musick & Wilson, 2003).

Financial planners need to ask boomers: Have you given much thought to what kind of job you want after you retire?

The goal of remaining engaged instead of seeking full-time retirement is likely to be financially inspired as well. Given the continued erosion of employer-sponsored defined benefit pension plans and retiree health benefits, and greater dependence on the more volatile investment income of defined contribution plans that prevail today, boomers believe they will likely remain at work longer than members of the previous generation (Mermin, Johnson, & Murphy, 2007). Scottrade (www.scottrade.com), an online investment brokerage firm based in St. Louis, commissioned the 2009 American Retirement Study and reported that nearly 75% of boomers felt that full retirement is not an option for them. The prospect of full-time retirement in the future took a particular beating during the last 3 months of 2008, when the net worth of American households fell by 9%, the largest quarterly decline since recordkeeping began in 1951.

Not everyone has the choice of working after age 65. There are health concerns, functional impairment, lack of job opportunities, age discrimination, caring for a spouse or other family member, and so forth. Nonetheless, the labor force participation rate among people older than age 65 rose from 11% in 1987 to 18% in 2012. Gallup polls conducted from 1996 to 2012 reflect that reality, with the average age at which working Americans expect to retire increasing from age 60 to age 67.

INSTITUTIONAL CHANGE

Business

Only 20% of employers offered flexible work arrangements that appeal to the needs of older workers, according to the Society for Human Resource Management, yet a majority of older employees were interested in this option. In contrast to the stereotype that older workers want to disengage from work, they are more satisfied with their jobs than younger workers, are more engaged in their work, have lower absenteeism, raise health care costs only 3% or less, and interact effectively with clients. The Bureau of Labor Statistics reports that the older a worker is when starting a job, the longer that person stays in the job. Older adults have the potential to be a financial bargain for their employers, as they may not need or seek a full salary.

Some employers have received the message that older adults are desirable employees and should be pursued. Home Depot, for instance, offers "snowbird specials," opportunities for older workers to do part-time summer work where they live in Maine, but also part-time winter work in Florida, where they are snowbirds (i.e., maintain a second residence or live for an extended period in a warmer climate during winter). Borders bookstores found that the turnover rate for employees age 50 and older was 10% of the rate for workers under 30. To attract older workers, they offered discounts on books and the opportunity to join reading and discussion groups.

Fifty percent of registered nurses are expected to retire in the next 15 years, just as boomers will step up the demand for nursing services. Hospitals and clinics are starting to find ways to reduce hours and change job responsibilities in order to take advantage of the experience and training of older nurses and extend their careers. Modifications in the work environment are also taking place. Florida Baptist Health in Coral Gables installed new patient beds that make it easier for older nurses to lift and move their patients.

Hospitals are getting more creative with recruiting older volunteers as well. They offer more flexible hours, free lunches or parking, and access to medical seminars. Older volunteers are given the opportunity to enjoy delivering positive results from hearing screenings to parents of newborns (while medical professionals deliver bad news). In exchange, older adults remain volunteers over a longer period of time than do young student volunteers. They also handle difficult situations in a calming manner, know how to offer emotional support to patients, and apply their maturity in a variety of ways.

Religious institutions may be considering older leadership more. Eliza Smith Brown, communications director of the Association of Theological Schools, reports that more than 20% of divinity school students are at least age 50. Ms. Brown thinks this trend is partly due to the aging process and a shifting interest in theology with age, and partly due to the comfort among congregation members toward a religious leader who has experienced the challenges and losses of aging and who communicates more effectively on these issues.

The *AARP National Employer Team* launched a website, www.aarp.org/work.html, to link job seekers who are 50 and older with employers who are older-worker friendly. These employers may provide such benefits as flexible hours, seasonal months-off programs, tuition assistance, older adult wellness programs, allocation of pretax earnings toward eldercare needs, large-screen computer monitors with ergonomic chairs, discounts on medications, or programs that pay grandparents to supervise play activities at on-site daycare facilities. When last checked, this AARP site listed 41 employers.

There are also companies that exclusively match people over age 50 with age-friendly businesses. *RetirementJobs.com, Inc.*(www.retirementjobs.com) is one such company, located at 204 2nd Ave., Waltham, MA 02451; 781-890-5050. Employee applicants pay for access to age-friendly employers, résumé editing, interviewing skills and other online workshops, job-seeking guides, self-employment and work-at-home opportunities, and other services. Businesses pay for job postings, for being designated an age-friendly company, and to gain access to employee applicants.

ReServe connects New York City retired professionals with opportunities in the workplace, particularly in service positions at nonprofit and public agencies. Retirees receive a standard $10 an hour stipend when hired, whereas employers pay $15 an hour to cover the employee stipend and administrative fees. In its first 2 years of operation, ReServe placed 275 older adults with 110 nonprofit organizations. It also has launched a joint program with AARP and won a contract to place people with city agencies. ReServe envisions itself as a model for other cities in the future, but it is currently focused on the NYC area and is located at ReServe Elder Service, Inc., 6 E. 39th St., Fl. 10, New York, NY 10016; 212-792-6205; www.reserveinc.org.

A surprisingly large number of baby boomers and older adults age 44–70 are interested in an *encore career*, according to a 2008 MetLife Foundation/Civic Ventures Encore Career Survey (www.metlife.com). An encore career combines income and personal meaning with social impact. Retirees move into jobs in such fields as education (30%), health care (23%), government (16%), and nonprofit organizations that serve a public good (9%). Almost 10% of the age 44 to 70 population surveyed were already engaged in encore careers, and almost half of the remaining surveyed (45%) were interested. To find out more about later-life shifting to careers that are meaningful and help the common good, see *Encore: Finding Work that Matters in the Second Half of Life* (Freedman, 2007).

Government and Foundations

Government and foundations can create more opportunities for older adults to contribute. The *Foster Grandparent Program* is an excellent government program that pays a small stipend to 30,000 older adults who help 275,000 young children and teenagers at physical and emotional risk. Foster grandparents serve 20 hours per week at $2.65 an hour, in schools, hospitals, correctional institutions, daycare facilities, and Head Start centers. This program could expand many times over, and help prevent many more of the young from becoming a burden on society.

Experience Corps is a foundation-supported program that has placed 2,000 older adults as tutors and mentors with 20,000 low-income children in urban public elementary schools and after-school programs in 23 cities. These programs not only boost the academic performance of students, but also enhance the physical and mental health of the older volunteers in the process (Fried et al., 2004; Rebok et al., 2004; Tan et al., 2009). Much work remains, as two thirds of the nation's fourth-graders in major urban areas are reading below basic levels for their grade. For more information, contact Experience Corps, 2120 L St. NW, #610, Washington, DC 20037; 202-478-6190; www.experiencecorps.org.

Shortly before he died, Senator Ted Kennedy sponsored the *Serve America Act*, which became law in April of 2009. Two components of this legislation are the *Encore Fellowships*, for persons age 55 and over who are willing to serve 1 year in areas of national need such as education and the environment, and the *Silver Scholars Program*, for individuals age 55 and over who will receive a $1,000 educational award after contributing 350 hours of service in the public or nonprofit sector. On a state level, the New York state legislature is considering similar legislation, entitled the Senior Property Tax Work-Off initiative, whereby homeowners who volunteer in preapproved public service positions would receive property tax reductions.

History professor Jack Hexter was forced to retire from Yale at age 65, then continued his academic career for another decade at Washington University in St. Louis. At the age of 80 he realized that the U.S. armed forces were being downsized after the first Gulf War, and perhaps many who were retiring from the army in their late 40s and early 50s might want to help fill the acute need for public-school teachers. Hexter persuaded then-Senator John Danforth to obtain federal money for his creative idea, *Troops to Teachers*. Several years later, the 3,000 retired veterans who transitioned into teaching surpassed the retention rates of traditional education graduates (Freedman & Moen, 2005).

According to the National Commission on Teaching and America's Future, a third of the nation's 3.2 million teachers could retire in the near future. Although tough economic times may mitigate this decline somewhat, the report is based on carefully examined attrition rates at both ends of the traditional teaching career. Beginners get discouraged by the hard work, frustrating working conditions, and low pay and status. Accomplished veterans are moved out by obsolete retirement policies that impose a financial penalty for continuing to work while receiving a pension. Senator Susan Collins of Maine has introduced a bill to Congress that could be applied to teachers that would allow retired federal workers to work part time without enduring the pension penalty that now exists.

The 629 Area Agencies on Aging are examples of local government agencies that could use reengagement counselors (or student volunteers) to help assess the local community's needs for the talents and experience of older adults, catalog these needs, publicize these work and volunteer opportunities, and, finally, recruit and help match older adults with these opportunities. Businesses and nonprofit organizations may also do this on their own—screen older adults, match them to needed tasks, and design ways to support them through ongoing training, recognition, and perhaps a stipend.

Education

Higher education can provide a venue for exploring creative retirement opportunities. The *Osher Lifelong Learning Institute* (OLLI) (formerly the North Carolina Center for Creative Retirement [NCCCR]), for instance, has just such a course: Creative Retirement in Uncertain Times. Through lectures, case studies, discussion groups, and community activities, older participants explore their image of retirement, their ability to revitalize themselves, and their plan of action. With the help of a civic engagement grant from the National Council on Aging, NCCCR created a Leadership Training Program for Older Persons. It enables low-income older adults age 50 and older to gain the skills and confidence necessary to advocate for their peers by becoming effective leaders in community organizations that rarely include representatives from low-income groups.

The OLLI is located at the University of North Carolina at Asheville, Reuter Center, COP #5000, One University Heights, Asheville, NC 28804; 828-251-6140; www.unca.edu/ncccr. For information about demonstration grants awarded to encourage civic engagement, contact the National Council on Aging, 300 D St. SW, #801, Washington, DC 20024; 202-479-1200; www.ncoa.org.

The American Association of Community Colleges is developing a nationwide program to retrain adults age 50 and older who want to find new work after traditional retirement age. The organization represents 1,200 community colleges and has received a $3.2 million grant from the Atlantic Philanthropies (AP) to develop such a program. AP believes that retraining older adults at community colleges is a good idea; the classes are relatively inexpensive and a nationwide infrastructure is already in place. In 2009, 388,000 students aged 50 and up were enrolled in community colleges, about 6% of community college enrollment.

According to the National Center for Education Statistics, 635,000 people age 50 and older were enrolled in degree-granting colleges in 2003, 80% of whom were part-time students. A large number of older adults also attend non-degree-granting programs at institutes of higher education. For instance, the Fromm Institute at the University of San Francisco (USF) is an educational program for retired persons taught by retired professors. The institute presents about 50 courses each year over three 8-week sessions. Program participants not only enjoy being in class with their peers, but they also have the opportunity to interact intergenerationally with more traditional students at the USF campus. Contact the Fromm Institute for Lifelong Learning, University of San Francisco, 2130 Fulton St., San Francisco, CA 94117; 415-422-6805; www.usfca.edu/fromm/contact.html.

The Plato Society of UCLA is another such non-degree-granting program in which a community of retired or semi retired men and women study topics in interactive groups where everyone participates. Contact the Plato Society of UCLA, 1083 Gayley Ave., 2nd Floor, Los Angeles, CA 90024; 310-794-0231; www.unex.ucla/plato. The Renaissance Society at California State University–Sacramento is a center for learning in retirement in which members choose to study topics proposed by their peers, who coordinate the seminars. Contact the Renaissance Society, CSU Sacramento, Foley Hall, Room 234, Sacramento, CA 95819; 916-278-7834; www.csus.edu/org/rensoc.

These programs represent just a few examples of older-adult peer-led lecture and discussion courses hosted at institutes of higher education. Contact nearby colleges and universities to find out if they offer similar educational programs.

Rosabeth Moss Kanter, a professor at the Harvard Business School, envisions a future where going to a university in your 50s or 60s is the norm, not the exception, in order to make a transition from the primary income-earning career to subsequent years of flexible service. No idea would be too idealistic for these older college students, from raising literacy rates to ending poverty to helping to reverse global warming.

Kanter envisions the development of these graduate programs at colleges and universities around the country, designed for older students who want to serve and solve problems. These students would be financially supported by foundations, employers, and government through scholarships and tax breaks. Kanter refers to this opportunity as "even higher" education.

Conclusion

Many boomers are entering a period during which they will get to shape their lives and live more in tune with their values and desires than perhaps at any other period of their lives. Moreover, the areas that older adults feel most passionate about—teaching, health care, environmental advocacy, and other nonprofit work and volunteer opportunities—happen to coincide with the greatest labor shortages.

It was not a trivial gesture when the American Association of Retired Persons changed its name to its initials, AARP. The organization thought it was misleading the public by having the term "retired" in its title. Former AARP CEO Bill Novelli described the institution of retirement as "the cultural agreement that, at a certain age, one stops working." In historical perspective, this cultural agreement has been relatively brief. Perhaps it's time to reinvent retirement and call it *reengagement.*

CREATIVE CAREER OPPORTUNITY: REENGAGEMENT COUNSELOR

The *reengagement counselor* helps older adults navigate postretirement work and volunteer opportunities. This job can be structured as an independent consultant for individuals or businesses, coordinated through an Area Agency on Aging, linked with a university or a Roads Scholar-type of educational program, or incorporated into human resource services at larger businesses. A large corporation, for instance, might want to retain some of their retiring workers by arranging for flexible work hours, new job responsibilities, and salary levels that are advantageous to both older employees and employers.

WELLNESS CENTER

Senior centers nationwide were established almost a half century ago primarily as nutrition programs, with the serving of a hot lunch in combination with nutrition education, which was often ignored by older adults as they were eating. The senior centers were typically located in a somewhat dreary institutional setting and would offer a bingo game and perhaps another diversion or two.

Some politicians have concluded that many senior centers have not advanced much from their unimaginative pasts and are now declining in relevance and attendance. New York City Mayor Michael Bloomberg, for instance, reported that if senior centers are to remain relevant for the coming cohort of boomers, they will need to emphasize health, education, and culture programs (Chen, 2008). Already losing popularity in New York City, 44% of the 329 senior centers are substantially underutilized. This comes at a time when a dramatic rise in the number of older adults is predicted in the coming decades, along with gloomy city and state budget forecasts.

Thus, there is great need for more attractive and efficient senior center operations, perhaps relying on boomers and older adults themselves to help figure out how to realize their own goals. Mayor Bloomberg was asking senior centers to submit plans to reinvent themselves as *wellness centers* and to attract more, as well as younger, people (i.e., boomers). The city plans to measure each center's success through benchmarks such as attendance, number of flu shots, and medical screenings.

Nationwide, there seems to be an emerging trend toward giving up the term *senior center.* Mather LifeWays (www.matherlifeways.com) in Chicago, for instance, has created the Café Plus concept, a community venue for older adults that rids itself of institutional stigma. Although this model focuses on older adults, it does not use old-age terms, and it patterns itself after the café model, with Internet access that is popular with the young.

Combining innovative restaurant food with affordable prices and innovative learning and wellness programs, the cafés are open to an ageless public. As noted in one of their brochures, "*Mather Café* is not a senior center. It is a restaurant, gathering place, learning center and health club—that happens to have customers who may range in age from 50 to 90, and even this may change." At one of its facilities there is a fitness center, a sculpture studio, classrooms, a café, and a sunny atrium.

In Butler County, Ohio, the agency Senior Citizens, Inc. changed its name to Partners in Prime. Furthermore, the organization's three senior centers have been renamed "Prime Clubs." The club activities are focused on wellness, with wireless Internet access, notebook computers, and new Prime Cafes. The board of directors believes the name change and wellness makeover will "help people live life at its prime." The Poway Senior Center in California is considering a name change, but in the meantime it has created an intergenerational lounge for Wii video games, added sushi and fusion dishes to its food menu, and lowered its membership eligibility age to 50. New names, updated programs, and upscale campus-like facilities are replacing senior centers in specific locations around the country.

Can community centers successfully attract older adults without using terms related to older adults or aging? What are the advantages and disadvantages of disassociating senior centers from the word *senior* and related aging terms? What are the advantages and disadvantages of making the senior center of the future more intergenerational?

CREATIVE CAREER OPPORTUNITY: WELLNESS CENTER DIRECTOR

In 2010 there were an estimated 15,000 senior centers in the United States. Only a few are well on their way to addressing the needs and desires of the boomer generation. There are wonderful opportunities to launch innovative new programs, to renovate existing sites or find more advantageous locations, to attract older adults with more creative food options, to adopt the latest fitness ideas and wellness initiatives, to brainstorm over new center names, and to consider exciting new intergenerational opportunities.

Given the challenging economic times that we live in, it is probably safe to assume that local and state governments will not fully fund these new ventures. Thus, entrepreneurial-oriented wellness center directors have three options to explore:

1. Hone their fundraising skills in the local community to help subsidize new ventures
2. Link some of these high-quality programs to a fee schedule, preferably on a sliding-scale basis
3. Inspire more boomers to take on new volunteer efforts, or expand their existing volunteer efforts, at wellness centers

PHYSICAL HEALTH

As a former general, President Dwight Eisenhower was very concerned about the emergence of a military-industrial complex that would dominate society and take over the budget. At the time little did he, or anyone else, realize that a few decades later the military-industrial complex would be left in the dust by the medical-industrial complex. By the turn of the century, the medical-industrial complex was four times larger than the military-industrial complex.

Driven by the advent of Medicare, an aging society, and an endless discovery of technological inventions—machines, equipment, procedures, drugs, lab tests—that improve medical care and raise costs, medical care inflation has been doubling overall inflation for decades now. And there is no end in sight. Health care (overwhelmingly medical care) has steadily increased to 17.6% of the gross domestic product, and economists are predicting the percentage increase will continue to rise dramatically in the coming decade if nothing is done about it.

At the same time we are unsuccessfully grappling with rising health care costs, there is ample evidence that it is not buying us more longevity relative to other countries or, even more important, healthy aging in late life. Many other countries spend far less than we do and keep their elderly not only living longer, but sustaining healthy years of life longer than we do.

So what do we do about it? One thing we need to do is recognize that as American society ages, health care is moving—or should be moving—from an emphasis on acute care to one of chronic care. The medical model for acute care is dominated by expensive equipment, tests, and surgery, and by health care professionals who engage in diagnosing, treating, and prescribing. This is a very expensive and controlling system, with insurance administrators and health professionals in charge and patients in a passive and compliant role.

In the chronic-care model that is developing, this approach can change. Chronic conditions wax and wane, but rarely disappear. Among today's Medicare beneficiaries, 87% have at least one chronic condition, such as arthritis, heart disease, diabetes, or a certain type of cancer, and a majority have more than one chronic condition. Twenty percent have five or more chronic conditions. Instead of focusing on a cure, chronic care needs to be focused on ongoing function and quality of life.

Individuals with chronic conditions need to be alert for symptoms that lead to the adjusting or changing of medications; experiment with nutrition, exercise, and stress management; and play a much more active role in the daily management of their chronic disease. These individuals need to also manage the social roles affected by their chronic condition, and the range of emotions that are triggered by the challenges of chronic disease.

How does one learn about managing chronic conditions? There are books to read, such as *Living a Healthy Life with Chronic Conditions* (Lorig et al., 2006); professional organizations like the Arthritis Foundation (www.arthritis.org) that provide written materials and community programs; and educational programs to attend, like the chronic disease self-management program developed by Kate Lorig and colleagues at Stanford University (http://patienteducation.stanford.edu/programs/cdsmp.html). The *chronic disease self-management* program is designed to be led by lay persons with chronic diseases, and to focus on the medical, social, and emotional management of chronic conditions.

Medical management refers to the ability to communicate effectively with health professionals, being educated about relevant medications, adhering to appropriate diets and exercise programs, and being an educated consumer of medical tests, interventions, equipment, and supplies.

Social management refers to learning how to maintain satisfying roles while living with chronic disease. If you are an avid gardener, how do you continue this hobby with bad knees? If your grandchildren have boundless energy and you do not, how do you reconcile this discrepancy so you still get to play with them? If you would like to organize a holiday dinner at home but have limited financial means and physical energy, how do you get others to share in the responsibility? Are there transportation resources that can alleviate your dependence on family members?

Emotional management refers to managing the emotions that accompany chronic conditions over time. How do you deal with the sadness, frustration, and anger that emerge from your physical condition? How do you ask for help when you need it, while minimizing the guilt of being unable to do things for others that you once did? Are there local support groups for emotional, informational, and practical support? Where can you find out about relaxation training and other types of stress management?

The chronic disease self-management program is taught by volunteer lay leaders who receive 20 hours of training. The course typically consists of seven weekly sessions each 2.5 hours in length, with 10 to 15 participants. The location can be a senior center, a church, a retirement community, or another site that will not charge for space.

Lorig's research over the years has demonstrated that participants wind up with more energy, fewer debilitating days, and fewer visits to physicians and emergency rooms (Lorig et al., 2001). Beginning in 2003 and continuing to 2009, there have been two 3-year evidence-based disease self-management initiatives launched by the Administration on Aging (AOA) to help local aging and health networks implement and evaluate health programs, such as the chronic disease self-management program, which empower older individuals.

The second AOA grant-funded initiative took place in 12 states and over 30 local communities, and involved state units on aging; the relevant Area Agencies on Aging; state health departments; and local community organizations such as senior centers, nutrition programs, senior housing projects, religious organizations, and adult day centers. The goal was to mobilize public/private partnerships at the state and community levels to implement and sustain the delivery of evidence-based programs. The National Council on Aging's Center for Healthy Aging (www.healthyagingprograms.com) served as the resource center for the successful grantees.

The active self-management of chronic diseases is associated with many challenges, such as depression, pain, fatigue, lack of support from family, and poor communication with physicians (Jerant, von Friederichs-Fitzwater, & Moore, 2005). A meta-analysis of 112 interventions to improve self-care for persons with chronic illnesses, however, led the researchers to conclude that there were beneficial effects on clinical outcomes and process of care (Tsai, Morton, Mangione, & Keeler, 2005). Another meta-analysis of 53 programs found clinically important benefits for self-management interventions with diabetes and hypertension, but less so with osteoarthritis (Chodosh et al., 2005).

Chronic disease self-management can also be adapted to the primary care clinic and home setting for the severely impaired older adult. The *Guided Care* program is coordinated by a trained nurse who focuses on 50 to 60 older patients with complex, comorbid conditions (Boyd et al., 2007). In addition to chronic disease management, the intervention includes lifestyle modification, caregiver education and support, and evaluation and treatment by a geriatrician. Guided Care begins with a comprehensive home assessment, which is followed by regular subsequent monitoring by a trained registered nurse. The model is designed to keep older adults in their homes and reduce the need for costly hospital care. There is evidence that a demonstration program was successful in accomplishing this objective (Leff et al., 2009).

CREATIVE CAREER OPPORTUNITY: CHRONIC DISEASE MANAGEMENT COORDINATOR

The *chronic disease management coordinator* helps older adults organize into groups to promote self-management. This job can be structured as an independent consultant for individuals; focused on older workers in a large corporate setting; or coordinated through an Area Agency on Aging, retirement community, senior center, or other local aging or health organization. The coordinator can also work with physicians and other clinicians in medical clinics, helping to organize small groups of patients with chronic conditions into ongoing health education and support groups. For those who are severely impaired, primary care clinic-based programs can be launched by geriatric nurses and physicians.

MENTAL HEALTH

Getting joy and having a kind of wisdom in your golden years—it's all tripe. I've gained no insight, no mellowing. I would make the same mistakes again.

—Woody Allen

I like to describe Woody Allen as a philosopher/humorist. But I really think he is a much better humorist than philosopher. The evidence is beginning to accumulate, despite what Woody says, that with age does come some insight and mellowing, though perhaps it is too soon to call that wisdom. We also need to caution, in a way that Woody Allen would approve: Sometimes wisdom comes with age, sometimes age just comes alone.

Typically, aging is viewed as a time of loss and decline. Not surprisingly, the overwhelming majority of research studies substantiate this process of accumulating decrements with age in the physical, social, and cognitive domains. However, there are an increasing number of researchers who now suggest that old age may also be a time of development, particularly in the emotional realm.

Laura Carstensen and colleagues (2000), for instance, asked 184 people between the ages of 18 and 94 to carry a beeper for a week. When the beeper went off they recorded their emotional state in a journal. After collecting the journals and analyzing the data, the researchers found some surprising results. Older people were less likely than younger people to experience persistent negative emotional states. In addition, they were more likely to maintain highly positive emotional states for a longer period of time.

When remembering the past, older adults are more likely than younger adults to focus on positive experiences (Kennedy et al., 2004). They have more emotionally gratifying memories of past choices and other autobiographical information than younger adults (Mather & Carstensen, 2005). The authors of a summary of research studies conducted on the adaptive value of life review with respect to mental health in later life reported on the tendency of older adults to interpret memories in terms of growth, their capacity to transform negative life events into good outcomes, and their ability to focus on positive events during shared life reviews (Cappeliez & O'Rourke, 2006).

There may be a biological basis for older adults' preference for the positive. In the aging brain of older adults—but not in younger adults—the amygdala showed decreased reactivity to negative information along with maintained, or increasing, reactivity to positive information (Mather et al., 2004). There may also be changes with age in the orbitofrontal cortex, impairing anger recognition (Ruffman, Sullivan, & Edge, 2006).

Psychology may play an even larger role in this shift toward an emotionally positive focus, specifically in the individual's reaction to the perception that there is a limited amount of time left to live. As one comes to recognize time as finite, the regulation of one's emotional state in the present becomes more important than other goals (Carstensen, 2006). Present-oriented goals regarding psychological well-being are prioritized over future-oriented goals aimed at acquiring information and achieving instrumental objectives (Lockenhoff & Carstensen, 2004).

Studies show that there is a bias in which older adults pay more attention than younger adults to positive information and less attention to negative information. Older adults also select people and situations that will maximize positive emotions and minimize negative ones (Mroczek & Spiro, 2005). Other studies support similar findings:

1. When reminiscing, older adults are more likely to focus on positive emotions than younger adults (Pasupathi & Carstensen, 2003).
2. When shown images on a computer screen, followed by a distraction task, older adults recall more positive and fewer negative images than do younger and middle-aged adults (Charles, Mather, & Carstensen, 2003).

3. When shown a series of faces portraying positive, negative, and neutral emotions, eye-tracking technology reveals that older subjects gaze longer on happy faces, and younger subjects on fearful faces (Isaacowitz, Wadlinger, Goren, & Wilson, 2006).

4. When examining facial expressions, older adults are less likely than younger adults to give a negative rating to individuals who may look dangerous (Ruffman et al., 2006).

5. Older adults tend to act less confrontationally when problems come up in their relationships. They regulate their reactions to problems better than do younger persons, arguing less and picking their battles more carefully (Birditt & Fingerman, 2005; Birditt et al., 2005).

6. A Gallup phone survey of 340,000 adults ages 18 to 85 reported that older adults experience negative emotions, such as anger and stress, less frequently than younger adults. Enjoyment and happiness decrease gradually until we hit age 50, then rise steadily for the next 25 years (Stone, Schwartz, Broderick, & Deaton, 2010).

7. Older adults appear to be less driven by emotional impulsivity, and less likely to respond thoughtlessly to negative emotional stimuli because their brains have slowed down compared to younger persons (Jeste & Harris, 2010).

8. Older adults were best at reinterpreting negative images in positive ways, that is, use positive reappraisal, which is a coping mechanism that draws heavily on life experience and lessons learned (Shiota & Levenson, 2009).

9. In late life, individuals become increasingly sensitized to sadness, which does not lead to a higher risk for depression but instead leads to greater intimacy in interpersonal relationships (Seider, Shiota, Whalen, & Levenson, 2011).

10. When asked to change a negative reaction to viewing a disgusting television clip into positive feelings and then to perform on a memory game, older adults were able to regulate their negative emotions without a subsequent decrease in memory performance, while younger adults were less able to do this (Scheibe & Blanchard-Fields, 2009).

Two overviews of the research literature, including some of the studies that I have summarized above, concluded that emotional experience improves with age (Carstensen et al., 2011; Scheibe & Carstensen, 2010).

Despite the likelihood of physical and emotional losses accumulating in old age, the old, according to psychiatrist Gene Cohen, become connoisseurs of "deep pleasure and satisfaction, especially in relationships with family and significant others." Or, as a psychologist and her colleagues state it: "Facing relatively shorter futures . . . older adults prioritize emotional goals because they are realized in the moment of contact rather than banked for some nebulous future time" (Carstensen et al., 2000). Lockenhoff and Carstensen (2004) label this process, whereby there is an increasing awareness of the boundaries on time that leads to a greater appreciation of emotional experience in the present, *socioemotional selectivity*.

Other theories pertain to this development as well. Tornstam (1989) posits in his theory of *gerotranscendence* that aging individuals become less interested in the material and the superfluous, and more selective in their social engagement and spiritual pursuits. Levenson, Jennings, Aldwin, and Shiraishi (2005), using the idea of *self-transcendence*, report a greater openness to experience, more agreeableness, increasing spirituality, and a connectedness to past and future generations.

Erik Erikson's (1950) theory of *stages of psychosocial development* describes a process whereby psychologically mature older adults have a greater need to contribute to the lives of others, referred to as *generativity*, as well as to seek a basic acceptance of one's own life, labeled *ego integrity*. Referring to ego integrity, Erikson directly addresses the importance of conducting a life review during the last stage of life in order to help foster this (Haber, 2006). One quasi-experimental study of 106 older adults with depressive symptoms offered insights into how this might occur. The researchers reported that a completed life review resulted in an increase in positive evaluations of social relations and of one's past, and a decline in negative evaluations of oneself and one's future (Bohlmeijer, Westerhof, & Emmerik-de Jong, 2008).

A *life review* is a structured and systematic review of one's life that often takes place in a paired encounter or in a group, through a series of questions involving the important domains of one's life. Family themes range from childhood, to the experience of being a parent, to being a grandparent. Work themes range from one's first job, to one's major life' work, to retirement. Once started, each life review interview can take more than an hour, depending on the fatigue level of the older adult; interviews may be conducted over several weeks.

Taking the time to conduct life review interviews, however, stands in stark contrast to lives based on time efficiency and productivity. A description of one day in my own life can serve as an example. One Sunday afternoon I went to the supermarket and scanned my goods, not interacting with anyone. I then went to the automatic teller machine and withdrew money, no teller necessary. I followed that up by grabbing a quick bite to eat at a drive-through restaurant, exchanging a minimum of words with a disembodied voice and spending a few seconds of time with a cashier. I then went home for the rest of the afternoon and sat in front of a computer screen to catch up on some work.

That evening, though, I met with an older person and worked with her on her life review. I learned about the important challenges in her life, some of which were met successfully, others not so successfully. I learned from interesting anecdotes about the historical context in which these challenges took place. I asked questions such as: What was it like growing up in your family in the late 1930s? Tell me about your experiences raising children in the 1950s. What were the highlights of your work career? What hobbies have given you great satisfaction? What spiritual activities give your life purpose and meaning? What has been your most significant health challenge, and how have you been dealing with it?

From an afternoon that focused on time efficiency and the avoidance of "unnecessary" human interaction, I experienced an enjoyable evening feeling connected to another human being. That evening was followed by several more evenings, until we completed an abbreviated version of her life story. The older woman I partnered with also felt a greater sense of connectedness, not only while working with me, but also when she shared the completed written product with her family and friends.

Life reviews are increasingly being done in community settings, as group projects or as multiple individual interviews. One-page summaries of these reviews can be posted on a centrally located bulletin board in a retirement community or senior center, or outside the doors of individual rooms in a nursing home. The result of these postings can be greater socialization among residents and visitors, and better relationships between them and staff. In short, this type of project can have a positive impact on the culture of a place, and on the friendliness of residents and their willingness to share important aspects of their lives. People start to know each other better and treat each other more personally.

The research on the emotional strength of older persons may be linked to research that demonstrates that aging persons who engage in life review may be able to improve their ability to manage their emotional health even more effectively (Haber, 2006). Additional benefits may accrue to daughters and sons, granddaughters and grandsons, and students who want to learn about life and history (Haber, 2008a). Young adults may gain insight into their own maturational process, and life reviews can foster intergenerational bonding in an era when many younger and older people are living age-segregated lives.

CREATIVE CAREER OPPORTUNITY: LIFE REVIEW SPECIALIST

The *life review specialist* helps older adults, on an individual or group basis, to record their life stories (mostly written, but also recording with audio and video). A growing number of professionals are launching careers in life review (Haber, 2008a). This career opportunity can be structured as an independent consultant for individuals, or it can be focused on residents in retirement communities, older adults at senior centers, older congregation members, or even family members and friends of the terminally ill or the deceased in coordination with a hospice or funeral home.

The specialist, for instance, can approach a retirement home administrator and offer to conduct life reviews or to train staff to conduct life reviews, and to help in the editing process. A completed review is given to the resident, who can share it with friends and family. For those who are also willing, a one-page abbreviated written version can be posted in a heavily trafficked location to create conversations and more supportive social interactions. Staff themselves can participate, including the administrator, and relationships between residents and staff can become more personal as commonalities are discovered, achievements admired, and communities developed.

SUPPORTIVE HOUSING

Supportive housing for aging people is typically informally organized within a private home, with reliance on family members, friends, neighbors, and connections with religious organizations. If affordable, paid caregiving is used to compensate for inadequate family caregiving resources or the declining health of the care recipient.

More formal arrangements outside of the home include congregate housing options with oversight of meal planning, housekeeping, laundry, medication usage, and personal or health care services. There are no standard terms to describe these arrangements, but they are typically identified as assisted living facilities, residential care facilities, and adult foster care homes—services that fall short of what is needed for nursing home care. These facilities tend to be locally defined with inconsistent terminology, policies, scope of services, and design features across (and sometimes within) states.

Many of these residencies fall short of providing all of the following features:

1. Private sleeping areas and bathrooms
2. Resident empowerment with respect to the timing and content of meals, hygiene schedule, and social activities
3. A homelike, versus an institutional-looking, setting with the option of having pets and allowing overnight guests
4. A sufficient number of well-trained staff who are available when needed
5. The opportunity to age in place until, and including, time of death

By 2021, when the leading edge of boomers will turn 75, there will likely be a rapid growth in supportive housing to meet not only these needs, but something more: the need to live with like-minded people who share interests, values, or philosophies. There are innovative housing options emerging, and they are likely to be more fully developed by boomers unwilling to be unnecessarily institutionalized, bureaucratized, or medicalized in late life, and wanting to be surrounded by caring people and with the opportunity for purposeful activities. A few such innovations are summarized next.

ELDER COHOUSING

If you are in your 50s or 60s, you may have a conversation with friends centered around the following question: Wouldn't it be neat if several of us who share similar values could get together in retirement and live out our remaining days together in a supportive community? The details vary, of course. Some boomers discuss buying homes near each other. Others discuss taking over a large home, dividing it up, and figuring out ways to live together and share expenses.

Well, some people are starting to do something about it. There is a new housing concept, called cohousing, in which adults figure out how to live interdependently as housemates or neighbors. The concept was imported from Denmark in the early 1990s, and the number of cohousing communities in the United States had grown to about 113 in 2008 (Thomas & Blanchard, 2009). There are cohousing organizations (e.g., www .cohousingpartners.com) that provide ideas on shared visions and values; strategies for architectural innovation, such as designs to enhance the sense of community that allow both common areas and privacy; and approaches to shared management and decision making. Cohousing refers to privately owned homes that are socially and architecturally innovative with resident input, in a caring, noninstitutional environment.

The cohousing concept has been extended to *elder cohousing*, which is designed to help older people not only live more communally in late life, but live in these homes until they die. The term *aging in place* can be a misnomer, because sooner or later a substantial majority of people leave their homes and wind up dying in a hospital or nursing home.

One cohousing organization, called the *Elder Cohousing Network*, is based in Boulder, Colorado, and has helped 85 individuals or groups to develop these innovative housing options. It began in 1991 in Davis, California, and focused on persons 55 and older. In August 2004 this network registered as a nonprofit organization to help existing groups figure out how to implement their housing ideas. They also help to network individuals in the same area who might want to consider forming a group for cohousing. For more information, contact the Elder Cohousing Network, 1460 Quince Ave., #102, Boulder, CO 80304; 303-413-8066; www.eldercohousing.org.

One such cohousing project, facilitated by the Elder Cohousing Network, began in 2002 and called itself the *Glacier Circle Community* (Karidis, 2007). About two dozen people in their 70s and 80s, mostly friends from a Unitarian Universalist Church in Davis, California, hired lawyers and architects to help them create a small cooperative-style housing community of seniors. The members of the community participated in facilitation training at the local university in order to enhance their communication skills with each other in the planning of their vision.

They came up with a plan for eight townhomes, ranging in size from 1,000 to 1,400 square feet and designed for energy efficiency with skylights and suntubes. There is a common garden that includes fruit trees, vegetables, and flowering plants, and a common house with an affordable second-floor apartment that is offered to an individual or couple in exchange for help with cooking and maintenance as the residents age in place. For additional information, contact Glacier Circle Senior Community, 2358 Glacier Place, Davis, CA 95616.

Elderspirit is also one of the first senior cohousing communities, founded by former nuns who left their order over philosophical differences. They wanted to build their own community dedicated to personal growth, mutual support, and the deepening of spirit in later life. This model project has now grown to 29 homes of mixed-income housing for individuals at least 55 years of age who share the values of spiritual growth and emotional support. The development is built along a scenic trail within easy walking distance of shops and downtown Abingdon, Virginia. For more information contact Elderspirit Development Corporation, P.O. Box 665, Abingdon, VA 24212; 276-628-8908; www.elderspirit.net.

GREEN HOUSE

For people who are frail, William Thomas has created the *Green House,* an innovative long-term care home—not facility—that does not succumb to the problems of institutionalization and the medical model. In traditional nursing homes, residents are viewed as sick and dependent, which fosters learned helplessness and induced disability. For example, wheelchair dependency may be encouraged to serve the needs of staff members, who must transport residents and are pressed for time. Dressing, feeding, bathing, and toileting need to be routinized and sped up for aides needing to stay on schedule. A staff member is more likely to rely on incontinence briefs than to take the time to develop individualized toileting routines.

A 2001 survey by the Kaiser Family Foundation reported that 43% of Americans stated that the idea of being placed in a nursing home is totally unacceptable. This discontent has triggered a nationwide movement toward culture change in nursing homes (Rahman & Schnelle, 2008). The effort to radically transform the nation's nursing homes is being focused on smaller residences and the empowerment of residents and staff. The best example of this is the Green House movement.

Green Houses are licensed as nursing homes, but look like surrounding homes in a residential community. They are homes, not homelike, though they are bigger than the average home. The first ones were constructed in Tupelo, Mississippi, in 2003 and were 6,400 square feet in area. The rooms in these homes include extra-expense items, such as ceiling lifts, but these innovations can save costs over the long term by reducing back injuries, employee turnover, and worker's compensation.

Green House workers are paid more and are better trained than nursing home staff, but the extra costs are offset by employee empowerment that reduces staff turnover and additional training expenses. The annual turnover rate in the average nursing home is 75%, whereas it was less than 10% in the first Green House in Tupelo. Moreover, not one staff person left during the first 3 years of its existence.

About 10 people live in a Green House, each having a private room and bath and access to a central hearth where cooking and socializing are done. There is a surrounding garden for contemplative walks and for growing vegetables and flowers. Doors can be opened to view the garden and hearth from an individual room, or closed for privacy. With the circular nature of the individual rooms, both the garden and the central hearth are within 30 feet. Strategically placed furniture help residents "cruise" to central areas and contribute to gains in mobility.

Green Houses promote autonomy. Residents get up, eat, and go to bed when they want. They decide on which foods to eat, which may even include pizza, wine, or ice cream. Medications are locked in individual rooms rather than distributed by a cart that is wheeled from room to room. There are few features that differ from the typical home. Those features that are unusual are deemphasized, such as a ceiling lift that is recessed and used only when needed for transfer. Induction cooking in the kitchen prevents residents from burning themselves on a stove. Stoves have shutoff valves, with pot trappers to prevent hot pots from burning residents. A safety gate around the kitchen can be used when necessary.

People in the first 10 Green Houses were selected from nursing homes in an attempt to represent a typical nursing home population. Of the first 40 selected, 12 had advanced dementia (a percentage lower than a typical nursing home), and all Green House residents had an array of physical and cognitive limitations and medical challenges associated with the average nursing home resident.

Decision making lies with residents and workers, unless there are safety or budget issues that cannot be handled at that level. Aides are called *shahbazim*, derived from the mythical Persian royal falcon that protected the king in ancient times, with the primary job responsibility to protect, nurture, and sustain.

The desired staff-to-resident ratio is 1:5; the nurse-to-house ratio is 1:2 houses (or 1:20 people), and one administrator (and one assistant) is allotted for every 12 houses (or 1:120 people). Staff find replacements for themselves if they are sick, either through a substitute pool or through other staff working overtime (which is managed within the allowable budget).

Shahbazim receive 120 hours of additional training in areas such as cardiopulmonary resuscitation first aid, culinary skills, safe food handling, communication, and dementia care. They are better paid than the average long-term care worker (by about 40%), and are given rotating responsibilities (purchasing food and cooking, housekeeping, scheduling, budget, etc.). Unless the nonclinical work teams undermine safety or go over budget, administrators cannot overrule their decisions.

Every one of the early Green Houses implemented had been fully staffed, never a day understaffed. Wheelchair use declined, and strength of residents increased. Residents have had the option to eat in a group or alone, with an individualized menu and pleasant surroundings—referred to as a *convivium*. A local cookbook is assembled to cater to the tastes of people born in a particular region. Shahbazim can eat with residents and participate in activities with them, along with family and friends. Most of these ideas are summarized in William Thomas' (2004) book *What Are Old People For?*

In another publication, called *CNS SeniorCare*, Thomas sums up his philosophy: "Old age, like all the other phases of our lives, should be about life and living. Treating aging as a medical condition that must be managed with the professional distance prescribed by the medical model is wrong and leads to terrible suffering. For decades we have organized the life of the elder or disabled individual in a skilled nursing facility around the needs of the institution, rather than individuals who live there."

One 2-year longitudinal study compared Green House residents to residents at a traditional nursing home with the same owner (Kane, Lum, Cutler, Degenholtz, & Yu, 2007). The Green House residents reported a higher quality of life, better emotional well-being, and a lower incidence of decline in late-loss ADL (activities of daily living) functioning. Unfortunately, this type of research on culture change nursing homes is in short supply (Rahman & Schnelle, 2008).

The Robert Wood Johnson Foundation provided a $10 million grant (between 2006 and 2010) to establish Green Houses around the United States, and to allow other long-term care owners and administrators to replicate them through training support and up to $125,000 in predevelopment loans. In 2011 the Green House concept had spread to over 100 homes operating on 43 campuses in 27 states. To find out more information about Green Houses, visit www.ncbcapitalimpact.org/thegreenhouse. To receive a free copy of the *Green House Project Guide Book* or the 8-hour orientation workshops, contact: The Green House Project, NCB Capital Impact, 2011 Crystal Dr., #800, Arlington, VA 22202; 703-302-8000.

VIRTUAL VILLAGES

Virtual villages are nonprofit, dues-paying, membership communities to help older residents stay in their own homes for as long as possible. These communities are often not self-sufficient and depend on local donors to subsidize the services they provide.

Lower-income communities, however, rely on support from the aging network, and are referred to as *Naturally Occurring Retirement Communities* (NORCs).

Services in virtual villages and NORCs are prescreened, and hourly rates are low because of the volume offered to providers. The services typically include home maintenance, home repairs, home health care, transportation, and other support unique to the community. Sometimes these communities also organize an exchange of donated volunteer hours among residents that can also be accumulated in volunteer credit hours that are formally recorded.

The virtual village idea began with the Beacon Hill Village in Boston in 2001. Several friends and neighbors developed a plan to help each other stay in their homes. They used a nonprofit organization to screen and organize programs and services to help accomplish the goal of aging in place. At Beacon Hill Village, residents are charged an annual membership fee of $600 for an individual and $850 for a couple, with discounts for those in financial need (Thomas & Blanchard, 2009).

Almost a decade later, the Beacon Hill Village model is spreading to other parts of the country, such as Cambridge, Massachusetts; Palo Alto, California; Washington, DC; and New Canaan, Connecticut. There were at least 60 village communities across the country in early 2011 and over 90 groups in the process of creating them (Scharlach, Graham, & Lehning, 2012). These supportive communities have the virtue of allowing older residents to remain in the same environs with long-standing neighbors and friends, as well as having a more natural intergenerational neighborhood. Residents are also less dependent on their grown children, who are often dispersed around the country and have their own families to support. For more information, visit www.beaconhillvillage.org.

NICHE RETIREMENT COMMUNITIES

Niche retirement communities refer to specialized retirement housing organized around a hobby, culture, religion, or some other belief, activity, or interest that the older residents share in common.

For instance, there are university-based retirement communities (UBRC) that offer retirees the opportunity to attend nearby campus activities, like athletic events, nationally recognized speakers, art exhibits, plays, and the like. Occasionally, the resource can come to the retirement facility. At a retirement community named Kendal, near Oberlin College in Ohio, the school sends string quarters to perform at the retirement facility.

Moreover, there is usually an opportunity for the older residents to sit in on certain classes at the university without being tested or graded. About half of the residents of the UBRC are alumni or former faculty and staff, the other half are interested in this type of living arrangement even without a former affiliation.

There are more than 25 UBRCs in existence, with a larger number in development. The UBRC are a win–win–win situation. The older adults gain an educational and culturally enriched lifestyle, the college students gain an intergenerational component to their educational experience, and the university can receive assets from the estates of grateful older residents who appreciated their retirement years at a nearby retirement facility.

There are artistically oriented niche retirement communities. The Burbank Senior Artists Colony in Burbank, California, for instance, attracts persons interested in painting, writing, or other artistic endeavors in their retirement years. This 141-unit community has a 40-seat performance theater, artist studios, art display galleries, and classrooms.

Rocinante, named after Don Quixote's horse, is a niche retirement community for aging hippies. Located in Summertown, Tennessee, it is led by Stephen Gaskin, its now-79-year-old founder. Astronomy lovers can select Chiefland Astronomy Village in Chiefland, Florida, where the skies are not affected by light pollution as much as other locations. Also, nearly every home has a built-in telescope. Nalcrest, a letter carriers' retirement community, about 70 miles east of Tampa, prohibits dogs that bite, a former occupational hazard.

Fox Hills Club in Bethesda, Maryland, is a wellness retirement community that offers gyms, spas, health-conscious restaurants, an organic herb garden, outdoor walking trails, and onsite personal trainers and physical therapists. The Ridge at Chukker Creek in Aiken, South Carolina, attracts retired equestrians with horse pastures, horseback trails, and community-shared barns to house the horses.

SMART HOMES AND TELEHEALTH

Smart homes are residences equipped with technology designed to enhance older residents' safety and independence, and to monitor their health status in their homes. *Telehealth* refers to health information transmitted electronically from the person's home to a physician's office, ambulatory care setting, or other medical location.

The Oregon Center for Aging and Technology (OCAT) at Oregon Health & Science University tests technology in more than 350 homes, apartments, and retirement communities. The goal is to find out how to keep aging adults safely in their homes. Motion sensors, for example, are installed throughout a home to alert people if help is needed. The sensors can reveal answers to the following questions: Did the person get out of bed? Did s/he open their refrigerator? Did s/he fall on the floor? Did s/he open their pillbox and take the proper medication?

With another experiment, OCAT raised other questions: Can Celia the Robot, who has a video screen that can be operated remotely by a faraway family member, reduce the isolation and improve the mental health of the older adult? Or would it be too intrusive? A Thai company called Dinsow 2 developed an even more impressive robot that can act as a personal health care assistant. It can serve medicine and food, and pick up and carry items. An older user can also say "Dinsow, come here" and then touch a menu on the robot's head in order to automatically call a family member, doctor, or another contact.

Paro, the robotic seal, has fur, big eyes, and responds to voice commands. This low-cost companion was developed at the AgeLab at Massachusetts Institute of Technology in order to calm older adults with dementia.

The Mayo Clinic Robert and Arlene Kogod Center on Aging sponsors a laboratory called HAIL (Healthy Aging and Independent Living). The researchers asked the following set of questions: Will older participants take their blood pressure and communicate through a tablet computer with video messaging to a health coach, and then follow suggestions on how to improve their blood pressure? Would it be intrusive to wear a band-aid-size cardiac sensor on the chest that transmits real-time information about heart health to a caregiving team?

As the evidence accumulates regarding the effectiveness of smart homes and telehealth, the bottom line will be, well, the bottom line. Will these gerotechnologies save money? Will the cost of widespread implementation be offset by reduced institutionalization, hospitalization, emergency room visits, and other medical costs? In addition, ethical issues such as privacy and confidentiality must be addressed.

For a review of 10 "nana" technologies, that is, technologies that your grandmother might use, access www.usatoday.com/tech/graphics/nana_tech/flash.htm.

Another website is run by the Center for Aging Services Technologies and it reviews new technologies that are commercially available or in development for older adults and their caregivers. Contact www.agingtech.org.

One final note. There is a movie I want to see, called *Robot & Frank*. It's a silly premise, but sometimes I like silly. Frank Langella (a favorite actor of mine who is age 74) in the movie starts to have memory problems and his children purchase a robot for him, similar to Dinsow 2. Frank, initially resistant to this robot companion, forms an unusual bond with him. He finds the robot useful in picking locks and casing a home to burgle (as I said, sounds silly). *Robot & Frank* won the Alfred P. Sloan Foundation prize at the 2012 Sundance Film Festival, an award for films that explore themes of science and technology.

CREATIVE CAREER OPPORTUNITY: SUPPORTIVE HOUSING SPECIALIST

The *supportive housing specialist* helps create housing alternatives for older adults needing assistance to remain as independent, autonomous, and socially connected as possible. This career path can be structured as an independent consultant for individuals interested in intentional communities, or it can be a government position that will likely be created to help find cost-effective and home-like alternatives for an aging population that will double in size between 2000 and 2030. There will be positions for supportive housing specialists in the creation of financial support to launch innovative housing alternatives, or for the design, marketing, or management of these facilities.

These new career opportunities in housing may be interrelated with the other topics previously described, as there will likely be a need for innovative physical health programming (such as chronic disease self-management) and mental health programming (such as life reviews) at these newly developed supportive housing sites.

CONCLUSION OF A GLIMPSE INTO THE FUTURE

The most succinct way to conclude this section of the chapter is to quote the late Peter Drucker (1909–2005), an innovative thinker, a productive author on the topic of work, and a person who retained a spirited personality and lifestyle into his mid-90s. He declared: "The best way to predict the future is to create it."

AND A LOOK BACK

I worked for a decade at Ball State University, David Letterman's alma mater, which got me thinking. If I look back at this entire book, what would be *my* Top Ten List, not of jokes, but of health promotion priorities. Then, I got to thinking a little more. Ten's a big number, and this book is already big enough. Besides, Letterman's telling jokes, which are easy to breeze through. So, let's be more realistic. What would be my top three health promotion priorities that I would pursue as President Haber (perhaps an unlikely prospect).

I list them in my order of importance (rather than in reverse order, as Letterman does). The third priority may be a surprise because it was only briefly mentioned in this book prior to now. As you read them, consider your own top three priorities, regardless of whether they appear in this book.

And now, "Paul (referring to Paul Shaffer, Letterman's musical sidekick) . . . drum roll please. . . ."

#1   Life Stories

I would strongly encourage (dare I say require?) every high school principal to challenge all seniors at their school to conduct a life review with an older adult. The senior may choose a family member if one is available and willing. Or, teachers and administrators can come up with a way to enlist older volunteers in the community. I would set 65 as a minimum age, because the life story is too incomplete prior to that.

I call this top priority "life stories" because it sounds more fun and spontaneous than the life review I describe in this book. I would ask students to help come up with several of the best stories that the older adult has to offer, about two pages long each, or longer if it comes easily.

First, I would ask the student and the older adult to examine hundreds of questions, beginning with the ones that I have stolen from many authors (who, in turn, stole most of them from other authors). I organized them in a similar fashion to the way James Birren did in his book: (1) family of origin; (2) marriage, children, and grandchildren; (3) career and work; (4) major historical event, or technology, or event of nature that influenced your life; (5) retirement or being an older adult; (6) health, body, and/or sexuality; (7) money, and its influence on your choices or opportunities; (8) meaning, purpose, or spirituality; (9) aging and death; and (10) a major turning point in your life. Let the older adult decide the categories of interest and also which questions within each category to address.

You can contact me for the list of questions at haberd@wou.edu, in the Gerontology Department at Western Oregon University. There are also many popular workbooks that just consist of life story questions that you can access at any bookstore. (I encourage you to enter these places before they disappear, even though I know how convenient online shopping is.)

Then, once you have the questions you want to pursue, let the person begin unfettered, without further instruction. At some point, though, to flesh out more details ask her or him who else (if anyone) plays a role in this story? What else did you or they do? Where were you or them? When did this happen? What was the historical context (if relevant)? How did this happen to come about? Why was it important? Some of these questions, if relevant, can further enrich a story.

Or you may ask another set of questions, for additional probing, that involve the senses: What did you see at this event or activity? What did you hear? What did you smell? What did you touch or who touched you? What did you taste?

There are other venues I might have chosen besides public high schools for implementing this priority. It could be encouraged, for instance, at every retirement center or other location where older adults congregate. The administrator at each facility can make this one of the essential services that it provides. Or, I could suggest that this activity takes place at every willing religious institution in the country. Most have a large segment of older congregants and they can be paired up with younger ones. This type of intergenerational exercise can be enriching at both ends of the life cycle as well as strengthen the bonds among members of a church, synagogue, mosque, or other religious site.

So why did I choose high schools? Because life stories cover so many important educational disciplines that all high school students can benefit from. This strategy is an exercise in *history*. But unlike reading a textbook (probably like this one, a bit on the dull side), this history lesson is gained firsthand, from someone's real-life experience. Fewer and fewer older adults have had direct experience with the Great Depression, but their parents certainly did. There are fewer and fewer who served in World War II, but most were affected by it. They were all old enough to remember where they were and their emotional reaction to President Kennedy's assassination. There are countless other historical events to explore with an older adult.

It is also an exercise in *psychology*. How has this person coped with loss? How did she or he navigate emotional challenges or transitions in career or family? How did she or he demonstrate resiliency and what lessons does he or she have to offer others?

It is also an exercise in *English*. Grammar, spelling, the ability to write good paragraphs in a meaningful sequence, and so forth—these are all important skills. These skills are eroding due to the shorthand conventions of texting and tweeting and other innovations in technology.

In addition, this is an exercise in *communication*. The student may choose to write the life stories with an older person, or perhaps record them through video or auditory modalities. Perhaps even conduct the life story through performance, maybe stage it in a theater. This is already being done in many parts of the country. If a group of older persons share their stories through performance, who will be in the audience? At minimum, family and friends of the students and the older adults. It could take place in a high school auditorium, perhaps at the participating school, with the best stories (come up with your own selection process) acted out or recited by the older adults and/or the students, in front of their peers.

How will you communicate most effectively with your audience? Do you want it to be humorous or serious, or both? Do you want it to tell life lessons or be lighter in style, letting the audience members draw their own lessons?

Depending on the interests and experience of the older adult you interview, you can wander into other important academic disciplines as well, like *science, religion, medicine*, and so forth. When I think of all the disciplines this exercise touches upon, and the intergenerational aspect of this strategy, it is clearly number one for me.

#2   Exercise

The old bromide is true: If exercise could be encapsulated in a pill, it would be the single most important medicine we could take. If you are not active as you age, it affects not only your physical health but your emotional health and your cognitive acuity as well. Even older adults in wheelchairs can increase their flexibility, strength, and endurance, and enhance their lives.

I would direct this priority, though, toward the majority of older adults who are mobile. Walking is the most popular form of exercise, and if it is done briskly and regularly it provides tremendous health benefits. It can be done in a beautiful natural setting and enrich one's spiritual life at the same time. It can be done with friends and family and enrich one's emotional life. It can be done alone and in a contemplative manner. It can be done with a pedometer, with meticulous record keeping.

I think one of the U.S. surgeon generals described the ideal regularity for this strategy well, to aim to exercise most days of the week. If the goal is every day, then every day that it is not done feels like a failure, and after several failures, one may feel like a loser. There will likely be days that you do not feel well, or are too busy, or just do not want to do it. Fine. But the old-fashioned "3 days a week" no longer makes sense. Exercise should be part of the daily routine as much as possible. But forget perfection.

Aerobics is a good beginning, but most people are now adding on strength building and flexibility, perhaps focusing on the core (stomach and back) or balance. My schedule is to do about 40 minutes of jogging about every other day, 30 minutes of strength building every other day, and 10 minutes of flexibility and balance every day that I can. If I miss a day, say jogging, then the next day I resume with jogging. I do not associate a particular type of exercise with a particular day of the week.

I like to break this routine sometimes with a hike, or a low-key athletic event that I participate in, or a type of exercise I do not normally do. I am very careful to be modest in my efforts when I move my body in a new way. If not, I make mistakes and pay for them with aches and stiffness. I added a few one-legged, half-knee bends a while back and the next day my butt was so sore I could not sit down without pain. I am a creature of habit who likes occasional variety. You may be a creature of variety who barely tolerates consistency. Either way, motivation is the key.

I was fortunate enough to grow up with a chronic health problem (yes, this sounds strange) that I believed required near-daily exercise to function at an acceptable level, so it is not a difficult habit for me in late life. Perhaps an older adult does not have this motivation, and has years of exercise neglect to deal with. Then you need to think about what spurs you to action. Do you need scenery? Do you need a fitness center? Do you need a friend? Do you need a bike? Do you need a pool? Do you like to dance? Can you turn housework into brisk activity? Pay attention to motivation.

You also need to figure out duration. Be modest at first. Start with a period of time that is easy to accomplish. We have good evidence that cumulative exercise is effective too, so you do not have to come up with one long time period. Also pay attention to your breathing (which should speed up) and your body heat (warmer, maybe beads of sweat). This lets you know if you are getting to a sufficient intensity level.

Not a particularly original topic to include in my top three. But a very close second in priority. Now to the surprising number three priority.

#3   Horticulture and Community Gardening

How can you go wrong listening to Michael Pollan, the Knight Professor of Journalism at University of California, Berkeley, one of *Time* magazine's 100 most influential people in the world, and the author of several popular books on food? In his book, *Food Rules*, Pollan (2011) recommends that you plant a vegetable garden if you have the space, a window box if you do not. In addition to communing with nature, your garden produces the freshest, most nutritious produce possible. He also notes the side benefits: being outside, getting exercise, saving money (a $70 dollar investment yields $600 worth of food, according to Pollen).

But the real inspiration for this choice has been Michelle Obama. On March 20, 2009, a hopeful gardener began to plant in her backyard. Not just any backyard, but the South Lawn of the White House. Not just any gardener, but the First Lady. Michelle Obama had come up with yet another project to foster one of her goals, improving the health of Americans. She had lots of questions, besides whether she would be allowed to do this to the White House grounds, such as: Was the soil fertile enough? Was the sunlight sufficient? Was her gardening inexperience too much of a barrier? Did she have enough time?

Ms. Obama had more on her mind than eating fresh vegetables. She wanted to send a message about the food we eat and the lives we live. Her first plan of action was to recruit 23 fifth-graders from a local elementary school to help plant the lettuce, peas, spinach, broccoli, kale, and collard greens. After three successful crops, Ms. Obama wrote about her experience in *American Grown: The Story of the White House Kitchen Garden and Gardens Across America* (Obama, 2012). Her goal in writing (with assistance) this book was to inspire families, schools, and communities to try their hands at gardening and "enjoy all the gifts of health, discovery, and connection a garden can bring" (p. 19).

Perhaps you do not have space comparable to the White House grounds, nor the array of expertise that she was able to marshall to help. If viable soil is inaccessible, plant in raised beds or on a sunny windowsill, patio, or balcony. You do not get the exercise of using hoes and shovels, tilling the ground until soft, but you do get the fruits and vegetables.

If expertise cannot come to you at your command, read a book, go to a garden event in your community and learn from master gardeners. You will have to learn about what is best to plant in your area, when to plant, what amounts of sun and water are needed, soil management and plant nutrients, how to control weeds, what to watch out for—pests, birds, rabbits, deer, soil erosion, the least toxic approach to pest control, and many other interesting and challenging topics.

Ms. Obama said her first crop cost $200 for soil, seeds, seedlings and soil nutrients, and produced 740 pounds of produce—not a bad financial pay-off. Whereas fresh food is generally more expensive than convenience food (thanks to misdirected government subsidies that I had hoped her husband would help do something about), not so when you grow your own.

Your produce can make thoughtful gifts and strengthen your emotional connections to others. You can also work with others on an individual garden, or work with others on a community garden. Community gardens can be intergenerational, involving local youth and older adults. There are about 18,000 community gardens in the United States and Canada, reclaiming empty or neglected land and changing it into crops.

Many examples of community gardens are provided by Michelle Obama in her book. The most ambitious one is in Seattle, Washington, where there are 76 gardens on 23 acres with 4,700 gardeners, about a third of whom donate their harvest to food banks and feeding centers. In 2010, 21,000 pounds of fresh produce were given away. There is an American Community Garden Association (www.communitygarden.org), which informs you about existing community gardens in your area or how to start your own.

Farmers' markets are a kind of community garden that you can participate in by buying your produce there. There are more than 7,000 farmers' markets nationwide. It is an opportunity to meet the people who grow our food and to eat fresh fruits and vegetables without participating in the work involved to grow them.

In the early 1900s it was estimated that there were 75,000 school gardens across America. They were also once considered nature study programs and part of the educational curriculum in America. School gardening experienced a resurgence in popularity during World War II, when victory gardens were often grown on school grounds. Afterward, they pretty much disappeared, only to make a small but growing (pun intended) comeback in the past few years.

Finally, consider working on your garden intergenerationally. This way my third priority, and the last sentence of this book on aging, become gerontologically relevant.

REFERENCES

AARP. (2001). *Global aging: Achieving its potential.* AARP Public Policy Institute report. Washington, DC: AARP.

Abelson, R. (2008, April 7). Medicare finds how hard it is to save money. *New York Times,* p. 24.

Abete, P., Ferrara, N., Cacciatore, F., Sagnelli, E., Manzi, M., Carnovale, V., . . . Rengo, F. (2001). High level of physical activity preserves the cardioprotective effect of preinfarction angina in elderly patients. *Journal of the American College of Cardiology, 38,* 1357–1367.

Abramson, J., Williams, S. A., Krumholz, H. M., & Vaccarino, V. (2001). Moderate alcohol consumption and risk of heart failure among older persons. *Journal of the American Medical Association, 285,* 1971–1977.

Ackerman, R., Cheadle, A., Sandhu, N., Madsen, L., Wagner, E. H., & LoGerfo, J. P. (2003). Community exercise program use and changes in health care costs for older adults. *American Journal of Preventive Medicine, 25,* 232–237.

Adachi, M., Ishihara, K., Abe, S., Okuda, K., & Ishikawa, T. (2002). Effect of professional oral health care on the elderly living in nursing homes. *Oral Medicine, 94,* 191–195.

Adams, D. (2006, March 27). Web sites let patients find like-minded physicians. *American Medical News, 49*(12), 1.

Address, R. (2005). *To honor and respect: A program and resource guide for congregations on sacred aging.* New York, NY: URJ Press.

Agatston, A. (2003). *The South Beach diet.* New York, NY: Random House.

Age, hearing loss and hearing aids. (2000, November). *Harvard Health Letter,* pp. 4–5.

Ahlquist, D., Skoletsky, J. E., Boynton, K. A., Harrington, J. J., Mahoney, D. W., Pierceall, W. E., . . . Shuber, A. P. (2000). Colorectal cancer screening by detection of altered human DNA in stool: Feasibility of a multitarget assay panel. *Gastroenterology, 119,* 1219–1227.

Ai, A., Peterson, C., Bolling, S. F., & Koenig, H. (2002). Private prayer and optimism in middle-aged and older patients awaiting cardiac surgery. *Gerontologist, 42,* 70–81.

Ajani, U., Ford, E. S., Greenland, K. J., Giles, W. H., & Mokdad, A. H. (2006). Aspirin use among U.S. adults behavioral risk factor surveillance system. *American Journal of Preventive Medicine, 30,* 74–77.

Ajzen, I. (1988). *Attitudes, personality, and behavior.* Chicago, IL: Dorsey Press.

Akincigil, A., Olfson, M., Siegel, M., Zurlo, K. A., Walkup, J. T., & Crystal, S. (2012). Race and ethnic disparities in deperssion care in community-dwelling elderly in the United States. *American Journal of Public Health, 102,* 319–328.

Albert, M., Jones, K., Savage, C. R., Berkman, L., Seeman, T., Blazer, D., & Rowe, J. W. (1995). Predictors of cognitive change in older persons: MacArthur studies of successful aging. *Psychology and Aging, 10*, 578–586.

Albertazzi, P. (2006). A review of non-hormonal options for the relief of menopausal symptoms. *Treatment Endocrinology, 5*, 101–113.

Alberts, D., Martínez, M. E., Roe, D. J., Guillén-Rodríguez, J. M., Marshall, J. R., van Leeuwen, J. B., . . . Sampliner, R. E. (2000). Lack of effect of a high-fiber cereal supplement on the recurrence of colorectal adenomas. *New England Journal of Medicine, 342*, 1156–1162.

Alexopoulos, G. S., Reynolds, C. F., 3rd., Bruce, M. L., Katz, I. R., Raue, P. J., Mulsant, B. H., . . . Prospect Group. (2009). Reducing suicidal ideation and depression in older primary care patients. *American Journal of Psychiatry, 166*, 882–890.

Algra, A. M., & Rothwell, P. M. (2012). Effects of regular aspirin use on long-term cancer incidence and metastasis. *Lancet Oncology, 13*, 518–527.

Almeida, D. M., Wethington, E., & Kessler, R. C. (2002). The daily inventory of stressful events: An interview-based approach for measuring daily stressors. *Assessment, 9*, 41–55.

Altman, L. (2001, November 14). Cholesterol fighters lower heart attack risk, study finds. *New York Times*, p. A14.

Ambady, N., Laplante, D., Nguyen, T., Rosenthal, R., Chaumeton, N., & Levinson, W. (2002). Surgeons' tone of voice: A clue to malpractice history. *Surgery, 132*, 5–9.

American Medical News. (1993, February 8). p. 31.

American Psychiatric Association. (1952). *Diagnostic and statistical manual of mental disorders*. Washington, DC: Author.

American Psychiatric Association. (2000). *Diagnostic and statistical manual of mental disorders* (4th ed., text rev.). Washington, DC: Author.

Andersen, L. F., Jacobs, D. R., Jr., Carlsen, M. H., & Blomhoff, R. (2006). Consumption of coffee is associated with reduced risk of death attributed to inflammatory and cardiovascular diseases in the Iowa Women's Health Study. *American Journal of Clinical Nutrition, 83*, 1039–1046.

Anderson, J. W., Konz, E. C., Frederich, R. C., & Wood, C. L. (2001). Long-term weight-loss maintenance: A meta-analysis of US studies. *American Journal of Clinical Nutrition, 74*, 579–584.

Anderson, L. (2008). *Aging even tougher for gays and lesbians*. Retrieved from http://www.chicagotribune.com/news/nationworld/chi-gay_elderlyoct21,0,2552870.story

Andrade, S. E., Majumdar, S. R., Chan, K. A., Buist, D. S., Go, A. S., Goodman, M., . . . Gurwitz, J. H. (2003). Low frequency of treatment of osteoporosis among postmenopausal women following a fracture. *Archives of Internal Medicine, 163*, 2052–2057.

Andren, S., & Elmstahl, S. (2008). Effective psychosocial intervention for family caregivers lengthens time elapsed before nursing home placement of individuals with dementia: A 5-year follow-up study. *International Psychogeriatrics, 20*, 1177–1192.

Andriole, G. L., Crawford, E. D., Grubb, R. L., 3rd., Buys, S. S., Chia, D., Church, T. R., . . . PLCO Project Team. (2009). Mortality results from a randomized prostate cancer screening trial. *New England Journal of Medicine, 360*, 1310–1319.

Angadi, S. S., Weltman, A., Watson-Winfield, D., Weltman, J., Frick, K., Patrie, J., & Gaesser, G. A. (2012). Effect of fractionized versus continuous, single-session exercise on blood pressure in adults. *Journal of Human Hypertension, 24*, 300–302.

Angell, M. (2004). *The truth about the drug companies: How they deceive us and what to do about it*. New York, NY: Random House.

Ansell, B. (2002). Should physicians be recommending statins for most older Americans? *Clinical Geriatrics, 10*, 33–40.

Antonioli, C., & Reveley, M. (2005). Randomised controlled trial of animal facilitated therapy with dolphins in the treatment of depression. *British Medical Journal, 331*, 1231.

Appel, L. J., Champagne, C. M., Harsha, D. W., Cooper, L. S., Obarzanek, E., Elmer, P. J., . . . Writing Group of the PREMIER Collaborative Research Group. (2003). Effects of comprehensive lifestyle modification on blood pressure control: Main results of the PREMIER clinical trial. *Journal of the American Medical Association, 289,* 2131–2132.

Ardell, D. (2000, November 10). The hierarchy of wellness. *Ardell Wellness Report,* pp. 1–3.

Aronow, W. (2005). Should the NCEP III guidelines be changed in elderly and younger persons at high risk for cardiovascular events? *Journal of Gerontology: Medical Sciences, 60A,* 591–592.

Asch, S. M., Sloss, E. M., Hogan, C., Brook, R. H., & Kravitz, R. L. (2000). Measuring underuse of necessary care among elderly Medicare beneficiaries using inpatient and outpatient claims. *Journal of the American Medical Association, 284,* 2325–2333.

Astin, J. A., Pelletier, K. R., Marie, A., & Haskell, W. L. (2000). Complementary and alternative medicine use among elderly persons: One-year analysis of a Blue Shield Medicare supplement. *Journal of Gerontology: Medical Sciences, 55A,* M4–M9.

Aston, G. (2002, July 1). Medicare's mindfield. *American Medical News,* pp. 5–6.

Atchley, R. (1998). Long-range antecedents of functional capability in later life. *Journal of Aging and Health, 10,* 3–19.

Atchley, R. (2009). *Spirituality and aging.* Baltimore, MD: Johns Hopkins University Press.

Atkins, R. (1992). *Dr. Atkins' new diet revolution.* New York, NY: Harper Collins.

Attracted to magnets? (2000, June 2). *Consumer Reports on Health.*

Auchincloss, A. H., Diez Roux, A. V., Mujahid, M. S., Shen, M., Bertoni, A. G., & Carnethon, M. R. (2009). Neighborhood resources for physical activity and healthy foods and incidence of type 2 diabetes mellitus. *Archives of Internal Medicine, 169,* 1698–1704.

Autier, P., & Gandini, S. (2007). Vitamin D supplementation and total mortality. *Archives of Internal Medicine, 167,* 1730–1737.

Avenell, A., Campbell, M. K., Cook, J. A., Hannaford, P. C., Kilonzo, M. M., McNeill, G., . . . Vale, L. D. (2005). Effect of multivitamin and multimineral supplements on morbidity from infections in older people. *British Medical Journal, 331,* 324–327.

Baby boomers turning to yoga for spiritual workouts. (2000, October 12). *Houston Chronicle,* pp. 1D, 3D.

Bach, P. B., Pham, H. H., Schrag, D., Tate, R. C., & Hargraves, J. L. (2004). Primary care physicians who treat Blacks and Whites. *New England Journal of Medicine, 351,* 575–584.

Bachmann, J., et al. (2012, May 10). *Fitness in middle age lowers medical costs later.* Presentation at the American Heart Association annual meeting. Atlanta, Georgia.

Badgwell, B. D., Giordano, S. H., Duan, Z. Z., Fang, S., Bedrosian, I., Kuerer, H. M., . . . Babiera, G. (2008). Mammography before diagnosis among women age 80 years and older with breast cancer. *Journal of Clinical Oncology, 26,* 2482–2488.

Bailey, C. (1996). *Smart eating.* Boston, MA: Houghton-Mifflin.

Baker, D., et al. (2007). Health literacy and mortality among elderly persons. *Archives of Internal Medicine, 167,* 1503–1509.

Baker, D., & Sudano, J. (2005). Health insurance coverage during the years preceding Medicare eligibility. *Archives of Internal Medicine, 165,* 770–776.

Baker, K. R., Nelson, M. E., Felson, D. T., Layne, J. E., Sarno, R., & Roubenoff, R. (2001). The efficacy of home based progressive strength training in older adults with knee osteoarthritis: A randomized clinical trial. *Journal of Rheumatology, 28,* 1655–1665.

Ballard, C. G., O'Brien, J. T., Reichelt, K., & Perry, E. K. (2002). Aromatherapy as a safe and effective treatment for the management of agitation in severe dementia: The results of a double-blind, placebo-controlled trial with Melissa. *Journal of Clinical Psychiatry, 63,* 553–558.

Balsalm, K., & D'Augelli, A. (2006). The victimization of older LGBT adults. In D. Kimmel, et al. (Eds.), *Lesbian, gay, bisexual, and transgender aging* (pp. 110–130). New York, NY: Columbia University Press.

Bandura, A. (1977). *Social learning theory*. Englewood Cliffs, NJ: Prentice-Hall.

Bandura, A. (1997). *Self-efficacy: The exercise of control*. New York, NY: W. H. Freeman.

Banks, M., & Banks, W. (2002). The effects of animal-assisted therapy on loneliness in an elderly population in long-term care facilities. *Journal of Gerontology: Biological and Medical Sciences, 57*, M428–M432.

Barnes, D. E., Yaffe, K., Satariano, W. A., & Tager, I. B. (2003). A longitudinal study of cardiorespiratory fitness and cognitive function in healthy older adults. *Journal of the American Geriatrics Society, 51*, 459–465.

Barnes, P. M., Bloom, B., & Nahin, R. (2008, December). *CDC National Health Statistics Report #12. Complementary and alternative medicine use among adults and children: United States, 2007*. Washington, DC: USDHHS.

Barrett, B. P., Brown, R. L., Locken, K., Maberry, R., Bobula, J. A., & D'Alessio, D. (2002). Treatment of the common cold with unrefined Echinacea. *Annals of Internal of Medicine, 137*, 939–946.

Bartholomew, J. B., Morrison, D., & Ciccolo, J. T. (2005). Effects of acute exercise on mood and well-being in patients with major depressive disorder. *Medical Science & Sports Exercise, 37*, 2032–2037.

Bauldoff, G. S., Hoffman, L. A., Zullo, T. G., & Sciurba, F. C. (2002). Exercise maintenance following pulmonary rehabilitation: Effect of distractive stimuli. *Chest, 122*, 948–954.

Bazzini, D. G., McIntosh, W. D., Smith, S. M., Cook, S., & Harris, C. (1997). The aging woman in popular film: Underrepresented, unattractive, unfriendly, and unintelligent. *Sex Roles, 36*, 531–543.

Beattie, M. S., Lane, N. E., Hung, Y. Y., & Nevitt, M. C. (2005). Association of statin use and development and progression of hip osteoarthritis in elderly women. *Journal of Rheumatology, 32*, 106–110.

Beck, A., Scott, J., Williams, P., Robertson, B., Jackson, D., Gade, G., & Cowan P. (1997). A randomized trial of group outpatient visits for chronically ill older HMO members: The cooperative health care clinic. *Journal of the American Geriatrics Society, 45*, 543–549.

Beckett, N. S., Peters R., Fletcher, A. E., Staessen, J. A., Liu, L., Dumitrascu, D., . . . HYVET Study Group. (2008). Treatment of hypertension in patients 80 years of age or older. *New England Journal of Medicine, 358*, 1887–1898.

Beekman, A. T., Geerlings, S. W., Deeg, D. J., Smit, J. H., Schoevers, R. S., de Beurs, E., . . . van Tilburg, W. (2002). The natural history of late-life depression: A 6-year prospective study in the community. *Archives of General Psychiatry, 59*, 605–611.

Beers, M., & Berkow, R. (2000). *The Merck manual of geriatrics* (3rd ed.). Whitehouse Station, NJ: Merck Research Laboratories.

Bellizzi, K. M., Breslau, E. S., Burness, A., & Waldron, W. (2011). Prevalence of cancer screening in older, racially diverse adults. *Archives of Internal Medicine, 17*, 2031–2037.

Benner, J. S., Glynn, R. J., Mogun, H., Neumann, P. J., Weinstein, M. C., & Avorn, J. (2002). Long-term persistence in use of statin therapy in elderly patients. *Journal of the American Medical Association, 288*, 455–461.

Benson, H. (1984). *Beyond the relaxation response*. New York, NY: Times Books.

Benson, H., Dusek, J. A., Sherwood, J. B., Lam, P., Bethea, C. F., Carpenter, W., . . . Hibberd, P. L. (2006). Study of the therapeutic effects of intercessory prayer in cardiac bypass patients. *American Heart Journal, 151*, 934–942.

Bent, S., Kane, C., Shinohara, K., Neuhaus, J., Hudes, E. S., Goldberg, H., & Avins, A. L. (2006). Saw palmetto for benign prostatic hyperplasia. *New England Journal of Medicine, 354,* 557–566.

Berger, J. S., Roncaglioni, M. C., Avanzini, F., Pangrazzi, I., Tognoni, G., & Brown, D. L. (2006). Aspirin for the primary prevention of cardiovascular events in women and men. *Journal of the American Medical Association, 295,* 306–313.

Berkman, L. (1983). *Health and ways of living: Findings from the Alameda county study.* New York, NY: Oxford University Press.

Berman, B. M., Lao, L., Langenberg, P., Lee, W. L., Gilpin, A. M., & Hochberg, M. C. (2004). Effectiveness of acupuncture as adjunctive therapy in osteoarthritis of the knee. *Annals of Internal Medicine, 141,* 901–910.

Betancourt, J., & Carrillo, J. (2002). *Cultural competence in health care: Emerging frameworks and practical approaches.* New York, NY: The Commonwealth Fund.

Beverly, E. A., Miller, C. K., & Wray, L. A. (2008). Spousal support and food-related behavior change in middle-aged and older adults living with type 2 diabetes. *Health Education and Behavior, 35,* 707–720.

Bhargava, A., & Du, X. (2009). Racial and socioeconomic disparities in adjuvant chemotherapy for older women with lymph node-positive, operable breast cancer. *Cancer, 115,* 2999–3008.

Biesada, A. (2000, June). Rx for trouble. *Texas Monthly,* pp. 72–76.

Binstock, R. (2009). Older voters and the 2008 election. *Gerontologist, 49,* 697–701.

Binstock, R., & Quadagno, J. (2001). Aging and politics. In R. Binstock & L. George (Eds.), *Aging and the social sciences* (pp. 333–350). San Diego, CA: Academic Press.

Birch, B. (1995). *Power yoga: The total wellness workout for mind and body.* New York, NY: Fireside.

Birditt, K., & Fingerman, K. (2005). Do we get better at picking our battles? *Journal of Gerontology: Psychological and Social Sciences, 60,* P121–P128.

Birditt, K. S., Fingerman, K. L., & Almeida, D. M. (2005). Age differences in exposure and reactions to interpersonal tensions. *Psychology and Aging, 20,* 330–340.

Birren, J., & Cochran, K. (2001). *Telling the stories of life through guided autobiography groups.* Baltimore, MD: Johns Hopkins University Press.

Birren, J., & Deutchman, D. (1991). *Guiding autobiography groups for older adults.* Baltimore, MD: Johns Hopkins University Press.

Birren, J., Kenyon, G., Ruth, J. E., Shroots, J. J. F., & Svendson, J. (1996). *Aging and biography: Explorations in adult development.* New York, NY: Springer.

Bischoff-Ferrari, H. A., Willett, W. C., Orav, E. J., Lips, P., Meunier, P. J., Lyons, R. A., . . . Dawson-Hughes, B. (2012). A pooled analysis of vitamin D dose requirements for fracture prevention. *New England Journal of Medicine, 367,* 77–78.

Bjelakovic, G., Nikolova, D., Gluud, L. L., Simonetti, R. G., & Gluud, C. (2008). Antioxidant supplements for prevention of mortality in health participants and patients with various diseases. *Cochrane Database Systematic Review, 16*(2), CD007176.

Black, D. M., Bauer, D. C., Schwartz, A. V., Cummings, S. R., & Rosen, C. J. (2012). Continuing bisphosphonate treatment for osteoporosis—For whom and for how long? *New England Journal of Medicine, 366,* 2051–2053.

Blackman, M. R., Sorkin, J. D., Münzer, T., Bellantoni, M. F., Busby-Whitehead, J., Stevens, T. E., . . . Harman, S. M. (2002). Growth hormone and sex steroid administration in healthy aged women and men: A randomized controlled trial. *Journal of the American Medical Association, 288,* 2282–2292.

Blair, G. (2001, fall/winter). The many faces I see. *Newsweek* [special issue], p. 64.

Blair, S. N., Kohl, H. W., 3rd., Paffenbarger, R. S., Jr., Clark, D. G., Cooper, K. H., & Gibbons, L. W. (1989). Physical fitness and all-cause mortality: A prospective study of healthy men and women. *Journal of the American Medical Association, 262,* 2395–2401.

Blake, H., Mo, P., Malik, S., & Thomas, S. (2009). How effective are physical activity interventions for alleviating depressive symptoms in older people? A systematic review. *Clinical Rehabilitation, 23,* 873–877.

Blank, T. O., Asencio, M., Descartes, L., & Griggs, J. (2009). Aging, health and GLBTQ family and community life. *Journal of GLBT Family Studies, 5,* 9–34.

Blendon, R. J., DesRoches, C. M., Benson, J. M., Brodie, M., & Altman, D. E. (2001). Americans' views on the use and regulation of dietary supplements. *Archives of Internal Medicine, 161,* 805–810.

Blittner, M., Goldberg, J., & Merbaum, M. (1978). Cognitive self-control factors in the reduction of smoking behavior. *Behavior Therapy, 9,* 553–561.

Bloom, S., et al. (2011, Spring). Picking up the PACE. *Generations,* pp. 53–55.

Blumenthal, J. A., Babyak, M. A., Moore, K. A., Craighead, W. E., Herman, S., Khatri, P., . . . Krishnan, K. R. (1999). Effects of exercise training on older patients with major depression. *Archives of Internal Medicine, 159,* 2349–2356.

Boehmer, U. (2002). Twenty years of public health research: Inclusion of lesbian, gay, bisexual, and transgender populations. *American Journal of Public Health, 92,* 1125–1130.

Bogner, H. R., Dahlberg, B., de Vries, H. F., Cahill, E., & Barg, F. K. (2008). Older patients' views on the relationship between depression and heart disease. *Family Medicine, 40,* 652–657.

Bohlmeijer, E. T., Westerhof, G, J., Emmerik-de Jong, M. (2008). The effects of integrative reminiscence on meaning in life. *Aging and Mental Health, 12,* 639–646.

Boling, R. (2000, March–April). A shot of youth. *Modern Maturity,* pp. 70–71.

Bolland, M., Grey, A., Avenell, A., Gamble, G. D., & Reid, I. R. (2011). Calcium supplements and myocardial infarction: The evidence grows. *British Medical Journal, 342,* d2040.

Boltri, J. M., Davis-Smith, Y. M., Seale, J. P., Shellenberger, S., Okosun, I. S., & Cornelius, M. E. (2008). Diabetes prevention in a faith-based setting. *Journal of Public Health Management and Practice, 14,* 29–32.

Bonita, R., Duncan, J., Truelsen, T., Jackson, R. T., & Beaglehole, R. (1999). Passive smoking as well as active smoking increases the risk of acute stroke. *Tobacco Control, 8,* 156–160.

Bonvicini, K., & Perlin, M. (2003). The same but different: Clinician-patient communication with gay and lesbian patients. *Patient Education and Counseling, 51,* 115–122.

Booth, K. M., Pinkston, M. M., & Poston, W. S. (2005). Obesity and the built environment. *Journal of the American Dietetic Association, 105,* S110–S117.

Borg, G. (1982). Psychophysical bases of perceived exertion. *Medicine and Science in Sports and Exercise, 14,* 377–381.

Bosworth, H. B., Powers, B., Grubber, J. M., Thorpe, C. T., Olsen, M. K., Orr, M., & Oddone, E. Z. (2008). Racial differences in blood pressure control. *Journal of General Internal Medicine, 23,* 692–698.

Boult, C., Reider, L., Leff, B., Frick, K. D., Boyd, C. M., Wolff, J. L., . . . Scharfstein, D. O. (2011). The effect of guided care teams on the use of health services. *Archives of Internal Medicine, 171,* 460–467.

Bowman, G. L., Silbert, L. C., Howieson, D., Dodge, H. H., Traber, M. G., Frei, B., . . . Quinn, J. F. (2012). Nutrient biomarker patterns, cognitifve function and MRI measures of brain aging. *Neurology, 78,* 241–249.

Boyd, C. M., Boult, C., Shadmi, E., Leff, B., Brager, R., Dunbar, L., . . . Wegener S. (2007). Guided care for multimorbid older adults. *Gerontologist, 47,* 697–704.

Brady, C. B., Spiro, A., 3rd., & Gaziano, J. M. (2005). Effects of age and hypertension status on cognition: The Veterans Affairs Normative Aging Study. *Neuropsychology, 19,* 770–777.

Bratton, R. L., Montero, D. P., Adams, K. S., Novas, M. A., McKay, T. C., Hall, L. J., . . . Maurer, M. S. (2002). Effect of "ionized" wrist bracelets on musculoskeletal pain: A randomized, double-blind, placebo-controlled trial. *Mayo Clinic Proceedings, 77,* 1164–1168.

Bravata, D. M., Smith-Spangler, C., Sundaram, V., Gienger, A. L., Lin, N., Lewis, R., . . . Sirard, J. R. (2007). Using pedometers to increase physical activity and improve health: A systematic review. *Journal of the American Medical Association, 298,* 2296–2304.

Brenes, G. A., Penninx, B. W., Judd, P. H., Rockwell, E., Sewell, D. D., & Wetherell, J. L. (2008). Anxiety, depression and disability across the lifespan. *Aging and Mental Health, 12,* 158–163.

Briggs, B. (2002, April 7). What is race? Color lines are blurring as more Americans proclaim mixed heritage. *Denver Post,* pp. 1L, 4L.

Broad, W. (2012). *The science of yoga.* New York, NY: Simon & Schuster.

Broadening your view of health. (2000, November). *Dr. Andrew Weil's Self Healing.* p. 2.

Broderick, J. E., Junghaenel, D. U., & Schwartz, J. E. (2005). Written emotional expression produces health benefits in fibromyalgia patients. *Psychosomatic Medicine, 67,* 325–334.

Brody, J. (1998, February 15). Cretan diet rich in fruits, vegetables, grains proves heart-healthy. *Houston Chronicle,* p. 5F.

Bross, M. H., Hartwig, L. C., & Herring, J. (1993, November). *Health promotion and disease prevention: A survey of rural family physicians.* Presentation at Society of Teachers of Family Medicine, Orlando, FL.

Brown, S. L., Smith, D. M., Schulz, R., Kabeto, M. U., Ubel, P. A., Poulin, M., . . . Langa, K. M. (2009). Caregiving behavior is associated with decreased mortality risk. *Psychological Science, 20,* 488–494.

Bruce, B., Fries, J. F., & Lubeck, D. P. (2005). Aerobic exercise and its impact on musculoskeletal pain in older adults: A 14 year prospective, longitudinal study. *Arthritis Research and Therapy, 7,* R1263–R1270.

Buchhave, P., Minthon, L., Zetterberg, H., Wallin, A. K., Blennow, K., & Hansson, O. (2012). Cerebro-spinal fluid levels of beta-amyloid 1–42, but not of tau, are fully changed already 5 to 10 years before the onset of Alzheimer's dementia. *Archives of General Psychiatry, 69,* 98–106.

Buchwald, A. (2006). *Too soon to say goodbye.* New York, NY: Random House.

Burkeman, O. (2012). *The antidote: Happiness for people who can't stand positive thinking.* New York, NY: Faber & Faber.

Burns, D. (1980). *Feeling good: The new mood therapy.* New York, NY: William Morrow.

Buscemi, N., Vandermeer, B., Hooton, N., Pandya, R., Tjosvold, L., Hartling, L., . . . Baker, G. (2006). Efficacy and safety of exogenous melatonin for secondary sleep disorders. *British Medical Journal, 332,* 385–393.

Buszewicz, M., Rait, G., Griffin, M., Nazareth, I., Patel, A., Atkinson, A., . . . Haines, A. (2006). Self management of arthritis in primary care: Randomised controlled trial. *British Medical Journal, 333,* 879–882.

Butler, R. (1995). Foreword: The life review. In B. Haight & J. Webster (Eds.), *The art and science of reminiscing* (pp. xvii–xxi). Washington, DC: Taylor and Francis.

Butler, R. N., Lewis, M. I., & Sunderland, T. (1998). *Aging and mental health: Positive psychosocial and biomedical approaches* (5th ed.). Needham Heights, MA: Allyn & Bacon.

Butler, S. (2012). Home care work: The companionship that was exempted. *Gerontologist*, *52*, 433–436.

Cahalin, L. P., Braga, M., Matsuo, Y., & Hernandez, E. D. (2002). Efficacy of diaphragmatic breathing in persons with chronic obstructive pulmonary disease: A review of the literature. *Journal of Cardiopulmonary Rehabilitation*, *22*, 7–21.

Caine, E., Lyness, J., & Conwell, Y. (1996). Diagnosis of late-life depression: Preliminary studies in primary care settings. *American Journal of Geriatric Psychiatry*, *4*, S45–S50.

Calfas, K. J., Long, B. J., Sallis, J. F., Wooten, W. J., Pratt, M., & Patrick, K. (1996). A controlled trial of physician counseling to promote the adoption of physical activity. *Preventive Medicine*, *25*, 225–233.

California cigarette sales fall due to stiff new tax. (1999, September 27). *American Medical News*, p. 9.

Callahan, D. (2000). *Promoting healthy behavior: How much freedom? Whose responsibility?* Washington, DC: Georgetown University Press.

Callahan, E. J., Bertakis, K. D., Azari, R., Robbins, J. A., Helms, L. J., & Chang, D. W. (2000). The influence of patient age on primary care resident physician-patient interaction. *Journal of the American Geriatrics Society*, *48*, 30–35.

Calle, E. E., Thun, M. J., Petrelli, J. M., Rodriguez, C., & Heath, C. W., Jr. (1999). Body-mass index and mortality in a prospective cohort of U.S. adults. *New England Journal of Medicine*, *341*, 1097–1105.

Camp, C., & Skrajner, M. (2004). Resident-assisted Montessori programming: Training persons with dementia to serve as group activity leaders. *Gerontologist*, *44*, 426–431.

Campbell, A. J. Robertson, M. C., Gardner, M. M., Norton, R. N., Tilyard, M. W., & Buchner, D. M. (1997). Randomised controlled trial of a general practice programme of home based exercise to prevent falls in elderly women. *British Medical Journal*, *315*, 1065–1069.

Cappeliez, P., & O'Rourke, N. (2006). Empirical validation of a model of reminiscence and health in later life. *Journal of Gerontology: Psychological Sciences*, *61B*, P237–P244.

Cardinal, B., & Engels, H. (2001). Ginseng does not enhance psychological well-being in healthy, young adults: Results of a double-blind, placebo-controlled, randomized clinical trial. *Journal of the American Dietetic Association*, *101*, 655–660.

Carey, B. (2012, Jaunary 10). Nicotine gum and skin patch face new doubt. *The New York Times*, pp. A1, A3.

Caro, F., & Morris, R. (2001). Maximizing the contributions of older people as volunteers. In S. Levkoff, et al. (Eds.), *Aging in good health* (pp. 341–356). New York, NY: Springer.

Carroll, M., et al. (2012). Trends in lipids and lipoproteins in U.S. adults: 1988–2010. *Journal of the American Medical Association*, *308*, 1545–1554.

Carstensen, L. (2006). The influence of a sense of time on human development. *Science*, *312*, 1913–1915.

Carstensen, L. L., Pasupathi, M., Mayr, U., & Nesselroade, J. R. (2000). Emotional experience in everyday life across the adult life span. *Journal of Personality and Social Psychology*, *79*, 644–655.

Carstensen, L. L., Turan, B., Scheibe, S., Ram, N., Ersner-Hershfield, H., Samanez-Larkin, G. R., . . . Nesselroade, J. R. (2011). Emotional experience improves with age. *Psychology and Aging*, *26*, 21–33.

Carter, D. (2004). *Stonewall: The riots that sparked the gay revolution*. New York, NY: St. Martin's Press.

Casado, B. L., Resnick, B., Zimmerman, S., Nahm, E. S., Orwig, D., Macmillan, K., & Magaziner, J. (2009). Social support for exercise by experts in older women post-hip fracture. *Journal of Women and Aging*, *21*, 48–62.

Cassel, C. (2002). Use it or lose it. *Journal of the American Medical Association*, *288*, 2333–2335.

Castillo-Richmond, A., Schneider, R. H., Alexander, C. N., Cook, R., Myers, H., Nidich, S., . . . Salerno, J. (2000). Effects of stress reduction on carotid atherosclerosis in hypertensive African Americans. *Stroke, 31,* 568–573.

Centers for Disease Control and Prevention. (2002). Prevalence of health-care providers asking older adults about their physical activity levels-United States, 1998. *Morbidity and Mortality Weekly Report, 51,* 412–414.

Chan, E. C., Vernon, S. W., O'Donnell, F. T., Ahn, C., Greisinger, A., & Aga, D. W. (2003). Informed consent for cancer screening with prostate-specific antigen. *American Journal of Public Health, 93,* 779–785.

Chandra, R. (1992). Effect of vitamin and trace-element supplementation on immune responses and infection in elderly subjects. *Lancet, 340,* 1124–1127.

Chandra, R. (1997). Graying of the immune system: Can nutrient supplements improve immunity in the elderly? *Journal of the American Medical Association, 277,* 1398–1399.

Chandra, R. (2001). Effect of vitamin and trace-element supplementation on cognitive function in elderly subjects. *Nutrition, 17,* 709–712.

Chang, P. P., Ford, D. E., Meoni, L. A., Wang, N. Y., & Klag, M. J. (2002). Anger in young men and subsequent premature cardiovascular disease: The precursors study. *Archives of Internal Medicine, 162,* 901–906.

Charles, S. T., Mather, M., & Carstensen, L. L. (2003). Aging and emotional memory. *Journal of Experimental Psychology: General, 132,* 310–324.

Chaufan, C., Hong, G. H., & Fox, P. (2009). Taxing "sin foods": Obesity prevention and public health policy. *New England Journal of Medicine, 361,* 113.

Chen, D. (2008, June 30). Bloomberg's next battle: Revamping senior centers. *The New York Times,* p. 17.

Chen, K. M., Chen, M. H., Lin, M. H., Fan, J. T., Lin, H. S., & Li, C. H. (2010). Effects of yoga on sleep quality and depression in elders in assisted living facilities. *Journal of Nursing Research, 18,* 53–61.

Chen, R. C., Sheets, N. C., Goldin, G. H., Holmes, J. A., Meyer, A. M., . . . Sturmer, T. (2012). Intensity-modulated therapy, proton therapy, or conformal radiation therapy and morbidity and disease control in localized prostate cancer. *Journal of the American Medical Association, 307,* 1611–1620.

Cheng, I., Witte, J. S., McClure, L. A., Shema, S. J., Cockburn, M. G., John, E. M., & Clarke, C. A. (2009, June 13). Socioeconomic status and prostate cancer incidence and mortality rates among the diverse population of California. *Cancer Causes Control* (e-publication).

Cheng, S. P., Tsai, T. I., Lii, Y. K., Yu, S., Chou, C. L., & Chen, I. J. (2009). The effects of a 12-week walking program on community-dwelling older adults. *Research Quarterly on Exercise and Sport, 80,* 524–532.

Cheng, S. T., Fung, H. H., & Chan, A. C. (2009). Self-perception and psychological well-being: The benefits of foreseeing a worse future. *Psychology and Aging, 24,* 632–633.

Cherkin, D. C., Eisenberg, D., Sherman, K. J., Barlow, W., Kaptchuk, T. J., Street, J., & Deyo, R. A. (2001). Randomized trial comparing traditional Chinese medical acupuncture, therapeutic massage, and self-care education for chronic low back pain. *Archives of Internal Medicine, 161,* 1081–1088.

Chiva-Blanch, G., Urpi-Sarda, M., Ros, E., Arranz, S., Valderas-Martínez, P., Casas, R., . . . Estruch, R. (2012). Dealcoholized red wine dcreases systolic and diastolicblood pressure. *Circulation Research.* doi:10.11611/circresaha.112.275636.

Chodosh, J., Morton, S. C., Mojica, W., Maglione, M., Suttorp, M. J., Hilton. L., . . . Shekelle, P. (2005). Meta-analysis: Chronic disease self-management programs for older adults. *Annals of Internal Medicine, 143,* 427–438.

Cholesterol-lowering drugs less effective than in studies. (2001, November 12). *Star Press*, p. 8C.

Chou, R., Dana, T., & Bougatsos, C. (2009). Screening older adults for impaired visual acuity: A review of the evidence for the USPSTF. *Annals of Internal Medicine, 151,* 44–58.

Christakis, N., & Allison, P. (2006). Mortality after the hospitalization of a spouse. *New England Journal of Medicine, 354,* 719–730.

Christakis, N., & Fowler, J. (2007). The spread of obesity in large social network over 32 years. *New England Journal of Medicine, 357,* 370–379.

Christen, W. G., Glynn, R. J., Chew, E. Y., & Buring, J. E. (2008). Vitamin E and age-related cataract in a randomized trial of women. *Ophthalmology, 115,* 822–829.

Christensen, K., Doblhammer, G., Rau, R., & Vaupel, J. (2009). Ageing populations: The challenges ahead. *Lancet, 374,* 1196–1208.

Christensen, K., McGue, M., Petersen, I., Jeune, B., & Vaupel, J. W. (2008, August 18). Exceptional longevity does not result in excessive levels of disability. *Proceedings of the National Academy of Science, 105,* 13274–13279 (e-publication).

Chu, Q. D., Smith, M. H., Williams, M., Panu, L., Johnson, L. W., Shi, R., . . . Glass, J. (2009). Race/ethnicity has no effect on outcome for breast cancer patients treated in an academic center with a public hospital. *Cancer Epidemiology Biomarkers Prevention, 18,* 2157–2161.

Chung, M., & Barfield, J. (2002). Knowledge of prescription medications among elderly emergency department patients. *Annals of Emergency Medicine, 39,* 605–608.

Ciatto, S. (2008). Recommending mammography screening beyond 80 years of age: A time for caution. *Women's Health, 4,* 353–355.

Clancy, D. E., Cope, D. W., Magruder, K. M., Huang, P., & Wolfman, T. E. (2003). Evaluating concordance to American Diabetes Association standards of care for type 2 diabetes through group visits in an uninsured or inadequately insured population. *Diabetes Care, 26,* 2032–2036.

Clark, A., Seidler, A., & Miller, M. (2001). Inverse association between sense of humor and coronary heart disease. *International Journal of Cardiology, 80,* 87–88.

Clark, C. E., Taylor, R. S., Shore, A. C., Ukoumunne, O. C., & Campbell, J. L. (2012). Association of a difference in systolic blood pressure between arms with vascular disease and mortality. *Lancet, 379,* 905–914.

Clark, R., & Kraemer, T. (2009). Clinical use of Nintendo Wii bowling simulation to decrease fall risk in an elderly resident of a nursing home. *Journal of Geriatric Physical Therapy, 32,* 174–180.

Clegg, D. O., Reda, D. J., Harris, C. L., Klein, M. A., O'Dell, J. R., Hooper, M. M., . . . Williams, H. J. (2006). Glucosamine, chondroitin sulfate, and the two in combination for painful knee osteoarthritis. *New England Journal of Medicine, 354,* 795–808.

Clemson, L., Fiatarone Singh, M. A., Bundy, A., Cumming, R. G., Manollaras, K., O'Loughlin, P., & Black, D. (2012). Integration of balance and strength-training into daily life activity to reduce rate of falls in older people. *British Medical Journal, 345,* e547.

Coakley, A., & Mahoney, E. (2009). Creating a therapeutic and healing environment with a pet therapy program. *Complementary Therapeutic Practices, 15,* 141–146.

Cohen, C. A., Colantonio, A., & Vernich, L. (2002a). Complementary and alternative medicine (CAM) use by older adults: A comparison of self-report and physician chart documentation. *Journal of Gerontology: Medical Sciences, 57A,* M223–M227.

Cohen, C. A., Colantonio, A., & Vernich, L. (2002b). Positive aspects of caregiving: Rounding out the caregiver experience. *International Journal of Geriatric Psychiatry, 17,* 184–188.

Colangelo, R. M., Stillman, M. J., Kessler-Fogil, D., & Kessler-Hartnett, D. (1997). The role of exercise in rehabilitation patients with end-stage renal disease. *Rehabilitation Nursing, 22,* 288–292, 302.

Colcombe, S. J., Erickson, K. I., Raz, N., Webb, A. G., Cohen, N. J., McAuley, E., & Kramer, A. F. (2003). Aerobic fitness reduces brain tissue loss in aging humans. *Journal of Gerontology: Series A, 58*, 176–180.

Collacott, E. A., Zimmerman, J. T., White, D. W., & Rindone, J. P. (2000). Bipolar permanent magnets for the treatment of chronic low back pain: A pilot study. *Journal of the American Medical Association, 283*, 1322–1325.

Collins, H., & Pancoast, D. (1976). *Natural helping networks: A strategy for prevention*. Washington, DC: National Association of Social Workers.

Colman, R. J., Anderson, R. M., Johnson, S. C., Kastman, E. K., Kosmatka, K. J., Beasley, T. M., . . . Weindruch, R. (2009). Caloric restriction delays disease onset and mortality in rhesus monkeys. *Science, 325*, 201–204.

Comfort, A. (1972). *The joy of sex*. New York, NY: Simon & Schuster.

Comondore, V. R., Devereaux, P. J., Zhou, Q., Stone, S. B., Busse, J. W., Ravindran, N. C., . . . Guyatt, G. H. (2009). Quality of care in for-profit and not-for-profit nursing homes. *British Medical Journal, 339*, 2732.

Concato, J., Wells, C. K., Horwitz, R. I., Penson, D., Fincke, G., Berlowitz, D. R., . . . Peduzzi, P. (2006). The effectiveness of screening for prostate cancer: A nested case-control study. *Archives of Internal Medicine, 166*, 38–43.

Connolly, C. (2001, May 17). Living longer, independently: A new study shows that more older Americans are avoiding chronic impairment. *The Washington Post*, p. D1.

Connor, S. P., Pyenson, B., Fitch, K., Spence, C., & Iwasaki, K. (2007). Comparing hospice and nonhospice patient survival among patients who die within a three-year window. *Journal of Pain Symptom Management, 33*, 238–246.

Constantino, G., Malgady, R. G., & Primavera, L. H. (2009). Congruence between culturally competent treatment and cultural needs of older Latinos. *Journal of Consulting and Clinical Psychology, 77*, 941–949.

Cook, J. M., Pearson, J. L., Thompson, R., Black, B. S., & Rabins, P. V. (2002). Suicidality in older African Americans: Findings from the EPOCH study. *American Journal of Geriatric Psychiatry, 10*, 437–446.

Cooper, G., & Kou, T. (2007). Underuse of colorectal cancer screening in a cohort of Medicare beneficiaries. *Cancer, 1112*, 293–299.

Cooper, J., & Feder, M. (2004). Inaccurate information about Lyme disease on the Internet. *Pediatric Infectious Diseases, 23*, 1105–1108.

Cooper, K. (1994). *Dr. Kenneth H. Cooper's antioxidant revolution*. Nashville, TN: Thomas Nelson.

Cooper, L. A., Roter, D. L., Johnson, R. L., Ford, D. E., Steinwachs, D. M., & Powe, N. R. (2003). Patient-centered communication, ratings of care, and concordance of patient and physician race. *Annals of Internal Medicine, 139*, 907–915.

Cornelis, M. C., El-Sohemy, A., Kabagambe, E. K., & Campos, H. (2006). Coffee, CYPIA2 genotype, and risk of myocardial infarction. *Journal of the American Medical Association, 295*, 1135–1141.

Cornu, J. N., Cancel-Tassin, G., Ondet, V., Girardet, C., & Cussenot, O. (2011). Olfactory detection of prostate cancer by dogs sniffing urine. *European Urology, 59*, 183–216.

Cornwell, B., Laumann, E. O., & Schumm, L. P. (2008). The social connectedness of older adults. *American Sociological Review, 73*, 185–203.

Corrada, M. M., Kawas, C. H., Mozaffar, F., & Paganini-Hill, A. (2006). Association of body mass index and weight change with all-cause mortality in the elderly. *American Journal of Epidemiology, 163*, 938–949.

Cotter, K., & Sherman, A. (2008). Love hurts: The influence of social relations on exercise self-efficacy for older adults with osteoarthritis. *Journal of Aging and Physical Activity, 16*, 465–483.

Cottreau, C. M., Ness, R. B., & Kriska, A. M. (2000). Physical activity and reduced risk of ovarian cancer. *Obstetrics and Gynecology, 96,* 609–614.

Counting on food labels. (2000, January 10). *Washington Post National Weekly,* p. 32.

Courtney, C., Farrell, D., Gray, R., Hills, R., Lynch, L., Sellwood, E., . . . AD2000 Collaborative Group. (2004). Long-term donepezil treatment in 565 patients with Alzheimer's disease. *Lancet, 363,* 2105–2115.

Coyne, J., Pajak, T. F., Harris, J., Konski, A., Movsas, B., Ang, K., . . . Radiation Therapy Oncology Group. (2007). Emotional well-being does not predict survival in head and neck cancer patients. *Cancer, 110,* 2568–2575.

Cram, P., Fendrick, A. M., Inadomi, J., Cowen, M. E., Carpenter, D., & Vijan, S. (2003). The impact of a celebrity promotional campaign on the use of colon cancer screening: The Katie Couric effect. *Archives of Internal Medicine, 163,* 1601–1605.

Crawford, M. J., Patton, R., Touquet, R., Drummond, C., Byford, S., Barrett, B., . . . Henry, J. A. (2004). Screening and referral for brief intervention of alcohol-misusing patients in an emergency department. *Lancet, 364,* 1334–1339.

Cress, M. E. Buchner, D. M., Prohaska, T., Rimmer, J., Brown, M., Macera, C., . . . Chodzko-Zajko, W. (2005). Best practices for physical activity programs and behavior counseling in older adult populations. *Journal of Aging and Physical Activity, 13,* 61–74.

Crimmins, E., & Beltran-Sanchez, H. (2010). Mortality and morbidity trends: Is there compression of morbidity? *Journal of Gerontology: Social Sciences, 66B,* 75–86.

Crossette, B. (2000, June 5). U.S. ranks far down on "healthy life" list. *The New York Times,* pp. 1A, 9A.

Curb, J. D., et al. (2000). Serum lipid effects of a high-monounsaturated fat diet based on macademia nuts. *Archives of Internal Medicine, 160,* 1154–1158.

Curtis, L. H., Østbye, T., Sendersky, V., Hutchison, S., Dans, P. E., Wright, A., . . . Schulman, K. A. (2004). Inappropriate prescribing for elderly Americans in a large outpatient population. *Archives of Internal Medicine, 164,* 1621–1625.

Dahl, A., Hassing, L. B., Fransson, E., Berg, S., Gatz, M., Reynolds, C. A., & Pedersen, N. L. (2010). Being overweight in midlife is associated with lower cognitive ability and steeper cognitive decline in later life. *Journal of Gerontology: Medical Sciences, 65A,* 57–62.

Dale, K. M., Coleman, C. I., Henyan, N. N., Kluger, J., & White, C. M. (2006). Statins and cancer risk: A meta-analysis. *Journal of the American Medical Association, 295,* 74–80.

D'Amico, A. V., Chen, M. H., Roehl, K. A., & Catalona, W. J. (2004). Preoperative PSA velocity and the risk of death from prostate cancer after radical prostatectomy. *New England Journal of Medicine, 351,* 125–135.

Danner, D. D., Snowdon, D. A., & Friesen, W. V. (2001). Positive emotions in early life and longevity: Findings from the nun study. *Journal of Personality and Social Psychology, 80,* 804–813.

Dass, R. (2000). *Still here: Embracing aging, changing and dying.* New York, NY: Riverhead Books.

Datti, B., & Carter, M. (2006). The effect of direct-to-consumer advertising on prescription drug use by older adults. *Drugs and Aging, 23,* 71–81.

Davis, M., Eshelman, E. R., & McKay, M. (2000). *The relaxation and stress management workbook.* Oakland, CA: New Harbinger Publications.

Davison, K. P., Pennebaker, J. W., & Dickerson, S. S. (2000). Who talks? The social psychology of illness support groups. *American Psychologist, 55,* 205–217.

Day, L., Fildes, B., Gordon, I., Fitzharris, M., Flamer, H., & Lord, S. (2002). Randomised factorial trial of falls prevention among older people living in their own homes. *British Medical Journal, 325,* 128–131.

Dean, A., Kolody, B., & Wood, P. (1990). Effects of social support from various sources on depression in elderly persons. *Journal of Health and Social Behavior, 31,* 148–161.

DeGuire, S., Gevirtz, R., Hawkinson, D., & Dixon, K. (1996). Breathing retraining: A three-year follow-up study of treatment for hyperventilation syndrome and associated functional cardiac symptoms. *Biofeedback Self-Regulation, 21,* 191–198.

Delany, S. L., Delany, A. E., & Hearth, A. H. (1993). *Having our say: The Delany sisters' first 100 years.* New York, NY: Kodansha International.

de Lorgeril, M., Salen, P., Martin, J. L., Monjaud, I., Delaye, J., & Mamelle, N. (1999). Mediterranean diet, traditional risk factors, and the rate of cardiovascular complications after myocardial infarction: Final report of the Lyon Diet Heart Study. *Circulation, 99,* 779–785.

Demling, R. (1999). Growth hormone therapy in critically ill patients. *New England Journal of Medicine, 341,* 837–839.

Deuster, L., Christopher, S., Donovan, J., & Farrell, M. (2008). A method to quantify residents' jargon use during counseling of standardized patients about cancer screening. *Journal of General Internal Medicine, 23,* 1947–1952.

Diem, S. J., Blackwell, T. L., Stone, K. L., Yaffe, K., Haney, E. M., Bliziotes, M. M., & Ensrud, K. E. (2007). Use of antidepressants and rates of hip bone loss in older women. *Archives of Internal Medicine, 167,* 1240–1245.

Dietary fat makes a comeback. (2001, July). *Tufts University Health & Nutrition Letter,* pp. 4–5.

Dieting. (2002, June). *Consumer Reports, 67,* 26–31.

Dimou, A., Syrigos, K. N., & Saif, M. W. (2009). Disparities in colorectal cancer in African-Americans vs. Whites: Before and after diagnosis. *World Journal of Gastroenterology, 15,* 3734–3743.

Dirx, M. J., Voorrips, L. E., Goldbohm, R. A., & van den Brandt, P. A. (2001). Baseline recreational physical activity, history of sports participation, and postmenopausal breast carcinoma risk in the Netherlands Cohort Study. *Cancer, 92,* 1638–1649.

Dittrick, G. W., Thompson, J. S., Campos, D., Bremers, D., & Sudan, D. (2005). Gallbladder pathology in morbid obesity. *Obesity Surgery, 15,* 238–242.

Dobkin, L. (2002). Senior wellness project secures health care dollars. *Innovations, 2,* 16–20.

Dolan, P. (2007a, March 5). The health whisperer. *American Medical News,* pp. 18–19.

Dolan, P. (2007b, August 6). More than sympathy. *American Medical News,* pp. 15–16.

Dorgo, S., Robinson, K. M., & Bader, J. (2009). The effectiveness of a peer-mentored older adult fitness program on perceived physical, mental, and social function. *Journal of the American Academy of Nurse Practitioners, 21,* 116–122.

Dorsey, E. R., Deuel, L. M., Beck, C. A., Gardiner, I. F., Scoglio, N. J., Scott, J. C., . . . Biglan, K. M. (2011). Group patient visits for Parkinson disease. *Neurology, 76,* 1542–1547.

Dosa, D. (2007). A day in the life of Oscar the cat. *New England Journal of Medicine, 357,* 4.

Douglas, R. M., Hemilä, H., Chalker, E., & Treacy, B. (2007, July 18). Vitamin C for preventing and treating the common cold. *Cochrane Database Systematic Review,* (3), CD000980.

Dr. Koop to cease operation. (2002, January 14). *American Medical News,* p. 12.

Dubois, M. (1999). Legal planning for gay, lesbian, and non-traditional elders. *Albany Law Review, 63,* 263–332.

Duenwald, M. (2002, May 7). Religion and health: New research revives an old debate. *The New York Times,* pp. D1–D4.

Duffy, J. F., Zeitzer, J. M., Rimmer, D. W., Klerman, E. B., Dijk, D. J., & Czeisler, C. A. (2002). Peak of circadian melatonin rhythm occurs later within the sleep of older subjects. *American Journal of Physiology: Endocrinology and Metabolism, 282,* E297–E303.

Duffy, S. W., Tabár, L., & Smith, R. A. (2002). The mammographic screening trials: Commentary on the recent work by Olsen and Gotzsche. *Cancer, 52,* 68–71.

Duffy, S. W., Tabár, L., Chen, H. H., Holmqvist, M., Yen, M. F., Abdsalah, S., . . . Holmberg, L. (2002). Impact of organized mammography service screening on breast carcinoma mortality in seven Swedish counties. *Cancer, 93*, 458–469.

Duhigg, C. (2007a, May 25). Congress putting long-term care under scrutiny. *The New York Times*, p. 17.

Duhigg, C. (2007b, September 23). At many homes, more profit and less nursing. *The New York Times*, pp. 1, 20, 21.

Duncan, P., Richards, L., Wallace, D., Stoker-Yates, J., Pohl, P., Luchies, C., . . . Studenski, S. (1998). A randomized, controlled pilot study of a home-based exercise program for individuals with mild and moderate stroke. *Stroke, 29*, 2055–2060.

Dunstan, D. W., Daly, R. M., Owen, N., Jolley, D., De Courten, M., Shaw, J., & Zimmet, P. (2002). High-intensity resistance training improves glycemic control in older patients with type 2 diabetes. *Diabetes Care, 25*, 1729–1736.

Dunstan, D. W., Kingwell, B. A., Larsen, R., Healy, G. N., Cerin, E., Hamilton, M. T., . . . Owen, N. (2012). Breaking up long sitting reduces postprandial glucose and insulin responses. *Diabetes Care, 35*, 971–983.

Ebersole, P., & Hess, P. (1990). *Toward healthy aging: Human needs and nursing response.* St. Louis, MO: C.V. Mosby.

Edinger, J. D., Wohlgemuth, W. K., Radtke, R. A., Marsh, G. R., & Quillian, R. E. (2001). Cognitive behavioral therapy for treatment of chronic primary insomnia: A randomized controlled trial. *Journal of the American Medical Association, 285*, 1856–1864.

Egede, L. (2003). Implementing behavioral counseling interventions in primary care to modify cardiovascular disease risk in adults with diabetes. *Cardiovascular Reviews & Reports, 24*, 306–312.

Ehman, J. W., Ott, B. B., Short, T. H., Ciampa, R. C., & Hansen-Flaschen, J. (1999). Do patients want physicians to inquire about their spiritual or religious beliefs if they become gravely ill? *Archives of Internal Medicine, 159*, 1803–1806.

Ehrenreich, B. (2009). *Bright-sided: How the relentless promotion of positive thinking has undermined America.* New York, NY: Henry Holt.

Eisenberg, A. (2002, April 18). Such a comfort to grandma, and he runs on double-A's. *The New York Times*, pp. D1, D4.

Eisner, M. D., Smith, A. K., & Blanc, P. D. (1998). Bartenders' respiratory health after establishment of smoke-free bars and taverns. *Journal of the American Medical Association, 280*, 1909–1914.

Elder, J. P., Williams, S. J., Drew, J. A., Wright, B. L., & Boulan, T. E. (1995). Longitudinal effects of preventive services on health behaviors among an elderly cohort. *American Journal of Preventive Medicine, 11*, 354–359.

Elkin, E. B., Kim, S. H., Casper, E. S., Kissane, D. W., & Schrag, D. (2007). Desire for information and involvement in treatment decisions. *Journal of Clinical Oncology, 25*, 5275.

Elliott, V. (2001a, December 10). Statins found to work better in studies than in practice. *American Medical News*, pp. 1–2.

Elliot, V. (2001b, September). Health of rural, urban residents lags behind suburbanites. *American Medical News*, p. 39.

Elliott, V. (2002, October 21). Aftermath of HRT study: Patient-by-patient re-evaluation. *American Medical News*, p. 35.

Elliott, V. (2007, February 7). Melanoma screening is worth the money, study shows. *American Medical News*, pp. 32–33.

Ellis, J. J., Erickson, S. R., Stevenson, J. G., Bernstein, S. J., Stiles, R. A., & Fendrick, A. M. (2004). Suboptimal statin adherence and discontinuation in primary and secondary prevention populations. *Journal of General Internal Medicine, 19*, 638–645.

Elmer, P. J., Obarzanek, E., Vollmer, W. M., Simons-Morton, D., Stevens, V. J., Young, D. R., . . . PREMIER Collaborative Research Group. (2006). Effects of comprehensive lifestyle modification on diet, weight, physical fitness, and blood pressure control. *Annals of Internal Medicine, 144*, 485–495.

Elmore, J. G., Barton, M. B., Moceri, V. M., Polk, S., Arena, P. J., & Fletcher, S. W. (1998). Ten-year risk of false positive screening mammograms and clinical breast examinations. *New England Journal of Medicine, 338*, 1089–1096.

Elwert, F., & Christakis, N. (2006). Widowhood and race. *American Sociological Review, 71*, 16–41.

Emanuel, E., & Pearson, S. (2012, January 3). It costs more, but is it worth more? *The New York Times*, p. 1.

Emery, C. F., Kiecolt-Glaser, J. K., Glaser, R., Malarkey, W. B., & Frid, D. J. (2005). Exercise accelerates wound healing among healthy older adults: A preliminary investigation. *Journal of Gerontology: Biological/Medical Sciences, 60*, 1432–1436.

End of debate: Fiber's great. (1996, July/August). *Health*, p. 16.

Eng, P. M., Rimm, E. B., Fitzmaurice, G., & Kawachi, I. (2002). Social ties and change in social ties in relation to subsequent total and cause-specific mortality and coronary heart disease incidents in men. *American Journal of Epidemiology, 155*, 700–709.

Engelhart, M. J., Geerlings, M. I., Ruitenberg, A., van Swieten, J. C., Hofman, A., Witteman, J. C., & Breteler, M. M. (2002). Dietary intake of antioxidants and risk of Alzheimer disease. *Journal of the American Medical Association, 287*, 3223–3229.

Engels, H., & Wirth, J. (1997). No ergogenic effects of ginseng during graded maximal aerobic exercise. *Journal of the American Dietetic Association, 97*, 1110–1115.

Erikson, E. (1950). *Childhood and society*. New York, NY: W.W. Norton.

Erikson, E. H., Erikson, J. M., & Kivnick, H. Q. (1987). *Vital involvement in old age*. New York, NY: W.W. Norton.

Eskin, S. (2001). Dietary supplements and older consumers. *AARP Public Policy Institute Data Digest, 66*, 1–8.

Espiritu, J. (2008). Aging-related sleep changes. *Clinical Geriatric Medicine, 24*, 1–14.

Etzioni, R., Penson, D. F., Legler, J. M., di Tommaso, D., Boer, R., Gann, P. H., & Feuer, E. J. (2002). Overdiagnosis due to prostate-specific antigen screening: Lessons from U.S. prostate cancer incidence trends. *Journal of the National Cancer Institute, 94*, 981–990.

Euroscreen Working Group. (2012). Summary of the evidence of breast cancer service screening outcomes in Europe and first estimate of the benefit and harm balance sheet. *Journal of Medical Screenings, 19*, 5–13.

Expert Panel on Detection, Evaluation, and Treatment of High Blood Cholesterol in Adults. (2001). Executive summary of the third report of the National Cholesterol Education Program (NCEP) Expert Panel on Detection, Evaluation, and Treatment of High Blood Cholesterol in Adults (Adult Treatment Panel III). *Journal of the American Medical Association, 285*, 2486–2497.

Falba, T., & Sindelar, J. (2008). Spousal concordance in health behavior change. *Health Services Research, 43*, 96–116.

Feart, C., Samieri, C., Rondeau, V., Amieva, H., Portet, F., Dartigues, J. F., . . . Barberger-Gateau, P. (2009). Adherence to a Mediterranean diet, cognitive decline, and risk of dementia. *Journal of the American Medical Association, 302*, 638–648.

Fedder, D. O., Koro, C. E., & L'Italien, G. J. (2002). New National Cholesterol Education Program III Guidelines for primary prevention lipid-lowering drug therapy. *Circulation, 105*, 152–156.

Federal Interagency Forum on Aging-Related Statistics. (2000). *Older Americans 2000: Key indicators of well-being*. Indicator 29: Use of Health Care Services (p. 44). Hyattsville, MD: Author.

Federal Interagency Forum on Aging-Related Statistics. (2012). *Older Americans 2012: Key indicators of well-being.* Hyattsville, MD: Author.

Feigelson, H. S., Patel, A. V., Teras, L. R., Gansler, T., Thun, M. J., & Calle, E. E. (2006, May 22). Adult weight gain and histopathologic characteristics of breast cancer among post-menopausal women. *Cancer* (e-publication).

Feinglass, J., Thompson, J. A., He, X. Z., Witt, W., Chang, R. W., & Baker, D. W. (2005). Effect of physical activity on functional status among older middle-age adults with arthritis. *Arthritis and Rheumatism, 53,* 879–885.

Feldstein, A. C., Nichols, G. A., Elmer, P. J., Smith, D. H., Aickin, M., & Herson, M. (2003). Older women with fractures. *Journal of Bone and Joint Surgery, 85-A,* 2294–2302.

Ferraro, K., & Koch, J. (1994). Religion and health among Black and White adults: Examining social support and consolation. *Journal for the Scientific Study of Religion, 33,* 362–375.

Feskanich, D., Willett, W., & Colditz, G. (2002). Walking and leisure-time activity and risk of hip fracture in postmenopausal women. *Journal of the American Medical Association, 288,* 2300–2306.

Fiatarone, M. A. Marks, E. C., Ryan, N. D., Meredith, C. N., Lipsitz, L. A., & Evans, W. J. (1990). High-intensity strength training in nonagenarians: Effects on skeletal muscle. *Journal of the American Medical Association, 263,* 3029–3034.

Fichtenberg, C., & Glantz, S. (2000). Association of the California Tobacco Control Program with declines in cigarette consumption and mortality from heart disease. *New England Journal of Medicine, 343,* 1772–1777.

Finestone, A. (2009). Definition of hypertension for the "old-old." *Journal of Gerontology: Medical Sciences, 64,* 1097.

Finkelstein, E. A., Trogdon, J. G., Cohen, J. W., & Dietz, W. (2009). Annual medical spending attributable to obesity: Payer-and service-specific estimates. *Health Affairs, 28,* 822–831.

Fiore, M. C., Novotny, T. E., Pierce, J. P., Giovino, G. A., Hatziandreu, E. J., Newcomb, P. A., … Davis, R. M. (1990). Methods used to quit smoking in the United States: Do cessation programs help? *Journal of the American Medical Association, 263,* 2760–2765.

Firestone, A. (2000). Exercise stress testing for older persons starting an exercise program. *Journal of the American Medical Association, 284,* 2591–2592.

Fishbein, M., & Ajzen, I. (1975). *Belief, attitude, intention and behavior: An introduction to theory and research.* Reading, MA: Addison-Wesley.

Fisman, D. N., Abrutyn, E., Spaude, K. A., Kim, A., Kirchner, C., & Daley, J. (2006). Prior pneumococcal vaccination is associated with reduced death, complications, and length of stay among hospitalized adults with community-acquired pneumonia. *Clinical Infectious Disease, 42,* 1093–1101.

Fitzgerald, F. (1994). The tyranny of health. *New England Journal of Medicine, 331,* 196–198.

Flaherty, J. H., Takahashi, R., Teoh, J., Kim, J. I., Habib, S., Ito, M., & Matsushita, S. (2001). Use of alternative therapies in older outpatients in the United States and Japan: Prevalence, reporting patterns, and perceived effectiveness. *Journal of Gerontology: Medical Sciences, 56A,* M650–M655.

Flegal, K. M., Carroll, M. D., Ogden, C. L., & Curtin, L. R. (2010). Prevalence and trends in obesity among US adults, 1999-2008. *Journal of the American Medical Association, 303,* 235–241.

Flegal, K. M., Carroll, M. D., Ogden, C. L., & Johnson, C. L. (2002). Prevalence and trends in obesity among US adults. *Journal of the American Medical Association, 288,* 1723–1727.

Flegal, K. M., Graubard, B. I., Williamson, D. F., & Gail, M. H. (2005). Excess deaths associated with underweight, overweight, and obesity. *Journal of the American Medical Association, 293,* 1861–1867.

Flegal, K. M., Troiano, R. P., Pamuk, E. R., Kuczmarski, R. J., & Campbell, S. M. (1995). The influence of smoking cessation on the prevalence of overweight in the United States. *New England Journal of Medicine, 333*, 1165–1170.

Fleisher, A., et al. (2012). Florbetapir PET analysis of amyloid-β deposition in the presenilin 1 E280A autosomal dominant Alzheimer's disease kindred. *Lancet Neurology, 11*, 1057–1065.

Fleming, M. F., Mundt, M. P., French, M. T., Manwell, L. B., Stauffacher, E. A., & Barry, K. L. (2000). Benefit-cost analysis of brief physician advice with problem drinkers in primary care settings. *Medical Care, 38*, 7–18.

Fletcher, A. (1994). *Thin for life*. Boston, MA: Houghton Mifflin.

Fletcher, R., & Fairfield, K. (2002). Vitamins for chronic disease prevention in adults: Clinical applications. *Journal of the American Medical Association, 287*, 3127–3129.

Fligor, B., & Cox, L. (2004). Output levels of commercially available portable compact disc players and the potential risk to hearing. *Ear and Hearing, 25*, 513–527.

Foody, J. M., Rathore, S. S., Galusha, D., Masoudi, F. A., Havranek, E. P., Radford, M. J., & Krumholz, H. M. (2006). Hydroxymethylglutaryl-CoA reductase inhibitors in older persons with acute myocardial infarction. *Journal of the American Geriatrics Society, 54*, 421–430.

Foster, G. D., Wyatt, H. R., Hill, J. O., McGuckin, B. G., Brill, C., Mohammed, B. S., . . . Klein, S. (2001). Evaluation of the Atkins diet: A randomized controlled trial. *Obesity Research, 9*(Suppl. 3), 132.

Franco, O. H., Bonneux, L., de Laet, C., Peeters, A., Steyerberg, E. W., & Mackenbach, J. P. (2004). The polymeal: A more natural, safer, and probably tastier (than the polypill) strategy to reduce cardiovascular disease by more than 75%. *British Medical Journal, 329*, 1447–1450.

Franco, O. H., de Laet, C., Peeters, A., Jonker, J., Mackenbach, J., & Nusselder, W. (2005). Effects of physical activity on life expectancy with cardio vascular disease. *Archives of Internal Medicine, 165*, 2355–2360.

Frank, L. D., Andresen, M. A., & Schmid, T. L. (2004). Obesity relationships with community design, physical activity, and time spent in cars. *American Journal of Preventive Medicine, 27*, 87–96.

Fredriksen-Goldsen, K. I., Kim, H. J., & Barkan, S. E. (2012). Disability among lesbian, gay, and bisexual adults. *American Journal of Public Health, 102*, e16–e21.

Free, C., Knight, R., Robertson, S., Whittaker, R., Edwards, P., Zhou, W., . . . Roberts, I. (2011). Smoking cessation support delived via mobile phone text messaging. *Lancet, 378*, 49–55.

Freedman, M. (1999). *Prime time: How baby boomers will revolutionize retirement and transform America*. New York, NY: Public Affairs.

Freedman, M. (2002, March–April). Prime time author answers his older critics on retirement. *Aging Today*, pp. 3, 6.

Freedman, M. (2007). *Encore: Finding work that matters in the second half of life*. New York, NY: Public Affairs.

Freedman, M., & Moen, P. (2005, April 29). Academics pioneer "the Third Age." *Chronicle of Higher Education*.

Freedman, N. D., Park, Y., Abnet, C. C., Hollenbeck, A. R., & Sinha, R. (2012). Association of coffee-drinking with total and cause-specific mortality. *New England Journal of Medicine, 366*, 1891–1904.

Freeman, E. E., Gange, S. J., Muñoz, B., & West, S. K. (2006). Driving status and risk of entry into long-term care in older adults. *American Journal of Public Health, 96*, 1254–1259.

Freitag, M. H., Peila, R., Masaki, K., Petrovitch, H., Ross, G. W., White, L. R., & Launer, L. J. (2006). Midlife pulse pressure and incidence of dementia: The Honolulu–Asia aging study. *Stroke, 37*, 33–37.

Fried, L. P. Carlson, M. C., Freedman, M., Frick, K. D., Glass, T. A., Hill, J., . . . Zeger, S. (2004). A social model for health promotion for an aging population. *Journal of Urban Health, 81,* 64–78.

Friedan, B. (1993). *The fountain of age.* New York, NY: Simon & Schuster.

Friedland, R. P., Fritsch, T., Smyth, K. A., Koss, E., Lerner, A. J., Chen, C. H., . . . Debanne, S. M. (2001). Patients with Alzheimer's disease have reduced activities in midlife compared with healthy control-group members. *Proceedings of the National Academy of Sciences, 98,* 3440–3445.

Friedman, D. (2008). *Jewish visions for aging.* Woodstock, VT: Jewish Lights.

Fries, J. (1989). *Aging well: A guide for successful seniors.* Reading, MA: Addison-Wesley.

Fritsch, T., McClendon, M. J., Smyth, K. A., Lerner, A. J., Chen, C. H., Petot, G. J., . . . Friedland, R. P. (2001). Effects of educational attainment on the clinical expression of Alzheimer's disease: Results from a research registry. *American Journal of Alzheimer's Disease and Other Dementias, 16,* 369–376.

Fuhrman, B., Rosenblat, M., Hayek, T., Coleman, R., & Aviram, M. (2000). Ginger extract consumption reduces plasma cholesterol, inhibits LDL oxidation and attenuates development of atherosclerosis in atherosclerotic, apolipoprotein E-deficient mice. *Journal of Nutrition, 130,* 1124–1131.

Fuller-Thompson, E., Nuru-Jeter, A., Minkler, M., & Guralnik, J. M. (2009). Black-White disparities in disability among older Americans. *Journal of Aging and Health, 21,* 677–698.

Gallagher, D., Heymsfield, S. B., Heo, M., Jebb, S. A., Murgatroyd, P. R., & Sakamoto, Y. (2000). Healthy percentage body fat ranges: An approach for developing guidelines based on body mass index. *American Journal of Clinical Nutrition, 72,* 694–701.

Gallo, J. J., Ryan, S. D., & Ford, D. E. (1999). Attitudes, knowledge, and behavior of family physicians regarding depression in late life. *Archives of Family Medicine, 8,* 249–256.

Gambert, S. (2002). The promise of statins. *Clinical Geriatrics, 10,* 15–16.

Gangwisch, J. E., Heymsfield, S. B., Boden-Albala, B., Buijs, R. M., Kreier, F., Opler, M. G., . . . Malaspina, D. (2008). Sleep duration associated with mortality in elderly. *Sleep, 31,* 1087–1096.

Gangwisch, J. E., Heymsfield, S. B., Boden-Albala, B., Buijs, R. M., Kreier, F., Pickering, T. G., . . . Malaspina, D. (2006). Short sleep duration as a risk factor for hypertension. *Hypertension, 47,* 833–839.

Gangwisch, J. E., Malaspina, D., Boden-Albala, B., & Heymsfield, S. B. (2005). Inadequate sleep as a risk factor for obesity. *Sleep, 10,* 1217–1220.

Ganz, P. A., Farmer, M. M., Belman, M. J., Garcia, C. A., Streja, L., Dietrich, A. J., . . . Kahn, K. L. (2005). Results of a randomized controlled trial to increase colorectal cancer screening in a managed care health plan. *Cancer, 104,* 2072–2083.

Ganzini, L., Goy, E. R., & Dobscha, S. K. (2009). Oregonians' reasons for requesting physician aid in dying. *Archives of Internal Medicine, 169,* 489–492.

Ganzini, L., Harvath, T. A., Jackson, A., Goy, E. R., Miller, L. L., & Delorit, M. A. (2002). Experiences of Oregon nurses and social workers with hospice patients who requested assistance with suicide. *New England Journal of Medicine, 347,* 582–588.

Gardner, C. D., Kiazand, A., Alhassan, S., Kim, S., Stafford, R. S., Balise, R. R., . . . King, A. C. (2007). Comparison of the Atkins, Zone, Ornish, and LEARN diets. *Journal of the American Medical Association, 297,* 969–977.

Gardner, C. D., Lawson, L. D., Block, E., Chatterjee, L. M., Kiazand, A., Balise, R. R., & Kraemer, H. C. (2007). Effect of raw garlic vs. commercial garlic supplements on plasma lipid concentrations in adults with moderate hypercholesterolemia. *Archives of Internal Medicine, 167,* 346–353.

Garibotto, V., Borroni, B., Kalbe, E., Herholz, K., Salmon, E., Holtoff, V., . . . Perani, D. (2008). Education and occupation as proxies for reserve in aMCI converters and AD: FDG-PET evidence. *Neurology, 71,* 1342–1349.

Garlic: Case unclosed. (2000, October). *Nutrition Action Healthletter,* pp. 8–9.

Gauvin, L., Richard, L., Kestens, Y., Shatenstein, B., Daniel, M., Moore, S. D., . . . Payette, H. (2012). Living in a well-serviced urban area is associated with maintenance of frequent walking among seniors in the VoisiNuAge Study. *Journal of Gerontology: Psychological Sciences and Social Sciences, 67,* 76–88.

Gaziano, J., et al. (2012). Multivitamins in the prevention of cancer in men. *Journal of the American Medical Association, 308,* 1871–1880.

Gearon, C. (2000). Going online . . . for health. *AARP Bulletin, 41,* 4, 14–15.

Gehlbach, S. H., Fournier, M., & Bigelow, C. (2002). Recognition of osteoporosis by primary care physicians. *American Journal of Public Health, 92,* 271–273.

Gellert, C., Schöttker, B., & Brenner, H. (2012). Smoking and all-cause mortality in older people. *Archives of Internal Medicine, 172,* 837–844.

Gelo, F. (2008, Summer). Invisible individuals. *Aging Well,* pp. 36–40.

George, L. (1986, Spring). Life satisfaction in later life. *Generations,* pp. 5–8.

Geruso, M. (2012). Black–white disparities in life expectancy. *Demography, 49,* 553–574.

Getting a boost from insurers. (1999, June). *American Medical News,* pp. 13–14.

Gielen, S., Schuler, G., & Hambrecht, R. (2001). Benefits of exercise training for patients with chronic heart failure. *Clinical Geriatrics, 9,* 32–45.

Giles, L., Glonek, G. F., Luszcz, M. A., & Andrews, G. R. (2005). Effect of social networks on 10 year survival in very old Australians. *Journal of Epidemiology and Community Health, 59,* 574–579.

Gill, T. M., Robison, J. T., Williams, C. S., & Tinetti, M. E. (1999). Mismatches between the home environment and physical capacity among community-living older persons. *Journal of the American Geriatrics Society, 47,* 88–92.

Glass, J., Lanctôt, K. L., Herrmann, N., Sproule, B. A., & Busto, U. E. (2005). Sedative hypnotics in older people with insomnia. *British Medical Journal, 331,* 1169–1173.

Glass, T., de Leon, C. M., Marottoli, R. A., & Berkman, L. F. (1999). Population based study of social and productive activities as predictors of survival among elderly Americans. *British Medical Journal, 319,* 478–483.

Glazer, S. D., Redmon, E. L., & Robinson, K. L. (2005). Continuing the connection: Emeriti/retiree centers on campus. *Educational Gerontology, 31,* 363–383.

Goldstein, M. G., Pinto, B. M., Marcus, B. H., Lynn, H., Jette, A. M., Rakowski, W., . . . Tennstedt, S. (1999). Physician-based physical activity counseling for middle-aged and older adults: A randomized trial. *Annals of Behavioral Medicine, 21,* 40–47.

Goodwin, J. S., Hunt, W. C., Key, C. R., & Samet, J. M. (1987). The effect of marital status on stage, treatment, and survival of cancer patients. *Journal of the American Medical Association, 258,* 3125–3130.

Goodwin, P. J., Leszcz, M., Ennis, M., Koopmans, J., Vincent, L., Guther, H., . . . Hunter, J. (2001). The effect of group psychosocial support on survival in metastatic breast cancer. *New England Journal of Medicine, 345,* 1719–1726.

Gotzsche, P., & Nielsen, M. (2009, October 7). Screening for breast cancer with mammography. *Cochrane Database Systematic Reviews, 4,* CD001877.

Gotzsche, P., & Olsen, O. (2000). Is screening for breast cancer with mammography justified? *Lancet, 355,* 129–134.

Gould, K. L., Ornish, D., Scherwitz, L., Brown, S., Edens, R. P., Hess, M. J., . . . Billings, J. (1995). Changes in myocardial perfusion abnormalities by positron emission tomography after long-term, intense risk factor modification. *Journal of the American Medical Association, 274,* 894–901.

Gould, R. L. Coulson, M. C., & Howard, R. J. (2012). Efficacy of cognitive behavioral therapy for anxiety disorders in older people. *Journal of the American Geriatrics Society, 60*, 218–229.

Gourlay, M. L., Fine, J. P., Preisser, J. S., May, R. C., Li, C., Lui, L. Y., . . . Study of Osteoporotic Fractures Research Group. (2012). Bone-density testing interval and transition to osteoporosis in older women. *New England Journal of Medicine, 366*, 225–233.

Gozalo, P., Teno, J. M., Mitchell, S. L., Skinner, J., Bynum, J., Tyler, D., & Mor, V. (2011). End-of-life transitions among nursing home residents with cognitive issues. *New England Journal of Medicine, 365*, 1212–1221.

Grabowski, D. C., Campbell, C. M., & Morrisey, M. A. (2004). Elderly licensure laws and motor vehicle fatalities. *Journal of the American Medical Association, 23*, 2840–2846.

Grandjean, A. C., Reimers, K. J., Bannick, K. E., & Haven, M. C. (2000). The effect of caffeinated, non-caffeinated, caloric and non-caloric beverages on hydration. *Journal of the American College of Nutrition, 19*, 591–600.

Grasso, P., & Haber, D. (1995). A leadership training program at a senior center. *Activities, Adaptation and Aging, 20*, 13–24.

Gravlee, C., & Mulligan, C. (2012). Education and genetic ancestry and blood pressure in African-Americans. *American Journal of Public Health, 102*, 1559–1565.

Green, L. (2005). Prospects and possible pitfalls of a preventive polypill: Confessions of a health promotion convert. *European Journal of Clinical Nutrition, 59*(Suppl.), S4–S8.

Green, L., & Kreuter, M. (1999). *Health promotion planning: An educational and ecological approach* (3rd ed.). Mountain View, CA: Mayfield.

Greenwood, R. (2002a). The PACE program: Rooted in community-based organizations. *Innovations, 3*, 29–34.

Greenwood, R. (2002b). The PACE model. *Center for Medicare Education, 2*, 1–8.

Greiner, K. A., Murray, J. L., & Kallail, K. J. (2000). Medical student interest in alternative medicine. *Journal of Alternative and Complementary Medicine, 6*, 231–234.

Gross, J. (2008, March 6). New generation gap emerges as older addicts seek help. *The New York Times*, pp. A1, A20.

Grossman, A., D'Augelli, A., & O'Connell, T. (2001). Being lesbian, gay, bisexual, and 60 or older in North America. *Journal of Gay and Lesbian Social Services, 13*, 23–40.

Grover, S. A., Lowensteyn, I., Joseph, L., Kaouache, M., Marchand, S., Coupal, L., . . . Cardiovascular Health Evaluation to Improve Compliance and Knowledge Among Uninformed Patients (CHECK-UP) Study Group. (2007). Patient knowledge of coronary risk profile improves the effectiveness of dyslipidemia therapy. *Archives of Internal Medicine, 167*, 2296.

Gueyffier, F., Bulpitt, C., Boissel, J. P., Schron, E., Ekbom, T., Fagard, R., . . . Coope, J. (1999). Antihypertensive drugs in very old people: A subgroup meta-analysis of randomized controlled trials. *Lancet, 353*, 793–796.

Gurwitz, J. H., Field, T. S., Harrold, L. R., Rothschild, J., Debellis, K., Seger, A. C., . . . Bates, D. W. (2003). Incidence and preventability of adverse drug events among older persons in the ambulatory setting. *Journal of the American Medical Association, 289*, 1107–1116.

Haber, D. (1979, November/December). Old age in China. *Aging*, pp. 7–9.

Haber, D. (1983a). Yoga as a preventive health care program. *International Journal of Aging and Human Development, 17*, 169–176.

Haber, D. (1983b). Promoting mutual help groups among older persons. *Gerontologist, 23*, 251–253.

Haber, D. (1984). Church-based programs for caregivers of non-institutionalized elders. *Journal of Gerontological Social Work, 7*, 43–55.

Haber, D. (1986). Health promotion to reduce blood pressure level among older Blacks. *Gerontologist, 26*, 119–121.

Haber, D. (1988a). A health promotion program in ten nursing homes. *Activities, Adaptation and Aging, 2,* 73–82.

Haber, D. (1988b). The interfaith volunteer caregivers program. *Journal of Religion & Aging, 3,* 151–156.

Haber, D. (1989). *Health care for an aging society: Cost conscious community care and self-care approaches.* New York, NY: Hemisphere/Taylor and Francis Group.

Haber, D. (1992). Self-help groups and aging. In A. Katz, et al. (Eds.), *Self-help: Concepts and applications* (pp. 295–298). Philadelphia, PA: Charles Press.

Haber, D. (1996). Strategies to promote the health of older persons: An alternative to readiness stages. *Family and Community Health, 19,* 1–10.

Haber, D. (1999). Minority access to hospice. *American Journal of Hospice and Palliative Care, 16,* 386–390.

Haber, D. (2001a). Medicare prevention: Movement toward research-based policy. *Journal of Aging and Social Policy, 13,* 1–14.

Haber, D. (2001b). Promoting readiness to change behavior through health assessments. *Clinical Gerontologist, 23,* 152–158.

Haber, D. (2002a). Health promotion and aging: Educational and clinical initiatives by the federal government. *Educational Gerontology, 28,* 1–11.

Haber, D. (2002b). Wellness General of the United States: A creative approach to promote family and community health. *Family and Community Health, 25,* 71–82.

Haber, D. (2004). Health and aging. In *AGHE brief bibliography: A selected annotated bibliography for gerontology instruction* (CD-ROM). Washington, DC: Association for Gerontology in Higher Education.

Haber, D. (2005a). Cultural diversity among older adults: Address health education. *Educational Gerontology, 31,* 683–697.

Haber, D. (2005b). Medicare prevention update. *Journal of Aging & Social Policy, 17,* 1–6.

Haber, D. (2006). Life review: Implementation, theory, and future direction. *International Journal of Aging & Human Development, 63,* 153–171.

Haber, D. (2007). Health contract in the classroom. *Gerontology & Geriatrics Education, 27,* 41–54.

Haber, D. (2008a). Guided life reviews by students with older adults in an assisted living facility. *Journal of Aging, Humanities, and the Arts, 2,* 113–125.

Haber, D. (2008b). Using today's headlines for teaching gerontology. *Educational Gerontology, 34,* 477–488.

Haber, D. (2009). Gay aging. *Gerontology & Geriatrics Education, 30,* 267–280.

Haber, D. (2011). Jewish aging: Model programs in social service, adult learning, intergenerational exchange, and research. *Journal of Religion, Spirituality & Aging, 23,* 304–317.

Haber, D., & George, J. (1981–1982). A preventive health care program with Hispanic elders. *Journal of Minority Aging, 6,* 1–11.

Haber, D., Hinman, M., Utsey, C., Babola, K., & Looney, C. (1997). Impact of a geriatric health promotion elective on occupational and physical therapy students. *Gerontology & Geriatrics Education, 18,* 65–76.

Haber, D., & Lacy, M. (1993). A socio-behavioral health promotion intervention with older adults. *Behavior, Health, and Aging, 3,* 73–85.

Haber, D., & Looney, C. (2000). Health contract calendars: A tool for health professionals with older adults. *Gerontologist, 40,* 235–239.

Haber, D., & Looney, C. (2003). Health promotion directory: Development, distribution, and utilization. *Health Promotion Practice, 4,* 72–77.

Haber, D., Looney, C., Babola, K., Hinman, M., & Utsey, C. J. (2000). Impact of a health promotion course on inactive, overweight, or physically limited older adults. *Family and Community Health, 22,* 48–56.

Haber, D., & Rhodes, D. (2004). Health contract with sedentary older adults. *Gerontologist,* *44,* 827–835.

Haber, D., & Wicht, J. (1987). Worksite wellness and aging. *Journal of Individual, Family, and Community Wellness, 4,* 31–34.

Hackney, M., & Earhart, G. (2009). Effects of dance on movement control in Parkinson's disease: A comparison of Argentine tango and American ballroom. *Journal of Rehabilitative Medicine, 41,* 475–481.

Hafner, K. (2012, August 12). In ill doctor, a surprise reflection of who picks assisted suicide. *The New York Times,* pp. 1, 4.

Haggstrom, D. A., Klabunde, C. N., Smith, J. L., & Yuan, G. (2012, June 1). Variations in primary care physicians' colorectal cancer screening recommendations by patient age and comorbidity. *Journal of General Internal Medicine* (online). doi:10.1007/s11606-012-2083-6

Haight, B. K., Michel, Y., & Hendrix, S. (1998). Life review: Preventing despair in newly relocated nursing home residents: Short- and long-term effects. *International Journal of Aging and Human Development, 47,* 119–142.

Hall, K., & Luepker, R. (2000). Is hypercholesterolemia a risk factor and should it be treated in the elderly? *American Journal of Health Promotion, 14,* 347–356. ·

Halm, E. A., Tuhrim, S., Wang, J. J., Rojas, M., Rockman, C., Riles, T. S., & Chassin, M. R. (2009). Racial and ethnic disparities in outcomes and appropriateness of carotid endarterectomy. *Stroke, 40,* 2493–2501.

Haney, D. (1999, November 25). The latest thing in fine dining: Food that is also medicine. *(Galveston, TX) Daily News,* p. A22.

Haney, E. M., Chan, B. K., Diem, S. J., Ensrud, K. E., Cauley, J. A., Barrett-Connor, E., . . . for the Osteoporotic Fractures in Men Study Group. (2007). Association of low bone density with SSRI use by older men. *Archives of Internal Medicine, 167,* 1246–1251.

Hanoch, Y., Rice, T., Cummings, J., & Wood, S. (2009). How much choice is too much? The case of the Medicare prescription drug benefit. *Health Services Research, 44,* 1157–1168.

Hansen, J. (2008). Community and in-home models. *Journal of Social Work Education, 44,* 83–87.

Hara, A. K., Leighton, J. A., Sharma, V. K., & Fleischer, D. E. (2004). Small bowel: Preliminary comparison of capsule endoscopy with barium study and CT. *Radiology, 230,* 260–265.

Hardy, D., Liu, C. C., Xia, R., Cormier, J. N., Chan, W., White, A., . . . Du, X. L. (2009). Racial disparities and treatment trends in a large cohort of elderly Black and White patients with nonsmall cell lung cancer. *Cancer, 115,* 2199–2211.

Harrington, C., Woolhandler, S., Mullan, J., Carrillo, H., & Himmelstein, D. U. (2001). Does investor ownership of nursing homes compromise the quality of care? *American Journal of Public Health, 91,* 1452–1455.

Harris, M. (2007). *Grave matters.* New York, NY: Scribner.

Harris, W. S. Gowda, M., Kolb, J. W., Strychacz, C. P., Vacek, J. L., Jones, P. G., . . . McCallister, B. D. (1999). A randomized, controlled trial on the effects of remote, intercessory prayer on outcomes in patients admitted to the coronary care unit. *Archives of Internal Medicine, 159,* 2273–2278.

Harvath, T. (2008). What if Maslow was wrong? *American Journal of Nursing, 108,* 11.

Harwood, J. (2007). *Understanding communication and aging.* Los Angeles, CA: Sage.

Haug, C. (2009). The risks and benefits of HPV vaccination. *Journal of the American Medical Association, 302,* 795–796.

Hawkley, L. C., Masi, C. M., Berry, J. D., & Cacioppo, J. T. (2006). Loneliness is a unique predictor of age-related differences in systolic blood pressure. *Psychology of Aging, 21,* 152–164.

Hayward, A. C., Harling, R., Wetten, S., Johnson, A. M., Munro, S., Smedley, J., . . . Watson, J. M. (2006). Effectiveness of an influenza vaccine programme for care home staff to prevent death, morbidity, and health service use among residents. *British Medical Journal, 333,* 1241.

Hazzard, W. (2005). The conflict between biogerontology and antiaging medicine. *Journal of the American Geriatrics Society, 53,* 1434–1435.

Head, D., Singh, T., & Bugg, J. M. (2012). The moderating role of exercise on stess-related effects on the hippocampus and memory in later adulthood. *Neuropsychology, 26,* 133–143.

Health promotion interchange. (1997, Fall). *Texas Department of Health Newsletter, 2,* 3.

Health Resources and Services Administration. (2002). *Women's health USA 2002.* Washington, DC: Health Resources and Services Administration, USDHHS.

Heart Outcomes Prevention Evaluation Study Investigators. (2000). Vitamin E supplementation and cardiovascular events in high-risk patients. *New England Journal of Medicine, 342,* 154–160.

Heart Protection Study Collaborative Group. (2002). MRC/BHF Heart Protection Study of cholesterol lowering simvastatin in 20,536 high-risk individuals: A randomized placebo-controlled trial. *Lancet, 360,* 7–22.

Hebert, P. L., Sisk, J. E., Wang, J. J., Tuzzio, L., Casabianca, J. M., Chassin, M. R., . . . McLaughlin, M. A. (2008). Cost-effectiveness of nurse-led disease management for heart failure in an ethnically diverse urban community. *Annals of Internal Medicine, 149,* 540–548.

Hedberg, K., Hopkins, D., & Southwick, K. (2002). Legalized physician-assisted suicide in Oregon. *New England Journal of Medicine, 346,* 450–452.

Heffernan, V. (2011, June 1). A prescription for fear. *The New York Times Magazine,* pp. 14, 16.

Heinonen, O. P., Albanes, D., Virtamo, J., Taylor, P. R., Huttunen, J. K., Hartman, A. M., . . . Edwards, B. K. (1998). Prostate cancer and supplementation with alpha-tocopherol and beta-carotene: Incidence and mortality in a controlled trial. *Journal of the National Cancer Institute, 90,* 440–446.

Henschke, C. I., International Early Lung Cancer Action Program Investigators, Yip, R., & Miettinen, O. S. (2006). Women's susceptibility to tobacco carcinogens and survival after diagnosis of lung cancer. *Journal of the American Medical Association, 296,* 180–184.

Herbert, R., & Gabriel, M. (2002). Effects of stretching before and after exercising on muscle soreness and risk of injury: Systematic review. *British Medical Journal, 325,* 468–470.

Hernandez, M. T., Rubio, T. M., Ruiz, F. O., Riera, H. S., Gil, R. S., & Gómez, J. C. (2000). Results of a home-based training program for patients with COPD. *Chest, 118,* 106–114.

Hernandez-Reif, M. (2001). Evidence-based medicine and massage. *Pediatrics, 108,* 1053.

Hernandez-Reif, M., Field, T., Krasnegor, J., & Theakston, H. (2001). Lower back pain is reduced and range of motion increased after massage therapy. *Neuroscience, 106,* 131–145.

Heroux, M., et al. (2009, April 20). Dietary patterns and the risk of mortality. *International Journal of Epidemiology* (e-publication).

Hertzman-Miller, R. P., Morgenstern, H., Hurwitz, E. L., Yu, F., Adams, A. H., Harber, P., & Kominski, G. F. (2002). Comparing the satisfaction of low back pain patients randomized to receive medical or chiropractic care. *American Journal of Public Health, 92,* 1628–1633.

Heschel, J. (1951). *The sabbath.* New York, NY: Farrar, Straus, and Giroux.

Heshka, S., Anderson, J. W., Atkinson, R. L., Greenway, F. L., Hill, J. O., Phinney, S. D., . . . Pi-Sunyer, F. X. (2003). Weight loss with self-help compared with a structured commercial program: A randomized trial. *Journal of the American Medical Association, 289,* 1792–1798.

Hess, T. M., Hinson, J. T., & Hodges, E. A. (2009). Moderators of and mechanisms underlying stereotype threat effects on older adults' memory performance. *Experimental Aging Research, 35,* 153–177.

High, K. (2001). Nutritional strategies to boost immunity and prevention infection in elderly individuals. *Clinical Infectious Disease, 33,* 1892–1900.

Hill, S., Blakely, T., Kawachi, I., & Woodward, A. (2004). Mortality among "never smokers" living with smokers. *British Medical Journal, 328,* 988–989.

Himes, J. (2001). Prevalence of individuals with skin-folds too large to measure. *American Journal of Public Health, 91,* 154–155.

Hinely, P. (2009, June 11). Wii-hab may enhance Parkinson's treatment. *Medical College of Georgia News,* pp. 1–2.

Hinman, M. R., Ford, J., & Heyl, H. (2002). Effects of static magnets on chronic knee pain and physical function: A double-blind study. *Alternative Therapies, 8,* 50–55.

Hires, B., Ham, S., & Forsythe, H. (2005). Comparison of websites offering nutrition services managed by registered dietitians and sites managed by non-dietitian nutrition consultants. *Journal of the American Dietetic Association, 105,* A-37.

Hodis, H. N., Mack, W. J., LaBree, L., Mahrer, P. R., Sevanian, A., Liu, C. R., . . . VEAPS Research Group. (2002). Alpha-tocopherol supplementation in healthy individuals reduces low-density lipoprotein oxidation but not atherosclerosis: The Vitamin E Atherosclerosis Prevention Study. *Circulation, 106,* 1453–1459.

Hohl, C. M., Dankoff, J., Colacone, A., & Afilalo, M. (2001). Polypharmacy, adverse drug-related events, and potential adverse drug interactions in elderly patients presenting to an emergency department. *Annals of Emergency Medicine, 38,* 666–671.

Hollenberg, N. (2006). The influence of dietary sodium on blood pressure. *Journal of the American College of Nutrition, 25,* 240S–246S.

Hollis, J. F., Gullion, C. M., Stevens, V. J., Brantley, P. J., Appel, L. J., Ard, J. D., . . . Weight Loss Maintenance Trial Research Group. (2008). Weight loss during the intensive intervention phase of the weight-loss maintenance trial. *American Journal of Preventive Medicine, 35,* 118–126.

Holmes, M. D., Chen, W. Y., Feskanich, D., Kroenke, C. H., & Colditz, G. A. (2005). Physical activity and survival after breast cancer diagnosis. *Journal of the American Medical Association, 293,* 2479–2486.

Holmes, T., & Rahe, R. (1967). The Social Readjustment Rating scale. *Journal of Psychosomatic Research, 11,* 213–218.

Holt-Lunstad, J., Smith, T. B., & Layton, J. B. (2010). Social relationships and mortality risk: A meta-analytic review. *PLoS Med, 7*(7), e1000316. doi:10.1371/journal/pmed.1000316.

Hooker, E. (1957). The adjustment of the male overt homosexual. *Journal of Projective Techniques, 21,* 18–31.

Hooyman, N., & Kiyak, H. (2011). *Social gerontology* (9th ed.). Boston, MA: Allyn & Bacon.

HOPE Trial. (2005). Effects of long-term vitamin E supplementation on cardiovascular events and cancer: A randomized controlled trial. *Journal of the American Medical Association, 293,* 1338–1347.

Horrocks, S., Anderson, E., & Salisbury, C. (2002). Systematic review of whether nurse practitioners working in primary care can provide equivalent care to doctors. *British Medical Journal, 324,* 819–823.

Horwath, C. (1991). Nutrition goals for older adults: A review. *Gerontologist, 31,* 811–821.

House, J. S., Landis, K. R., & Umberson, D. (1988). Social relationships and health. *Science, 241,* 540–545.

Howard, B. V., Manson, J. E., Stefanick, M. L., Beresford, S. A., Frank, G., Jones, B., . . . Prentice, R. (2006). Low-fat dietary pattern and weight change over 7 years: The Women's Health Initiative. *Journal of the American Medical Association, 295,* 39–49.

Howard, R. J., Juszczak, E., Ballard, C. G., Bentham, P., Brown, R. G., Bullock, R., . . . CALM-AD Trial Group. (2007). Donepezil for the treatment of agitation in Alzheimer's disease. *New England Journal of Medicine, 357,* 1382–1392.

Howley, E., & Franks, B. (1997). *Health fitness instructor's handbook* (3rd ed.). Champaign, IL: Human Kinetics.

How McNuggets changed the world. (2001, January 22). *U.S. News & World Report,* p. 54.

Hrobjartsson, A., & Gotzsche, P. (2001). Is the placebo powerless? An analysis of clinical trials comparing placebo with no treatment. *New England Journal of Medicine, 344,* 1594–1602.

Hsu, Y., & Wang, J. (2009). Physical, affective, and behavioral effects of group reminiscence on depressed institutionalized elders in Taiwan. *Nursing Research, 58,* 294–299.

Hu, F. B., Sigal, R. J., Rich-Edwards, J. W., Colditz, G. A., Solomon, C. G., Willett, W. C., . . . Manson, J. E. (1999). Walking compared with vigorous physical activity and risk of type 2 diabetes in women. *Journal of the American Medical Association, 282,* 1433–1439.

Hu, F. B., Stampfer, M. J., Solomon, C., Liu, S., Colditz, G. A., Speizer, F. E., . . . Manson, J. E. (2001). Physical activity and risk for cardiovascular events in diabetic women. *Annals of Internal Medicine, 134,* 96–105.

Hu, F. B., Willett, W. C., Li, T., Stampfer, M. J., Colditz, G. A., & Manson, J. E. (2004). Adiposity as compared with physical activity in predicting mortality among women. *New England Journal of Medicine, 26,* 2694–2703.

Hu, G., Sarti, C., Jousilahti, P., Silventoinen, K., Barengo, N. C., & Tuomilehto, J. (2005). Leisure time, occupational, and commuting physical activity and the risk of stroke. *Stroke, 36,* 1994–1999.

Huang, A. J., Subak, L. L., Thom, D. H., Van Den Eeden, S. K., Ragins, A. I., Kuppermann, M., . . . Brown, J. S. (2009). Sexual function and aging in racially and ethnically diverse women. *Journal of the American Geriatrics Society, 57,* 1362–1368.

Huffman, M. (2007). Health coaching. *Home Healthcare Nurse, 25,* 271–274.

Humphrey, L. L., Helfand, M., Chan, B. K., & Woolf, S. H. (2002). Breast cancer screening: A summary of the evidence for the U.S. preventive services task force. *Annals of Internal Medicine, 137*(5 Pt. 1), 347–360.

Hurwitz, E. L., Morgenstern, H., Harber, P., Kominski, G. F., Belin, T. R., Yu, F., . . . University of California-Los Angeles. (2002). A randomized trial of medical care with and without physical therapy and chiropractic care. *Spine, 27,* 193–204.

Husaini, B. A., Reece, M. C., Emerson, J. S., Scales, S., Hull, P. C., & Levine, R. S. (2008). A church-based program on prostate cancer screening for African American men. *Ethnic Disability, 18*(Suppl. 2), 179–184.

Hyman, D., & Pavlik, V. (2001). Characteristics of patients with uncontrolled hypertension in the United States. *New England Journal of Medicine, 345,* 479–486.

Hypericum Depression Trial Study Group. (2002). Effect of *Hypericum perforatum* (St. John's wort) in major depressive disorder: A randomized controlled trial. *Journal of the American Medical Association, 287,* 1807–1814.

Idler, E., & Kasl, S. (1992). Religion, disability, depression, and the timing of death. *American Journal of Sociology, 97,* 1052–1079.

Idler, E. L., McLaughlin, J., & Kasl, S. (2009). Religion and the quality of life in the last year of life. *Journal of Gerontology: Psychological Sciences, 64,* 528–537.

Ionica, N., Sourwine, M., Steinle, N. I., & Rochester, C. D. (2012). Vitamin B_{12}: Considerations for maintaining optimum health for elders. *Clinicial Geriatrics, 20,* 22–27.

Irwin, M. R., Olmstead, R., & Motivala, S. J. (2008). Improving sleep quality in older adults with moderate sleep complaints: A randomized, controlled trial of Tai Chi. *Sleep, 31,* 1001–1008.

Irwin, M. R., Olmstead, R., & Oxman, M. N. (2007). Augmenting immune responses to varicella zoster virus in older adults: A randomized, controlled trial of Tai Chi. *Journal of the American Geriatrics Society, 55,* 511–517. p. 435

Isaac, V., Stewart, R., Artero, S., Ancelin, M. L., & Ritchie, K. (2009). Social activity and improvement in depressive symptoms in older people: A prospective community cohort study. *American Journal of Geriatric Psychiatry, 17,* 688–696.

Isaacowitz, D. M., Wadlinger, H. A., Goren, D., Wilson, H. R. (2006). Selective preference in visual fixation away from negatives in old age. *Psychology and Aging, 21,* 40–48.

Is "change in the wind" for entertainment industry's ageism? (2009, January–February). *Aging Today,* pp. 11, 15.

Israel, B. (1985). Social networks and social support: Implications for natural helper and community level interventions. *Health Education Quarterly, 12,* 65–80.

Is this the right way to test supplements? (2000, September). *UC Berkeley Wellness Letter, 16,* 1–2.

Jackevicius, C. A., Mamdani, M., & Tu, J. V. (2002). Adherence with statin therapy in elderly patients with and without acute coronary syndromes. *Journal of the American Medical Association, 288,* 462–467.

Jackson, N. C., Johnson, M. J., & Roberts, R. (2008). The potential impact of discrimination fears of older gays, lesbians, bisexuals and transgender individuals living in small- to moderate-sized cities on long-term health care. *Journal of Homosexuality, 54,* 325–339.

Jackson, R. D., LaCroix, A. Z., Gass, M., Wallace, R. B., Robbins, J., Lewis, C. E., . . . Women's Health Initiative Investigators. (2006). Calcium and vitamin D supplementation and the risk of fractures. *New England Journal of Medicine, 354,* 669–683.

Jacob. J. (2002, March). Wellness programs help companies save on health costs. *American Medical News,* pp. 32–33.

Jacobs, E. J., Rodriguez, C., Brady, K. A., Connell, C. J., Thun, M. J., & Calle, E. E. (2006). Cholesterol-lowering drugs and colorectal cancer incidence in a large United States cohort. *Journal of the National Cancer Institute, 98,* 69–72.

Jacobson, M., & Brownell, K. (2000). Small taxes on soft drinks and snack foods to promote health. *American Journal of Public Health, 90,* 854–857.

Jakes, R. W. Khaw, K., Day, N. E., Bingham, S., Welch, A., Oakes, S., . . . Wareham, N. J. (2001). Patterns of physical activity and ultrasound attenuation by heel bone among Norfolk cohort of European Prospective Investigation of Cancer. *British Medical Journal, 322,* 140–143.

Jampol, L. M., et al. (2001). Antioxidants, zinc and age-related macular degeneration: Results and recommendations. *Archives of Ophthalmology, 119,* 1533–1534.

Janson, C., Chinn, S., Jarvis, D., Zock, J. P., Torén, K., Burney, P., & European Community Respiratory Health Survey. (2001). Effect of passive smoking on respiratory symptoms, bronchial responsiveness, lung function, and total serum IgE in the European Community Respiratory Health Survey: A cross-sectional study. *Lancet, 358,* 2103–2109.

Janz, N. K., Mujahid, M. S., Hawley, S. T., Griggs, J. J., Alderman, A., Hamilton, A. S., . . . Katz, S. J. (2009, September 16). Racial/ethnic differences in quality of life after diagnosis of breast cancer. *Journal of Cancer Survivors* (e-publication).

Jefferson, T., Rivetti, D., Rivetti, A., Rudin, M., Di Pietrantonj, C., & Demicheli, V. (2005). Efficacy and effectiveness of influenza vaccines in elderly people: A systematic review. *Lancet, 366,* 1165–1174.

Jensen, M. K., Koh-Banerjee, P., Franz, M., Sampson, L., Grønbaek, M., & Rimm, E. B. (2006). Whole grains, bran, and germ in relation to homocysteine and markers of glycemic control, lipids, and inflammation. *American Journal of Clinical Nutrition, 83,* 275–283.

Jerant, A. F., von Friederichs-Fitzwater, M. M., & Moore, M. (2005). Patients' perceived barriers to active self-management of chronic conditions. *Patient Education and Counseling, 57,* 300–307.

Jeste, D., & Harris, J. (2010). Wisdom—A neuroscience perspective. *Journal of the American Medical Association, 304,* 1602–1603.

Jette, A. M., Lachman, M., Giorgetti, M. M., Assmann, S. F., Harris, B. A., Levenson, C., . . . Krebs, D. (1999). Exercise—It's never too late: The Strong for Life program. *American Journal of Public Health, 89,* 66–72.

Jiang, B., Kronenberg, F., Nuntanakorn, P., Qiu, M. H., & Kennelly, E. J. (2006). Evaluation of the botanical authenticity and phytochemical profile of black cohosh. *Journal of Agricultural Food Chemistry, 54,* 3242–3253.

Jiang, W., Babyak, M., Krantz, D. S., Waugh, R. A., Coleman, R. E., Hanson, M. M., . . . Blumenthal, J. A. (1996). Mental stress-induced myocardial ischemia and cardiac events. *Journal of the American Medical Association, 275,* 1651–1656.

Jick, H., Zornberg, G. L., Jick, S. S., Seshadri, S., & Drachman, D. A. (2000). Statins and the risk of dementia. *Lancet, 356,* 1627–1631.

Johnson-Kozlow, M., Roussos, S., Rovniak, L., & Hovell, M. (2009). Colorectal cancer test use among Californians of Mexican origin: Influence of language barriers. *Ethnicity and Disease, 19,* 315–322.

Jolicoeur, D., Ewy, B. M., Ockene, J. K., Pbert, L., & Abrams, D. B. (2009). Addressing tobacco use and dependence. In S. A. Shumaker, J. K. Ockene, & K. A. Riekert (Eds.), *The handbook of health behavior change* (pp. 59–84). New York, NY: Springer.

Jonas, S. (2000). *Talking about health and wellness with patients.* New York, NY: Springer.

Joseph, C. N., Porta, C., Casucci, G., Casiraghi, N., Maffeis, M., Rossi, M., & Bernardi, L. (2005). Slow breathing improves arterial baroflex sensitivity and decreases blood pressure in essential hypertension. *Hypertension, 46,* 714–718.

Kalia, N. K., Miller, L. G., Nasir, K., Blumenthal, R. S., Agrawal, N., & Budoff, M. J. (2006). Visualizing coronary calcium is associated with improvements in adherence to statin therapy. *Atherosclerosis, 185,* 394–399.

Kaline, K., Bornstein, S. R., Bergmann, A., Hauner, H., & Schwarz, P. E. (2007). The importance and effect of dietary fibers in diabetes prevention with particular consideration of whole grain products. *Hormonal Metabolic Research, 39,* 687–693.

Kane, R. (2001). Long-term care and a good quality of life: Bringing them closer to together. *Gerontologist, 41,* 293–304.

Kane, R. A., Lum, T. Y., Cutler, L. J., Degenholtz, H. B., & Yu, T. C. (2007). Resident outcomes in small-house nursing homes: A longitudinal evaluation of the initial Green House program. *Journal of the American Geriatrics Society, 55,* 832–839.

Kane, R. L., Homyak, P., Bershadsky, B., & Flood, S. (2006). Variations on a theme called PACE. *Journal of Gerontology: Medical Sciences, 61A,* 689–693.

Kanji, N., White, A. R., & Ernst, E. (2004). Autogenic training reduces anxiety after coronary angioplasty. *American Heart Journal, 147,* E10.

Kannus, P., Parkkari, J., Niemi, S., Pasanen, M., Palvanen, M., Järvinen, M., & Vuori, I. (2000). Prevention of hip fracture in elderly people with use of a hip protector. *New England Journal of Medicine, 343,* 1506–1513.

Kant, A. (2000). Consumption of energy-dense, nutrient-poor foods by adult Americans: Nutritional and health implications. The third National Health and Nutrition Examination Survey, 1988–1994. *American Journal of Clinical Nutrition, 72,* 929–936.

Karidis, A. (2007). Building a new way to age. *Innovations, 3,* 8–11.

Katzmarzyk, P. T., Church, T. S., Craig, C. L., & Bouchard, C. (2009). Sitting time and mortality from all-causes, cardiovascular disease and cancer. *Medicine & Science in Sports & Exercise, 41,* 998–1005.

Kawachi, I., Colditz, G. A., Speizer, F. E., Manson, J. E., Stampfer, M. J., Willett, W. C., & Hennekens, C. H. (1997). A prospective study of passive smoking and coronary heart disease. *Circulation, 95,* 2374–2379.

Kazel, R. (2004, June 28). Dieting for dollars. *American Medical News,* pp. 17–18.

Keenan, P. (2009). Smoking and weight change after new health diagnoses in older adults. *Archives of Internal Medicine, 163,* 237–242.

Keitel, W. A., Atmar, R. L., Cate, T. R., Petersen, N. J., Greenberg, S. B., Ruben, F., & Couch, R. B. (2006). Safety of high doses of influenza vaccine and effect on antibody responses in elderly persons. *Archives of Internal Medicine, 166,* 1121–1127.

Keller, M. B., McCullough, J. P., Klein, D. N., Arnow, B., Dunner, D. L., Gelenberg, A. J., . . . Zajecka, J. (2000). A comparison of nefazodone, the cognitive behavioral-analysis system of psychotherapy, and their combination for the treatment of chronic depression. *New England Journal of Medicine, 342,* 1462–1470.

Kelley, G. (2001, October 22). *Low-impact exercise can increase bone mass in women.* Paper presented at Massachusetts General Hospital Institute of Health Professions, American Public Association Annual Meeting, Atlanta, Georgia.

Kelley, G., & Kelley, K. (2000). Progressive resistance exercise and resting blood pressure: A meta-analysis of randomized controlled trials. *Hypertension, 35,* 838–843.

Kenchaiah, S., Evans, J. C., Levy, D., Wilson, P. W., Benjamin, E. J., Larson, M. G., . . . Vasan, R. S. (2002). Obesity and the risk of heart failure. *New England Journal of Medicine, 347,* 305–313.

Kennedy, Q., Mather, M., & Carstensen, L. L. (2004). The role of motivation in the age-related positivity effect in autobiographical memory. *Psychological Science, 15,* 208–214.

Kennelly, B. (2001). Suffering in deference: A focus group study of older cardiac patients' preferences for treatment and perceptions of risk. *Quality Health Care, 10*(Suppl. 1), i23–i28.

Kershaw, S. (2003, October 20). Immigrants now embrace homes for elderly. *The New York Times,* pp. A1, A10.

Kessler, D. (2009). *The end of overeating.* New York, NY: Rodale.

Khatri, P., Blumenthal, J. A., Babyak, M. A., Craighead, W. E., Herman, S., Baldewicz, T., . . . Krishnan, K. R. (2001). Effects of exercise training on cognitive functioning among depressed older men and women. *Journal of Aging and Physical Activity, 9,* 43–57.

Kiecolt-Glaser, J. K., Dura, J. R., Speicher, C. E., Trask, O. J., Glaser, R. (1991). Spousal caregivers of dementia victims: Longitudinal changes in immunity and health. *Psychosomatic Medicine, 53,* 345–362.

Kiel, D. P., Magaziner, J., Zimmerman, S., Ball, L., Barton, B. A., Brown, K. M., . . . Birge, S. J. (2007). Efficacy of a hip protector to prevent hip fracture in nursing home residents. *Journal of the American Medical Association, 298,* 413–422.

Kim, K. K., Horan, M. L., Gendler, P., & Patel, M. K. (1991). Development and evaluation of the Osteoporosis Health Belief Scale. *Research in Nursing and Health, 14,* 155–163.

King, A. C., Ahn, D. K., Oliveira, B. M., Atienza, A. A., Castro, C. M., & Gardner, C. D. (2008). Promoting physical activity through hand-held computer technology. *American Journal of Preventive Medicine, 34,* 138–142.

King, A. C., Baumann, K., O'Sullivan, P., Wilcox, S., & Castro, C. (2002). Effects of moderate-intensity exercise on physiological, behavioral, and emotional responses to family caregiving: A randomized controlled trial. *Journal of Gerontology: Medical Sciences, 57A,* M26–M36.

King, A. C., Oman, R. F., Brassington, G. S., Bliwise, D. L., & Haskell, W. L. (1997). Moderate-intensity exercise and self-rated quality of sleep in older adults. *Journal of the American Medical Association, 277*, 32–37.

King, W. C., Brach, J. S., Belle, S., Killingsworth, R., Fenton, M., & Kriska, A. M. (2003). The relationship between convenience of destinations and walking levels in older women. *American Journal of Health Promotion, 18*, 74–82.

Kivipelto, M., Ngandu, T., Fratiglioni, L., Viitanen, M., Kåreholt, I., Winblad, B., . . . Nissinen, A. (2005). Obesity and vascular factors at midlife and the risk of dementia and Alzheimer's disease. *Archives of Neurology, 62*, 1556–1560.

Klatsky, A. L., Morton, C., Udaltsova, N., & Friedman, G. D. (2006). Coffee, cirrhosis, and transaminase enzymes. *Archives of Internal Medicine, 166*, 1190–1195.

Klein, B. E., Klein, R., Lee, K. E., & Grady, L. M. (2006). Statin use and incident nuclear cataract. *Journal of the American Medical Association, 295*, 2752–2758.

Klein, E., et al. (2011). Vitamin E and the risk of prostate cancer: The Selenium and Vitamin E Cancer Prevention Trial. *Journal of the American Medical Association, 306*, 1549–1556.

Klem, M. L., Wing, R. R., McGuire, M. T., Seagle, H. M., & Hill, J. O. (1997). A descriptive study of individuals successful at long-term maintenance of substantial weight loss. *American Journal of Clinical Nutrition, 66*, 239–246.

Klesges, R. C., Johnson, K. C., & Somes, G. (2006). Varenicline for smoking cessation: Definite promise, but no panacea. *Journal of the American Medical Association, 296*, 94–95.

Kling, E., & Kimmel, D. (2006). SAGE: New York City's pioneer organization for LGBT elders. In D. C. Kimmel, T. Rose, & S. David (Eds.), *Lesbian, gay, bisexual, and transgender aging* (pp. 265–276). New York, NY: Columbia University Press.

Knauer, N. (2009). LGBT elder law: Toward equity in aging. *Harvard Journal of Law & Gender, 32*, 1–58.

Knoops, K. T., de Groot, L. C., Kromhout, D., Perrin, A. E., Moreiras-Varela, O., Menotti, A., & van Staveren, W. A. (2004). Mediterranean diet, life style factors, and 10-year mortality in elderly European men and women. *Journal of the American Medical Association, 292*, 1433–1439.

Knowler, W. C., Barrett-Connor, E., Fowler, S. E., Hamman, R. F., Lachin, J. M., Walker, E. A., . . . Diabetes Prevention Program Research Group. (2002). Reduction in the incidence of type 2 diabetes with lifestyle intervention or metformin. *New England Journal of Medicine, 346*, 393–403.

Ko, C., & Sonnenberg, A. (2005). Comparing risks and benefits of colorectal cancer screening in elderly patients. *Gastroenterology, 129*, 1163–1170.

Koch, K. (1977). *I never told anybody*. New York, NY: Random House.

Koenig, H. (2000). Religion, spirituality, and medicine: Application to clinical practice. *Journal of the American Medical Association, 284*, 1708.

Koenig, H. G., Cohen, H. J., George, L. K., Hays, J. C., Larson, D. B., & Blazer, D. G. (1997). Attendance at religious services, interleukin-6, and other biological parameters of immune function in older adults. *International Journal of Psychiatry in Medicine, 27*, 233–250.

Koenig, H. G., Hays, J. C., Larson, D. B., George, L. K., Cohen, H. J., McCullough, M. E., . . . Blazer, D. G. (1999). Does religious attendance prolong survival? A six-year follow-up study of 3,968 older adults. *Journal of Gerontology: Biological/Medical Sciences, 54*, M370–M376.

Koepsell, T., McCloskey, L., Wolf, M., Moudon, A. V., Buchner, D., Kraus, J., & Patterson, M.(2002). Crosswalk markings and the risk of pedestrian-motor vehicle collisions in older pedestrians. *Journal of the American Medical Association, 288*, 2136–2143.

Koepsell, T. D., Wolf, M. E., Buchner, D. M., Kukull, W. A., LaCroix, A. Z., Tencer, A. F., . . . Larson, E. B. (2004). Footwear style and risk of falls in older adults. *Journal of the American Geriatrics Society, 52,* 1495–1501.

Kolata, G. (2009, March 19). Prostate cancer screening found to save few, if any, lives. *The New York Times,* p. 27.

Kolata, G. (2012, July 10). In dieting, magic isn't a substitute for science. *The New York Times,* pp. D5–D6.

Kolata, G., & Moss, M. (2002, February 11). X-ray vision in hindsight: Science, politics and the mammogram. *The New York Times,* p. A23.

Kominski, G. F., Heslin, K. C., Morgenstern, H., Hurwitz, E. L., & Harber, P. I. (2005). Economic evaluation of four treatment for low-back pain. *Medical Care, 43,* 428–435.

Kostis, J. B., Cabrera, J., Cheng, J. Q., Cosgrove, N. M., Deng, Y., Pressel, S. L., & Davis, B. R. (2011). Association between chlorthalidone treatment of systolic hypertension and long-term survival. *Journal of the American Medical Association, 306,* 2588–2593.

Kotecki, J. E., Elanjian, S. I., & Torabi, M. R. (2000). Health promotion beliefs and practices among pharmacists. *Journal of the American Pharmaceutical Association, 40,* 773–779.

Kottke, T. E., Battista, R. N., DeFriese, G. H., & Brekke, M. L. (2000). Attributes of successful smoking cessation interventions in medical practice: A meta-analysis of 42 controlled trials. *Journal of the American Medical Association, 259,* 2883–2889.

Kraus, W. E., Houmard, J. A., Duscha, B. D., Knetzger, K. J., Wharton, M. B., McCartney, J. S., . . . Slentz, C. A. (2002). Effects of the amount and intensity of exercise on plasma lipoproteins. *New England Journal of Medicine, 347,* 1483–1492.

Krause, N. (2002). Church-based social support and health in old age: Exploring variations by race. *Journal of Gerontology: Social Sciences, 57B,* S332–S347.

Krause, N. (2008). *Aging in the church.* West Conshohocken, PA: Templeton Foundation Press.

Krause-Parello, C. (2008). The mediating effect of pet attachment support between loneliness and general health in older females living in the community. *Journal of Community Health Nursing, 25,* 1–14.

Kreuzer, M., Krauss, M., Kreienbrock, L., Jöckel, K. H., & Wichmann, H. E. (2000). Environmental tobacco smoke and lung cancer: A case-control study in Germany. *American Journal of Epidemiology, 151,* 241–250.

Kristal, A. R., Littman, A. J., Benitez, D., & White, E. (2005). Yoga practice is associated with attenuated weight gain in healthy, middle-aged men and women. *Alternative Therapy and Health Medicine, 4,* 28–33.

Kritz-Silverstein, D., Barrett-Connor, E., & Corbeau, C. (2001). Cross-sectional and prospective study of exercise and depressed mood in the elderly: The Rancho Bernardo Study. *American Journal of Epidemiology, 153,* 596–603.

Kruger, J., et al. (2002, May 17). Prevalence of health-care providers asking older adults about their physical activity levels-United States, 1998. *Morbidity and Mortality Weekly Report, 51,* 412–414.

Kuehn, B. (2012). USPSTF: Taking vitamin D and calcium doesn't prevent fractures in older women. *Journal of the American Medical Association, 308,* 225–226.

Kukell, W., et al. (2002). Dementia and Alzheimer's disease incidence: A prospective cohort study. *Archives of Neurology, 59,* 1737–1746.

Kupfer, D., & Frank, E. (2002). Placebo in clinical trials for depression: Complexity and necessity. *Journal of the American Medical Association, 287,* 1853–1854.

Kurlowicz, L. (1997). Nursing standard of practice protocol: Depression in elderly patients. *Geriatric Nursing, 18,* 192–200.

Kushi, L. H., Folsom, A. R., Prineas, R. J., Mink, P. J., Wu, Y., & Bostick, R. M. (1996). Dietary antioxidant vitamins and death from coronary heart disease in postmenopausal women. *New England Journal of Medicine, 334,* 1156–1162.

Lachman, M. (1986). Personal control in later life: Stability, change and cognitive correlates. In M. Baltes & P. Baltes (Eds.), *The psychology of control and aging*. Hillsdale, NJ: Erlbaum.

Lachman, M., & Andreoletti, C. (2006). Strategy use mediates the relationship between control beliefs and memory performance for middle-aged and older adults. *Journal of Gerontology: Psychological/Social Sciences, 61*, P88–P94.

LaCroix, A. Z., Leveille, S. G., Hecht, J. A., Grothaus, L. C., & Wagner, E. H. (1996). Does walking decrease the risk of cardiovascular disease hospitalization and death in older adults? *Journal of the American Geriatrics Society, 44*, 113–120.

LaGesse, D. (2002, August 26/September 2). Swallowing air. *U.S. News & World Report*, p. 72.

Lai, H., & Good, M. (2006). Music improves sleep quality in older adults. *Journal of Advanced Nursing, 53*, 134.

Lamy, P. (1988, Summer). Actions of alcohol and drugs in older people. *Generations*, pp. 9–13.

Lan, C., Chen, S. Y., Lai, J. S., & Wong, M. K. (1999). The effect of Tai Chi on cardiorespiratory function in patients with coronary artery bypass surgery. *Medical Science Sports Exercise, 31*, 634–638.

Landers, S. (2001, June 18). Beyond cholesterol: New uses for statins. *American Medical News*, pp. 32–33.

Landrum, M. B., Meara, E. R., Chandra, A., Guadagnoli, E., & Keating, N. L. (2008). Is spending more always wasteful? The appropriateness of care and outcomes among colorectal cancer patients. *Health Affairs, 27*, 159–168.

Lang, F. (2001). Regulation of social relationships in later adulthood. *Journal of Gerontology: Psychological Sciences, 56B*, P321–P326.

Langer, E., & Rodin, J. (1976). The effects of choice and enhanced personal responsibility for the aged: A field experiment in an institutional setting. *Journal of Personality and Social Psychology, 34*, 191–198.

Langlois, J. A., Keyl, P. M., Guralnik, J. M., Foley, D. J., Marottoli, R. A., & Wallace, R. B. (1997). Characteristics of older pedestrians who have difficulty crossing the street. *American Journal of Public Health, 87*, 393–397.

Lantz, M. (2002). Depression in the elderly: Recognition and treatment. *Clinical Geriatrics, 10*, 18–24.

LaRosa, J. C., Grundy, S. M., Waters, D. D., Shear, C., Barter, P., Fruchart, J. C., . . . Treating to New Targets (TNT) Investigators. (2005). Intensive lipid lowering with atorvastatin in patients with stable coronary disease. *New England Journal of Medicine, 352*, 1425–1435.

Larson, D. (1995). Faith: The forgotten factor in healthcare. *American Journal of Natural Medicine, 2*, 10–15.

Larson, E. B., Wang, L., Bowen, J. D., McCormick, W. C., Teri, L., Crane, P., & Kukull, W. (2006). Exercise is associated with reduced risk for incident dementia among persons 65 years of age and older. *Annals of Internal Medicine, 144*, 73–81.

Lau, D., & Kirby, J. (2009). The relationship between living arrangement and preventive care use among community-dwelling elderly persons. *American Journal of Public Health, 99*, 1315–1321.

Lavretsky, H., Alstein, L. L., Olmstead, R. E., Ercoli, L. M., Riparetti-Brown, M., Cyr, N. S., & Irwin, M. R. (2011). Complementary use of Tai Chi Chih augments escitalopram in the treatment of geriatric depression. *American Journal of Geriatric Psychiatry, 19*, 839–850.

Lavretsky, H., Epel, E. S., Siddarth, P., Nazarian, N., Cyr, N. S., Khalsa, D. S., . . . Irwin, M. R. (2012, March 11). A pilot study of yogic meditation for family dementia caregivers with depressive symptoms. *International Journal of Geriatric Psychiatry*. (online). doi:10.1002/gps3790

Lawlor, D., & Hopker, S. (2001). The effectiveness of exercise as an intervention in the management of depression: Systematic review and meta-regression analysis of randomized controlled trials. *British Medical Journal, 322,* 763–767.

Lazar, S. W., Kerr, C. E., Wasserman, R. H., Gray, J. R., Greve, D. N., Treadway, M. T., . . . Fischl, B. (2005). Meditation experience is associated with increased cortical thickness. *Neuroreport, 16,* 1893–1897.

Lazarus, R., & Folkman, S. (1984). *Stress, appraisal and coping.* New York, NY: Springer.

Le Bars, P. L., Katz, M. M., Berman, N., Itil, T. M., Freedman, A. M., & Schatzberg, A. F. (1997). A placebo-controlled trial of Ginkgo biloba. *Journal of the American Medical Association, 278,* 1327–1332.

Ledikwe, J. H., Blanck, H. M., Kettel Khan, L., Serdula, M. K., Seymour, J. D., Tohill, B. C., & Rolls, B. J. (2006). Dietary energy density is associated with energy intake and weight status in US adults. *American Journal of Clinical Nutrition, 83,* 1362–1368.

Lee, A., & Beaver, H. (2003). Visual loss in the elderly. *Clinical Geriatrics, 11,* 46–53.

Lee, C., Ayers, S. L., & Kronenfeld, J. J. (2009). The association between perceived provider discrimination, healthcare utilization and health status in racial and ethnic minorities. *Ethnicity and Disease, 19,* 330–337.

Lee, C. D., Blair, S. N., & Jackson, A. S. (1999). Cardiorespiratory fitness, body composition, and all-cause and cardiovascular disease mortality in men. *American Journal of Clinical Nutrition, 69,* 373–380.

Lee, G., & Cassidy, M. (1986). Family and kin relations of the rural elderly. In R. Coward & G. Lee (Eds.), *The elderly in rural society* (pp. 151–170). New York, NY: Springer.

Lee, I. M., Cook, N. R., Gaziano, J. M., Gordon, D., Ridker, P. M., Manson, J. E., . . . Buring, J. E. (2005). Vitamin E in the primary prevention of cardiovascular disease and cancer: The Women's Health Study. *Journal of the American Medical Association, 294,* 56–65.

Lee, I. M., Sesso, H. D., Oguma, Y., & Paffenbarger, R. S., Jr. (2003). Relative intensity of physical activity and risk of coronary heart disease. *Circulation, 107,* 1110–1116.

Lee, J., Soeken, K., & Picot, S. J. (2007). A meta-analysis of interventions for informal stroke caregivers. *Western Journal of Nursing Research, 29,* 344–356.

Lee, M., & Ernst, E. (2011). Systematic reviews of t'ai chi. *British Journal of Sports Medicine.* Retrieved from http://dx.doi.org/10.1136/bjsm.2010.080622

Lee, S. J., Sudore, R. L., Williams, B. A., Lindquist, K., Chen, H. L., & Covinsky, K. E. (2009). Functional limitations, socioeconomic status, and all-cause mortality in moderate alcohol drinkers. *Journal of the American Geriatrics Society, 57,* 1110–1112.

Leeb, B. F., Schweitzer, H., Montag, K., & Smolen, J. S. (2000). A meta-analysis of chondroitin sulfate in the treatment of osteoarthritis. *Journal of Rheumatology, 27,* 205–211.

Leff, B., & Novak, T. (2011, Spring). It takes a team. *Generations,* pp. 60–63.

Leff, B., Reider L., Frick, K.D., Scharfstein, D.O., Boyd, C.M., Frey, K., . . . Boult, C. (2009). Guided care and cost of complex healthcare. *American Journal of Managed Care, 15,* 555–559.

Lehtinen, M., & Paavonen, J. (2004). Vaccination against human papillomaviruses shows great promise. *Lancet, 364,* 1731–1732.

Leigh, J. P., Tancredi, D. J., & Kravitz, R. L. (2009). Physician career satisfaction within specialties. *BMC Health Services Research, 16,* 166.

Leipzig, R. M., Whitlock, E.P., Wolff, T.A., Barton, M.B., Michael, Y.L., Harris, R., . . . US Preventive Services Task Force Geriatric Workgroup. (2010). Reconsidering the approach to prevention recommendations for older adults. *Annals of Internal Medicine, 153,* 809–814.

Lenz, M., Richter, T., & Mühlhauser, I. (2009). The morbidity and mortality associated with overweight and obesity in adulthood. *Deutsches Arzteblatt International, 106,* 641–648.

Leonhardt, D. (2009, July 7). In health reform, a cancer offers an acid test. *The New York Times,* pp. 7–8.

Leveille, S. G., Wagner, E. H., Davis, C., Grothaus, L., Wallace, J., LoGerfo, M., & Kent, D. (1998). Preventing disability and managing chronic illness in frail older adults: A randomized trial of a community-based partnership with primary care. *Journal of the American Geriatrics Society, 46,* 1191–1198.

Leveille, S. G., Wee, C. C., & Iezzoni, L. I. (2005). Trends in obesity and arthritis among baby boomers and their predecessors, 1971–2002. *American Journal of Public Health, 95,* 398–399.

Levenson, M. R., Jennings, P. A., Aldwin, C. M., & Shiraishi, R. W. (2005). Self-transcendence: Conceptualization and measurement. *International Journal of Aging and Human Development, 60,* 127–143.

Levine, J. A., Lanningham-Foster, L. M., McCrady, S. K., Krizan, A. C., Olson, L. R., Kane, P. H., . . . Clark, M. M. (2005). Interindividual variation in posture allocation: Possible role in human obesity. *Science, 307,* 584–586.

Levy, B. R., Slade, M. D., Kunkel, S. R., & Kasl, S. V. (2002). Longevity increased by positive self-perceptions of aging. *Journal of Personality and Social Psychology, 83,* 261–270.

Lewis, C. (1988). Disease prevention and health promotion practices of primary care physicians in the United States. *American Journal of Preventive Medicine, 4*(Suppl. 4), 9–16.

Li, F., Fisher, K. J., Brownson, R. C., & Bosworth, M. (2005). Multilevel modeling of built environment characteristics related to neighborhood walking activity in older adults. *Journal of Epidemiology and Community Health, 59,* 558–564.

Li, F., Fisher, K. J., & Harmer, P. (2005). Improving physical function and blood pressure in older adults through cobblestone mat walking: A randomized trial. *Journal of the American Geriatrics Society, 53,* 1305–1312.

Li, G., Higdon, R., Kukull, W.A., Peskind, E., Van Valen Moore, K., Tsuang, D., . . . Larson, E. B. (2004). Statin therapy and risk of dementia in the elderly. *Neurology, 63,* 1624–1628.

Li, Y. (2007). Recovering from spousal bereavement in later life: Does volunteer participation play a role? *Journal of Gerontology, 62B,* S257–S266.

Liberman, U. A., Weiss, S. R., Bröll, J., Minne, H. W., Quan, H., Bell, N. H., . . . Favus, M. (1995). Effect of oral alendronate on bone mineral density and the incidence of fractures in postmenopausal osteoporosis. *New England Journal of Medicine, 333,* 1437–1443.

Lichtenberg, P. (2009). Controversy and caring: An update on current issues in dementia. *Generations, 33,* 5–10.

Liddon, N. C., Leichliter, J. S., & Markowitz, L. E. (2012). Human papillomavirus vaccine and sexual behavior among adolescent and young women. *American Journal of Preventive Medicine, 42,* 44–52.

Liebman, B. (2008, July/August). Fiber free-for-all. *Nutrition Action Healthletter,* pp. 3–5.

Lien, C. Y., Lin, H. R., Kuo, I. T., & Chen, M. L. (2009). Perceived uncertainty, social support and psychological adjustment in older patients with cancer being treated with surgery. *Journal of Clinical Nursing, 18,* 2311–2319.

Lightwood, J., & Glantz, S. (2009, September 21). Declines in acute myocardial infarction after smoke-free laws and individual risk attributable to secondhand smoke. *Circulation* (e-publication).

Lin, F. R., & Ferrucci, L. (2012). Hearing loss and falls among older adults in the United States. *Archives of Internal Medicine, 72*, 369–371.

Lin, I., & Brown, S. (2012). Unmarried boomers confront old age: A national portrait. *Gerontologist, 52*, 153–165.

Lin, L. C., Yang, M. H., Kao, C. C., Wu, S. C., Tang, S. H., & Lin, J. G. (2009). Using acupressure and Montessori-based activities to decrease agitation for residents with dementia. *Journal of the American Geriatrics Society, 57*, 1022–1029.

Lin, J. S., Eder, M., & Weinmann, S. (2011). Behavioral counseling to prevent skin cancer. *Annals of Internal Medicine, 154*, 190–201.

Lin, O. S., Kozarek, R. A., Schembre, D. B., Ayub, K., Gluck, M., Drennan, F., . . . Rabeneck, L. (2006). Screening colonoscopy in very elderly patients: Prevalence of neoplasia and estimated impact on life expectancy. *Journal of the American Medical Association, 295*, 2357–2365.

Lindau, S. T., Schumm, L. P., Laumann, E. O., Levinson, W., O'Muircheartaigh, C. A., & Waite, L. J. (2007). A study of sexuality and health among older adults in the United States. *New England Journal of Medicine, 357*, 752–764.

Linden, W., Lenz, J. W., & Con, A. H. (2001). Individualized stress management for primary hypertension. *Archives of Internal Medicine, 161*, 1071–1080.

Lindquist, L. A., Cameron, K. A., Messerges-Bernstein, J., Friesema, E., Zickuhr, L., Baker, D. W., & Wolf, M. (2012). Hiring and screening practices of agencies supplying paid caregivers to older adults. *Journal of the American Geriatrics Society, 60*, 1253–1259.

Link, C., & McKinlay, J. (2009). Disparities in the prevalence of diabetes: Is it race/ethnicity or socioeconomic status? *Ethnicity and Disease, 19*, 288–292.

Liu, H., Bravata, D. M., Olkin, I., Nayak, S., Roberts, B., Garber, A. M., & Hoffman, A. R. (2007). Systematic review: The safety and efficacy of growth hormone in the healthy elderly. *Annals of Internal Medicine, 146*, 104–115.

Liu-Ambrose, T., Khan, K. M., Eng, J. J., Gillies, G. L., Lord, S. R., & McKay, H. A. (2005). The beneficial effects of group-based exercises on fall risk profile and physical activity persist 1 year postintervention in older women with low bone mass. *Journal of the American Geriatrics Society, 53*, 1767–1773.

Liu-Ambrose, T., Nagamatsu, L. S., Graf, P., Beattie, B. L., Ashe, M. C., & Handy, T. C. (2010). Resistance training and executive function. *Archives of Internal Medicine, 170*, 170–178.

Lockenhoff, C., & Carstensen, L. (2004). Socioemotional selectivity theory, aging, and health. *Journal of Personality, 72*, 1395–1424.

Loeb, S., Metter, E. J., Kan, D., Roehl, K. A., & Catalona, W. J. (2012). Prostate-specific antigen velocity (PSAV) risk count improves the specificity of screening for clinically significant prostate cancer. *British Journal of Urology International, 109*, 508–513.

Logue, E., Sutton, K., Jarjoura, D., & Smucker, W. (2000). Obesity management in primary care: Assessment of readiness to change among 284 family practice patients. *Journal of the American Board of Family Practice, 13*, 164–171.

Looney, C., & Haber, D. (2001). Interest in hosting an exercise program for older adults at African-American churches. *Journal of Religious Gerontology, 13*, 19–29.

Lopez, C. N., Martinez-Gonzalez, M. A., Sanchez-Villegas, A., Alonso, A., Pimenta, A. M., & Bes-Rastrollo, M. (2009). Costs of Mediterranean and Western dietary patterns. *Journal of Epidemiology and Community Health, 63*, 920–927.

Lorig, K., Chastain, R. L., Ung, E., Shoor, S., & Holman, H. R. (1989). Development and evaluation of a scale to measure perceived self-efficacy in people with arthritis. *Arthritis and Rheumatism, 32*, 37–44.

Lorig, K. (1992). *Patient education: A practical approach*. St. Louis, MO: Mosby-Year Book.

Lorig, K., et al. (2006). *Living a healthy life with chronic conditions* (3rd ed.). Palo Alto, CA: Bull.

Lorig, K. R., Ritter, P., Stewart, A. L., Sobel, D. S., Brown, B. W., Jr., Bandura, A., . . . Holman, H. R. (2001). Chronic disease self-management program. *Medical Care, 39,* 1217–1223.

Lorig, K. R., Sobel, D. S., Stewart, A. L., Brown, B. W., Jr., Bandura, A., Ritter, P., . . . Holman, H. R. (1999). Evidence suggesting that a chronic disease self-management program can improve health status while reducing hospitalization: A randomized trial. *Medical Care, 37,* 5–14.

Lucas, F., et al. (2006). Black patients are more likely to die after major surgery than White patients. *Annals of Surgery, 243,* 281–286.

Lutwack-Bloom, P., Wijewickrama, R., & Smith, B. (2005). Effects of pets versus people visits with nursing home residents. *Journal of Gerontological Social Work, 44,* 137–159.

Ma, J., Drieling, R., & Stafford, R. S. (2006, May 25). US women desire greater professional guidance on hormone and alternative therapies for menopause symptom management. *Menopause* (e-publication).

Maison, P., Balkau, B., Simon, D., Chanson, P., Rosselin, G., & Eschwège, E. (1998). Growth hormone as a risk for premature mortality in healthy subjects: Data from the Paris prospective study. *British Medical Journal, 316,* 1132–1133.

Maison, P., Byrne, C. D., Hales, C. N., Day, N. E., & Wareham, N. J. (2001). Do different dimensions of the metabolic syndrome change together over time? Evidence supporting obesity as the central feature. *Diabetes Care, 10,* 1758–1763.

Manheimer, M. (2009). Gearing up for the big show: Lifelong learning programs are coming of age. In R. Hudson (Ed.), *The boomers and their future* (Vol. 2, pp. 99–112). Santa Barbara, CA: Praeger Press.

Manson, J. E., Greenland, P., LaCroix, A. Z., Stefanick, M. L., Mouton, C. P., Oberman, A., . . . Siscovick, D. S. (2002). Walking compared with vigorous exercise for the prevention of cardiovascular events in women. *New England Journal of Medicine, 347,* 716–725.

Manson, J. E., Hu, F. B., Rich-Edwards, J. W., Colditz, G. A., Stampfer, M. J., Willett, W. C., . . . Hennekens, C. H. (1999). A prospective study of walking as compared with vigorous exercise in the prevention of coronary heart disease in women. *New England Journal of Medicine, 341,* 650–658.

Manton, K. G., Gu, X., & Lamb, V. L. (2006). Change in chronic disability from 1982 to 2004/05. *Proceedings of the National Academy of Science, 103,* 18374–18379.

Manton, K. G., Stallard, E., & Corder, L. S. (1998). The dynamics of dimensions of age-related disability 1982–1994 in the U.S. elderly population. *Journal of Gerontology: Biological Sciences, 53A,* B59–B70. p. 486.

Many suffer from anti-gay violence. (2008, December 24). *The Star Press,* p. 7. Retrieved from http://www.thestarpress.com

Maraldi, C., Volpato, S., Penninx, B. W., Yaffe, K., Simonsick, E. M., Strotmeyer, E. S., . . . Pahor, M. (2007). Diabetes mellitus, glycemic control, and incident depressive symptoms among 70- to 79-year-old persons: The health, aging, and body composition study. *Archives of Internal Medicine, 167,* 1137–1144.

Marcus, B. H. Albrecht, A. E., King, T. K., Parisi, A. F., Pinto, B. M., Roberts, M., . . . Abrams, D. B. (1999). The efficacy of exercise as an aid for smoking cessation in women: A randomized controlled trial. *Archives of Internal Medicine, 159,* 1229–1234.

Margolin, A., Kleber, H. D., Avants, S. K., Konefal, J., Gawin, F., Stark, E., . . . Vaughan, R. (2002). Acupuncture for the treatment of cocaine addiction: A randomized controlled trial. *Journal of the American Medical Association, 287,* 55–63.

Martin, L. G., Freedman, V. A., Schoeni, R. F., & Andreski, P. M. (2009). Health and functioning among baby boomers approaching 60. *Journal of Gerontology: Social Sciences, 64B,* 369–377.

Maruta, T., Colligan, R. C., Malinchoc, M., & Offord, K. P. (2000). Optimists vs. pessimists: Survival rate among medical patients over a 30-year period. *Mayo Clinic Proceedings, 75*, 140–143.

Marziali, E., & Garcia, L. (2011). Dementia caregivers' responses to 2 internet-based intervention programs. *American Journal of Alzheimer's Disease and other Dementias, 26*, 36–43.

Maskarinec, G., Erber, E., Grandinetti, A., Verheus, M., Oum, R., Hopping, B. N., . . . Kolonel, L. N. (2009). Diabetes incidence based on linkages with health plans. *Diabetes, 58*, 1732–1738.

Maskarinec, G., Grandinetti, A., Matsuura, G., Sharma, S., Mau, M., Henderson, B. E., & Kolonel, L. N. (2009b). Diabetes prevalence and body mass index differ by ethnicity. *Ethnicity and Disease, 19*, 49–55.

Mason, D. (2001). Editorial: An apple a day. *American Journal of Nursing, 101*, 7.

Masoro, E. (2005). Overview of caloric restriction and ageing. *Mechanisms of Ageing Development, 126*, 913–922.

Masse, I., Bordet, R., Deplanque, D., Al Khedr, A., Richard, F., Libersa, C., & Pasquier, F. (2005). Lipid lowering agents are associated with a slower cognitive decline in Alzheimer's disease. *Journal of Neurology, Neurosurgery, and Psychiatry, 76*, 1611–1613.

Mather, M., & Carstensen, L. (2005). Aging and motivated cognition: The positivity effect in attention and memory. *Trends in Cognitive Science, 10*, 496–502.

Mather, M., Canli, T., English, T., Whitfield, S., Wais, P., Ochsner, K., . . . Carstensen, L. L. (2004). Amygdala responses to emotionally valenced stimuli in older and younger adults. *Psychological Sciences, 15*, 259–263.

Mather, M., Gorlick, M. A., & Lighthall, N. R. (2009). To brake or accelerate when the light turns yellow? Stress reduces older adults' risk taking in a driving game. *Psychological Sciences, 20*, 174–176.

Mattison, J. A., et al. (2012). Impact of caloric restriction on health and survival in rhesus monkeys from the NIA study. *Nature, 489*, 318–321.

Mausbach, B. T., Coon, D. W., Depp, C., Rabinowitz, Y. G., Wilson-Arias, E., Kraemer, H. C., . . . Gallagher-Thompson, D. (2004). Ethnicity and time to institutionalization of dementia patients. *Journal of the American Geriatrics Society, 52*, 1077–1084.

Mazieres, B., Combe, B., Phan Van, A., Tondut, J., & Grynfeltt, M. (2001). Chondroitin sulfate in osteoarthritis of the knee: A prospective, double blind, placebo controlled multicenter clinical study. *Journal of Rheumatology, 28*, 173–181.

McAlindon, T. E., LaValley, M. P., Gulin, J. P., & Felson, D. T. (2000). Glucosamine and chondroitin for treatment of osteoarthritis: A systematic quality assessment and meta-analysis. *Journal of the American Medical Association, 283*, 1469–1475.

McAuley, E., & Courneya, K. (1993). Adherence to exercise and physical activity as health promoting behaviors: Attitudinal and self-efficacy influences. *Applied and Preventive Psychology, 2*, 65–77.

McCarthy, E. P., Burns, R. B., Freund, K. M., Ash, A. S., Shwartz, M., Marwill, S. L., & Moskowitz, M. A. (2000). Mammography use, breast cancer stage at diagnosis, and survival among older women. *Journal of the American Geriatrics Society, 48*, 1226–1233.

McCormack, G., Giles-Corti, B., & Milligan, R. (2006). Demographic and individual correlates of achieving 10,000 steps/day: Use of pedometers in a population-based study. *Health Promotion Journal of Australia, 17*, 43–47.

McCormick, K. A., Cochran, N. E., Back, A. L., Merrill, J. O., Williams, E. C., & Bradley, K. A. (2006). How primary care providers talk to patients about alcohol. *Journal of General Internal Medicine, 21*, 966–972.

McCoy, S. L., Tun, P. A., Cox, L. C., Colangelo, M., Stewart, R. A., & Wingfield, A. (2005). Hearing loss and perceptual effort: Downstream effects on older adults' memory for speech. *Journal of Experimental Psychology, 58,* 22–33.

McCullough, M., Jezierski, T., Broffman, M., Hubbard, A., Turner, K., & Janecki, T. (2006). Diagnostic accuracy of canine scent detection in early- and late-stage lung and breast cancers. *Integrative Cancer Therapy, 5*(1), 30–39.

McFarland, K., Rhoades, D., Roberts, E., & Eleazer, P. (2006). Teaching communication and listening skills to medical students using life review with older adults. *Gerontology & Geriatrics Education, 27,* 81–94.

McGinnis, J., & Foege, W. (1993). Actual causes of death in the United States. *Journal of the American Medical Association, 270,* 2207–2212.

McGinnis, J. M., Williams-Russo, P., & Knickman, J. R. (2002). The case for more active policy attention to health promotion. *Health Affairs, 21,* 78–93.

McGinnis, S., & Zoske, F. (2008). The emerging role of faith community nurses in prevention and management of chronic disease. *Policy and Politics for Nurse Practitioners, 9,* 173–180.

McGuire, K. M., Greenberg, M. A., & Gevirtz, R. (2005). Autonomic effects of expressive writing in individuals with elevated blood pressure. *Journal of Health Psychology, 10,* 197–209.

McGuire, L., Kiecolt-Glaser, J. K., & Glaser, R. (2002). Depressive symptoms and lymphocyte proliferation in older adults. *Journal of Abnormal Psychology, 111,* 192–197.

McGwin, G., Jr., Sarrels, S. A., Griffin, R., Owsley, C., & Rue, L. W., 3rd. (2008). The impact of a vision screening on older driver fatality rates. *Archives of Ophthalmology, 1126,* 1544–1547.

McMurray, J. (1990). Creative arts with older people. *Activities, Adaptation and Aging, 14*(1/2), entire issue.

McNicholas, J., Gilbey, A., Rennie, A., Ahmedzai, S., Dono, J. A., & Ormerod, E. (2005). Pet ownership and human health. *British Medical Journal, 331,* 1252–1254.

McPherson, C. P., Swenson, K. K., & Lee, M. W. (2002). The effects of mammographic detection and comorbidity on the survival of older women with breast cancer. *Journal of the American Geriatrics Society, 50,* 1061–1068.

McTiernan, A., et al. (2002, July). *Exercise and breast cancer rates.* Presentation at the International Cancer Congress, Oslo.

McWhinney-Morse, S. (2009). Beacon Hill Village. *Generations, 33,* 85–86.

Meier, K., & Licari, M. (1997). The effect of cigarette taxes on cigarette consumption, 1955 through 1994. *American Journal of Public Health, 87,* 1126–1130.

Melchart, D., Linde, K., Fischer, P., & Kaesmayr, J. (2000). Echinacea for preventing and treating the common cold. *Cochrane Database System Review,* (2), CD000530.

Melchart, D., Streng, A., Hoppe, A., Brinkhaus, B., Witt, C., Wagenpfeil, S., . . . Linde, K. (2005). Acupuncture in patients with tension-type headache: Randomised controlled trial. *British Medical Journal, 331,* 376–379.

Mellin, L., Croughan-Minihane, M., & Dickey, L. (1997). The solution method: 2-year trends in weight, blood pressure, exercise, depression, and functioning of adults trained in development skills. *Journal of the American Dietetic Association, 97,* 1133–1138.

Mellinger, G., & Balter, M. (1983). *Collaborative project* (GSMIRSB Report). Washington, DC: National Institute of Mental Health.

Melnikow, J., Kohatsu, N. D., & Chan, B. K. (2000). Put prevention into practice: A controlled evaluation. *American Journal of Public Health, 90,* 1622–1625.

Merck Company Foundation. (2007). *The state of aging and health in America 2007.* Whitehouse Station, NJ: Author.

Mermin, G. B., Johnson, R. W., & Murphy, D. P. (2007). Why do boomers plan to work longer? *Journal of Gerontology: Social Sciences, 62B*, S286–S294.

Merrick, E. L., Horgan, C. M., Hodgkin, D., Garnick, D. W., Houghton, S. F., Panas, L., . . . Blow, F. C. (2008). Unhealthy drinking patterns in older adults. *Journal of the American Geriatrics Society, 56*, 1769–1770.

Metlife Mature Market Institute. (2006). *Out and aging: The Metlife study of lesbian and gay baby boomers.* New York, NY: Metropolitan Life Insurance Company.

Mettler, M. (1997). Unpublished update on the *Healthwise Handbook* program. Boise, ID: Healthwise.

Meydani, S. N., Meydani, M., Blumberg, J. B., Leka, L. S., Siber, G., Loszewski, R., . . . Stollar, B. D. (1997). Vitamin E supplementation and in vivo immune response in healthy elderly subjects. *Journal of the American Medical Association, 277*, 1380–1386.

Michael, Y. L., Berkman, L. F., Colditz, G. A., & Kawachi, I. (2001). Living arrangements, social integration, and change in function: Health status. *American Journal of Epidemiology, 153*, 123–131.

Michels, K. B., Giovannucci, E., Joshipura, K. J., Rosner, B. A., Stampfer, M. J., Fuchs, C. S., . . . Willett, W. C. (2000). Prospective study of fruit and vegetable consumption and incidence of colon and rectal cancers. *Journal of the National Cancer Institute, 92*, 1740–1752.

Milch, C. E., Edmunson, J. M., Beshansky, J. R., Griffith, J. L., & Selker, H. P. (2004). Smoking cessation in primary care. *Preventive Medicine, 38*, 284–294.

Miller, A. B., To, T., Baines, C. J., & Wall, C. (2002). The Canadian national breast screening study. *Annals of Internal Medicine, 137*(5 Pt. I), 305–312.

Miller, E. R., 3rd., Pastor-Barriuso, R., Dalal, D., Riemersma, R. A., Appel, L. J., & Guallar, E. (2005). Meta-analysis: High-dosage vitamin E supplementation may increase all-cause mortality. *Annals of Internal Medicine, 142*, 37–46.

Mintzes, B., Barer, M. L., Kravitz, R. L., Bassett, K., Lexchin, J., Kazanjian, A., . . . Marion, S. A. (2003). How does direct-to-consumer advertising affect prescribing? *Canadian Medical Association Journal, 169*, 405–412.

Mitchell, C. (2012, April 30). *With weights, you can lighten your load.* McMaster University Research News release, Hamilton, Ontario.

Mitrou, P. N., Kipnis, V., Thiébaut, A. C., Reedy, J., Subar, A. F., Wirfält, E., . . . Schatzkin, A. (2007). Mediterranean dietary pattern and prediction of all-cause mortality in a US population. *Archives of Internal Medicine, 167*, 2461–2468.

Mittelman, M. S., Roth, D. L., Coon, D. W., & Haley, W. E. (2004). Sustained benefit of supportive intervention for depressive symptoms in caregivers of patients with Alzheimer's disease. *American Journal of Psychiatry, 161*, 850–856.

Monaghan, E. (2006, April 24). United States fares poorly in international patient survey. *American Medical News*, pp. 5, 7.

Monsivais, P., & Drewnowski, A. (2007). The rising cost of low-energy-density foods. *Journal of the American Dietary Association, 107*, 2071–2076.

Montamat, S., & Cusack, B. (1992). Overcoming problems with polypharmacy and drug misuse in the elderly. In G. Omenn (Ed.), *Clinics in geriatric medicine* (pp. 143–158), Philadelphia, PA: W. B. Saunders.

Montgomery, P. (2002). Treatments for sleep problems in elderly people. *British Medical Journal, 325*, 1049.

Moore, A. A., Seeman, T., Morgenstern, H., Beck, J. C., & Reuben, D. B. (2002). Are there differences between older persons who screen positive on the CAGE questionnaire and the Short Michigan Alcoholism Screening Test-geriatric version? *Journal of the American Geriatrics Society, 50*, 858–862.

More people lifting weights—and getting injured. (2000). *Health & Nutrition Letter* (Tufts University), *18*, 1, 8.

Morewedge, C. K., Huh, Y. E., & Vosgerau, J. (2010). Thought for food. *Science, 330*, 1530–1533.

Morgan, D. (1993, May 24/31). The best prescription might be just taking time to care. *American Medical News*, p. 9.

Moriarity, J. P., Branda, M. E., Olsen, K. D., Shah, N. D., Borah, B. J., Wagie, A. E., . . . Naessens, J. M. (2012). The effects of incremental costs of smoking and obesity on health care costs among adults. *Journal of Occupational and Environmental Medicine, 54*, 286–289.

Morin, C. M., Colecchi, C., Stone, J., Sood, R., & Brink, D. (1999). Behavioral and pharmacological therapies for late-life insomnia: A randomized controlled trial. *Journal of the American Medical Association, 281*, 991–999.

Morley, J. (2002). Drugs, aging and the future. *Journal of Gerontology: Medical Sciences, 57A*, M2–M6.

Morris, M. C., Evans, D. A., Bienias, J. L., Tangney, C. C., & Wilson, R. S. (2002). Vitamin E and cognitive decline in older persons. *Archives of Neurology, 59*, 1125–1132.

Morrow-Howell, N., Hinterlong, J., Rozario, P. A., & Tang, F. (2002). Effects of volunteering on the well-being of older adults. *Journal of Gerontology, 58B*, S137–S145.

Morrow-Howell, N., Hinterlong, J., Rozario, P. A., & Tang, F. (2003). Effects of volunteering on the well-being of older adults. *Journal of Gerontology: Psychological Sciences, 58*, S137–S145.

Morrow-Howell, N., Hong, S. I., & Tang, F. (2009). Who benefits from volunteering? *Gerontologist, 49*, 91–102.

Mostofsky, E., Maclure, M., Sherwood, J. B., Tofler, G. H., Muller, J. E., & Mittleman, M. A. (2012). Risk of acute myocardial infarction after the death of a significant person in one's life. *Circulation, 125*, 491–496.

Most patients don't see excess weight as health danger. (1999, November 8). *American Medical News*, pp. 26–27.

Mroczek, D., & Spiro, A. (2005). Change in life satisfaction during adulthood. *Journal of Personality and Social Psychology, 88*, 189–202.

Mukamal, K. J., Conigrave, K. M., Mittleman, M. A., Camargo, C. A., Jr., Stampfer, M. J., Willett, W. C., & Rimm, E. B. (2003). Roles of drinking pattern and type of alcohol consumed in coronary heart disease in men. *New England Journal of Medicine, 348*, 109–118.

Mukamal, K. J., Maclure, M., Muller, J. E., Sherwood, J. B., & Mittleman, M. A. (2001). Prior alcohol consumption and mortality following acute myocardial infarction. *Journal of the American Medical Association, 285*, 1965–1970.

Mullan, F. (1992). Rewriting the social contract in health. In A. Katz, et al. (Eds.), *Self-help: Concepts and applications* (pp. 61–67). Philadelphia, PA: Charles Press.

Munnell, A., & Wu, A. (2012, October). Are aging baby boomers squeezing young workers out of jobs? *Center for Retirement Research*, 12–18.

Murphy, M., Nevill, A., Neville, C., Biddle, S., & Hardman, A. (2002). Accumulating brisk walking for fitness, cardiovascular risk, and psychological health. *Medical Science & Sports Exercise, 34*, 1468–1474.

Musick, M., & Wilson, J. (2003). Volunteering and depression: The role of psychological and social resources in different age groups. *Social Science Medicine, 56*, 259–269.

Myers, J., Prakash, M., Froelicher, V., Do, D., Partington, S., & Atwood, J. E. (2002). Exercise capacity and mortality among men referred for exercise testing. *New England Journal of Medicine, 346*, 793–801.

Naegle, M. (2008). Screening for alcohol use and misuse in older adults: Using the short michigan alcoholism screening text-geriatric version. *American Journal of Nursing, 108,* 50–58.

Nagamatsu, L. S., Handy, T. C., Hsu, C. L., Voss, M., & Liu-Ambrose, T. (2012). Resistance training promotes cognitive functioning brain plasticity in seniors with mild cognitive impairment. *Archives of Internal Medicine, 172,* 666–668.

Napoli, M. (2001). Overdiagnosis and overtreatment. *American Journal of Nursing, 101,* 11.

Nasvadi, G., & Wister, A. (2009). Do restricted driver's licenses lower crash risk among older drivers? *Gerontologist, 49,* 474–484.

National Council on the Aging. (2002). *American perceptions of aging in the 21st century.* Sampling, Interviewing and Data Preparation by Harris Interactive, Inc. Retrieved from http://www.ncoa.org

National Institutes of Health Consensus Development Panel on Acupuncture. (1998). Acupuncture. *Journal of the American Medical Association, 280,* 1518–1524.

Neergaard, L. (1998, February 23). Dietary supplement users are advised to use caution. *Houston Chronicle,* p. 3.

Negoianu, D., & Goldfarb, S. (2008). Just add water. *Journal of the American Society of Nephrology, 19,* 1041–1043.

Nelson, H. D., Walker, M., Zakher, B., & Mitchell, J. (2012). Menopausal hormone therapy for the primary prevention of chronic conditions. *Annals of Internal Medicine, 15,* 104–113.

Nestle, M. (2002). *Food politics.* Los Angeles: University of California Press.

Neuhouser, M. L. Wassertheil-Smoller, S., Thomson, C., Aragaki, A., Anderson, G. L., Manson, J. E., . . . Prentice, R. L. (2009). Multivitamin use and risk of cancer and cardiovascular disease in the Women's Health Initiative cohorts. *Archives of Internal Medicine, 169,* 294–304.

Neuner, J. M., Binkley, N., Sparapani, R. A., Laud, P. W., & Nattinger, A. B. (2006). Bone density testing in older women and its association with patient age. *Journal of the American Geriatrics Society, 54,* 485–489.

Neville, K. (2000). Sugar: How do I disguise thee? *Environmental Nutrition, 23,* 2.

Newbould, J., Taylor, D., & Bury, M. (2006). Lay-led self-management in chronic illness: A review of the evidence. *Chronic Illness, 2,* 249–261.

Newcomer, J. W., Selke, G., Melson, A. K., Hershey, T., Craft, S., Richards, K., & Alderson, A. L. (1999). Decreased memory performance in healthy humans induced by stress-level cortisol treatment. *Archives of General Psychiatry, 56,* 527–533.

Newcomer, R. J., Kang, T., & Doty, P. (2012). Allowing spouses to be paid personal care providers. *Gerontologist, 52,* 517–530.

The new diet pill. (2000). *Berkeley Wellness Letter, 16,* 2.

Newton, K. M., Reed, S. D., LaCroix, A. Z., Grothaus, L. C., Ehrlich, K., & Guiltinan, J. (2006). Treatment of vasomotor symptoms of menopause with black cohosh, multibotanicals, soy, hormone therapy, or placebo. *Annals of Internal Medicine, 145,* 869–879.

Nichol, K. L., Nordin, J., Mullooly, J., Lask, R., Fillbrandt, K., & Iwane, M. (2003). Influenza vaccination and reduction in hospitalizations for cardiac disease and stroke among the elderly. *New England Journal of Medicine, 348,* 1322–1332.

Nielsen, S., & Popkin, B. (2003). Patterns in trends in food portion sizes, 1977–1998. *Journal of the American Medical Association, 289,* 450–453.

Nguyen, N. T., Hohmann, S., Slone, J., Varela, E., Smith, B. R., & Hoyt, D. (2010). Improved bariatric surgery outcomes for Medicare beneficiaries after implementation of the Medicare national coverage determination. *Archives of Surgery, 145,* 72–78.

NIH State-of-the-Science Panel. (2006). National Institutes of Health Conference statement. *Annals of Internal Medicine, 145,* 839–844.

Nissen, S. E., Nicholls, S. J., Sipahi, I., Libby, P., Raichlen, J. S., Ballantyne, C. M., . . . ASTEROID Investigators. (2006). Effect of very high-intensity statin therapy on regression of coronary atherosclerosis. *Journal of the American Medical Association, 295,* 1583–1584.

Noble, H. (1999, September 5). Some say Koop sold out on Web by blurring line between ads, facts. *Houston Chronicle,* p. 16A.

Nordin, J., Mullooly, J., Poblete, S., Strikas, R., Petrucci, R., Wei, F., . . . Nichol, K. L. (2001). Influenza vaccine effectiveness in preventing hospitalizations and deaths in persons 65 years or older in Minnesota, New York, and Oregon: Data from 3 health plans. *Journal of Infectious Diseases, 184,* 665–670.

Nualnim, N., Parkhurst, K., Dhindsa, M., Tarumi, T., Vavrek, J., & Tanaka, H. (2012). Effects of swimming training on blood pressure vascular function in adults >50 years of age. *The American Journal of Cardiology, 109,* 1005–1010.

Nutting, P. (1987). Community-oriented primary care: From principle to practice. In P. Nutting (Ed.), *Community-oriented primary care* (pp. xv–xxv). Albuquerque, NM: University of New Mexico Press.

Obama, M. (2012). *American grown: The story of the White House kitchen garden and gardens across America.* New York, NY: Crown Publishers.

Oberman, A., & Kreisberg, R. (2002). Lipid management in older patients. *Clinical Geriatrics, 10,* 41–50.

Obisesan, T., & Gillum, R. (2009). Cognitive function, social integration and mortality in a U.S. national cohort study of older adults. *BMC Geriatrics, 9,* 33.

Oboler, S. K., Prochazka, A. V., Gonzales, R., Xu, S., & Anderson, R. J. (2002). Public expectations and attitudes for annual physical examinations and testing. *Annals of Internal Medicine, 136,* 652–659.

O'Connor, M. B., O'Connor, C., & Walsh, C. H. (2008). A dog's detection of low blood sugar: A case report. *Ireland Journal of Medical Science, 177,* 155–157.

Offit, P. (2012). Studying complementary and alternative therapies. *Journal of the American Medical Association, 307,* 1803–1804.

Olfson, M., & Marcus, S. (2009). National patterns in antidepressant medication treatment. *Archives of General Psychiatry, 66,* 848–856.

Oliveria, S. A., Lapuerta, P., McCarthy, B. D., L'Italien, G. J., Berlowitz, D. R., & Asch, S. M. (2002). Physician-related barriers to the effective management of uncontrolled hypertension. *Archives of Internal Medicine, 162,* 413–420.

Olsen, O., & Gotzsche, P. (2001). Cochrane review on screening for breast cancer with mammography. *Lancet, 358,* 1340–1342.

Olson, E. (2012, March 8). Wanted: Health professionals to treat the aging. *The New York Times,* p. F8.

Orel, N. (2004). Gay, lesbian, and bisexual elders. *Journal of Gerontological Social Work, 43,* 57–77.

Ornish, D. (2001). *Eat more, weigh less.* New York, NY: Harper Collins.

Ornish, D., Scherwitz, L. W., Billings, J. H., Brown, S. E., Gould, K. L., Merritt, T. A., . . . Brand, R. J. (1998). Intensive lifestyle changes for reversal of coronary heart disease. *Journal of the American Medical Association, 280,* 2001–2007.

Ornstein, R., & Sobel, D. (1989). *Healthy pleasures.* Reading, MA: Addison-Wesley.

O'Rourke, R. W., Andrus, J., Diggs, B. S., Scholz, M., McConnell, D. B., & Deveney, C. W. (2006). Perioperative morbidity associated with bariatric surgery: An academic center experience. *Archives of Surgery, 141,* 262–268.

Osborne, N. H., Upchurch, G. R., Jr., Mathur, A. K., & Dimick, J. B. (2009). Explaining racial disparities in mortality after abdominal aortic aneurysm repair. *Journal of Vascular Surgery, 50,* 709–713.

Ostir, G. V., Goodwin, J. S., Markides, K. S., Ottenbacher, K. J., Balfour, J., & Guralnik, J. M. (2002). Differential effects of premorbid physical and emotional health on recovery from acute events. *Journal of the American Geriatrics Society, 50,* 713–718.

Ostir, G. V., Markides, K. S., Peek, M. K., & Goodwin, J. S. (2001). The association between emotional well-being and the incidence of stroke in older adults. *Psychosomatic Medicine, 63,* 210–215.

Ostir, G. V., Markides, K. S., Black, S. A., & Goodwin, J. S. (2000). Emotional well-being predicts subsequent functional independence and survival. *Journal of the American Geriatrics Society, 48,* 473–478.

Oswald, R., & Masciadrelli, B. (2008). Generative ritual among nonmetropolitan lesbians and gay men. *Journal of Marriage & Family, 70,* 1060–1073.

Ott, B. R., Heindel, W. C., Papandonatos, G. D., Festa, E. K., Davis, J. D., Daiello, L. A., & Morris, J. C. (2008). A longitudinal study of drivers with Alzheimer's disease. *Neurology, 70,* 1171–1178.

Otte, C., Zhao, S., & Whooley, M. A. (2012). Statin use and risk of depression in patients with coronary heart disease. *Journal of Clinical Psychiatry, 73,* 610–615.

Palmore, E. (2000). Ageism in gerontological language. *Gerontologist, 40,* 645.

Palombo, R., et al. (2002). *The aging states project: Promoting opportunities for collaboration between the public health aging networks.* Washington, DC: Association of State and Territorial Chronic Disease Program and the National Association of State Units on Aging.

Papp, K. V., Walsh, S. J., & Snyder, P. J. (2009). Immediate and delayed effects of cognitive interventions in healthy elderly. *Alzheimer's and Dementia, 5,* 50–60.

Pargament, K. I., Koenig, H. G., Tarakeshwar, N., & Hahn, J. (2001). Religious struggle as a predictor of mortality among medically ill elderly patients: A 2-year longitudinal study. *Annals of Internal Medicine, 161,* 1881–1885.

Park, M., & Unutzer, J. (2011). Geriatric depression in primary care. *Psychiatry Clinics of North America, 34,* 469–487.

Park, Y., Hunter, D. J., Spiegelman, D., Bergkvist, L., Berrino, F., van den Brandt, P. A., . . . Smith-Warner, S. A. (2005). Dietary fiber intake and risk of colorectal cancer: A pooled analysis of prospective cohort studies. *Journal of the American Medical Association, 294,* 2849–2857.

Parker, C., Muston, D., Melia, J., Moss, S., & Dearnaley, D. (2006). A model of the natural history of screen-detected prostate cancer, and the effect of radical treatment on overall survival. *British Journal of Cancer, 94,* 1361–1368.

Pashayan, N., Powles, J., Brown, C., & Duffy, S. W. (2006, July 11). Excess cases of prostate cancer and estimated overdiagnosis associated with PSA testing in East Anglia. *British Journal of Cancer* (e-publication).

Pasternak, R. C., Smith, S. C., Jr., Bairey-Merz, C. N., Grundy, S. M., Cleeman, J. I., Lenfant, C., . . . National Heart, Lung and Blood Institute. (2002). ACC/AHA/NHLBI clinical advisory on the use and safety of statins. *Circulation, 106,* 1024–1028.

Pasupathi, M., & Carstensen, L. (2003). Age and emotional experience during mutual reminiscing. *Psychology and Aging, 18,* 430–442.

Patel, N. R., Rollison, D. E., Barnholtz-Sloan, J., Mackinnon, J., Green, L., & Giuliano, A. R. (2009). Racial and ethnic disparities in the incidence of invasive cervical cancer in Florida. *Cancer, 115,* 3991–4000.

Paterna, S., Gaspare, P., Fasullo, S., Sarullo, F. M., & Di Pasquale, P. (2008). Normal-sodium diet compared with low-sodium diet in compensated congestive heart failure: Is sodium an old enemy or a new friend? *Clinical Science, 114,* 221–230.

Paul-Labrador, M., Polk, D., Dwyer, J. H., Velasquez, I., Nidich, S., Rainforth, M., ... Merz, C. N. (2006). Effects of a randomized controlled trial of transcendental meditation on components of the metabolic syndrome in subjects with coronary heart disease. *Archives of Internal Medicine, 166,* 1218–1224.

Paulson, R. J., Boostanfar, R., Saadat, P., Mor, E., Tourgeman, D. E., Slater, C. C., ... Jain, J. K. (2002). Pregnancy in the sixth decade of life: Obstetric outcomes in women of advanced reproductive age. *Journal of the American Medical Association, 288,* 2320–2323.

Pear, R. (2002, February 28). Nine in 10 nursing homes lack adequate staff, study finds. *The New York Times,* pp. A1, A11.

Peeters, A., Barendregt, J. J., Willekens, F., Mackenbach, J. P., Al Mamun, A., Bonneux, L., NEDCOM, the Netherlands Epidemiology and Demography Compression of Morbidity Research Group. (2003). Obesity in adulthood and its consequences for life expectancy: A life-table analysis. *Annals of Internal Medicine, 138,* 24–32.

Peikes, D., Chen, A., Schore, J., & Brown, R. (2009). Effects of care coordination on hospitalization, quality of care, and health care expenditures among Medicare beneficiaries. *Journal of the American Medical Association, 301,* 603–618.

Pelletier, K. (1996). A review and analysis of the health and cost-effective outcome studies of comprehensive health promotion and disease prevention programs at the worksite: 1993–1995 update. *American Journal of Health Promotion, 10,* 380–388.

Pelletier, K. (2009). A review and analysis of the clinical and cost-effectiveness studies of comprehensive health promotion and disease management programs at the worksite. *Journal of Occupational and Environmental Medicine, 51,* 822–837.

Peng, X. D., Huang, C. Q., Chen, L. J., & Lu, Z. C. (2009). Cognitive behavioural therapy and reminiscence techniques for the treatment of depression in the elderly: A systematic review. *Journal of Internal Medicine Research, 37,* 975–982.

Penninx, B. (2000). A happy person, a healthy person? *Journal of the American Geriatrics Society, 48,* 590–592.

Penninx, B. W., Messier, S. P., Rejeski, W. J., Williamson, J. D., DiBari, M., Cavazzini, C., ... Pahor, M. (2001). Physical exercise and the prevention of disability in activities of daily living in older persons with osteoarthritis. *Archives of Internal Medicine, 161,* 2309–2316.

Penninx, B. W., Rejeski, W. J., Pandya, J., Miller, M. E., Di Bari, M., Applegate, W. B., & Pahor, M. (2002). Exercise and depressive symptoms: A comparison of aerobic and resistance exercise effects on emotional and physical function in older persons with high and low depressive symptomatology. *Journal of Gerontology: Psychological Sciences, 57B,* P124–P132.

Pereira, M. A., Kartashov, A. I., Ebbeling, C. B., Van Horn, L., Slattery, M. L., Jacobs, D. R., Jr., & Ludwig, D. S. (2005). Fast-food habits, weight gain, and insulin resistance. *Lancet, 365,* 36–42.

Peripheral vascular disease: What should you do if you have it? (2000, June 7). *Focus on Healthy Aging* (Mount Sinai School of Medicine).

Persky, T. (1998). Overlooked and underserved: Elders in need of mental health care. *Journal of the California Alliance for the Mentally Ill, 9,* 7–9.

Personal data on web sites are vulnerable. (2000, February). *American Medical News,* p. 6.

Petersen, M. (2001, November 21). Increased spending on drugs is linked to more advertising. *The New York Times,* Business, p. B1.

Petrella, R., & Bartha, C. (2000). Home based exercise therapy for older patients with knee osteoarthritis: A randomized clinical trial. *Journal of Rheumatology, 27,* 2215–2221.

Pezzin, L. E., Keyl, P. M., & Green, G. B. (2007). Disparities in the emergency department evaluation of chest pain patients. *Academic Emergency Medicine, 14,* 149–156.

Phelan, E. A., Williams, B., Leveille, S., Snyder, S., Wagner, E. H., & LoGerfo, J. P. (2002). Outcomes of a community-based dissemination of the health enhanced program. *Journal of the American Geriatrics Society, 50,* 1519–1524.

Philipp, M., Kohnen, R., & Hiller, K. O. (1999). Hypericum extract versus imipramine or placebo in patients with moderate depression: Randomized multicentre study of treatment for eight weeks. *British Medical Journal, 319,* 1534–1538.

Phipps, K. R., Orwoll, E. S., Mason, J. D., & Cauley, J. A. (2000). Community water fluoridation, bone mineral density, and fractures: Prospective study of effects in older women. *British Medical Journal, 321,* 860–864.

Pinquart, M., Duberstein, P. R., & Lyness, J. M. (2007). Effects of psychotherapy and other behavioral interventions on clinically depressed older adults: A meta-analysis. *Aging and Mental Health, 11,* 645–657.

Piper, M. E., Smith, S. S., Schlam, T. R., Fiore, M. C., Jorenby, D. E., Fraser, D., & Baker, T. B. (2008). A randomized, placebo-controlled clinical trial of five smoking cessation pharmacotherapies. *Archives of General Psychiatry, 66,* 1253–1262.

Politi, M. (2009). Patient-provider communication about sexual health among unmarried middle-aged and older women. *Journal of General Internal Medicine, 24,* 511–516.

Pollack, A. (2008, November 28). The minimal impact of a big hypertension study. *The New York Times,* pp. 13, 17.

Pollan, M. (2008). *In defense of food.* New York, NY: Penguin Press.

Pollan, M. (2007, April 22). You are what you grow. *The New York Times Magazine,* pp. 15–18.

Pollan, M. (2011). *Food rules.* New York, NY: Penguin Press.

Pope, E. (2012, January–February). Sitting: Hazardous to your health. *AARP Bulletin,* pp. 28, 30.

Porter, E. (2012, August 22). Rationing health care more fairly. *The New York Times,* pp. 1–2.

Porter, M. (2000). Resistance training recommendations for older adults. *Topics in Geriatric Rehabilitation, 15*(3), 60–69.

Powell, P., Bentall, R. P., Nye, F. J., & Edwards, R. H. (2001). Randomised controlled trial of patient education to encourage graded exercise in chronic fatigue syndrome. *British Medical Journal, 322,* 387–390.

The power of the placebo effect. (2000, November 3). *Focus on Healthy Aging* (Mount Sinai School of Medicine), *11,* 1, 6.

PPIP. (2000). *Put prevention into practice.* Agency for Healthcare Research and Quality. Retrieved from http://www.ahrq.gov/clinic/ppipix.htm

Preserving your sight. (2002, February). *Consumer Reports on Health,* pp. 1, 4–5.

Pribble, J. M., Goldstein, K. M., Fowler, E. F., Greenberg, M. J., Noel, S. K., & Howell, J. D. (2006). Medical news for the public to use? What's on local TV news. *American Journal of Managed Care, 12,* 170–176.

Priplata, A. A., Patritti, B. L., Niemi, J. B., Hughes, R., Gravelle, D. C., Lipsitz, L. A., . . . Collins, J. J. (2006). Noise-enhanced balance control in patients with diabetes and patients with stroke. *Annals of Neurology, 59,* 4–12.

Pritikin, N. (1984). The Pritikin diet. *Journal of the American Medical Association, 251,* 1160–1161.

Prochaska, J., Johnson, S., & Lee, P. (2009). The transtheoretical model of behavior change. In S. A. Shumaker, J. K. Ockene, & K. A. Riekert (Eds.), *The handbook of health behavior change* (pp. 59–84). New York, NY: Springer.

Prochaska, J. O., DiClemente, C. C., Velicer, W. F., & Rossi, J. S. (1993). Standardized, individualized, interactive, and personalized self-help programs for smoking cessation. *Health Psychology, 12*, 399–405.

Prochazka, A. V., Lundahl, K., Pearson, W., Oboler, S. K., & Anderson, R. J. (2005). Support of evidence-based guidelines for the annual physical examination: A survey of primary care providers. *Archives of Internal Medicine, 165*, 1347–1352.

Pronk, N. P., Goodman, M. J., O'Connor, P. J., & Martinson, B. C. (2000). Relationship between modifiable health risks and short-term health care charges. *Journal of the American Medical Association, 282*, 2235–2239.

Province, M. A., Hadley, E. C., Hornbrook, M. C., Lipsitz, L. A., Miller, J. P., Mulrow, C. D., . . . Wolf, S. L. (1995). The effects of exercise on falls in elderly patients: A preplanned meta-analysis of the FICSIT trials. *Journal of the American Medical Association, 273*, 1341–1347.

Pruchno, R. (2012). Not your mother's old age: Baby boomers at age 65. *Gerontologist, 52*, 149–152.

Pruchno, R., & McKenney, D. (2002). Psychological well-being of Black and White grandmothers raising grandchildren: Examination of a two-factor model. *Journal of Gerontology: Psychological/Social Sciences, 57*, 444–451.

Putnam, R. (2000). *Bowling alone: The collapse and revival of American community.* New York, NY: Simon & Schuster.

Pyke, S. D., Wood, D. A., Kinmonth, A. L., & Thompson, S. G. (1997). Change in coronary risk and coronary risk factor levels in couples following lifestyle intervention. *Archives of Family Medicine, 6*, 354–360.

Qato, D. M., Alexander, G. C., Conti, R. M., Johnson, M., Schumm, P., & Lindau, S. T. (2008). Use of prescription and over-the-counter medications and dietary supplements among older adults in the United States. *Journal of the American Medical Association, 300*, 2867–2878.

Quinn, M., & McNabb, W. (2001). Training lay health educators to conduct a church-based weight-loss program for African American women. *Diabetes Education, 27*, 231–238.

Rabin, R. (2007, July 17). Calorie labels may qualify options, not actions. *The New York Times*, p. 2.

Rabin, R. (2012, November 6). Reassessing flu shots as the season draws near. *The New York Times*, p. D5.

Raebel, M. A., Malone, D. C., Conner, D. A., Xu, S., Porter, J. A., & Lanty, F. A. (2004). Health services use and health care costs of obese and non-obese individuals. *Archives of Internal Medicine, 164*, 2135–2140.

Rahman, A., & Schnelle, J. (2008). The nursing home culture-change movement: Recent past, present, and future directions for research. *Gerontologist, 48*, 142–148.

Rakowski, W., Wells, B. L., Lasater, T. M., & Carleton, R. A. (1991). Correlates of expected success at health habit change and its role as a predictor in health behavior research. *American Journal of Preventive Medicine, 7*, 89–94.

Ramasubbu, K., & Mann, D. (2006). The emerging role of statins in the treatment of heart failure. *Journal of the American College of Cardiology, 47*, 342–344.

RAND. (2003). *Health risk appraisals and medicare.* Baltimore, MD: Centers for Medicare & Medicaid Services.

Rastas, S., Pirttilä, T., Viramo, P., Verkkoniemi, A., Halonen, P., Juva, K., . . . Sulkava, R. (2006). Association between blood pressure and survival over 9 years in a general population aged 85 and older. *Journal of the American Geriatrics Society, 54*, 912–918.

Rea, T. D., Breitner, J. C., Psaty, B. M., Fitzpatrick, A. L., Lopez, O. L., Newman, A. B., . . . Kuller, L. H. (2005). Statin use and the risk of incident dementia: The Cardiovascular Health Study. *Archives of Neurology, 62*, 1047–1051.

Rebok, G. W., Carlson, M. C., Glass, T. A., McGill, S., Hill, J., Wasik, B. A., . . . Rasmussen, M. D. (2004). Short-term impact of experience corps participation on children and schools. *Journal of Urban Health, 81*, 79–83.

Reeves, M., & Rafferty, A. (2005). Healthy lifestyle characteristics among adults in the United States, 2000. *Archives of Internal Medicine, 165*, 854–857.

Reginster, J. Y., Deroisy, R., Rovati, L. C., Lee, R. L., Lejeune, E., Bruyere, O., . . . Gossett, C. (2001). Long-term effects of glucosamine sulphate on osteoarthritis progression: A randomized, placebo-controlled clinical trial. *Lancet, 357*, 251–256.

Rehman, S. U., Nietert, P. J., Cope, D. W., & Kilpatrick, A. O. (2005). What to wear today? Effect of doctor's attire on the trust and confidence of patients. *American Journal of Medicine, 118*, 1279–1286.

Reichenbach, S., Sterchi, R., Scherer, M., Trelle, S., Bürgi, E., Bürgi, U., . . . Jüni, P. (2007). Chondroitin for osteoarthritis of the knee or hip. *Annals of Internal Medicine, 146*, 580–590.

Reid, J. (1995). Development in late life: Older lesbian and gay lives. In A. D'Augelli & J. Patterson (Eds.), *Lesbian, gay, and bisexual identities over the lifespan: Psychological perspectives* (pp. 215–240). New York, NY: Oxford University Press.

Rejeski, W. (2008). Mindfulness: Reconnecting the body and mind in geriatric medicine and gerontology. *Gerontologist, 48*, 135–141.

Renehan, A. G., Tyson, M., Egger, M., Heller, R. F., & Zwahlen, M. (2008). Body-mass index and incidence of cancer. *Lancet, 371*, 569–578.

Rexrode, K. M., Hennekens, C. H., Willett, W. C., Colditz, G. A., Stampfer, M. J., Rich-Edwards, J. W., . . . Manson, J. E. (1997). A prospective study of body mass index, weight change, and risk of stroke in women. *Journal of the American Medical Association, 277*, 1539–1545.

Reynolds, R. F., Walker, A. M., Obermeyer, C. M., Rahman, O., & Guilbert, D. (2001). Discontinuation of postmenopausal hormone therapy in a Massachusetts HMO. *Journal of Clinical Epidemiology, 54*, 1056–1064.

Reynolds, S. L., Saito, Y., & Crimmins, E. M. (2005). The impact of obesity on active life expectancy in older American men and women. *Gerontologist, 45*, 438–444.

Rhoden, E., & Morgentaler, A. (2004). Risks of testosterone-replacement therapy and recommendations for monitoring. *New England Journal of Medicine, 350*, 482–492.

Rhodes, E. C., Martin, A. D., Taunton, J. E., Donnelly, M., Warren, J., & Elliot, J. (2000). Effects of one year of resistance training on the relation between muscular strength and bone density in elderly women. *British Journal of Sports Medicine, 34*, 18–22.

Rice, V., & Stead, L. (2002). Nursing interventions for smoking cessation. *Cochrane Library*, issue 1. Oxford: Update Software.

Rich, J., & Black, W. (2000). When should we stop screening? *Effective Clinical Practice, 3*, 78–84.

Ricks, D. (2001, May 27). Study finds cholesterol drugs also cut risks of breast cancer. *Houston Chronicle*, p. 12A.

Rigaud, A., & Forette, B. (2001). Hypertension in older adults. *Journal of Gerontology: Medical Sciences, 56A*, M217–M225.

Ring-Dimitriou, S., Steinbacher, P., von Duvillard, S. P., Kaessmann, H., Müller, E., Sänger, A. M. (2009). Exercise modality and physical fitness in perimenopausal women. *European Journal of Applied Physiology, 105*, 739–747.

Ritchie, K., & Kildea, D. (1995). Is senile dementia "age-related" or "ageing-related"? Evidence from meta-analysis of dementia prevalence in the oldest old. *Lancet, 346*, 931–934.

Robertson, M. C., Devlin, N., Gardner, M. M., & Campbell, A. J. (2001). Effectiveness and economic evaluation of a nurse delivered home exercise programme to prevent falls: 1 and 2. *British Medical Journal, 322*, 697–704.

Roby, D. H., Nicholson, G. L., & Kominski, G. F. (2009, October). African Americans in commercial HMOs more likely to delay prescription drugs and use the emergency room. *Policy Brief, UCLA Center on Health Policy and Research*, pp. 1–12.

Rodin, J. (1986). Aging and health: Effects of the sense of control. *Science, 233*, 1271–1275.

Rodin, J., & Langer, E. (1977). Long-term effects of a control-relevant intervention with the institutionalized aged. *Journal of Personality and Social Psychology, 35*, 897–902.

Rosendahl, E., & Kirschenbaum, P. (1992, November). *Weight loss and mood among older adults*. Paper presentation at the 45th Gerontological Society of America Annual Meeting, Washington, DC.

Rosenstock, I. (1990). The health belief model: Explaining health behavior through expectancies. In K. Glanz, et al. (Eds.), *Health Behavior and Health Education: Theory, Research, and Practice* (pp. 39–61). San Francisco, CA: Jossey-Bass.

Rosenthal, E. (2008, September 24). Fast food hits Mediterranean: A diet succumbs. *The New York Times*.

Roszak, T. (1998). *America the wise*. Boston, MA: Houghton Mifflin.

Rothwell, P. M., Price, J. F., Fowkes, F. G., Zanchetti, A., Roncaglioni, M. C., Tognoni, G., . . . Meade, T. W. (2012). Short-term effects of daily aspirin on cancer incidence, mortality, and non-vascular death. *Lancet, 379*, 1602–1612.

Rotter, J. (1954). *Social learning and clinical psychology*. Englewood Cliffs, NJ: Prentice-Hall.

Rovio, S., Kåreholt, I., Helkala, E. L., Viitanen, M., Winblad, B., Tuomilehto, J., . . . Kivipelto, M. (2005). Leisure-time physical activity at midlife and the risk of dementia and Alzheimer's disease. *Lancet Neurology, 11*, 705–711.

Ruffman, T., Ng, M., & Jenkin, T. (2009). Older adults respond quickly to angry faces despite labeling difficulty. *Journal of Gerontology: Psychological Sciences, 64B*, 171–179.

Ruffman, T., Sullivan, S., & Edge, N. (2006). Differences in the way older and younger adults rate threat in faces but not situations. *Journal of Gerontology: Psychological Sciences, 61B*, P187–P194.

Ruggiero, K. J., Amstadter, A. B., Acierno, R., Kilpatrick, D. G., Resnick, H. S., Tracy, M., & Galea, S. (2009). Social and psychological resources associated with health status in a representative sample of adults affected by the 2004 Florida hurricanes. *Psychiatry, 72*, 195–210.

Ruitenberg, A., van Swieten, J. C., Witteman, J. C., Mehta, K. M., van Duijn, C. M., Hofman, A., & Breteler, M. M. (2002). Alcohol consumption and risk of dementia. *Lancet, 359*, 282–286.

Russell, R. M., Rasmussen, H., & Lichtenstein, A. H. (1999). Modified food guide pyramid for people over seventy years of age. *Journal of Nutrition, 129*, 751–753.

Rybarczyk, B., Lopez, M., Benson, R., Alsten, C., & Stepanski, E. (2002). Efficacy of two behavioral treatment programs for comorbid geriatric insomnia. *Psychology of Aging, 17*, 288–298.

Sacco, R. L., Elkind, M., Boden-Albala, B., Lin, I. F., Kargman, D. E., Hauser, W. A., . . . Paik, M. C. (1999). The protective effect of moderate alcohol consumption on ischemic stroke. *Journal of the American Medical Association, 281*, 53–60.

Sahyoun, N. R., Jacques, P. F., Zhang, X. L., Juan, W., & McKeown, N. M. (2006). Whole-grain intake is inversely associated with the metabolic syndrome and mortality in older adults. *American Journal of Clinical Nutrition, 83*, 124–131.

Salazar-Martinez, E., Willett, W. C., Ascherio, A., Manson, J. E., Leitzmann, M. F., Stampfer, M. J., & Hu, F. B. (2004). Coffee consumption and risk for type 2 diabetes mellitus. *Annals of Internal Medicine, 140*, 1–8.

Saliba, J., Wattacheril, J., & Abumrad, N. N. (2009, June 16). Endocrine and metabolic response to gastric bypass. *Current Opinion Clinical Nutrition Metabolic Care* (e-publication).

Salmon, J. (2007, January 29–February 4). God's (weight-loss) plan. *The Washington Post National Weekly Edition*, p. 31.

Salon, I. (1997). Weight control and nutrition: Knowing when to intervene. *Geriatrics, 52,* 33–41.

Samuel-Hodge, C. D., Keyserling, T. C., Park, S., Johnston, L. F., Gizlice, Z., & Bangdiwala, S. I. (2009). A randomized trial of a church-based diabetes self-management program for African Americans with type 2 diabetes. *Diabetes Education, 35,* 439–454.

Sankaranarayanan, R., Nene, B. M., Shastri, S. S., Jayant, K., Muwonge, R., Budukh, A. M., . . . Dinshaw, K. A. (2009). HPV screening for cervical cancer in rural India. *New England Journal of Medicine, 360,* 1385–1394.

Sano, M., Ernesto, C., Thomas, R. G., Klauber, M. R., Schafer, K., Grundman, M., . . . Thal, L. J. (1997). A controlled trial of selegiline, alpha-tocopherol, or both as treatment for Alzheimer's disease. *New England Journal of Medicine, 336,* 1216–1222.

Sareh, P., Sourwine, M., Rochester, C. D., Steinle, N. I., & Steinle, N. I. (2011, December). Viatmin D and calcium: Implications for healthy aging. *Clinical Geriatrics,* 29–34.

Sarkamo, T., Tervaniemi, M., Laitinen, S., Forsblom, A., Soinila, S., Mikkonen, M., . . . Hietanen, M. (2008). Music listening enhances cognitive recovery and mood after middle cerebral artery stroke. *Brain, 131,* 866–876.

Sauaia, A., Min, S. J., Lack, D., Apodaca, C., Osuna, D., Stowe, A., . . . Byers, T. (2007). Church-based breast cancer screening education. *Prevention and Chronic Disease, 4,* A99.

Saunders, C. (1977). Dying they live: St. Christopher's hospice. In H. Feifel (Ed.), *New meanings of death.* New York, NY: McGraw-Hill.

Sawaya, G. F., McConnell, K. J., Kulasingam, S. L., Lawson, H. W., Kerlikowske, K., Melnikow, J., . . . Washington, A. E. (2003). Risk of cervical cancer associated with extending the interval between cervical-cancer screenings. *New England Journal of Medicine, 349,* 1501–1509.

Sawitzke, A. D., Shi, H., Finco, M. F., Dunlop, D. D., Bingham, C. O., 3rd., Harris, C. L., . . . Clegg, D. O. (2008). The effect of glucosamine and/or chondroitin sulfate on the progression of knee osteoarthritis. *Arthritis and Rheumatism, 58,* 3183–3191.

Schachter-Shalomi, Z. (1995). *From age-ing to sage-ing.* New York, NY: Warner Books.

Schardt, D. (2000a, October). Glucosamine & chondroitin: Joint relief? *Nutrition Action Healthletter,* p. 10.

Schardt, D. (2000b, September). Palmetto and the prostate. *Nutrition Action Healthletter,* p. 9.

Scharlach, A., Graham, C., & Lehning, A. (2012). The "Village" model: A consumer-driven approach for aging in place. *Gerontologist, 52,* 418–427.

Schatzkin, A., Lanza, E., Corle, D., Lance, P., Iber, F., Caan, B., . . . Cahill, J. (2000). Lack of effect of low-fat, high-fiber diet on the recurrence of colorectal adenomas. *New England Journal of Medicine, 342,* 1149–1155.

Scheibe, S., & Blanchard-Fields, F. (2009). Effects of regulating emotions on cognitive performance: What is costly for young adults is not so costly for older adults. *Psychology and Aging, 24,* 217–223.

Scheibe, S., & Carstensen, L. (2010). Emotional aging: Recent findings and future trends. *Journal of Gerontology: Psychological Sciences, 65B,* 135–144.

Scheier, M. F., Matthews, K. A., Owens, J. F., Schulz, R., Bridges, M. W., Magovern, G. J., & Carver, C. S. (1999). Optimism and rehospitalization after coronary artery bypass graft surgery. *Archives of Internal Medicine, 159,* 829–835.

Schilling, L. M., Scatena, L., Steiner, J. F., Albertson, G. A., Lin, C. T., Cyran, L., . . . Anderson, R. J. (2002). The third person in the room: Frequency, role, and influence of companions during primary care medical encounters. *Journal of Family Practice, 51,* 685–690.

Schillinger, D., Grumbach, K., Piette, J., Wang, F., Osmond, D., Daher, C., . . . Bindman. A. B. (2002). Association of health literacy with diabetes outcomes. *Journal of the American Medical Association, 288,* 475–482.

Schlenker, R. E., Powell, M. C., & Goodrich, G. K. (2002). Rural-urban home health care differences before the Balanced Budget Act of 1997. *Journal of Rural Health, 18,* 359–372.

Schlosser, E. (2001). *Fast food nation.* Boston, MA: Houghton Mifflin.

Schmid, R. (2000, May 11). Study: Doctors often miss alcohol abuse symptoms. *Galveston Daily News,* p. 9.

Schmitt, C. (2002, September 30). Nursing home myth of old age. *U.S. News & World Report,* pp. 66–74.

Schneider, E. C., Cleary, P. D., Zaslavsky, A. M., & Epstein, A. M. (2001). Racial disparity in influenza vaccination. *Journal of the American Medical Association, 286,* 1455–1460.

Schneider, E. C., Zaslavsky, A. M., & Epstein, A. M. (2002). Racial disparities in the quality of care for enrollees in Medicare managed care. *Journal of the American Medical Association, 287,* 1288–1294.

Schneider, E. C., Zaslavsky, A. M., & Epstein, A. M. (2005). Quality of care in for-profit and not-for-profit health plans enrolling Medicare beneficiaries. *American Journal of Medicine, 118,* 1392–1400.

Schneider, R. H., Alexander, C. N., Staggers, F., Rainforth, M., Salerno, J. W., Hartz, A., . . . Nidich, S. I. (2005). Long-term effects of stress reduction on mortality in persons 55+ with systemic hypertension. *American Journal of Cardiology, 95,* 1060–1064.

Schoen, C., Osborn, R., How, S. K., Doty, M. M., & Peugh, J. (2009, November 13). In chronic conditions: Experiences of patients with complex health care needs, in eight countries, 2008. *Health Affairs, 28* (e-publication).

Schonberg, M. A., McCarthy, E. P., Davis, R. B., Phillips, R. S., & Hamel, M. B. (2004). Breast cancer screening in women aged 80 and older: Results from a national survey. *Journal of the American Geriatrics Society, 52,* 1688–1695.

Schulz, R. (1976). Effects of control and predictability on the physical and psychological well-being of the institutionalized aged. *Journal of Personality and Social Psychology, 33,* 563–573.

Schulz, R., Belle, S. H., Czaja, S. J., McGinnis, K. A., Stevens, A., & Zhang, S. (2004). Long-term care placement of dementia patients and care-giver health and well-being. *Journal of the American Medical Association, 292,* 961–967.

Schwartz, K. (2011, January 25). One in six seniors lives in poverty. *National Council on the Aging Press Release.*

Schwartz, L., & Woloshin. S. (2012). How the FDA forgot the evidence. *Clinical Research Education, 344,* e1086.

Scranton, R. E., Young, M., Lawler, E., Solomon, D., Gagnon, D., & Gaziano, J. M. (2005). Statin use and fracture risk: Study of a US veterans population. *Archives of Internal Medicine, 165,* 2007–2012.

Seals, D., et al. (2001). Blood pressure reductions with exercise and sodium restriction in postmenopausal women with elevated systolic pressure: Role of arterial stiffness. *Journal of the American College of Cardiology, 38,* 506–513.

Sears, B. (1995). *Entering the zone.* New York, NY: HarperCollins.

Sears, B. (1997). *Mastering the zone.* New York, NY: HarperCollins.

Seider, B. H., Shiota, M. N., Whalen, P., & Levenson, R. W. (2011). Greater sadness reactivity in late life. *Social Cognitive and Affective Neuroscience, 6,* 186–194.

Sellmeyer, D. E., Stone, K. L., Sebastian, A., & Cummings, S. R. (2001). A high ratio of dietary animal to vegetable protein increases the rate of bone loss and the risk of fracture in postmenopausal women. *American Journal of Clinical Nutrition, 73,* 118–122.

Seshasai, S. R., Wijesuriya, S., Sivakumaran, R., Nethercott, S., Erqou, S., Sattar, N., & Ray, K. K. (2012). Effect of aspirin on vascular and non-vascular outcomes. *Archives of Internal Medicine, 172,* 209–216.

Sesso, H., et al. (2012). Multivitamins in the prevention of cardiovascular disease in men. *Journal of the American Medical Association, 308,* 1751–1760.

Shai, I., Schwarzfuchs, D., Henkin, Y., Shahar, D. R., Witkow, S., Greenberg, I., . . . Dietary Intervention Randomized Controlled Trial (DIRECT) Group. (2008). Weight loss with a low-carbohydrate, Mediterranean, or low-fat diet. *New England Journal of Medicine, 359,* 229–241.

Shamblin, G. (1997). *The weigh down diet.* Franklin, TN: Weigh Down Workshop.

Shamblin, G. (2000). *Rise above.* Franklin, TN: Weigh Down Workshop.

Sheffet, A. M., Ridlen, S., & Louria, D. B. (2006). Baseline behavioral assessment for the New Jersey Health Wellness Promotion Act. *American Journal of Health Promotion, 20,* 401–410.

Shelton, D. (2000, April 10). Men avoid physician visits, often don't know whom to see. *American Medical News,* pp. 1, 33.

Shelton, R. C., Keller, M. B., Gelenberg, A., Dunner, D. L., Hirschfeld, R., Thase, M. E., . . . Halbreich, U. (2001). Effectiveness of St. John's wort in major depression: A randomized controlled trial. *Journal of the American Medical Association, 285,* 1978–1986.

Shen, J., Wenger, N., Glaspy, J., Hays, R. D., Albert, P. S., Choi, C., & Shekelle, P. G. (2000). Electroacupuncture for control of myeloablative chemotherapy-induced emesis: A randomized controlled trial. *Journal of the American Medical Association, 284,* 2755–2761.

Sherman, K. J., Cherkin, D. C., Erro, J., Miglioretti, D. L., & Deyo, R. A. (2005). Comparing yoga, exercise, and a self-care book for chronic low back pain: A randomized, controlled trial. *Annals of Internal Medicine, 143,* 849–856.

Shiota, M., & Levenson, R. (2009). Effects of aging on experimentally instructed detached reappraisal, positive reappraisal, and emotional suppression. *Psychology and Aging, 24,* 890–900.

Sierpina, V. (2001). *Integrative health care: Complementary and alternative therapies for the whole person.* Philadelphia, PA: F.A. Davis.

Simon, G. E., Ludman, E. J., Tutty, S., Operskalski, B., & Von Korff, M. (2004). Telephone psychotherapy and telephone care management for primary care patients starting antidepressant treatment. *Journal of the American Medical Association, 292,* 935–942.

Simon, S. R., Chan, K. A., Soumerai, S. B., Wagner, A. K., Andrade, S. E., Feldstein, A. C., . . . Gurwitz, J. H. (2005). Potentially inappropriate medication use by elderly persons in U.S. health maintenance organization, 2000–2001. *Journal of the American Geriatrics Society, 53,* 227–232.

Simons, M., Keller, P., Dichgans, J., & Schulz, J. B. (2001). Cholesterol and Alzheimer's disease. *Neurology, 57,* 1089–1093.

Sinaki, M., Itoi, E., Wahner, H. W., Wollan, P., Gelzcer, R., Mullan, B. P., . . . Hodgson, S. F. (2002). Stronger back muscles reduce the incidence of vertebral fractures: A prospective 10 year follow-up of postmenopausal women. *Bone, 30,* 836–841.

Singer, P. (2009, July 19). Why we must ration health care. *The New York Times Magazine,* pp. 38–44.

Singh, N. A., Clements, K. M., & Singh, M. A. (2001). The efficacy of exercise as a long-term antidepressant in elderly subjects: A randomized, controlled trial. *Journal of Gerontology: Medical Sciences, 56A,* M497–M504.

Sink, K. M., Covinsky, K. E., Barnes, D. E., Newcomer, R. J., & Yaffe, K. (2006). Caregiver characteristics are associated with neuropsychiatric symptoms of dementia. *Journal of the American Geriatrics Society, 54,* 796–803.

Sink, K. M., Holden, K. F., & Yaffe, K. (2005). Pharmacological treatment of neuropsychiatric symptoms of dementia. *Journal of the American Medical Association, 293,* 596–608.

Siris, E. S., Miller, P. D., Barrett-Connor, E., Faulkner, K. G., Wehren, L. E., Abbott, T. A., . . . Sherwood, L. M. (2001). Identification and fracture outcomes of undiagnosed low bone mineral density in postmenopausal women: Results from the national osteoporosis risk assessment. *Journal of the American Medical Association, 286*, 2815–2822.

Sivertsen, B., Omvik, S., Pallesen, S., Bjorvatn, B., Havik, O. E., Kvale, G., . . . Nordhus, I. H. (2006). Cognitive behavioral therapy vs. zopiclone for treatment of chronic primary insomnia in older adults. *Journal of the American Medical Association, 295*, 2851–2858.

Skinner, B. (1953). *Science and human behavior.* New York, NY: Macmillan.

Skoog, I., Lithell, H., Hansson, L., Elmfeldt, D., Hofman, A., Olofsson, B., . . . SCOPE Study Group. (2005). Effect of baseline cognitive function and antihypertensive treatment on cognitive and cardiovascular outcomes: Study on Cognition and Prognosis in the Elderly (SCOPE). *American Journal of Hypertension, 18*, 1052–1059.

Slivka, D., Raue, U., Hollon, C., Minchev, K., & Trappe, S. (2008). Single muscle fiber adaptations to resistance training in old (80+ yr) men: Evidence for limited skeletal muscle plasticity. *American Journal of Physiology, 295*, R273–R280.

Sloan, R., & Bagiella, E. (2002). Claims about religious involvement and health outcomes. *Annals of Behavioral Medicine, 24*, 14–21.

Small, G. (2002). What we need to know about age related memory loss. *British Medical Journal, 324*, 1502–1505.

Small, G. W., Silverman, D. H., Siddarth, P., Ercoli, L. M., Miller, K. J., Lavretsky, H., . . . Phelps, M. E. (2006). Effects of a 14-day healthy longevity lifestyle program on cognition and brain function. *American Journal of Geriatric Psychiatry, 14*, 538–545.

Smith, A. K., McCarthy, E., Weber, E., Cenzer, I. S., Boscardin, J., Fisher, J., & Covinsky, K. (2012). Half of older Americans seen in emergency departments in last month of life; most admitted to hospital, and many die there. *Health Affairs, 31*, 1277–1285.

Smith, D. B., Feng, Z., Fennell, M. L., Zinn, J. S., & Mor, V. (2007). Separate and unequal: Racial segregation and disparities in quality across U.S. nursing homes. *Health Affairs, 26*, 1448–1458.

Smyth, J. M., Stone, A. A., Hurewitz, A., & Kaell, A. (1999). Effects of writing about stressful experiences on symptom reduction in patients with asthma or rheumatoid arthritis: A randomized trial. *Journal of the American Medical Association, 281*, 1304–1309.

Sneaker-clad army wins battle of the mall. (2001, August 28). *New York Times*, pp. A1, A11.

Snitz, B. E., O'Meara, E. S., Carlson, M. C., Arnold, A. M., Ives, D. G., Rapp, S. R., . . . Ginkgo Evaluation of Memory (GEM) Study Investigators. (2009). Gingko biloba for preventing cognitive decline in older adults: A randomized trial. *Journal of the American Medical Association, 302*, 2663–2670.

Snowdon, D. A., Greiner, L. H., & Markesbery, W. R. (2000). Linguistic ability in early life and the neuropathology of Alzheimer's disease and cerebrovascular disease: Findings from the Nun study. *Annals of the New York Academy of Sciences, 903*, 34–38.

Snyder, P. (2001). Effects of age on testicular function and consequences of testosterone treatment. *Journal of Clinical Endocrinology Metabolism, 86*, 2369–2372.

Solberg, L. I., Asche, S. E., Boyle, R. G., Boucher, J. L., & Pronk, N. P. (2005). Frequency of physician-directed assistance for smoking cessation in patients receiving cessation medications. *Archives of Internal Medicine, 165*, 656–660.

Solis, H. (2011). Caring for our caregivers. Official blog of the U.S. Department of Labor. Retrieved from http://social.dol.gov/blog/careing-for-our-caregivers/

Solomon, P. R., Adams, F., Silver, A., Zimmer, J., & DeVeaux, R. (2002). Gingko for memory enhancement: A randomized controlled trial. *Journal of the American Medical Association, 288*, 835–840.

Sorbero, M. E., Saul, M. I., Liu, H., & Resnick, N. M. (2012). Are geriatricians more efficient than other physicians at managing inpatient care for elderly patients? *Journal of the American Geriatrics Society, 60,* 869–876.

Sperber, S. J., Shah, L. P., Gilbert, R. D., Ritchey, T. W., & Monto, A. S. (2004). Echinacea purpura for prevention of experimental rhinovirus colds. *Clinical Infectious Disease, 38,* 1367–1371.

Spiegel, D. (2001). Mind matters: Group therapy and survival in breast cancer. *New England Journal of Medicine, 345,* 1767–1768.

Spiegel, D., Bloom, J. R., Kraemer, H. C., & Gottheil, E. (1989). Effect of psychosocial treatment on survival of patients with metastatic breast cancer. *Lancet, 2,* 888–891.

Spira, J. (2001). Comparison of St. John's wort and imipramine: Study design casts doubt on St. John's wort in treating depression. *British Medical Journal, 322,* 493–494.

Spitzer, R. L., Terman, M., Williams, J. B., Terman, J. S., Malt, U. F., Singer, F., & Lewy, A. J. (1999). Jet lag: Clinical features, validation of a new syndrome-specific scale, and lack of response to melatonin in a randomized, double-blind trial. *American Journal of Psychiatry, 156,* 1392–1396.

Squires, S. (2002, October 14–20). We're fat and getting fatter. *The Washington Post National Weekly Edition,* p. 34.

Staessen, J. A., Fagard, R., Thijs, L., Celis, H., Birkenhäger, W. H., Bulpitt, C. J., . . . Zanchetti, A. (1998). Subgroup and per-protocol analysis of the randomized European trial on isolated systolic hypertension in the elderly. *Archives of Internal Medicine, 158,* 1681–1691.

Stafford, R. S., Drieling, R. L., & Hersh, A. L. (2004). National trends in osteoporosis visits and osteoporosis treatment, 1988–2003. *Archives of Internal Medicine, 164,* 1525–1530.

Stamatakis, E., Davis, M., Stathi, A., & Hamer, M. (2012). Association between multiple indicators of objectively-measured and self-rated cardiometabolic risk in older adults. *Preventive Medicine, 54,* 82–87.

Statin drugs: Benefits beyond cholesterol lowering. (2001, June). *Tufts University Health & Nutrition Letter,* p. 6.

Stead, L. F., Bergson, G., & Lancaster, T. (2008). Physician advice for smoking cessation. *Cochrane Database Systematic Review, 16,* CD000165.

Stearns, S. C., Bernard, S. L., Fasick, S. B., Schwartz, R., Konrad, T. R., Ory, M. G., & DeFriese, G. H. (2000). The economic implications of self-care: The effect of lifestyle, functional adaptations, and medical self-care among a national sample of Medicare beneficiaries. *American Journal of Public Health, 90,* 1608–1612.

Stefanek, M. E., Palmer, S. C., Thombs, B. D., & Coyne, J. C. (2009, October 15). Finding what is not there: Unwarranted claims of an effect of psychosocial intervention on recurrence and survival. *Cancer* (e-publication).

Steffen-Batey, L., Nichaman, M. Z., Goff, D. C., Jr., Frankowski, R. F., Hanis, C. L., Ramsey, D. J., & Labarthe, D. R. (2000). Change in level of physical activity and risk of all-cause mortality or reinfarction: The Corpus Christi Heart Project. *Circulation, 102,* 2204–2209.

Stephens, N. G., Parsons, A., Schofield, P. M., Kelly, F., Cheeseman, K., & Mitchinson, M. J. (1996). Randomised controlled trial of vitamin E in patients with coronary disease: Cambridge heart antioxidant study (CHAOS). *Lancet, 347,* 781–786.

Steward, H., et al. (1998). *Sugar busters.* New York, NY: Ballantine Books.

Stewart, K. J., Hiatt, W. R., Regensteiner, J. G., & Hirsch, A. T. (2002). Exercise training for claudication. *New England Journal of Medicine, 347,* 1941–1951.

St. John's wort and all. (2000, September). *Nutrition Action Healthletter,* pp. 6–8.

Stock, R. D., Reece, D., & Cesario, L. (2004). Developing a comprehensive interdisciplinary senior health-care practice. *Journal of the American Geriatrics Society, 52*, 2128–2133.

Stokols, D., Pelletier, K. R., & Fielding, J. E. (1995). Integration of medical care and worksite health promotion. *Journal of the American Medical Association, 273*, 1136–1142.

Stolberg, S. (2002). Minorities get inferior care, even if insured, study finds. *The New York Times*, pp. A1, A30.

Stone, A. A., Schwartz, J. E., Broderick, J. E., & Deaton, A. (2010). A snapshot of the age distribution of psychological well-being in the U.S. *Proceedings of the National Academy of Sciences, 107*, 9985–9990.

Stone, R. I., Bryant, N., & Barbarotta, L. (2009). Supporting culture change: Working toward smarter state nursing home regulation. *Commonwealth Fund, 68*, 1.

Stores, G., & Crawford, C. (1998). Medical student education in sleep and its disorders. *Journal of Royal College of Physicians (London), 32*, 149–153.

Strawbridge, W. J., Cohen, R. D., Shema, S. J., & Kaplan, G. A. (1997). Frequent attendance at religious services and mortality over 28 years. *American Journal of Public Health, 87*, 957–961.

Strawbridge, W. J., Deleger, S., Roberts, R. E., & Kaplan, G. A. (2002). Physical activity reduces the risk of subsequent depression for older adults. *American Journal of Epidemiology, 156*, 328–334.

Street, R. L., Jr., Gordon, H. S., Ward, M. M., Krupat, E., & Kravitz, R. L. (2005). Patient participation in medical consultations: Why some patients are more involved than others. *Medical Care, 43*, 960–969.

Study looks at patients' online use. (2002, May 6). *American Medical News*, p. 28.

Sturm, R., & Cohen, D. (2004). Suburban sprawl and physical and mental health. *Public Health, 118*, 488–496.

Sulmasy, D., & Rahn, M. (2001). I was sick and you came to visit me: Time spent at the bedsides of seriously ill patients with poor prognoses. *American Journal of Medicine, 111*, 385–389.

The surprising power of placebos. (2000, February). *Self Healing*, pp. 2–3.

Surwit, R. S., van Tilburg, M. A., Zucker, N., McCaskill, C. C., Parekh, P., Feinglos, M. N., . . . Lane, J. D. (2002). Stress management improves long-term glycemic control in type 2 diabetes. *Diabetes Care, 25*, 30–34.

Sutherland, J. M., Fisher, E. S., & Skinner, J. S. (2009). Getting past denial: The high cost of health care in the United States. *New England Journal of Medicine, 361*, 1227–1230.

Sutton, S. (2001). Back to the drawing board? A review of applications of the trans-theoretical model to substance use. *Addiction, 96*, 175–186.

Swan, J. (2005, December 14). *Physical activity of boomers compared to other age cohorts*. Paper presented at American Public Health Association Annual Meeting, Philadelphia.

Swoboda, F. (2001). Study challenges image of older drivers as dangerous. *The Washington Post*, p. E1.

Syme, L. (2003). Psychosocial interventions to improve successful aging. *Annals of Internal Medicine, 139*, 400–402.

Szabo, L. (2009, August 4). Number of Americans taking antidepressants doubles. *USA Today*, p. 3.

Tabar, L., Vitak, B., Chen, H. H., Yen, M. F., Duffy, S. W., & Smith, R. A. (2001). Beyond randomized controlled trials. *Cancer, 91*, 1724–1731.

Taguchi, A., Ohtsuka, M., Nakamoto, T., & Tanimoto, K. (2006). Screening for osteoporosis by dental panoramic radiographs. *Clinical Calcium, 16*, 67–73.

Tai-Seale, M., McGuire, T., Colenda, C., Rosen, D., & Cook, M. A. (2007). Two-minute mental health care for elderly patients. *Journal of the American Geriatrics Society, 55,* 1903–1911.

Tan, E. J., Rebok, G. W., Yu, Q., Frangakis, C. E., Carlson, M. C., Wang, T., . . . Fried, L. P. (2009). The long-term relationship between high-intensity volunteering and physical activity in older African American women. *Journal of Gerontology: Psychological/Social Sciences, 64,* 304–311.

Tanaka, H., Monahan, K. D., & Seals, D. R. (2001). Age-predicted maximal heart rate revisited. *Journal of the American College of Cardiology, 37,* 153–156.

Tanasescu, M., et al. (2003, April). Physical activity in relation to cardiovascular disease and total mortality among men with type 2 diabetes. *Circulation* (e-publication).

Tanasescu, M., Leitzmann, M. F., Rimm, E. B., Willett, W. C., Stampfer, M. J., & Hu, F. B. (2002). Exercise type and intensity in relation to coronary heart disease in men. *Journal of the American Medical Association, 288,* 1994–2000.

Tarn, D. M., Heritage, J., Paterniti, D. A., Hays, R. D., Kravitz, R. L., & Wenger, N. S. (2006). Physician communication when prescribing new medications. *Archives of Internal Medicine, 166,* 1855–1862.

Taylor, A., Jacques, P. F., Chylack, L. T., Jr., Hankinson, S. E., Khu, P. M., Rogers, G., . . . Willett, W. C. (2002). Long-term intake of vitamins and carotenoids and odds of early age-related cortical and posterior subcapsular lens opacities. *American Journal of Clinical Nutrition, 75,* 540–549.

Taylor, D. H., Jr., Hasselblad, V., Henley, S. J., Thun, M. J., & Sloan, F. A. (2002). Benefits of smoking cessation for longevity. *American Journal of Public Health, 92,* 990–996.

Taylor, H. R., Tikellis, G., Robman, L. D., McCarty, C. A., & McNeil, J. J. (2002). Vitamin E supplementation and macular degeneration: Randomised controlled trial. *British Medical Journal, 325,* 11–14.

Temel, J. S., Greer, J. A., Muzikansky, A., Gallagher, E. R., Admane, S., Jackson, V. A., . . . Lynch, T. J. (2010). Early palliative care for patients with metastic, non-small cell lung cancer. *New England Journal of Medicine, 363,* 733–742.

Teno, J. M., Fisher, E. S., Hamel, M. B., Coppola, K., & Dawson, N. V. (2002). Medical care inconsistent with patients' treatment goals: Association with 1-year Medicare resource use and survival. *Journal of the American Geriatrics Society, 50,* 496–500.

Terpenning, M. (2005). Geriatric orgal health and pneumonia risk. *Clinical Infectious Diseases, 40,* 1807–1810.

Thacker, S. B., Gilchrist, J., Stroup, D. F., & Kimsey, C. D., Jr. (2004). The impact of stretching on sports injury risk: A systematic review of the literature. *Medical Science & Sports Exercise, 36,* 371–378.

Theodosakis, J. (1997). *The arthritis cure.* New York, NY: St. Martin's Press.

Thomas, D. B., Gao, D. L., Ray, R. M., Wang, W. W., Allison, C. J., Chen, F. L., . . . Self, S. G. (2002). Randomized trial of breast self-examination in Shanghai: Final results. *Journal of the National Cancer Institute, 94,* 1445–1457.

Thomas, K. S., Muir, K. R., Doherty, M., Jones, A. C., O'Reilly, S. C., & Bassey, E. J. (2002). Home based exercise programme for knee pain and knee osteoarthritis: Randomised controlled trial. *British Medical Journal, 325,* 752.

Thomas, W. (1994). *The Eden Alternative.* Acton, MA: VanderWyk & Burnham.

Thomas, W. (1996). *Life worth living.* Acton, MA: VanderWyk & Burnham.

Thomas, W. (2004). *What are old people for?* Acton, MA: VanderWyk & Burnham.

Thomas, W., & Blanchard, J. (2009). Moving beyond place: Aging in community. *Generations, 33,* 12–17.

Thompson, I. M., Pauler, D. K., Goodman, P. J., Tangen, C. M., Lucia, M. S., Parnes, H. L., . . . Coltman, C. A., Jr. (2004). Prevalence of prostate cancer among men with a prostate-specific antigen level. *New England Journal of Medicine, 350,* 2239–2246.

Thompson, R., Haber, D., Chambers, C., Fanuiel, L., Krohn, K., & Smith, A. J. (1998). Orientation to community in a family medicine residency program. *Family Medicine, 30,* 22–26.

Thompson, R., Haber, D., Fanuiel, L., Krohn, K., & Chambers, C. (1996). COPC in a family medicine residency program. *Family Medicine, 28,* 326–330.

Thorogood, M., Simera, I., Dowler, E., Summerbell, C., & Brunner, E. (2007). A systematic review of population and community dietary interventions to prevent cancer. *Nutritional Research Review, 20,* 74–88.

Thorson, J. (2000). *Aging in a changing society.* New York, NY: Taylor & Francis.

Thun, M. J., Peto, R., Lopez, A. D., Monaco, J. H., Henley, S. J., Heath, C. W., Jr., & Doll, R. (1997). Alcohol consumption and mortality among middle-aged and elderly U.S. adults. *New England Journal of Medicine, 337,* 1705–1714.

Tilburt, J. C., Emanuel, E. J., Kaptchuk, T. J., Curlin, F. A., & Miller, F. G. (2008). Prescribing "placebo treatments": Results of national survey of US internists and rheumatologists. *British Medical Journal, 337,* 1938.

Time to deal with hearing loss? (2002). *Consumer Reports on Health, 14,* 1, 4–6.

Tornstam, L. (1989). Gero-transcendence. *Aging, 1,* 55–63.

Tough anti-tobacco effort cited for 14% decline in lung cancer. (2000, December 1). *Houston Chronicle,* p. 9A.

Trafford, A. (2000, July 3). What will people do with the extra decade? *Houston Chronicle,* p. 3C.

Trappe, S., Williamson, D., & Godard, M. (2002). Maintenance of whole muscle strength and size following resistance training in older men. *Journal of Gerontology: Biological Sciences, 57A,* B138–B143.

Trichopoulou, A., Orfanos, P., Norat, T., Bueno-de-Mesquita, B., Ocké, M. C., Peeters, P. H., . . . Trichopoulos, D. (2005). Modified Mediterranean diet and survival: EPIC-elderly prospective cohort study. *British Medical Journal, 330,* 991.

Trichopoulou, A., Vasilopoulou, E., & Lagiou, A. (1999). Mediterranean diet and coronary heart disease: Are antioxidants critical? *Nutrition Reviews, 57,* 253–255.

Tsai, A., & Wadden, T. (2005). Systematic review: An evaluation of major commercial weight loss programs in the United States. *Annals of Internal Medicine, 142,* 56–66.

Tsai, A. C., Morton, S. C., Mangione, C. M., & Keeler, E. B. (2005). A meta-analysis of interventions to improve care for chronic illnesses. *American Journal of Managed Care, 11,* 478–488.

Tseng, H. F., Chi, M., Smith, N., Marcy, S. M., Sy, L. S., & Jacobsen, S. J. (2012). Herpes zoster vaccine and the incidence of recurrent Herpes zoster in an immunocompetent elderly population. *Journal of Infectious Diseases, 206,* 190–196.

Tucker, K. L., Rich, S., Rosenberg, I., Jacques, P., Dallal, G., Wilson, P. W., & Selhub, J. (2000). Plasma vitamin B-12 concentrations relate to intake source in the Framingham Offspring Study. *American Journal of Clinical Nutrition, 71,* 514–522.

Tuomilehto, J., Lindström, J., Eriksson, J. G., Valle, T. T., Hämäläinen, H., Ilanne-Parikka, P., . . . Finnish Diabetes Prevention Study Group. (2001). Prevention of type 2 diabetes mellitus by changes in lifestyle among subjects with impaired glucose tolerance. *New England Journal of Medicine, 344,* 1343–1350.

Turner, R. B., Bauer, R., Woelkart, K., Hulsey, T. C., & Gangemi, J. D. (2005). An evaluation of *Echinacea angustifolia* in experimental rhinovirus infections. *New England Journal of Medicine, 353,* 341–348.

Uebelhack, R., Blohmer, J. U., Graubaum, H. J., Busch, R., Gruenwald, J., & Wernecke, K. D. (2006). Black cohosh and St. John's wort for climacteric com plaints: A randomized trial. *Obstetrical Gynecology, 107,* 247–255.

Umberson, D., Williams, K., Powers, D. A., Liu, H., & Needham, B. (2006). You make me sick: Marital quality and health over the life course. *Journal of Health and Social Behavior, 47*, 1–16.

Unutzer, J., Katon, W., Callahan, C. M., Williams, J. W., Jr., Hunkeler, E., Harpole, L., . . . Oishi, S. (2003). Depression treatment in a sample of 1,801 depressed older adults in primary care. *Journal of the American Geriatrics Society, 51*, 505–514.

Unutzer, J., & Park, M. (2012). Strategies to improve the management of depression in primary care. *Primary Care, 39*, 415–431.

USDHHS. (1979). *Healthy people: The surgeon general's report on health promotion and disease prevention.* Washington, DC: USGPO.

USPSTF. (1989). *Guide to clinical preventive services: An assessment of the effectiveness of 169 interventions.* Baltimore, MD: Williams & Wilkins.

USPSTF. (1996). *Guide to clinical preventive services.* Baltimore, MD: Williams & Wilkins.

USPSTF. (2000). Colon cancer screening (USPSTF recommendation). *Journal of the American Geriatrics Society, 48*, 333–335.

Vaillant, G. (2002). *Aging well: Surprising guideposts to a happier life from the landmark Harvard study of adult development.* Boston, MA: Little, Brown.

Vaillant, G., & Western, R. (2001). Healthy aging among inner-city men. *International Psychogeriatrics, 13*, 425–437.

Valcour, V. G., Masaki, K. H., & Blanchette, P. L. (2002). Self-reported driving, cognitive status, and physician awareness of cognitive impairment. *Journal of the American Geriatrics Society, 50*, 1265–1267.

Valenzuela, M. J., Matthews, F. E., Brayne, C., Ince, P., Halliday, G., Kril, J. J., . . . Medical Research Council Cognitive Function and Ageing Study. (2012). Multiple biological pathways link cognitive lifestyle to protection from dementia. *Biological Psychiatry, 71*, 783–791.

Valtin, H. (2008, June). In the drink: Do we really need 8 glasses of water a day? *Nutrition Action Healthletter,* pp. 12–13.

Van Dongen, M. C., van Rossum, E., Kessels, A. G., Sielhorst, H. J., & Knipschild, P. G. (2000). The efficacy of ginkgo for elderly people with dementia and age-associated memory impairment: New results of a randomized clinical trial. *Journal of the American Geriatrics Society, 48*, 1183–1194.

Van Leeuwen, R., Boekhoorn, S., Vingerling, J. R., Witteman, J. C., Klaver, C. C., Hofman, A., & de Jong, P. T. (2005). Dietary intake of antioxidants and risk of age-related macular degeneration. *Journal of the American Medical Association, 294*, 3101–3107.

Varghese, R., & Norman, P. (2004). Carotid endarterectomy in octogenarians. *New Zealand Journal of Surgery, 74*, 215–217.

Vasan, R. S., Beiser, A., Seshadri, S., Larson, M. G., Kannel, W. B., D'Agostino, R. B., & Levy, D. (2002). Residual lifetime risk for developing hypertension in middle-aged women and men: The Framingham Heart Study. *Journal of the American Medical Association, 287*, 1003–1010.

Vasan, R. S., Larson, M. G., Leip, E. P., Evans, J. C., O'Donnell, C. J., Kannel, W. B., & Levy, D. (2001). Impact of high-normal blood pressure on the risk of cardio vascular disease. *New England Journal of Medicine, 345*, 1291–1297.

Vickers, A. J. (2011). Empirical evaluation of guidelines on prostate-specific antigen velocity in prostate cancer detection. *Journal of the National Cancer Institute, 103*, 1635–1636.

Vickers, A. J., Rees, R. W., Zollman, C. E., McCarney, R., Smith, C. M., Ellis, N., . . . Van Haselen, R. (2004). Acupuncture for chronic headache in primary care: Large, pragmatic, randomized trial. *British Medical Journal, 328*, 744–747.

Viera, A. J., Kshirsagar, A. V., & Hinderliter, A. L. (2007). Lifestyle modification advice for lowering or controlling high blood pressure: Who's getting it? *Journal of Clinical Hypertension, 11*, 850–858.

Vik, S. A., Maxwell, C. J., & Hogan, D. B. (2004). Measurement, correlates, and health outcomes of medication adherence among seniors. *Annals of Pharmacotherapy, 38*, 303–312.

Vincent, K., & Braith, R. (2002). Resistance exercise and bone turnover in elderly men and women. *Medicine & Science in Sports & Exercise, 34*, 17–23.

Vincent, K. R., Braith, R. W., Feldman, R. A., Kallas, H. E., & Lowenthal, D. T. (2002b). Improved cardiorespiratory endurance following 6 months of resistance exercise in elderly men and women. *Archives of Internal Medicine, 162*, 673–678.

Vincent, K. R., Braith, R. W., Feldman, R. A., Magyari, P. M., Cutler, R. B., Persin, S. A., . . . Lowenthal, D. T. (2002). Resistance exercise and physical performance in adults aged 60 to 83. *Journal of the American Geriatrics Society, 50*, 1100–1107.

Vogelzangs, N., Kritchevsky, S. B., Beekman, A. T., Newman, A. B., Satterfield, S., Simonsick, E. M., . . . Penninx, B. W. (2008). Depressive symptoms and change in abdominal obesity in older persons. *Archives of General Psychiatry, 65*, 1386–1393.

Volandes, A. E., Brandeis, G. H., Davis, A. D., Paasche-Orlow, M. K., Gillick, M. R., Chang, Y., . . . Mitchell, S. L. (2012). A randomized controlled trial of a goals-of-care video for elderly patients admitted to skilled nursing facilities. *Journal of Palliative Medicine, 15*, 805–811.

Volandes, A. E., Paasche-Orlow, M., Gillick, M. R., Cook, E. F., Shaykevich, S., Abbo, E. D., & Lehmann, L. (2008). Health literacy, not race, predicts end-of-life care. *Journal of Palliative Medicine, 11*, 754–762.

Von Faber, M., Bootsma-van der Wiel, A., van Exel, E., Gussekloo, J., Lagaay, A. M., van Dongen, E., . . . Westendorp, R. G. (2001). Successful aging in the oldest old: Who can be characterized as aged? *Archives of Internal Medicine, 161*, 2694–2700.

Vorona, R. (2009). Sleep and sleep disorders in later life. *Activities in Geriatrics and Gerontology Education and Research* (Virginia Center on Aging), *24*, 1–5.

Waber, R. L., Shiv, B., Carmon, Z., & Ariely, D. (2008). Commercial features of placebo and therapeutic efficacy. *Journal of the American Medical Association, 299*, 1016–1017.

Waite, L. J., Laumann, E. O., Das, A., & Schumm, L. P. (2009). Sexuality: Measures of part-nerships, practices, attitudes, and problems in the national social life, health, and aging study. *Journal of Gerontology: Psychological/Social Sciences, 64*(Suppl.), 156–166.

Wakimoto, P., & Block, G. (2001). Dietary intake, dietary patterns, and changes with age: An epidemiological perspective. *Journal of Gerontology, Series A, 56A*(special issue II), 65–80.

Wald, D., & Wald, N. (2012). Implementation of a simple, age-based strategy in the prevention of cardiovascular disease: The Polypill approach. *Journal of Evaluation in Clinical Practice, 18*, 612–615.

Wald, N., & Law, M. (2003). A strategy to reduce cardiovascular disease by more than 80%. *British Medical Journal, 326*, 1419.

Wallace, S. P., Cochran, S. D., Durazo, E. M., & Ford, C. L. (2011, March). The health of aging lesbian, gay and bisexual adults in California. *California Health Interview Survey of the UCLA Center for Health Policy Research*, pp. 1–8.

Wallerstein, N., & Bernstein, E. (1988). Empowerment education: Freier's ideas adapted to health education. *Health Education Quarterly, 15*, 379–394.

Wallston, B. S., Wallston, K. A., Kaplan, G. D., & Maides, S. A. (1976). Development and validation of the health locus of control scale. *Journal of Consulting and Clinical Psychology, 44*, 580–585.

Wang, L., Larson, E. B., Bowen, J. D., & van Belle, G. (2006). Performance-based physical function and future dementia in older people. *Archives of Internal Medicine, 166,* 1115–1120.

Wannamethee, S. G., Shaper, A. G., & Walker, M. (2001). Physical activity and risk of cancer in middle-aged men. *British Journal of Cancer, 85,* 1311–1316.

Watson, K. H., Chandrasekran, S., & Steinle, N. I. (2012, February). Popular diets: Examining weight loss diets for geriatric patients. *Clinical Geriatrics,* 25–31.

Watt, L., & Cappeliez, P. (2000). Integrative and instrumental reminiscence therapies for depression in older adults. *Aging & Mental Health, 4,* 166–183.

Wechsler, H., Levine, S., Idelson, R. K., Rohman, M., & Taylor, J. O. (1983). The physician's role in health promotion: A survey of primary care practitioners. *New England Journal of Medicine, 308,* 97–100.

Wei, M., Gibbons, L. W., Kampert, J. B., Nichaman, M. Z., & Blair, S. N. (2000). Low cardiorespiratory fitness and physical inactivity as predictors of mortality in men with type 2 diabetes. *Annals of Internal Medicine, 132,* 605–611.

Weinstein, A. R., Sesso, H. D., Lee, I. M., Cook, N. R., Manson, J. E., Buring, J. E., & Gaziano, J. M. (2004). Relationship of physical activity vs. body mass index with type 2 diabetes in women. *Journal of the American Medical Association, 292,* 1188–1194.

Wen, C. P., Wai, J. P., Tsai, M. K., Yang, Y. C., Cheng, T. Y., Lee, M. C., . . . Wu, X. (2012). Minimum amount of physical activity for reduced mortality and extended life expectancy. *Lancet, 378,* 1244–1253.

Weuve, J., Kang, J. H., Manson, J. E., Breteler, M. M., Ware, J. H., & Grodstein, F. (2004). Physical activity, including walking, and cognitive function in older women. *Journal of the American Medical Association, 292,* 1454–1461.

Weyant, R. J., Newman, A. B., Kritchevsky, S. B., Bretz, W. A., Corby, P. M., Ren, D., . . . Harris, T. (2004). Periodontal disease and weight loss in older adults. *Journal of the American Geriatrics Society, 52,* 547–553.

Wheeler, J. A., Gorey, K. M., & Greenblatt, B. (1998). The beneficial effects of volunteering for older volunteers and the people they serve: A meta-analysis. *International Journal of Aging and Human Development, 47,* 69–79.

White, A. M., Philogene, G. S., Fine, L., & Sinha, S. (2009). Social support and self-reported health status of older adults in the United States. *American Journal of Public Health, 99,* 1872–1878.

Whitehead, M. (1997). Editorial: How useful is the "stages of change" model? *Health Education Journal, 56,* 111–112.

Whitmer, R. A., Gunderson, E. P., Barrett-Connor, E., Quesenberry, C. P., Jr., & Yaffe, K. (2005). Obesity in middle age and future risk of dementia: A 27 year longitudinal population based study. *British Medical Journal, 330,* 1339–1340.

Whitson, H. E., Heflin, M. T., & Burchett, B. M. (2006). Patterns and predictors of smoking cessation in an elderly cohort. *Journal of the American Geriatrics Society, 54,* 466–471.

Wieland, D., Lamb, V. L., Sutton, S. R., Boland, R., Clark, M., Friedman, S., . . . Eleazer, G. P. (2000). Hospitalization in the program of all-inclusive care for the elderly (PACE). *Journal of the American Geriatrics Society, 48,* 1529–1530.

Wierzalis, E., et al. (2006). Gay men and aging. In D. Kimmel et al. (Eds.), *Lesbian, gay, bisexual, and transgender aging* (pp. 91–109). New York, NY: Columbia University Press.

Willett, W. (2005). *Eat, drink, and be healthy.* Boston, MA: Free Press/Simon & Schuster.

Williams, J. W., Jr., Noël, P. H., Cordes, J. A., Ramirez, G., & Pignone, M. (2002). Rational clinical examination: Is this patient clinically depressed? *Journal of the American Medical Association, 287,* 1160–1167.

Williams, J. E., Nieto, F. J., Sanford, C. P., Couper, D. J., & Tyroler, H. A. (2002). The association between trait anger and incident stroke risk: The ARIC Study. *Stroke, 33,* 13–20.

Williams, J. E., Nieto, F. J., Sanford, C. P., & Tyroler, H. A. (2001). Effects of an angry temperament on coronary heart disease risk: The atherosclerosis risk in communities study. *American Journal of Epidemiology, 154,* 230–235.

Williams, K. N., Herman, R., Gajewski, B., & Wilson, K. (2009). Elderspeak communication: Impact on dementia care. *American Journal of Alzheimer's Disease and Other Dementias, 24,* 11–20.

Williams, M. (1996). Increasing participation in health promotion among older African-Americans. *American Journal of Health Behaviors, 20,* 389–399.

Williams, R. B., Barefoot, J. C., Califf, R. M., Haney, T. L., Saunders, W. B., Pryor, D. B., . . . Mark, D. B. (1992). Prognostic importance of social and economic resources among medically treated patients with angiographically documented coronary artery disease. *Journal of the American Medical Association, 267,* 520–524.

Willis, C. M., Church, S. M., Guest, C. M., Cook, W. A., McCarthy, N., Bransbury, A. J., . . . Church, J. C. (2004). Olfactory detection of human bladder cancer by dogs. *British Medical Journal, 329,* 712.

Wilson, D. (2007, April 15). Aging: Disease or business opportunity? *The New York Times,* pp. B1, B7.

Wilson, K. M., Kasperzyk, J. L., Rider, J. R., Kenfield, S., van Dam, R. M., Stampfer, M. J., . . . Mucci, L. A. (2011). Coffee consumption and prostate cancer risk and progression. *Journal of the National Cancer Institute, 103,* 876–884.

Wilson, M. (2005). Cholesterol and the aged: And the beat goes on. *Journal of Gerontology: Medical Sciences, 60A,* 600–602.

Wilson, R., Mendes De Leon, C. F., Barnes, L. L., Schneider, J. A., Bienias, J. L., Evans, D. A., & Bennett, D. A. (2002). Participation in cognitively stimulating activities and risk of incident Alzheimer's disease. *Journal of the American Medical Association, 287,* 742–748.

Wilt, T., Ishani, A., Stark, G., MacDonald, R., Lau, J., & Mulrow, C. (1998). Saw palmetto extracts for treatment of benign prostatic hyperplasia. *Journal of the American Medical Association, 280,* 1604–1609.

Wilt, T. J., & Brawer, M. K. (2012). The prostate cancer intervention versus observation trial. *New England Journal of Medicine.*

Wing, R., & Jeffery, R. (1999). Benefits of recruiting participants with friends and increasing social support for weight loss and maintenance. *Journal of Consulting Clinical Psychology, 67,* 132–138.

Wisconsin study describes rural obesity problem. (1996, April 1). *American Medical News,* p. 25.

Witt, C., Brinkhaus, B., Jena, S., Linde, K., Streng, A., Wagenpfeil, S., . . . Willich, S. N. (2005). Acupuncture in patients with osteoarthritis of the knee: A randomized trial. *Lancet, 366,* 136–143.

Woelk, H., et al. (2000). Comparison of St. John's wort and imipramine for treating depression: Randomised controlled trial. *British Medical Journal, 321,* 536–539.

Wolf, S. L., Barnhart, H. X., Kutner, N. G., McNeely, E., Coogler, C., & Xu, T. (1996). Reducing frailty and falls in older persons: An investigation of Tai Chi and computerized balance training. *Journal of the American Geriatrics Society, 44,* 489–497.

Wolff, J., & Greenberg, D. (2012). Going it together: Persistence of older adults' accompaniment to physician visits by a family companion, *Journal of the American Geriatrics Society, 60,* 106–112.

Wolff, J. L., Dy, S. M., Frick, K. D., & Kasper, J. D. (2007). End-of-life care. *Archives of Internal Medicine, 167,* 40–46.

Wolfson, L., Whipple, R., Derby, C., Judge, J., King, M., Amerman, P., . . . Smyers, D. (1996). Balance and strength training in older adults: Intervention gains and Tai Chi maintenance. *Journal of the American Geriatrics Society, 44,* 498–506.

Woods, B., Aguirre, E., Spector, A. E., & Orrell, M. (2012). Cognitive stimulation to improve cognitive functioning in people with dementia. *Cochrane Database of Systematic Reviews, 2,* 1469–1493x.

Woodward, N., & Wallston, B. (1987). Age and health care beliefs: Self-efficacy as a mediator of low desire for control. *Psychology and Aging, 2,* 3–8.

Woodward, W. A., Huang, E. H., McNeese, M. D., Perkins, G. H., Tucker, S. L., Strom, E. A., . . . Buchholz, T. A. (2006). African-American race is associated with a poorer overall survival rate for breast cancer patients treated with mastectomy and doxorubicin-based chemotherapy. *Cancer, 107,* 2662–2668.

Woolf, S., & Johnson, R. (2000). A one-year audit of topics and domains in the *Journal of the American Medical Association* and the *New England Journal of Medicine. American Journal of Preventive Medicine, 19,* 79–86.

Wu, C. H., Erickson, S. R., Piette, J. D., & Balkrishnan, R. (2012). Mental health resource utilization and health care costs associated with race. *Journal of the National Medical Association, 104,* 78–88.

Wynd, C. (2005). Guided health imagery for smoking cessation and long-term abstinence. *Journal of Nursing Scholarship, 37,* 245–250.

Yaffe, K., Barnes, D., Nevitt, M., Lui, L. Y., & Covinsky, K. (2001). A prospective study of physical activity and cognitive decline in elderly women: Women who walk. *Archives of Internal Medicine, 161,* 1703–1708.

Yaffe, K., Barrett-Connor, E., Lin, F., & Grady, D. (2002). Serum lipoprotein levels, statin use, and cognitive function in older women. *Archives of Neurology, 59,* 378–384.

Yaffe, K., Laffan, A. M., Harrison, S. L., Redline, S., Spira, A. P., Ensrud, K. E., . . . Stone, K. L. (2011). Sleep-disordered breathing, hypoxia, and risk of mild cognitive impairment and dementia in older women. *Journal of the American Medical Association, 306,* 613–619.

Yahnke, R. (2005). Heroes of their own stories: Expressions of aging in international cinema. *Gerontology & Geriatrics Education, 26,* 57–76.

Yancy, W. S., Guyton, J. R., Bakst, R. P., Tomlin, K. F., Bryson, W. H., Perkins, C. E., & Westman, E. C. (2001). A randomized controlled trial of a very-low carbohydrate diet with nutritional supplements versus a very-low-fat/low-calorie diet. *Obesity Research, 9*(Suppl. 3), 17.

Yanovski, J. A., Yanovski, S. Z., Sovik, K. N., Nguyen, T. T., O'Neil, P. M., & Sebring, N. G. (2000). A prospective study of holiday weight gain. *New England Journal of Medicine, 342,* 861–867.

Yarnall, K. S., Pollak, K. I., Østbye, T., Krause, K. M., & Michener, L. J. (2003). Primary care: Is there enough time for prevention? *American Journal of Public Health, 93,* 635–641.

Yudkin, P., Hey, K., Roberts, S., Welch, S., Murphy, M., & Walton, R. (2003). Abstinence from smoking eight years after participation in randomized controlled trial of nicotine patch. *British Medical Journal, 327,* 28–29.

Yueh, B., Collins, M. P., Souza, P. E., Boyko, E. J., Loovis, C. F., Heagerty, P. J., . . . Hedrick, S. C. (2010). Long-term effectiveness of screening for hearing loss. *Journal of the American Geriatrics Society, 58,* 427–434.

Yuen, H. K., Huang, P., Burik, J. K., & Smith, T. G. (2008). Impact of participating in volunteer activities for residents living in long-term-care facilities. *American Journal of Occupational Therapy, 62,* 71–76.

Yusuf, S., Hawken, S., Ounpuu, S., Bautista, L., Franzosi, M. G., Commerford, P., . . . INTERHEART Study Investigators. (2005). Obesity and the risk of myocardial infarction in 27,000 participants from 52 countries. *Lancet, 366,* 1640–1649.

Zandi, P. P., Sparks, D. L., Khachaturian, A. S., Tschanz, J., Norton, M., Steinberg, M., . . . Cache County Study investigators. (2005). Do statins reduce risk of incident dementia and Alzheimer disease? *Archives of General Psychiatry, 62,* 217–224.

Zarowitz, B., & Hauersperger, K. (2012). Changing recommendations for calcium supplementation. *Geriatric Nursing, 33,* 384–386.

Zauber, A. G., Winawer, S. J., O'Brien, M. J., Lansdorp-Vogelaar, I., van Ballegooijen, M., Hankey, B. F., . . . Waye, J. D. (2012). Colonoscopic polypectomy and long-term prevention of colorectal-cancer deaths. *New England Journal of Medicine, 366,* 687–696.

Zeni, A. L., Hoffman, M. D., & Clifford, P. S. (1996). Energy expenditure with indoor exercise machines. *Journal of the American Medical Association, 275,* 1424–1427.

Zhan, C., Sangl, J., Bierman, A. S., Miller, M. R., Friedman, B., Wickizer, S. W., & Meyer, G. S. (2001). Potentially inappropriate medication use in the community-dwelling elderly: Findings from the 1996 Medical Expenditure Panel Survey. *Journal of the American Medical Association, 286,* 2823–2829.

Zhan, W., Cruickshanks, K. J., Klein, B. E., Klein, R., Huang, G. H., Pankow, J. S., . . . Tweed, T. S. (2010). Generational differences in the prevalence of hearing impairment in older adults. *American Journal of Epidemiology, 171,* 260–266.

Zhang, Y., Cantor, K. P., Dosemeci, M., Lynch, C. F., Zhu, Y., & Zheng, T. (2006). Occupational and leisure-time physical activity and risk of colon cancer by subsite. *Journal of Occupational and Environmental Medicine, 48,* 236–243.

Zhu, S. H., Anderson, C. M., Tedeschi, G. J., Rosbrook, B., Johnson, C. E., Byrd, M., & Gutiérrez-Terrell, E. (2002). Evidence of real-world effectiveness of a telephone quitline for smokers. *New England Journal of Medicine, 347,* 1087–1093.

Zilberberg, M., & Tijia, J. (2011). Growth in dementia-associated hospitalization among the oldest old in the United States. *Archives of Internal Medicine, 171,* 850–851.

Zubieta, J. K., Bueller, J. A., Jackson, L. R., Scott, D. J., Xu, Y., Koeppe, R. A., . . . Stohler, C. S. (2005). Placebo effects mediated by endogenous opioid activity on mu-opioid receptors. *Journal of Neuroscience, 25,* 7754–7762.

INDEX